The Essential Clinical Handbook for the Foundation Programme

A comprehensive guide for Foundation doctors on how to achieve your e-portfolio core clinical competencies

Edited by

Rameen Shakur

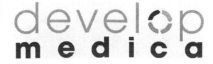

Published by Developmedica 2010
Castle Court
Duke Street
New Basford,
Nottingham, NG7 7JN
0845 838 0571
www.developmedica.com

Developmedica recommends that readers follow NICE and NHS guidelines, and the rules and guidelines of the institution in which they practise, in the performance of their day-to-day duties. The views expressed in this book are those of Developmedica and not those of the National Health Service. Developmedica is in no way associated with the National Health Service, the Foundation Programme or NICE.

Every effort has been made to ensure the accuracy of the material contained within this guide. However it must be noted that medical treatments, drug dosages/formulations, equipment, procedures and best practice are currently evolving within the field of medicine. Readers are therefore advised always to check the most up-to-date information relating to:

– The applicable drug manufacturer's product information and data sheets relating to recommended dose/formulation, administration and contraindications.
– The latest applicable local and national guidelines.
– Applicable local and national codes of conduct and safety protocols.

It is the responsibility of the practitioner, based on their own knowledge and expertise, to diagnose, treat and ensure the safety and best interests of the patient are maintained. To the fullest extent of the Law, the Publisher, Editor and Authors do not accept any responsibility or legal liability for any errors in the text or the misuse or misapplication of any of the material in this book.

Every effort has been made to contact the copyright holders of any material reproduced within this publication. If any have been inadvertently overlooked, the publishers will be pleased to make restitution at the earliest opportunity.

A catalogue record for this title is available from the British Library.

ISBN 978-1-906839-09-3

Typeset by Replika Press Pvt. Ltd. (India)

Printed by Bell and Bain, Glasgow

Cover design: 'Heart of the Matter' by Santron Sathasivam, London

1 2 3 4 5 6 7 8 9 10

Contents

Vimal Raj

7. Fluid management and shock. **315**

Mandeep Kaler, Ravivarma Balasubramaniam

8. DOPS: Direct observation of procedural skills **319**

John Apps, Tabitha Turner-Stokes, Christopher Yu, Santron Sathasivam, Rameen Shakur

9. Practical prescribing **357**

David Scott, Rameen Shakur

Foreword by Professor Lord Ara Darzi

The introduction of the Foundation Programme has been fundamental in helping bridge the gap for Foundation Year doctors, ensuring that high quality continuous education is provided with a rigorous curriculum.

This is a practical handbook of the Foundation Programme curriculum in medicine and surgery, incorporating current assessment tools used for postgraduate medical education as its basis, such as Directly Observed Procedures and Clinical Based Discussions. It provides Foundation Doctors with a valuable and practical clinical insight into their FY1 and FY2 years. It is clearly designed and laid out to aid the busy Foundation Year doctor and will enable them to successfully complete their e-portfolio to a high standard in order to achieve the best attainable scores. Key chapters include: Case Based Discussions of both core surgical and medical cases, supplemented by up-to-date guidelines from NICE; comprehensive illustrated step-by-step instructions on how to competently and safely carry out the major procedures one may experience during the Foundation training; and the Mini-Clinical Evaluation Exercise, which highlights the necessary clinical examination skills required for successful attainment of high scores in the assessments.

I have no doubt that this book will provide a valuable reference guide for medical students and junior doctors to completion of their Foundation training and their chosen postgraduate medical or surgical careers.

Professor Ara Darzi

Foreword by Sir Graeme Catto

Who knows what will be expected of doctors forty years from now? The science will have changed; society's expectations will have changed – but people will not have changed. They will trust us when most burdened by ill health and worries. That need for trust and humanity in medicine is unchanging but It Is conditional. It depends on our professionalism – our competence and our unfailing willingness to put the interests of our patients first.

The Foundation Programme is critically important in promoting both aspects of our professionalism. Not only does it allow the postgraduate student to integrate the knowledge, skills and behaviours acquired during the undergraduate years and provide the good quality clinical care patients expect, but it ensures a breadth of experience across a range of specialties. The well documented problems of the last few years have produced some significant benefits. Firstly they have emphasised the importance of postgraduate education in creating the well-informed, flexible medical workforce any health service will require In the years ahead. Secondly we now have a credible and creditable curriculum for the Foundation Programme in the UK.

This Handbook is not only *essential* but unique. It is the only text that covers the whole Foundation Programme curriculum, incorporating medical and surgical topics in a way that is practical and immediately relevant for the busy postgraduate student. The chapters on practical procedures and mini clinical evaluations provide detailed information and are particularly useful for doctors in training. Whatever specialty you choose to pursue, this Handbook provides the necessary basic information. Aimed at postgraduate students during the Foundation years, this text cannot but improve patient care and patient safety. Perhaps as importantly, it is an enjoyable read – for all postgraduate medical students whatever their age and stage.

Graeme Catto

Acknowledgements

Kindness is the language which the deaf can hear and the blind can see.

—Mark Twain

The production of a book of this scale has required the sustained hard work, dedication and help of many. This adventure began at the inception of the book in a curry house not too far from a CCU near you. I am sincerely grateful to all that have given their unyielding time and effort to this project. I have been particularly inspired by the seniors who have imparted to this book so much of their wisdom and expertise for the benefit of the next generation of Foundation doctors. Thank you Lord Darzi and Sir Graeme Catto for your guidance and words of support for this book. Thank you Dr. McElligott for taking the time to advise us constructively during the initial phases of the book and for the meticulous attention to detail.

I have been particularly touched by the hard work done by all the contributors, formatters and illustrators. You know who you are. Thank you particularly Chris and Santron for all your beaverish late nights getting all of the manuscript into publication format.

Mandeep, Prita, Simon, Ruth and Ravi: thank you guys, especially for putting up with my tireless emailing. I hope you will agree it was worth it. A big vote of thanks should also go to Matt Green and all at Developmedica, who have supported us admirably from the beginning. From a personal viewpoint I would like to thank my family, Mom, Dad and brother for putting up with my long nights of writing.

Finally, thank you, the reader. On behalf of all the team we sincerely hope that this book will enhance your medical/surgical career. This is a unique book, and we envisage it to be a practical companion to all Foundation doctors and clinical medical students in training. We look forward to your comments in regard to the book and hope this may inspire more to develop a keen interest in teaching and clinical medicine.

Bon Chance.

Dr. Rameen Shakur
The Royal Brompton and The London
Chest Hospitals
London, UK
2010

Acknowledgement of figures

Illustrations were provided by members of the team as follows:

Mr Christopher Yu: Figures 3.1, 3.2, 3.13, 3.24-3.26, 4.1, 4.21.

Mr Santron Sathasivam: Figures 3.2-3.4, 3.29, 3.30, 4.22, 4.24-4.31, 4.33, 7.1, 8.3-8.5, 8.9, 8.10, 8.12-8.14, 8.16, 8.17, 8.21-8.24, 8.27, 10.2-10.7.

Dr Sandeep Panniker: Figures 3.14-3.16, 3.33–3.38, 3.40-3.47, 3.49, 3.50, 3.55.

Dr Rashmi Patel: Figure 3.32.

Dr Vimal Raj: Figures 3.5-3.10, 3.12, 3.17, 3.18, 3.20-3.23, 3.27, 3.28, 3.31, 3.57, 3.58, 4.3-4.5, 4.7-4.9, 4.11-4.13, 4.18, 4.32, 4.34-4.37, 6.1-6.30, 8.20, 8.23, 8.26.

Dr Mandeep Kaler: Figures 4.6 and 8.18.

Mr Ravivarma Balasubramaniam: Figure 4.16.

Dr John Apps: Figures 8.1, 8.2, 8.11, 8.28.

Dr John Apps and Dr Tabitha Turner-Stokes: Figures 8.6, 8.7, 8.15, 8.19, 8.25.

Professor David Scott: Figures 9.1 and 9.2.

We also thank the National Institute for Health and Clinical Excellence (NICE); The Resuscitation Council UK; The United Kingdom Foundation Programme Office; The British Thoracic Society; Professor PA Routledge at the Cardiff University Therapeutics and Toxicology Centre; and Andrew Goldberg and Gerard Stansby; for kind permission to include illustrations from their publications, which are acknowledged in full where they appear.

Contributors

The Editor:

Dr Rameen Shakur is a run-through London Specialist Trainee in Cardiology at the London Chest hospital. He is also an honorary Cardiology research fellow at the Royal Brompton Hospital, National Heart and Lung Institute, London. He is a clinical teacher in medicine at Green Templeton College, University of Oxford. Dr Shakur trained at Cambridge, Oxford and Edinburgh medical schools. He has won numerous prizes and scholarships, most notably a Churchill Fellowship for Harvard Medical School for the application of genomic medicine in Cardiology, a Peter Kirk Fellowship, a Wellcome Trust scholarship for the Sanger Centre Genome Campus, Cambridge and a British Heart Foundation grant for cardiovascular research as a medical student. He is also a trainee representative for the Postgraduate Medical Education and Training Board (PMETB) committee. Dr Shakur is also a member of the General Medical Council's (GMC) Reference Community. He is the national chair of Medic-SHARE (Medical Doctors and Students Hospital Audit and Research Exchange).

Dr Shakur has also recently been selected as one of the youngest fellows of the Royal Society of the Arts (FRSA).

Editorial Co-ordinator:

Mr Christopher Yu is a 5th year medical student at Imperial College School of Medicine. He recently completed a BSc in Cardiovascular Sciences at the Royal Brompton Hospital, London.

Formatting and illustrating:

Mr Santron Sathasivam is a 4th year medical student at Bart's and The London School of Medicine and Dentistry. He is currently undertaking a BSc in Experimental Pathology and has produced the majority of the illustrations in the book.

Major contributors:

Dr Prita Rughani graduated from Bart's and The London School of Medicine and Dentistry. She is currently an ST1 Trainee in Paediatrics at Epsom University Hospital, London.

Dr Mandeep Kaler graduated from Bart's and The London School of Medicine and Dentistry. She is currently an ST1 Trainee in Obstetrics and Gynaecology at University College London Hospital, London.

Dr Simon Green graduated from Nottingham Medical School. He is a Higher Specialist Trainee in Geriatrics and General Internal Medicine on the North East Thames rotation. He is currently working at The North Middlesex University Hospital.

Dr Vimal Raj graduated from Bellary Medical College, India. He is currently a Radiology Fellow in Cardiothoracic Imaging at Papworth Hospital, Cambridge.

Mr Ravivarma Balasubramaniam graduated from Leeds University Medical School. He is currently an ST3 surgical trainee in the Midlands Deanery, doing General/Colorectal Surgery.

Dr John Apps graduated from Cambridge University (Pre-Clinical) and University of Oxford Medical School. He is currently an academic Foundation Year 2 doctor at University College London Hospital, London.

Dr Tabitha Turner-Stokes graduated from Cambridge University (Pre-Clinical) and University College London Medical School. She is currently an academic Foundation Year 2 doctor in the Rheumatology department at University College London Hospital, London.

Dr Sandeep Panikker graduated from Imperial College School of Medicine, London. He is currently a Cardiology SpR at St Bartholomew's Hospital, London.

Mrs Ruth Green graduated from the University of Portsmouth with a degree in Psychology before training as a Nurse. She has specialised in emergency and acute medical care. She is currently Unit Manager for the Emergency Department in a London hospital.

Contributors:

Dr. Abhishek Joshi graduated from Oxford University Medical School. He is currently a Foundation Year 2 doctor in Thoracic Surgery at Guy's Hospital, London

Dr Geraldine McElligott graduated from the Middlesex Hospital, London. She is currently a Consultant Geriatrician at Whipps Cross University Hospital.

Dr Rashmi Patel graduated from Cambridge University (Pre-Clinical) and University Oxford Medical School. He is currently an academic Foundation Year 2 doctor in Accident & Emergency at The Whittington Hospital, London.

Prof. David Scott did his undergraduate degree in Pharmacy and worked in several hospitals and universities before becoming Professor of Clinical Pharmacy in Nairobi. He has now returned to Oxford where he is a senior pharmacist in the Oxford Radcliffe Hospital and teaches in pharmacy and medicine.

About the publisher

Developmedica is a specialist provider of books, courses and eLearning solutions tailored to meet your career development needs. Visit our web site at www.developmedica.com and find out more.

Our approach is friendly and personal. Please telephone or email any time to discuss your requirements.

Tell us what you think

Developmedica are committed to publishing high quality books and would be delighted to hear your thoughts on how this book helped you, or your suggestions on any new topics we should be pursuing to support individuals in progressing their careers. Simply email your thoughts to publishing@developmedica.com.

Better still, please submit a testimonial to the website that you purchased this book from, and email us with a link to where you have placed the testimonial, and you will be entered into our monthly prize draw with the chance to win one of a range of prizes.

Free companion material available from the Developmedica web site

Wherever possible, Developmedica makes companion material relating to its books available on the Developmedica web site without charge.

Please visit www.developmedica.com and see what we have to offer.

Abbreviations

5HIAA – 5-hydroxyindoleacetic acid

5HT – 5-hydroxytryptamine

A&E – Accident & Emergency

AAA – Abdominal aortic aneurysm

ABC – Airway, breathing, circulation

ABCDE – Airway, breathing, circulation, disability, exposure

ABG – Arterial blood gas

ABPI – Ankle brachial pressure index

ABX – Abdominal X-ray

AC – Adenocarcinoma

ACE – Angiotensin converting enzyme

ACS – Acute coronary syndrome

ACTH – Adrenocorticotrophic hormone

ADAM 33 – ADAM metallopeptidase domain 33

ADH – Anti-diuretic hormone

ADLs – Activities of daily living

AEDs – Anti-epileptic drugs

AF – Atrial fibrillation

AFB – Acid fast bacillus

AFFIRM – Atrial fibrillation followup investigation of rhythm management

AFP – Serum α-feloprotein

AIDS – Acquired immunodeficiency syndrome

AL – Amyloid light chain

ALP – Alkaline phosphatase

ALS – Advanced Life Support

ALT – Alanine aminotransferase

AMA – Anti-mitochondrial antibodies

AMTS – Abbreviated mental test score

ANA – Antinuclear antibodies

ANCA – Antineutrophil cytoplasmic antibodies

Anti-LKM antibodies – Anti-liver/kidney/microsomal antibodies

Anti-SLA – Anti-soluble liver antigen

AP – Anterio-posterior

APTT – Activated partial thromboplastin time

APUD cells – Amine precursor uptake and decarboxylation cells

ARVC – Arrhythmogenic right ventricular cardiomyopathy

ASIS – Anterior superior iliac spine

ASO – Anti-streptolysin-O

AST – Aspartate aminotransferase

A–V – Arterio-venous

AVNRT – Atrioventricular nodal- re-entrant tachycardia

AVRT – Atrioventricular re-entrant tachycardia

AXR – Abdominal X-ray

BCC – Basal cell carcinoma

BCG – Bacille Calmette-Guérin

BD – Bis die (twice a day)

BE – Base excess

BIPAP – Biphasic positive airway pressure

BMI – Body mass index

BNF – British national formulary

BNP – Brain-type natriuretic peptide

BOOP – Bronchiolitis obliterans organising pneumonia

BP – Blood pressure

BPAG1 – Bullous pemphigoid antigens 1

BPH – Benign prostatic hyperplasia

Bpm – Beats per minute

BRCA – Breast cancer gene

BTS – British Thoracic Society

BXO – Balanitis xerotica obliterans

CA 19-9 – Carbohydrate antigen 19-9

CABG – Coronary artery bypass graft

CAGE – Cutting, annoyed, guilty, eye-opener

CARD – Caspase Recruitment Domain

CbDs – Case based Discussions

CBG – Capillary blood glucose

CCF – Congestive cardiac failure

CD – Crohn's disease

CEA – Carcinoembryonic antigen

Ch – French gauge

CHART – Continuous hyperfractionated accelerated radiotherapy

CHF – Congestive heart failure

CK – Creatinine kinase

CK-MB – Creatinine kinase muscle/brain type

CLL – Chronic lymphocytic leukaemia

CLO – Campylobacter-like organism

CML – Chronic myeloid leukaemia

CMV – Cytomegalovirus

CNS – Central nervous system

COPD – Chronic obstructive pulmonary disease

COX – Cyclo-oxygenase

CPAP – Continuous positive airway pressure

CPPD – Calcium pyrophosphate dehydrate

CPR – Cardiopulmonary resuscitation

CRH – Corticotrophin releasing hormone

CRP – C-reactive protein

CSF – Cerebrospinal fluid

CT – Computer tomography

CTPA – Computer tomography pulmonary angiogram

CVP – Central venous pressure

Cx – Circumflex artery

CXR – Chest X-ray

DC cardioversion – Direct current cardioversion

DCIS – Ductal carcinoma *in situ*

DCM – Dilated cardiomyopathy

DEXA – Dual energy X-ray absorptiometry

DIC – Disseminated intravascular coagulation

DMARDs – Disease modifying anti-rheumatic drugs

DMSA – Dimercaptosuccinic acid

DNA – Deoxyribonucleic acid

DNAR – Decision not to attempt resuscitation

DOB – Date of birth

DOPS – Direct observation of procedural skills

DOT – Directly observed therapy

DSH – Deliberate self-harm

DTs – Delirium Tremens

DVLA – Driver and Vehicle Licensing Agency

DVT – Deep vein thrombosis

EADs – Early after depolarisations

EAU – Emergency Assessment Unit

EBV – Epstein-Barr virus

ECG – Electrocardiogram

ED – Emergency Department

EEG – Electroencephalography

EF – Ejection fraction

ELISA – Enzyme-linked immunosorbent assay

EMF – Endomyocardial fibrosis

ENT – Ears, Nose, and Throat

ERCP – Endoscopic retrograde cholangiopancreatography

ERDS – End-stage renal failure

ESR – Erythrocyte sedimentation rate

ESWL – Extracorporeal shock wave lithotripsy

ET – Endotracheal

EVAR – Endovascular aneurysm repair

EVLA – Endovenous laser ablation

FAP – Familial adenomatous polyposis

FBC – Full Blood Count

FER – Forced expiratory ratio

FEV_1 – Forced expiratory volume in one second

FFP – Fresh frozen plasma

FNA – Fine needle aspiration

FVC – Forced vital capacity

FY – Foundation Year

G6PD – Glucose-6-phosphate dehydrogenase

GABA – Gamma-aminobutyric acid

GALS – Gait, arms, legs, and spine

GCS – Glasgow coma score

GGT – Gamma-glutamyl transferase

GHB – Gamma-hydroxybutyrate

GI – Gastrointestinal

GMC – General Medical Council

GOR – Gastro-oesophageal reflux

GORD – Gastro-oesophageal reflux disease

GP – General practitioner

GTN – Glyceryl trinitrate

GUM – genitourinary medicine

HAV – Hepatitis A virus

Hb – Haemoglobin

HBcAg – Core antigen

HBeAg – Pre-core antigen

HBsAg – Surface antigen

HBV – Hepatitis B virus

HCG – Human chorionic gonadotropin

HCM – Hypertrophic cardiomyopathy

HCV – Hepatitis C virus

HDU – High dependency unit

HDV – Hepatitis D virus

HER2 – Human epidermal growth factor receptor 2

HIV – Human immunodeficiency virus

HLA – Human leukocyte antigen

HNPCC – Hereditary non-polyposis colon cancer

HO – House officer

HPV – Human papilloma virus

HRT – Hormone replacement therapy

HSV – Herpes simplex virus

IBD – Inflammatory bowel disease

IBS – Irritable bowel syndrome

ICP – Intracranial pressure

ICU – Intensive care unit

Ig – Immunoglobulin

IHD – Ischaemic heart disease

ILS – Immediate life support

IM – Intramuscular

INR – International normalised ratio

ISDN – Isosorbide dinitrate

IUCD – Intrauterine coil device

IV – Intravenous

IVP – Intravenous pyelogram

IVU – Intravenous urogram

JVP – Jugular venous pressure

KUB – Kidneys-ureters-bladder

LA – Local anaesthetic

LAD – Left anterior descending artery

LBBB – Left bundle branch block

LCIS – Lobular carcinoma *in situ*

LDH – Lactate dehydrogenase

LFTs – Liver function tests

LHRH - luteinising-hormone releasing hormone

LMWH – Low molecular weight heparin

LOS – Lower oesophageal sphincter

LP – Lumbar puncture

LQTS – Long QT syndrome

LSD – Lysergic acid diethylamide

LV – Left ventricle

LVP – Large-volume paracentesis

MAO – Monoamine oxidase

MC+S – Microscopy, culture, and sensitivity

MCP – Metacarpophalangeal

MCV – Mean cell volume

MDCT – Multi-detector computer tomography

MDMA – 3,4-methylenedioxymethamphetamine ectasy

MDRTB – Multi-drug resistant TB

MDT   Multi-disciplinary team

MEN – Multiple endocrine neoplasia

MEWS – Modified early warning score

MHC – Major histocompatibility complex

MI – Myocardial infarction

Mini-CEX – Mini clinical evaluation exercise

Mini-PAT – Mini peer assessment tool

MMSE – Mini mental state examination

MRCP – Magnetic resonance Cholangiopancreatography

MRI – Magnetic resonance imaging

MRSA – Methicillin-resistant *Staphylococcus aureus*

MS – Multiple sclerosis

MST – Morphine sulphate tablets

MSU – Mid-stream urine

NAC – N-acetylcysteine

NAFLD – Non-alcoholic fatty liver disease

NAPQI – N-acetyl-p-benzoquinoneimine

NBM – Nil by mouth

Nd:YAG – Neodymium-doped yttrium aluminium garnet

NG – Nasogastric

NHS – National Health Service

NICE – National Institute for Health and Clinical Excellence

NIV – Non-invasive ventilation

NOD – Nucleotide-binding oligomerization domain

NSAID – Non-steroidal anti-inflammatory drug

NSCLC – Non-small-cell lung cancer

NSGCT – Non-seminomatous germ cell tumours

NSTEMI – Non-ST elevation myocardial infarction

NYHA – New York heart association

OCP – Oral contraceptive pill

OD – Omin die (once daily)

OGD – Oesophagogastroduodenoscopy

OGTT – Oral glucose tolerance test

OSCE – Objective Structured Clinical Examination

OTC – Over the counter

PA – Postero-anterior

PALS – Patient Advice and Liaison Services

PBC – Primary biliary cirrhosis

PCI – Percutaneous coronary intervention

PCNL – Percutaneous nephrolithotomy

PCP   *Pneumocystis carinii*

PCR – Polymerase chain reaction

PE – Pulmonary embolism

PEA – Pulseless electrical activity

PEF – Peak expiratory flow

PEFR – Peak expiratory flow rate

PET – Positron emission tomography

PIP – Proximal inter-phalangeal

PND – Paroxysmal nocturnal dyspnoea

PNS – Peripheral nervous system

PO – Per oral

PPI – Proton pump inhibitor

PR – Per rectum

PRN – Pro re nata (as needed)

PSA – Prostate specific antigen

PT – Prothrombin time

PTFE – Polytetrafluroethylene

PTH – Parathyroid hormone

PUO – Pyrexia of unknown origin

PUVA – Psoralens and ultraviolet A phototherapy

RA – Rheumatoid arthritis

RBBB – Right bundle branch block

RBC – Red blood cell

RCA – Right coronary artery

RCM – Restrictive cardiomyopathy

RCR – Royal College of radiologists

RIF – Right iliac fossa

RNA – Ribonucleic acid

ROSC – Return of spontaneous circulation

RTA – Road traffic accident

SA – Sino-atrial node

SAAG – Serum-ascitic albumin gradient

SAH – Subarachnoid haemorrhage

SANAD – Study of Standard and New Anti-Epileptic Drugs

SCC – Squamous cell carcinoma

SCLC – Small-cell lung cancer

SDH – Subdural haemorrhage

SHO – Senior house officer

SIADH – Syndrome of inappropriate antidiuretic hormone secretion

SIRS – Systemic inflammatory response syndrome

SLE – Systemic lupus erythematosus

SMA – Smooth muscle antibodies

SMR – Standard mortality ratio

SOB – Shortness of breath

SOL – Space occupying lesion

SpR – Specialist Registrar

SSRI – Selective serotonin reuptake inhibitors

ST – Specialist Trainee

STEMI – ST elevation myocardial infarction

SUDEP – Sudden unexplained death in epilepsy

SVT – Supra-ventricular tachycardia

SXR – Skull X-ray

TB – Tuberculosis

TCA – Tricyclic antidepressants

TDS – Ter die sumendus (three times a day)

TENS – Transcutaneous electrical nerve stimulator

TFT – Thyroid function tests

TGF – Tumour growth factor

TIA – Transient ischaemic attack

TIPSS – Transjugular intrahepatic portasystemic stent shunt

TNF – Tumor necrosis factors

TNM – Tumour-node-metastasis

TOE – Transoesophageal echocardiography

TP – Trombocytopenic purpura

tPA – Tissue plasminogen activator

TPN – Total parenteral nutrition

TRUS – Transrectal ultrasound scan

TSH – Thyroid stimulating hormone

tTGA – Tissue transglutaminase

TUR – Transurethral resection

TURBT – Transurethral resection of bladder tumour

TURP – Trans-urethral resection of the prostate

TWOC – Trial without catheter

U&Es – Urea and electrolytes

UA – Unstable angina

UC – Ulcerative colitis

UMN – Upper motor neuron

URTI – Upper respiratory tract infection

USS – Ultrasound scan

UTI – Urinary tract infection

V/Q scan – Ventilation perfusion

VF – Ventricular fibrillation

VT – Ventricular tachycardia

VZV – Varicella zoster virus

WBC – White blood cell

WCC – White cell count

WE – Wernicke's encephalopathy

WHO – World Health Organisation

WLE – Wide local excision

WPW – Wolff-Parkinson-White

XDRTB – Extremely drug resistant TB

How to use this book

This book, written by doctors, is intended for Foundation Year doctors, Medical students and Educational and Clinical supervisors. The book has been designed to cover the Foundation Programme curriculum. The top 20 symptoms/presentations mentioned in the curriculum are covered in the medical and surgical chapters of this book. A differential diagnosis table for each symptom/presentation exists at the beginning of each subchapter. **The differentials in bold are covered in the subchapter. Please note that the differentials not in bold may be covered in other subchapters of the book and thus you may need to refer to the index.**

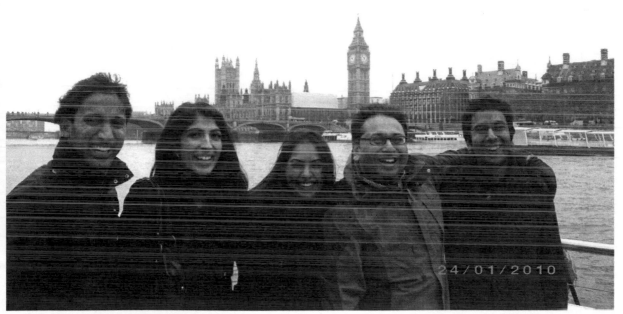

The Editor and some members of the authorial team celebrating publication. Left to right: Sandeep Panniker, Prita Rughani, Mandeep Kaler, Rameen Shakur, Abhishek Joshi.

Dedication

*I would like to dedicate this book to my beloved parents and my brother.
Thank you for your unyielding support.*

Rameen Shakur

Chapter 1   So you have finally made it: Doctor

"Doctors are men who prescribe medicines of which they know little, to cure diseases of which they know less, in human beings of whom they know nothing."

François-Marie Arouet ("Voltaire" 1694–1778)

Voltaire may not have been the best admirer of medics, but he does highlight an important point. Given the great strides medicine has and continues to make during history it is often too easy as doctors to believe that we have all the answers to the problems of the human body. Unfortunately, the humble truth is we do not. However, we are trying to find out. This is why the practice of medicine, although steeped in tradition, continues to evolve to reflect the dichotomy facing any medical practioner. Medicine is both a science and an art: it is all-important that the logical scientist and the illogical humanitarian combine to apply the knowledge of medicine within the context of humanity.

The Doctor

The road to success is long, tiring and full of difficult decisions; yet the study and practice of medicine continues to inspire the human spirit. The promise of heartfelt satisfaction when done well and the unyielding feeling of guilt and remorse when realising more could have been done, make the practice of medicine so enthralling. Never a dull moment, but never a time to take one's 'eyes off the ball' either. So congratulations if after all your endeavours you have joined this historical fraternity and welcome if you have decided to take the challenge recently. This book aspires to provide students and doctors essential medical and surgical knowledge to enable the successful completion of their Foundation training. The book also contains a number of practical step-by-step guides for the safe completion of essential procedures. We hope you find this book useful.

On the wards

Whether as a clinical student or as a junior doctor the majority of your time and efforts will be on the wards. It is here that you will experience the daily stresses and strains of caring for in-patients. At the end of the day no matter how much we have gained through knowledge or experience, it comes down to one thing: it is all for the patient. We as doctors are there to serve to the best of our ability all those who have entrusted us with their health during their times of illness. This trust has been gained through generations and generations of doctors across the globe all following the same code; that your patient comes first. Hence, with this in mind, be conscious of all that goes on with your patients and take this privilege to aid a member of humanity with the same dignity, patience and sincerity you would were it yourself on the other side.

There is no 'I' in team

One does not need to be a spelling bee champion to realise this fact, but it is an important point which is often not reiterated as coherently as it should be during medical training. The team (of which you are a member) shares all of its success and failures together. There are no individual winners or losers in this process, rather collective achievements. This may be a difficult concept to understand in a traditional training setting where the emphasis has always been on learning to improve oneself, but in essence the same applies here as well. Through your experiences and knowledge try and share this with others in the team so as to develop a sustainable and friendly environment for the exchange of knowledge. Although how well the team dynamics are established will depend very much on the guidance of the consultant and other senior members of the team, we all can still play our part.

Work, rest and play

Medics have always had a discernable reputation for being a hardworking and conscientious group, but this should not be the case at the expense of one's own health and wellbeing. A profession which takes pride in leading the fight against disease for the betterment of patients and humanity often neglects its own members. This is partly due to our reluctance to ask for help or to admit that we too are human. With the inception and now enforcement of the European Working Time Directive during all training of doctors, this should aid us all in having a better work–life balance. However, reality and the nature of the job may show us a different picture. Therefore it is important for all concerned to be aware of the stresses on each member of the team and to be aware of confidential services which can be accessed by all during times of need. The practice of medicine should be an enjoyable and fascinating experience for those willing to engage in this profession. It is therefore our collective responsibility that this should always remain so, now and tomorrow. Welcome.

"There are no incurable diseases – only the lack of will. There are no worthless herbs – only the lack of knowledge."

Ibn Sina (Avicenna, 981–1037)

Welcome to your Foundation years. The first years of practice as a doctor have always been challenging. You will have to adapt your theoretical knowledge to practical situations, often very quickly and under pressure of time. With the advent of new Foundation assessments, you will also have to prove that you are able to do this on a regular basis in order to progress. Whilst you will be using the knowledge and skills you gained in medical school, you will also need to acquire and exercise many new skills which have more to do with being effective in the workplace. Being well prepared and ready to enter the working world will enhance the amount of time you spend learning new skills and gaining clinical acumen. It will gain you the trust of your seniors, who will be more inclined to teach and allow you more independence to practice.

This chapter will cover some general and practical pieces of advice for a successful Foundation Programme. We hope you find it useful.

BEFORE YOU START

Things to learn whilst shadowing

Every Foundation Year (FY) doctor has passed their medical finals. What you need to do is make sure that you are ready to put that knowledge into practice. Making sure you have made the correct preparations will mean you can hit the ground running.

Many hospitals and medical schools arrange shadowing periods where one can prepare to start working in the job without having to immediately take on the responsibility. If your course does not offer this, try to arrange it yourself, the week before your attachment officially starts. Calling your Consultant's secretary and leaving a message to this effect should be a good start.

Know your hospital

Do you know your way around? Where are the wards where you have patients? Where is radiology? Where are theatres? Make sure you have a rough idea about the layout of the hospital. If you work in a big hospital, limit yourself to the areas relevant to your team before you arrive. These will include your wards, your consultant's and their secretary's office, the radiology department and any areas where specialist procedures might be taking place, e.g. theatres, endoscopy suite and cardiac catheterisation laboratory.

Know your job

Make sure you know exactly what your job entails. Are you going to a specialist gastroenterology unit in a tertiary referral centre, or are you going to an acute general medical ward? It is important to know the difference.

If you start somewhere very specialist, then you might be expected to know a bit more about the cutting edge medicine done in that environment. Essentially, you will need to know your area in a lot of depth, and might benefit from some preparatory reading of postgraduate literature. You might also find yourself being much more focused on administrative details, rather than the clinical picture. If you start in a less specialist unit, you might be expected to manage patients with a range of different conditions. For example, a geriatrics ward will present you with a broad spectrum of conditions to treat. In that case, it would be a good idea to make sure you are confident of all your general medical knowledge, without focusing too hard on a certain area.

You should also ensure you have a full timetable for the Firm activities. When are the theatre lists? When and where do multi-disciplinary team (MDT) meetings take place? Find out what your specific role in these activities is likely to be before you arrive late to the first one, and have no clue what to do!

Know your team

Make sure you introduce yourself formally to the entire team, and know everybody's name and role. A description of the various members of the team, and what they can do for you, appears below:

The Consultant

The 'Boss': a doctor who is, theoretically, completely trained to deliver care for anyone under his care. Consultants hold ultimate responsibility for the care of their patients, and therefore oversee your actions.

Your Consultant will be the person who undertakes your clinical induction and end-of-rotation meetings, and will have a hand in completing other Foundation assessments. He/she is responsible for your training on your placement with the firm.

Your Consultant's attitudes and preferences will closely dictate the way you do your job. Ask around other doctors in the hospital to see if they have any hints on what sort of things your Consultant likes. Does he/she get especially upset about anything? Does he/she often use specific management strategies that do not strictly adhere to the guidelines? The best people to ask, obviously, are your immediate predecessors in the job, and your immediate seniors in the team.

One of the worst mistakes you can make is to be so frightened of your Consultant that you fail to ask them any questions. It is your duty to implement their wishes, so ensure you understand their reasoning at all times.

Specialist Trainee (ST) doctors

Formerly Specialist Registrars (SpR), these doctors are training to be Consultants in a specific field. They are now referred to by the number of years of specialist training they have had. Registrars have usually completed at least three years of specialist training, so they are referred to as ST3, but you will still know them as 'the Reg'. They tend to be involved in all aspects of the patient's care, including out-patient clinics, performing procedures and operations, working on the wards and doing on-calls. They still have to answer to the Consultant, but they tend to make most of the day-to-day management decisions, and lead the daily ward-rounds.

When things begin to get frightening, for example an acutely unwell patient, your Registrar is the person to whom you should turn. They are experienced and skilled in dealing with problems, and are usually available to contact. Memorise their bleep numbers. Again, make sure you fully understand what they want you to do, and try to understand why. Registrars can also help you with Direct Observation of Procedural Skills (DOPS), Mini-Clinical Evaluation Exercises (Mini-CEXs) and Case-based Discussions (CbDs).

Sometimes firms will have Associate Specialists, Staff Grade or Clinical Fellows attached to them. They are often in equivalent Registrar positions, but with either non-training or research posts. They are often very useful for advice.

The Senior House Officer (SHO)

'SHO' is now a defunct term, and has been replaced with the more junior STs (ST1 and ST2) and often FY2 doctors as well. These doctors will be your first port of call for any help you may need. Their jobs are similar to yours, but they will, hopefully, be quicker, more efficient and more confident than you. They will be able to supervise DOPS, and will be able to explain useful short-cuts and strategies to you, to make you more effective and efficient. All STs can do DOPS and Mini-CEX, while CbDs should be done by ST3 and above.

The House Officer (HO)/Foundation Year 1 doctor:

This is where one begins. Although at the end of a long chain of command, at least there is only one way to go; up. (See our section below, 'How to be a good FY doctor'.)

The secretary

Your Consultant's secretary will know where most of the team are supposed to be in the hospital, and how to get hold of them. He/she might also help co-ordinate the team, and will be essential for getting your consultant's signature on things. Make sure you have a good relationship here, because they will be able to access information that you might not.

Know your ward

Obviously know where your ward is, but also make sure you know who is on it, and how they can help you. This section gives descriptions of the different professionals that work on the ward.

Nurses

The most important people to you in the hospital, they make the difference between things going smoothly, and things completely falling apart. It is absolutely essential to work to have them on your side.

Find out who is in charge of the ward (Senior Sister/Charge Nurse) and make a special effort to introduce yourself. This person will be incredibly useful to you both practically and educationally. They can solve problems that you might be having trouble with. Remember: you work on their ward, and they will know the systems and the other staff better than you do.

Ensure you know who the other nurses and healthcare assistants are, and what skills they have. This may take some time, but it means you can ask the right favour from the right person. Knowing the people you work with on a day to day basis will also make for a much easier start to your job.

You must get nurses to complete your Mini-Peer Assessment Tool (Mini-PAT), and they can also observe you completing DOPS assessments. However, they cannot perform Mini-CEX or CbD assessments.

Specialist nurses

These nurses are highly trained in a single field, e.g. cardiac, endoscopy, diabetes, cancer (MacMillan nurses). They work with consultant doctors in the same field. Use their experience in their specialist field as much as you can, and learn from them.

Pharmacists

The ward pharmacist knows the dosages and indications for drugs, and they can also tell you if a drug you want to prescribe is in the hospital formulary. Ask them if you are unsure. Pharmacists can also work directly with the hospital pharmacy, to get medications for your patients quickly, especially in emergency situations and prior to discharges. Look out for their green ink on your drug charts.

Physiotherapists

Physiotherapists use physical therapies such as breathing exercises, muscular training and motivational strategies to improve your patient's stability, strength, stamina and confidence. They often use frames and walking aids to get patients moving, especially after operations. They work in rehabilitation, and are an essential part of your discharge planning. They will also help in cases of acute pneumonia, and other respiratory illnesses.

Occupational therapists (OTs)

If your patient has any persisting difficulties after they have been treated for their illness, the OT will help them to find solutions for these issues, and suggest modifications to maximise your patient's independence. They can advise on changes to the home that a patient is going back to, or can suggest if a patient might need to move to new accommodation. They can also provide simple solutions to help patients look after themselves. They are an essential part of your discharge team. Getting a very thorough OT assessment will prevent premature discharges home.

Social workers

If your patient needs support when leaving hospital, the social worker will help to co-ordinate and find funding for it. They are invaluable when aiming to discharge elderly patients, who may need carers at home or funding for nursing home placements. Liaise with them about realistic discharge dates and update your team on their advice regarding patients' discharge.

Know your equipment

Equipment

Make sure you know where everything is on your ward. You will need to know the location of equipment quickly in emergency situations. Equipment that you should find and remember the location of:

- Tape
- Needles
- Syringes
- Cannulas and flushes
- Gauze and dressings
- Blood gas syringes
- Wound packs
- Request forms
- Continuation sheets

Practical procedures

Use your shadowing period to sharpen up your venepuncture, arterial puncture, cannulation and other practical skills. From now on, if someone else cannot perform these tasks, you will be called. Ensure you have a few tricks up your sleeve.

HOW TO BE A GOOD FOUNDATION YEAR DOCTOR

You have three things to achieve as an FY doctor.

1. You have the responsibility to learn and develop.
2. You must provide evidence that you have learned and developed.
3. You must ensure the smooth running of your team, and therefore the good clinical care of your patients.

The best FY doctors meet the "four Cs" criteria:

- Confident
- Competent
- Congenial
- Conventional

The best strategy, especially when you start, is to make sure the team runs smoothly, and the learning will follow. You need to be able to do what is required, and feel secure that you are doing it well. Be friendly and approachable to anyone who might want to talk to your team, from relatives to other Consultants. Always use accepted management practices, and recognise your limits.

Being organised

Your job will be to organise and ensure the smooth running of the ward round, making sure all the jobs and investigations are requested and done, and ensure that the results are known. You will need to keep track of the progress of all your Consultant's patients and know what the plans for their treatments are.

You will have to arrange their discharges and write their discharge letters. In addition, you will also be responsible for referring to other consultants and specialist services. Depending on who else is on your team, and how much they trust you, you will also be responsible for the early management of acutely ill patients, and deciding and prescribing basic therapeutics. Furthermore, you will be responsible for completing your own Foundation Programme assessments.

If you feel as if your organisational ability has not always been exemplary, now is the time to think very carefully about how you will be better. Here are some hints:

- Take an extra ten minutes before the day starts for planning and make your list.
- Write down everything in the same place.
- Get a clipboard to hold loose bits of paper and lists together.
- Always carry two spare pens (one will run out, one will go missing).

The ward round

The ward round usually happens in the morning, although this may vary from firm to firm, and sets the tone for your day. It is the time of day when your team reviews all the patients under your care, and moves the management onwards. Your job as an FY doctor is to ensure the ward round moves smoothly, that decisions and plans are documented, and that the jobs that are generated are done quickly and effectively. It is also important for you to document clearly all points from the ward round in patients' notes. There are various different ward rounds to be familiar with:

Types of ward rounds

- Consultant ward rounds: the team's Consultant sees all their patients. Decisions are made and management is moved forward. You should be very well prepared for this ward round. Your Consultant will have a limited amount of time, and needs to spend as much time as possible thinking and making decisions, not waiting for you to find yesterday's blood results, so have all information to hand.
- Post-take ward rounds: the new admissions are seen by the Consultant. If you have clerked the new patients, then you will be required to present the patient to the team on the round. This can be nerve-wracking, especially as you still have to do the rest of your job at the same time. The biggest mistake you can make on a post-take round is to miss a new patient off your List. Use every possible method to ensure you have got all of them.
- Business round: the most senior doctor, usually the Registrar,

takes a ward round to ensure that the management of patients is progressing.

There are a number of important factors which are beneficial for the FY doctor in preparing for a smooth ward round. These are summarised in the top tips table.

Top tips to be prepared for the ward round

- 'The List' – well organised
- The exact location of all your patients
- Blank request forms
- Continuation sheets for the notes
- The latest investigation results
- Easy access to the medical notes
- Easy access to the observation charts
- Easy access to the drug chart
- A nurse, to tell you of any recent changes, and to inform of management changes.

The List

The List is a list of all your patients, with the following:

- Patient's name
- Date of birth
- Hospital number
- Location in the hospital
- Presenting complaint and diagnosis
- Jobs that they need doing

Name	Number	DoB	Problem	Results	Jobs	Ward
Bloggs, J.	1234567	10/4/22	Chest pain	Trop-ve	Book ETT	A1
Doe, J.	7654321	11/11/18	Dark urine	Creatinine 450	Chase renal USS	B7
Huff, M.	456978	14/7/45	Off legs	White cells 11	Chase urine dip	C3

Figure 2.1: An example of a list

Make enough copies of the list for all the members of your team, and circulate these at the beginning of the ward round. Keeping a good list is probably the most important thing an FY doctor can do. If you do not know where your patients are, your team will find it difficult to look after them. Also remember to dispose of lists in the blue confidential waste bags at all times.

Some FY doctors prefer to do a 'pre-round', where they see the patients before the ward round. This allows you to be fully informed of location and progress before you start the ward round, and also allows you to ensure all the information you need is ready at hand when the Boss comes around. However, this may not always be practical due to time constraints.

During the round

Guide the team from patient to patient. As you arrive at each patient, you might offer a summary of their age, presenting complaint, the diagnosis and treatment, and then an update on any major changes since the last ward round. Inform the team of any notable blood results and update them on the Multi Disciplinary Team (MDT) feedback, i.e. for the physiotherapist, social services and other allied health professionals.

Whilst the team and the patient discuss the next steps you will need to present the observation chart, find the correct place in the notes and be ready to make changes to the drug chart. Be ready to act on any instructions you get at this point.

Then you will need to write down what happens on the round in the notes. Document the following:

- Any new complaints the patient has, or how he/she is feeling
- Any findings on examination at the bedside
- This morning's observations
- The impression on the ward round, e.g. getting better, new atrial fibrillation (AF), etc.
- The management plan

After the ward round

Sit down. Speak with your team about who is the most appropriate person to do the required jobs, and get help prioritising them. It might be that the ST4 is best placed to talk to another Consultant about a certain aspect of care. The FY doctor will probably end up with the lion's share of the jobs to do. Mention it to your team if you feel that your jobs list is too much for you to cope with. Remember to prioritise jobs and to be aware of when is the most appropriate time to do them.

Doing the jobs

Getting the jobs done after a ward round is more complex than it sounds. Rather than doing all the jobs in the order that you get them, or trying to do the ones that sound the most interesting first, you will have to prioritise. Develop a strategy for getting things done quickly, efficiently and to a high standard. Organise your tasks, so that you can do all the similar jobs at the same time. This will save you time; if you only have to sit down and request laboratory investigations once a day, you will only have to find the request forms once a day, too. Usually the jobs from a ward round break down into clear sections:

- Jobs that need to be done immediately
- Radiological investigations
- Laboratory investigations
- Referrals
- Discharges
- Other jobs

Setting priorities

Once you have categorised your jobs, you need to prioritise them. Working out what to do first is difficult. If you can, try to sit down with a senior and work out what order you should do things in. Use some basic rules for prioritising jobs:

- Know who your sickest patients are. Do jobs for them first.
- If you need an investigation done by the end of the day, focus on it early on.
- If you need to involve someone who works regular office hours, do these jobs before 5 pm.
- Do clinical jobs before clerical jobs.

Decide the order in which you are going to do the jobs, then do them, but try to be flexible. You never know when you are going to be bleeped about an emergency.

Immediate jobs

If you discover a sick patient on the ward round, or something needs to be done immediately, obviously you should do this first. If your team is big enough you may want to even drop off the ward round and do the job then and there, so long as someone else can carry on the usual jobs on the rounds.

Radiological Investigations

Find out very early on what your hospital's method for requesting radiological interventions are. Some hospitals use a computer based system, some use forms. You will need to know the quickest and the most effective ways of doing this very early on in your job. Note that there is often a quick way to request an investigation, but that this is rarely the quickest way to make the investigation actually happen. For example, you could send an electronic request, but this will never be quicker than going up to the radiology department yourself, and asking a Consultant radiologist for a scan.

Radiologists are legally responsible for the radiation dose they expose patients to. This means they need to justify the investigation in the same way that a physician must justify giving a drug. Add to this the fact that computer tomography (CT) and magnetic resonance imaging (MRI) machines are often under pressure to deliver more and more investigations, and you will find that getting an immediate scan can sometimes be a challenge.

Getting an urgent scan

Sometimes getting an urgent scan is a bit like trying to sell something. You have to convince the radiologist that interrupting their planned lists, and using their valuable scanner time, is clinically necessary now. When requesting an urgent scan, take time to go to see the Consultant radiologists in person. Tell them the history and the clinical picture of the patient, and mention any relevant investigations. Ask them to look at any previous images (always have your List, so you can tell them the hospital number) and then ask them what the next radiological step would be. The most useful piece of information you can offer is what immediate steps in the management depend on the results of the scan. For example, if the results of a CT scan will mean a patient goes to

theatre that afternoon, then the CT is more likely to happen than if it is to diagnose a chronic, non-emergency problem, in which case it can wait. Ask your team for this information before you speak with the radiologists.

Avoid speaking to the radiologists about every single scan, and making all of them sound extremely urgent. If you gain a reputation for only making sensible requests, then you will be more likely to get your urgent scans when you need them. If you label everything as urgent in an effort to get even routine things done quickly and impress your team, you are more likely to have difficulty when things are really serious. Be judicious (see Radiology chapter).

Laboratory investigations

By the end of your first day, you will already know how to request laboratory investigations. Make sure you do this properly, and follow your local guidelines. The commonly used laboratories are biochemistry, haematology and microbiology.

Find out how to contact these labs directly, both during office hours and on-call. Sometimes you might need a result quickly, or need advice about how to do a specific test. You can call the laboratory and ask for advice. Also find out how to request tests on samples for each laboratory. Learn which colour blood bottles are required for each test. This varies slightly from hospital to hospital. All samples sent to any laboratory should be sent labelled with:

- The patient's name
- Date of birth
- Unique identifying number
- Date and time

They should be accompanied by a request form with as much clinical detail as you can, and the exact nature of the test required.

If the result of a laboratory test is needed urgently, then you will have to make sure the sample is collected quickly, either by taking the blood yourself, or by asking the relevant professional to do it. If it is a blood test that can wait until the next day, then you can ask the phlebotomists to do it. You will need to know your local policy for requesting the phlebotomy team to take bloods for you. (See 'Ordering bloods/working with phlebotomists' on page 9).

In an emergency, the good FY doctor will know at least two ways of getting the most common laboratory tests done in an emergency. For example, you can test electrolytes by sending a laboratory sample, or by running some venous blood through a blood gas machine, for a guide to the result. Similarly, you can test serum haemoglobin in the lab, or get a more rough-and-ready reading by using a blood analyser, often found in Accident & Emergency (A&E) departments. You should find out where these machines are kept in your hospital before you have to use these strategies in an emergency.

Referrals

Referrals to other Consultants are the way your team can get other specialists' opinions on your patient's condition and management. They are an important part of the patient's care, because they ensure that the patient's management is optimal in all aspects. Often, you might make a referral because your team feels that their own expertise is not the most important, and that the patient would be better looked after by another team.

Referrals are strictly not clinical jobs and they are often regarded as being less urgent by the busy FY doctor, left until there is a more convenient time to do them. You might be able to do them later in the day, but remember; there will never be a 'more convenient' time, and this can delay important decisions. Make time and do your referrals so that they arrive at the Consultant in question's office by the next morning.

How to write a referral letter

Use a word processor to ensure that your letter is legible! Include the patient's name, date of birth and hospital number, as well as where they are in the hospital.

You will be referring for a reason; put the specific question you are trying to get answered in the first line of your letter. Then outline the patient's current admission. Start with the presenting complaint and characterise this. Describe physical findings and the results of investigations so far. If your team has made a diagnosis and initiated treatment, then describe these. Include any information that the specialist will want to know; make your referral relevant to that Consultant's specialty area. You should try to capture the interest of your reader. End your letter by restating your original request.

Print the letter on your hospital/departmental letter-headed paper and take it directly to the Consultant in question's secretary. If the referral is urgent, bleep the Consultant's Registrar and speak with them directly.

Discharges

When a patient leaves hospital, they need to go with medications, and a letter should be written to them and their General Practitioner (GP) summarising their hospital stay and any changes that may have occurred. There is usually a planned time for the patient to go home, and this will often be dictated by when the transport can be booked, when the drugs are available from pharmacy, and other social factors. This means you will be harassed by nurses to get discharge letters done on time.

It will help your reputation, if you get these letters done on time from the start. Try to anticipate discharges and write the letters in advance, so that you avoid writing them in a hurry whilst the ambulance drivers look at their watches.

How to write discharge letters

The letter is a communication from the hospital to the GP, informing him of what has happened to the patient whilst in hospital. It is the only record the GP will have, and so it is important that it is clear. Include the following information in the letter:

- Patient's name, date of birth and hospital number
- Presenting complaint
- Physical findings
- Results of investigations

- Diagnosis
- Management
- Medications on discharge
- Any follow-up planned by the hospital
- Any follow-up suggestions to the GP
- Your name and contact details

Other jobs

As the most junior member on the team, a lot of the odd jobs will fall to you. You might think that, as a highly trained doctor, they are beneath you, but there are many menial tasks that often need some medical knowledge to accomplish. Do these jobs cheerfully and view them as a contribution to the smooth working of the team, even if it is just buying the coffee.

How to be efficient

FY doctors have always had to work very hard. This is unlikely to change, and if you are not strategic and intelligent about the way in which you go about doing your job, you will quickly be snowed under by more and more work. This is depressing and stressful, and will also prevent you from learning from your job, which is your main aim as an FY doctor. This section will try to suggest ways in which you can ensure your working day runs smoothly and efficiently. This section provides some hints on how to be efficient. However, these are not hard and fast rules, and cannot replace the experience you will gain for yourself with your particular job.

Invest in your reputation

This is not as superficial as it seems. A reputation for being polite, kind, caring and considerate of the people around you, patients and professionals, will be your most useful asset for your Foundation year and beyond. If you obviously care for your patients and their relatives, then it is much more likely that the professionals around you will want to help you. This will help you with requesting services from other specialties, and will encourage other staff around you to support you in your work. A good reputation is easy to forge. Simply make sure that, each and every time, you are trying to do your best for your patients. If this manifests as spending an extra hour at work explaining something to a relative in your first couple of weeks at work, it will certainly pay dividends later on, when you need a favour from another member of the team. It is surprising how quickly and consistently public opinion spreads, and so long as you are genuine, having a good reputation keeps paying off. However, also comply with the European Working time directive where possible!

Delegate

You are the most junior member of the team, so any jobs that are delegated to you might seem like your problem to deal with alone. This is not strictly true. There are always nurses or other professionals around with the same technical skills as you. You might ask a nurse on the ward if he/she would not mind taking blood from a patient, or passing a nasogastric (NG) tube. Your low rank means you will have to ask these things as a favour, but if you have worked on your reputation early on, you will be more likely to get a positive response.

Ordering bloods/working with phlebotomists

Phlebotomists can save you huge amounts of time, if used correctly. Make sure you are aware of the methods of requesting blood tests, and exactly how to get these to the phlebotomy team. Do this on time! Then, ensure you have a good relationship with the phlebotomists on your ward. Simply introducing yourself and thanking them for taking blood is often a good start, and takes a minute. If you have a good relationship with phlebotomists, you might be able to add requests to their list if you have forgotten to request them earlier, or the need has just arisen.

The same rule goes for the 'intravenous (IV) teams' that some hospitals have for placing a cannula and other more complex IV access. Be polite, be grateful and be strategic.

Avoid overloading the phlebotomists with requests. Phlebotomists work to time not workload, and if there are bloods left over they will leave them for you, which means a crucial test might be delayed. Sick patients will need daily bloods, but stable patients might need them every three to four days while 'social' patients should be checked once a week.

Shortcuts

There are always shortcuts; either real physical shortcuts around the hospital, or through the systems that you have to negotiate. These will be specific to your particular job and hospital, but you should find them as they will save you valuable time. Try to devise new systems in your hospital work so you can build in your own shortcuts. However, you should never use a shortcut that might compromise patient care.

How to be effective

Getting your jobs done quickly is very different from doing them well. As mentioned above, there may be some jobs that can be done quickly and with minimal effort, and others that can be delegated. This might include getting a CT or ultrasound scan (USS) done on the same day, referring a patient so that they are taken over by another team, or getting an expert opinion either on the ward or on a telephone. These things each take a specific skill, but there are some general steps you can take in order to complete a task effectively.

As an FY doctor, most of the important tasks will not be done by you, so usually your most useful skill will be to get help from experts. Often, these people will be senior doctors, so you need an approach to dealing with them. Some effective strategies are described in this section.

Know your patient

Whenever you approach a senior about something, always know everything about the patient that you can possibly learn. Senior doctors will always know more medicine than you, but you might know about the patient, and the purpose of the

interaction is to get the best advice from them possible. Take a few minutes to read through the notes from the current admission. To get more background, avoid reading in-patient notes from the previous admission, look through previous discharge letters and correspondence. When you have a feel for the patient, you can set about performing the task.

Have a focused question

Focus on the most important aspects of the problem, and explain exactly what you need from the person you are talking to. Be clear about what you expect, and be prepared to justify the request. Consider the alternative options that the person you are talking to might suggest, and explain why your team have decided on this specific path.

Confirm the plan

After getting the opinion/agreeing on the next step, make sure you repeat it back to the person you are talking to, so that you are absolutely clear what you need to do next. This may take an extra minute, but it will eliminate any ambiguity in your communication, which is often where problems arise in patient management. Always remember to document all conversations regarding the patient's care in his or her medical notes.

Calling for help

Every doctor in the hospital, apart from the FY1 doctors, is more senior than you, so in theory you could ask any of them for help. In reality, you will limit your requests to members of your team. If you do not understand something, or are unable to complete a technical job, then bleep your immediate seniors.

If a patient is severely unwell, and you are alarmed, call your Registrar (or ST3, ST4, ST5) because they will need to know eventually. Do not be frightened to call these senior doctors: it is part of their job to support junior staff, and you will inevitably learn something from them.

There may be other specialist teams available to help, and you should consider if you need their help. For example, there may be an IV team who can help you with IV access, or there may be a urology specialist nurse to help with urinary catheterisations.

When to go home

Every day as an FY doctor will be tiring, and you will want to leave work on time. Here is a checklist to make sure you have done all the things that need to be done on the day:

- All changes documented in the notes, with a plan for treatment
- All jobs from the ward round done
- All new investigation results reviewed and acted on
- Any sick patients stabilised, or handed over to the on-call team
- All fluids prescribed for the night
- All monitored drugs prescribed e.g. warfarin, monitored antibiotics such as gentamicin, etc.

Once you are satisfied that you have done all these things, leave quickly before more work turns up!

Professionalism

It is very difficult to define professionalism, but it is obvious when someone is not professional. In the context of the Foundation Programme, professionalism roughly corresponds to the attitudes of the FY doctor, taken apart from his or her clinical knowledge and technical ability; you need good people in order to have good doctors. Here are some general rules:

- Be punctual
- Be honest
- Be polite
- Know your limits
- Be willing to admit to mistakes
- Be willing to improve

Whistle-blowing

If one of your colleagues or seniors is not up to scratch, is not coping with the job, or worse is lying or covering up mistakes, it is your professional duty to your patients to do something about it. Each trust has its own whistle-blowing procedures, so find out what your local policies are. As an FY doctor, however, your actions are fairly simple. Speak to your Consultant about what you think the problem is, and take his or her guidance on what to do next. If your Consultant is the problem, speak with another one that you get on with; this can be your educational supervisor.

If you are worried that no-one is taking your concern seriously, put it in writing to your Foundation Supervisor. This will give you a record of the communication, and will encourage action on the part of your seniors.

BEING ON-CALL

The on-call is where you will learn the most, so be well prepared and try to enjoy it. As an FY doctor, the requirements of on-calls break down into roughly three different categories:

- Clerking new patients: when new patients arrive in the hospital as part of the on-call admitting team
- Emergency Jobs: where a patient becomes acutely unwell
- Maintenance Jobs: where a job needs doing to continue a specific management plan or where a non-emergency change occurs

You will find different emphasis on these categories across rotations, but the main challenge of being on-call will remain the same, and that is unpredictability.

Dealing with unpredictability

When you are on-call as an FY doctor, you are the first port of call for any simple jobs that need to be done, and for assessing acutely ill patients and for seeing new admissions. The nature of the job means that you can never fully predict what will happen, and when. You will have to deal with an unpredictable work load. You will also have to attend acutely ill patients, and it will not always be clear what the diagnosis is. Again, you will have to learn how to work with uncertainty.

On-call work does not arrive in an organised manner, it is your job to organise it into a sensible order. Your bleep will bleep, and you will have more work to do. Prioritise your jobs. If they are emergencies or urgent, do them as soon as you can. If they are routine, then try to do them geographically. Write down the details of every phone call, so you remember everything you have been asked to do.

Before your on-call (be prepared)

Take a thorough handover of any jobs or the details of any sick patients that the day teams are worried about. You should be bleeped by each team, or else they will use the hospital's recognised handover system. Get each patient's name, identity number and location as well as their working diagnosis and what you need to do. Try to do this verbally as well as getting a written handover, because you can then ask questions about management whilst you talk about the patient.

At the beginning of your on-call

Find out who your seniors are for the on-call, and make contact with them early on. Establish that you will call them if you feel out of your depth.

The beginning of the on-call is the time to maximise your efficiency. Be proactive and visit all the wards you are responsible for, to discover what jobs the nurses have for you. Ask all the trained nurses on the ward if they need anything done and do these jobs as soon as you can. Usually, there will be some basic jobs such as:

- Prescribing fluids
- Prescribing warfarin
- Prescribing simple analgesia
- Rewriting drug charts
- Drug levels to check for monitoring

If you are on call for a weekend, then prescribe enough fluids or warfarin for each patient to last until the end of the on-call, if it is safe to do so.

If the nurses on a ward have not worked out what jobs they need doing, try to anticipate them. Do any of the patients have bags of fluids up now? If so, quickly check if there are more written up, saving yourself a trip back there later on. This sort of forward planning will help you greatly later in the on-call.

Find out what skills the nurses on the wards have. If you are on-call, it can be invaluable if you can find a nurse who will take any of the routine bloods on the ward.

It is unlikely that you will be able to anticipate all of the routine on-call jobs that you will need to do, but working hard to clear the routine work early on will give you more time to work when patients become sick.

If you are bleeped to attend a ward to do the jobs, tell the person bleeping you that you are coming round, and ask if there is anything urgent.

Dealing with the sick patient

Inevitably during your on-call, a nurse will bleep you and tell you about a patient they are worried about, and that they would like you to see them. It is almost impossible to judge how sick a patient is on the other end of a telephone, so never try to do it. Nevertheless, try to get as much information as you can from the first call. Does the patient have chest pain, breathlessness, abdominal pain or developing neurology?

It might be tempting to dismiss a bleep as somebody being overcautious, or as having very little substance, but remember that some nurses have a lot of experience and can recognise when someone is ill, whether the observations indicate it or not. Even if it is a gut feeling, take it seriously.

You will need to assess the patient for yourself, but ask the nurses to get a fresh set of observations and electrocardiogram (ECG), get the patient on high flow oxygen while you are on the way, and if the blood pressure is low, suggest getting a bag of fluids ready for when you arrive. Ask if they can find the notes, drug chart and observations and collect them together for you. Then head down to the ward as quickly as possible.

Rehearse the differentials for the presenting complaint in your head as you walk to the ward. Stay calm. When you arrive, make a quick airway, breathing, circulation (ABC) assessment and put out an immediate arrest call if any of these are compromised. (See Resuscitation chapter.)

If you are satisfied that the patient does not warrant an arrest call, look at the notes and familiarise yourself with the story, and then go back and assess the patient in this context. Get a swift history of the latest problem from the patient and nurses if possible, then examine the relevant system, form an impression and do some basic investigations, like taking bloods and ordering an X-ray. Always ensure you achieve IV access early on in a sick patient.

You may not know exactly what is wrong with the patient, but remember that there are often general measures that can be taken, especially by dealing with symptoms. Then, when you have put an interim plan in motion, call your senior and inform them of what has happened and what you are doing about it. They will instruct you on what to do next. If you ever feel unsure or out of your depth, call your seniors immediately. Never try to soldier on when you have any doubts about management

Two sick patients

If you have two patients that are sick, you are not going to be able to do everything for both of them. Call for help from your seniors and take their advice. They will help you prioritise your work and develop a strategy for dealing with both patients. As you become more confident, you will be better able to deal with having more than one sick patient.

Clerking new patients

You might have to clerk new patients whilst on-call, which is time consuming. As soon as you are bleeped, ask the nurse calling you what the basic presenting complaint is, what the observations are and whether the patient looks well or not. Then you might ask if anyone can take bloods from the patient.

You can then review the patient briefly and assess how unwell they are. If they are essentially stable, then you can work on other, more urgent jobs, and return when things are more settled. If they look acutely unwell, then you may have to break off and work on them now.

DEALING WITH DEATH

Death stalks the wards at all times. People in hospital are sick and some of them will die. You will need to get used to this. When a patient dies, you should quickly confirm their death, otherwise the rest of the hospital cannot get on with dealing with the death. You may also be required to write a death certificate and a cremation form.

How to confirm death

As an FY doctor, it will be your job to confirm their death. This is fairly simple. (See Table 2.1).

Confirming death:

1. Ask the nurses to ensure that any relatives have left the bedside
2. Check that the patient does not respond to verbal and pain stimuli
3. Feel for a central pulse for three minutes, whilst listening for heart sounds
4. Feel for respiratory effort for three minutes, whilst listening for breath sounds
5. Inspect the pupils and confirm that they are fixed and dilated
6. If you are unsure, you can look for 'rail-roading' in the retinal veins

---

Table 2.1: The process of confirming death.

When you are satisfied that the patient is dead, check if there is a pacemaker by feeling over the chest. Then write the time of death with your findings in the notes, and make sure to write out the patient's full name, date of birth and hospital number yourself, so that there can be no doubt.

Mention if you spoke to anyone present about the death and document whether or not they had any concerns, and make it clear whether or not there was a pacemaker present.

Writing a death certificate

Once your patient is confirmed dead, they need to have a certificate written so that their death can be registered and their funeral planned. You will often have to write this. Death certificates will require several pieces of information to be filled in. (See Table 2.2).

Part Ia

Deciding on the causes of death is often tricky. Always talk to your consultant about causes of death before you complete a

---

Information needed for the death certificate:

- The patient's name
- The place of death
- The last time you saw the patient alive
- The causes of death:
  - o Ia the immediate cause
  - o Ib the condition causing Ia
  - o Ic the condition causing Ib
  - o II conditions contributing to the death, but not directly causing it
- Your name and signature
- Your qualifications
- The consultant responsible for the patient's care

Table 2.2: The basic information needed to fill in the death certificate.

certificate. Remember that the mode of death is different from the cause of death. Your patient may have had a cardiac arrest; this is the mode of dying. The cause is likely to be something else, for example pneumonia or ventricular tachycardia. This is what you will write in part Ia.

Never use vernacular or vague terms. Use 'antero-lateral myocardial infarct' rather than 'big heart attack' or 'cerebrovascular accident' and 'bronchopneumonia' instead of 'stroke' and 'chest infection'. When people die of metastatic cancer, we often write 'carcinomatosis'.

You may sometimes have to make a decision between two possible causes of death, which were both present in the same patient, for example pneumonia and pulmonary oedema. If this is the case, see if you can use the observations charts and nursing notes as well as medical notes to guide you.

Parts Ib and Ic

These are the conditions that led directly to the immediate cause of death. For example, if your patient died of pulmonary oedema, then they most likely had left ventricular failure (Ib) which will have been caused by some form of cardiac disease, e.g. ischaemic heart disease or myocardial infarction (Ic). If your patient had a cerebrovascular event (Ia), then that may have been caused by AF (Ib) which may have been caused by thyrotoxicosis (Ic).

Part II

This is where you write the other conditions that your patients had which contributed, but were did not directly cause death. Often, conditions such as renal failure or dementia, that made treating the primary causes more difficult, are included here along with co-morbidities in the same organ system as the terminal illness. If your patient died of pneumonia, then their previous pulmonary fibrosis is included.

The Coroner's Office

You will have to discuss a case with the Coroner if:

1. Your patient has been in hospital less than 24 hours
2. Had an operation within the last year of life.

3. The patient's death is deemed to be in any way 'unnatural', i.e. violent, accidental, involving substance abuse, due to industrial disease. You will have to discuss this with the coroner's office.

4. If you cannot give a cause of death.

Call the Coroner's Office and discuss the case with them. Read the notes first, and know the case thoroughly! They may suggest what to write, or they may suggest talking to a pathologist about the case. Sometimes they will tell you a post-mortem is required.

Coroners make decisions on the cause of death if you cannot do so.

They may say the death was due to suicide, homicide, misadventure or natural causes, and then give a natural cause. As an FY doctor, if there is even the slightest suggestion that a death was due to anything other than natural causes, you must speak with the Coroner's Office.

Cremation forms

If a patient's family have decided that their relative is to be cremated, then you will have to write a cremation form to state that there is no reason why the body should not be cremated. Essentially, you are saying that there is no reason to suspect any foul-play in the patient's death, and so a cremation is legally acceptable. This is a big responsibility, and you should take it seriously.

As an FY doctor, you will only fill out Part A of the cremation form. This contains some more detailed information about the patient such as their address, occupation, time and place of death as well as some information about you, i.e. stating how you were responsible for their care, when you saw him/her before and after death, and how long you cared for him/her. You will also be required to state a time when you have inspected the body.

Then you are required to describe the evidence you have used to give the causes of death you have written on the death certificate. Give as much diagnostic information as possible: include elements from the history, ('central chest pain radiating between shoulder blades'), findings on examination, ('quiet heart sounds, diastolic murmur, difference in blood pressure in each arm'), and findings on investigations ('small complexes on ECG, CT showed pericardial effusion and aortic dissection). If you are including chronic conditions in parts Ib, Ic and II, then write 'previous diagnosis of X'.

You must include the names and addresses of any people nursing the patient, and anyone present at the moment of death, and note whether you have spoken to them and whether they have any concerns. If there was no-one present, or you have not spoken to these people, because the patient died during the night for example, then say so.

You must also state that there are no potentially explosive pacemakers, implants or prostheses that might damage a cremation oven, so be sure to inspect the body and be sure of this for yourself. If an oven explodes, you are responsible!

Once you have completed the form, a more senior doctor checks it. They may call you and other people you have mentioned on the death certificate, so as to discuss what was written and whether anyone has any concerns about the patient's death. This may feel a little like an interrogation, but so long as you have been as accurate as you can on the form, there is little to worry about. If you've written something stupid, it will be picked up on here.

THE FOUNDATION PROGRAMME ASSESSMENTS

Recall that the FY doctor's main role is to ensure the smooth running of the team. This task in itself will always be linked with learning new facts and skills in medicine. The difference between how things used to be and the new Foundation Programme is that you are now required to demonstrate that you have these skills. The tools used to demonstrate your competency in the task set out by the Foundation Programme curriculum are largely practical and professional, rather than knowledge-based. You will need to show that you can perform certain procedures (using DOPS), that you are clinically competent to assess and manage patients (using Mini-CEX), that you are developing your knowledge (using CbDs), and that you are working well within your team (using Mini-PAT).

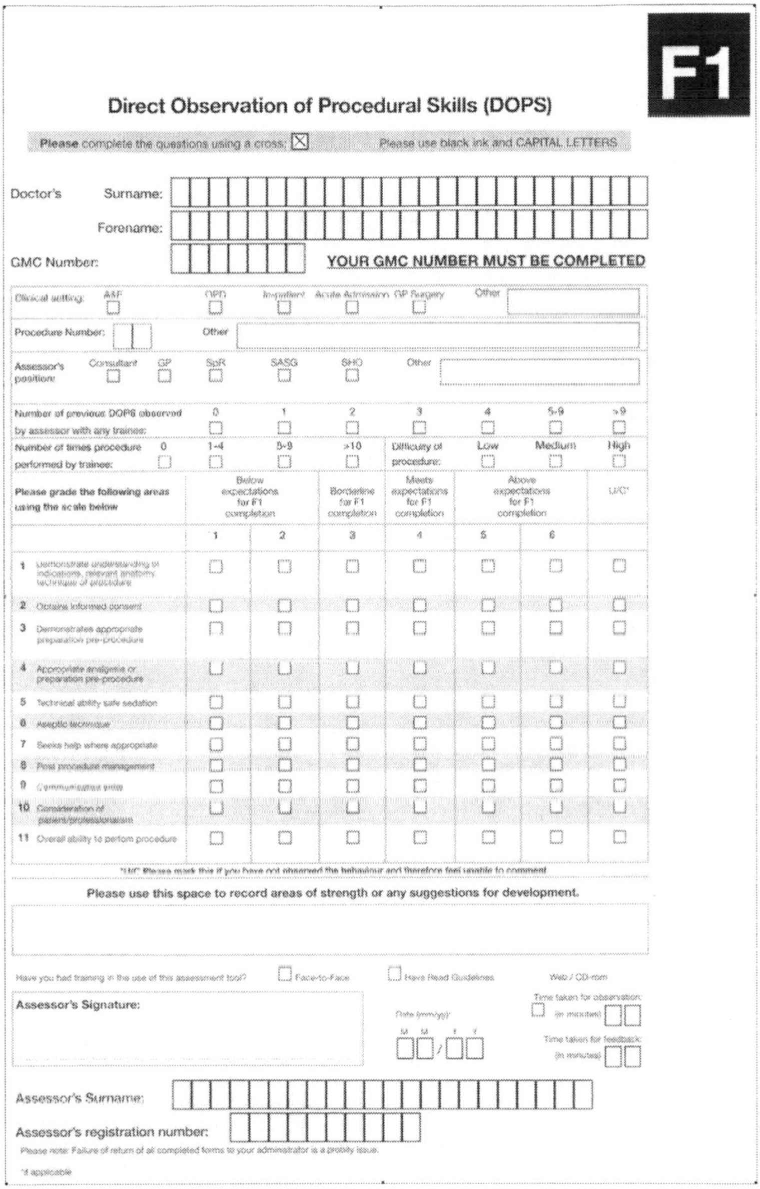

F1

Direct Observation of Procedural Skills (DOPS)

Please complete the questions using a cross: ☒ Please use black ink and CAPITAL LETTERS

Doctor's Surname:

Forename:

GMC Number: **YOUR GMC NUMBER MUST BE COMPLETED**

Clinical setting: A&E ☐ OPD ☐ In-patient ☐ Acute Admission ☐ GP Surgery ☐ Other

Procedure Number: Other

Assessor's position: Consultant ☐ GP ☐ SpR ☐ SASG ☐ SHO ☐ Other

Number of previous DOPS observed by assessor with any trainee: 0 ☐ 1 ☐ 2 ☐ 3 ☐ 4 ☐ 5-9 ☐ >9 ☐

Number of times procedure performed by trainee: 0 ☐ 1-4 ☐ 5-9 ☐ >10 ☐

Difficulty of procedure: Low ☐ Medium ☐ High ☐

Please grade the following areas using the scale below	Below expectations for F1 completion		Borderline for F1 completion	Meets expectations for F1 completion	Above expectations for F1 completion		U/C*
	1	2	3	4	5	6	
1 Demonstrate understanding of indications, relevant anatomy, technique of procedure	☐	☐	☐	☐	☐	☐	☐
2 Obtains informed consent	☐	☐	☐	☐	☐	☐	☐
3 Demonstrates appropriate preparation pre-procedure	☐	☐	☐	☐	☐	☐	☐
4 Appropriate analgesia or preparation pre-procedure	☐	☐	☐	☐	☐	☐	☐
5 Technical ability safe sedation	☐	☐	☐	☐	☐	☐	☐
6 Aseptic technique	☐	☐	☐	☐	☐	☐	☐
7 Seeks help where appropriate	☐	☐	☐	☐	☐	☐	☐
8 Post procedure management	☐	☐	☐	☐	☐	☐	☐
9 Communication skills	☐	☐	☐	☐	☐	☐	☐
10 Consideration of patient/professionalism	☐	☐	☐	☐	☐	☐	☐
11 Overall ability to perform procedure	☐	☐	☐	☐	☐	☐	☐

*U/C Please mark this if you have not observed the behaviour and therefore feel unable to comment

Please use this space to record areas of strength or any suggestions for development.

Have you had training in the use of this assessment tool? ☐ Face-to-Face ☐ Have Read Guidelines ☐ Web / CD-rom

Assessor's Signature:

Date (mm/yy): M M / Y Y

Time taken for observation: (in minutes)

Time taken for feedback: (in minutes)

Assessor's Surname:

Assessor's registration number:

Please note: Failure of return of all completed forms to your administrator is a probity issue.

*if applicable

Figure 2.2: The assessment form for DOPS. ***Courtesy of United Kingdom Foundation Programme Office***

Direct Observation of Procedural Skills

DOPS are assessments of practical skills, which demonstrate your ability to perform a certain skill, and identify strengths and areas for development. (See Direct Observation of Procedural Skills chapter). You will need to perform a minimum of six of these in each year of the Foundation Programme, selected from a core group.

The requirement for being an assessor for DOPS is that you are competent in the procedure yourself, so this means that many other professionals, not just doctors, can sign them. Nurses, in particular, are a good source of DOPS. Try to think about where you might get the opportunity to perform some of the procedures.

For example, drug rounds are good times to be observed while giving injections. Neurology clinics will most likely be the best place for lumbar punctures.

A DOPS involves being observed performing a procedure, and then the assessor providing feedback and suggesting improvements. They will need to fill out a form, which is currently stored electronically on your e-portfolio.

Mini-Clinical Evaluation Exercise

This is an assessment of your ability to perform a clinical evaluation of a patient; essentially taking a history, or examining

Figure 2.3 The assessment form for Mini-CEX. *Courtesy of United Kingdom Foundation Programme Office*

them, making a diagnosis and then deciding on a management plan. It is a core medical skill that only more senior doctors (STs and above) will be able to assess you on. You will need to complete six of these Mini-CEX assessments in each year of the Foundation Programme.

Your assessors will watch you perform the task, and then give feedback and fill out your assessment form.

On-calls or working in assessment units are good opportunities to get these forms signed off, as are post-take ward rounds, because they all require you to be demonstrating clinical judgement, which is an essential part of the assessment.

Case-based Discussions

This is an assessment of your developing clinical knowledge, to show that you are learning medical facts as well as skills. You will sit down with your Consultant and talk through a case that you have selected, using the medical notes as guidance. Your assessor will ask you about your knowledge of the case, and you will need to show that you know an appropriate amount about it, as well as demonstrating that you have learned from the specific case.

You will need to book a time with your Consultant for this

Figure 2.4: The assessment form for CbD. *Courtesy of United Kingdom Foundation Programme Office*

discussion, and request the notes from medical records. The best person to work with in doing both these things is your Consultant's secretary.

Mini-Peer Assessment Tool

This 360-degree assessment, where people you work with from all aspects of your job are required to give structured feedback on your work. You will be able to nominate these people, but they will have to be senior doctors, nurses and other healthcare professionals. You will get a rating and written feedback from these people, which in theory should be anonymous. This is the best form of assessing how good a team player you are and allows you to appreciate the role of the MDT and allied health professionals in the management of patients.

Rater Form mini-PAT (Peer Assessment Tool) F1

Please complete the questions using a cross: ☒   Please use black ink and CAPITAL LETTERS

Doctor's   Surname:

Forename:

GMC Number: YOUR GMC NUMBER MUST BE COMPLETED

How do you rate this Doctor in their:	Below expectations for F1 completion 1	2	Borderline for F1 completion 3	Meets expectations for F1 completion 4	Above expectations for F1 completion 5	6	U/C*
Good Clinical Care							
1 Ability to diagnose patient problems	☐	☐	☐	☐	☐	☐	☐
2 Ability to formulate appropriate management plans	☐	☐	☐	☐	☐	☐	☐
3 Awareness of their own limitations	☐	☐	☐	☐	☐	☐	☐
4 Ability to respond to psychological aspects of illness	☐	☐	☐	☐	☐	☐	☐
5 Appropriate utilisation of resources e.g. ordering investigations	☐	☐	☐	☐	☐	☐	☐
Maintaining good medical practice							
6 Ability to manage time effectively / prioritise	☐	☐	☐	☐	☐	☐	☐
7 Technical skills (appropriate to current practice)	☐	☐	☐	☐	☐	☐	☐
Teaching and Training, Appraisal and Assessing							
8 Willingness and effectiveness when teaching/training colleagues	☐	☐	☐	☐	☐	☐	☐
Relationship with Patients							
9 Communication with patients	☐	☐	☐	☐	☐	☐	☐
10 Communication with carers and/or family	☐	☐	☐	☐	☐	☐	☐
11 Respect for patients and their right to confidentiality	☐	☐	☐	☐	☐	☐	☐
Working with colleagues							
12 Verbal communication with colleagues	☐	☐	☐	☐	☐	☐	☐
13 Written communication with colleagues	☐	☐	☐	☐	☐	☐	☐
14 Ability to recognise and value the contribution of others	☐	☐	☐	☐	☐	☐	☐
15 Accessibility/Reliability	☐	☐	☐	☐	☐	☐	☐
16 Overall, how do you rate this doctor compared to a doctor ready to complete F1 training?	☐	☐	☐	☐	☐	☐	☐

Do you have any concerns about this doctor's probity or health?   [ ] Yes   [ ] No
If yes please state your concerns:

*U/C Please mark this if you have not observed the behaviour and therefore feel unable to comment.

Figure 2.5: Assessment form for Mini-PAT. *Courtesy of United Kingdom Foundation Programme Office*

Further reading and references

➤ The following sites will provide up to date information in regards to the Foundation Programme:

➤ www.foundationprogramme.nhs.uk

➤ www.rcplondon.ac.uk

➤ www.rcseng.ac.uk

ABDOMINAL PAIN

Differential diagnosis

System/Organ	Disease
Gut	Gastritis
	Gastro-oesophageal reflux disease (GORD)
	Peptic Ulcer
	Intestinal obstruction
	Diverticulitis
	Inflammatory bowel disease (IBD)
	Ulcerative colitis
	Crohn's disease
	Appendicitis
	Volvulus
	Gastroenteritis
	Strangulated hernia
	Constipation
	Irritable bowel syndrome (IBS)
Hepato-biliary	Cholecystitis
	Ascending cholangitis
Pancreatic	Acute pancreatitis
	Chronic pancreatitis
Splenic (referred to shoulder tip)	Infarction
	Rupture
Urinary tract	**Urinary tract Infection (UTI)/ pyelonephritis**
	Acute urinary retention
	Polycystic kidney (e.g. haemorrhage into cyst)
	Ureteric colic
Gynaecological	Ectopic pregnancy
	Ovarian cyst (rupture or torsion)
	Endometriosis
	Severe dysmenorrhea
Vascular	Aortic dissection
	Ischaemic colitis
Peritoneum	Peritonitis
Abdominal wall	Rectus sheath haematoma
Retroperitoneal	Retroperitoneal haemorrhage
Referred	Lower lobar pneumonia
	Myocardial infarction (MI)
	Thoracic spinal disease
Other	Hypercalcaemia
	Diabetic ketoacidosis (DKA)
	Porphyria
	Uraemia

Gastro-oesophageal reflux disease (GORD)

Epidemiology

Affects up to 30% of Western Populations. There is a higher incidence in the developed countries as obesity tends to be more common in these individuals.

Aetiology

The mechanism and precipitant of GORD is highlighted in Table 3.1:

Mechanism	Precipitant
Reduced clearance from oesophagus	Poor posture, post-prandial, systemic sclerosis
Reduced pressure of the lower oesophageal sphincter	Foods with a high fat content, alcohol, caffeine, smoking, pregnancy, nitrates and channel blockers
Direct damage to the mucosa of the oesophagus	Alcohol, hot drinks, acidic stomach contents, bile, non-steroidal anti-inflammatory drugs (NSAID)
Increased production of gastric acids	Zollinger-Ellison syndrome
Damage to the anti-reflux mechanism	Hiatus hernia
Delayed gastric emptying	Pyloric stenosis, gastric atony
Increased intra-abdominal pressure	With increased abdominal girth such as in obesity, ascites, tight clothing and pregnancy

Table 3.1: Causes of GORD.

Pathophysiology

A small amount of post-prandial reflux is physiologically normal. However GORD involves the passage of acidic gastric contents into the distal portion of the oesophagus which causes symptoms and impairs quality of life. It usually occurs in patients where there is dysfunction of the lower oesophageal sphincter (LOS). The LOS consists of an intrinsic muscular band around the lower 4 centimeters of the oesophagus and the crural diaphragm surrounding the proximal 2 centimeters of this.

Oesophagitis may be evident macroscopically or microscopically but correlates poorly with symptoms experienced by the patient. Around two thirds of patients with symptoms of heartburn have no evidence of oesophagitis on endoscopy.

Microscopically there is an initial hypertrophy of the epithelial layer of the oesophagus. Subsequently, there is an infiltration of inflammatory cells resulting in macroscopic inflammation,

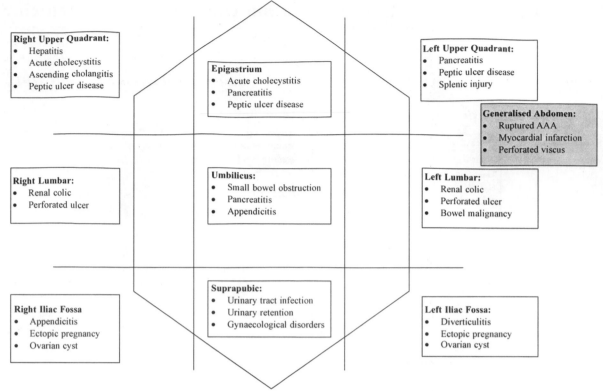

Figure 3.1: Potential diagnoses of pain in each area of the abdomen.

erosions and mucosal ulceration. As healing occurs strictures may form.

With prolonged exposure to acid there is metaplasia of the normal stratified squamous epithelium and Barrett's oesophagus develops.

Key features in the history/examination

- Epigastric or retrosternal burning pain. It can be worse on lying flat, bending down or on straining.
- Symptoms of acid reflux mostly occur after meals and there is some symptomatic relief with the use of antacids.
- Exacerbation of symptoms with large, fatty meals and tight clothing.
- Waterbrash: the excessive production of saliva and bitter taste in the mouth due to acidic gastric contents refluxing into the oespohagus.
- Recurrent chest infections caused by nocturnal aspiration.
- Chronic cough or wheeze.
- Dysphagia or odynophagia due to ulcers of the oesophageal mucosa and any resultant strictures.
- Patients with oesophageal ulceration may present with an upper GI bleed .
- Nausea and vomiting may be a feature.

- Typically, the only sign on examination may be epigastric tenderness.
- It may be difficult to distinguish between the symptoms of GORD and those of cardiac ischaemia clinically, as both may be provoked by exercise and relieved by the use of glyceryl trinitrate spray.
- The following features in the history should cause 'alarm' and require further investigation.

Alarm symptoms requiring further investigation
Weight loss
Haematemesis
Dysphagia
Odynophagia

Table 3.2: Alarm symptoms requiring further investigations

Investigations

Blood tests:

- Full blood count (FBC): if there is anaemia then add haematinics too.
- Urea & electrolytes (U&E's).
- Clotting screen.

Endoscopy:

- An endoscopy is not indicated as a routine investigation in those presenting with symptoms of dyspepsia without any alarming features.

- In those who present at 55 years or over, with a new onset of symptoms of dyspepsia without an obvious precipitant, must be investigated urgently by endoscopy.

- Other indications for endoscopy are symptoms persisting for over 4 weeks and patients more than 40 years old who have features such as dysphagia or unintentional weight loss.

- Endoscopy findings are normal in more than half of patients with GORD with some showing features of oesophagitis.

Other:

- A barium meal: is not always useful as it may illustrate gastro-oesophageal reflux even in asymptomatic individuals. It can demonstrate a hiatus hernia.

- Oesophageal pH and manometry studies: with a pH electrode positioned 5 centimeters above the LOS, can be performed in those patients where the gastroscopy is normal despite typical features of GORD or if symptoms are unresponsive to treatment. The total exposure of the oesophagus to acid is measured over a 24-hour period with time spent with pH<4 of significance. A relationship between low pH and symptoms is sought.

  With no erosions on endoscopy, the presence of a positive 24-hour pH study gives a diagnosis of non-erosive reflux disease (NERD) but a negative study gives a diagnosis of 'functional heartburn.'

- Cardiac investigations may be required for atypical pain.

Management

➤ Advice on lifestyle measures: to stop smoking, lose weight, avoid any drugs which precipitate symptoms, avoid fatty/spicy foods, alcohol, eating large meals late at night, and hot drinks such as coffee and tea. If night-time dyspepsia is a problem elevation of the head of the bed by 15 cm at night may help.

➤ Antacids such as magnesium and aluminium hydroxide or alginates (e.g. gaviscon).

➤ Drugs to suppress acid production such as proton pump inhibitors (e.g. omeprazole) and H_2 receptor antagonists (e.g. ranitidine).

➤ Prokinetic drugs are effective in relief of nausea and vomiting, e.g. metoclopramide and domperidone and are used in conjunction with acid suppressing agents.

➤ Patients who do not respond or are intolerant to medical therapy may require surgical management: the most common procedure is the laparoscopic Nissen fundoplication, where the fundus of the stomach is sutured around the end of the distal oesophagus. This results in a region of high-pressure at the lower oesophagus reducing the volume of acid reflux.

Prognosis:

➤ Approximately 50% of patients are successfully treated with weight loss and the prescribing of simple antacids.

Peptic ulcer disease

Epidemiology

Peptic ulceration is now decreasing in the developed world due to effective treatment of *Helicobacter pylori*. H. *pylori* is a gram-negative microaerophilic flagellated bacillus which is contracted in childhood. The incidence is 40% in the developed world and up to 80% in the developing world. It is associated with a lower socio-economic background and overcrowded living conditions.

Males are more commonly affected than females with a ratio of 4:1. Duodenal ulcers are 3–4 times more common than gastric ulcers. Duodenal ulcers are most likely between 20 to 60 years of age whereas gastric ulcers tend to present more in the elderly population.

Aetiology

The major causes are *Helicobacter pylori* infection and NSAID use. Other causes include gastric cancers (adenocarcinoma and lymphoma), gastrinoma (Zollinger-Ellison Syndrome), hyperparathyroidism, radiation and severe systemic illness.

Smoking, chronic alcohol use and stress increase the likelihood of peptic ulceration.

Pathophysiology

Peptic ulcers form due to a breach in the mucosa in the stomach and duodenum. Duodenal ulcers tend to develop due to impairment in the production of gastric acid. Gastric ulcers usually result from the affects of cytotoxins produced by bacteria such as H. pylori and the resultant stimulation of an immune response.

Key features in the history/examination

- Epigastric pain, related to meal times, with symptoms of nausea, heartburn, chest pain and acid reflux, bloating, haematemesis (including coffee-ground vomiting) and malaena. There may be epigastric tenderness on examination.

- Gastric ulcers classically present with epigastric pain precipitated by food. Associated symptoms of anorexia, vomiting and weight loss are common and more pronounced if there is an underlying malignant ulcer.

- Duodenal ulcers classically present with pain 1–3 hours after food and during the night. The pain is often relieved by milk or other neutral foods. The pain may radiate to the back in the case of a posterior ulcer.

- Symptoms respond to antacid treatment.

- Vomiting may relieve the symptoms of pain.

- A gastric carcinoma should be excluded if an epigastric mass is palpable.

Look for complications:

- Perforation (more commonly associated with duodenal ulcers) with signs of peritonitis.

- Upper GI bleeding with pallor or a more acute haemorrhage with malaena on digital rectal examination.
- Gastric outlet obstruction (pre-pyloric or duodenal ulcer) with projectile vomiting and a succession splash.

H. *pylori*	Chronic use of Aspirin and NSAID
• Was first described by Marshall and Warren in their landmark 1983 paper (winning the Nobel prize in 2005) • Accounts for the development of 70% of gastric ulcers and 95% of duodenal ulcers. • The bacteria invade the gastric mucosal layer causing inflammation, which is usually asymptomatic. Only 15% of those infected develop an ulcer. • A link exists between H. *pylori* infection and the development of B-cell gastric lymphomas of mucosa-associated lymphoid tissue.	• Reduce the mucosal defence mechanisms by inhibiting the cyclo-oxygenase (COX) enzymes COX-1 and COX-2 (constitutively expressed in the stomach). COX-1 is responsible for the production of prostaglandins from the gastric mucosa which increase the secretion of bicarbonate and mucous and blood flow to the gastric mucosa.

Table 3.3: How H. *Pylori* and NSAID/Aspirin leads to peptic ulcer disease.

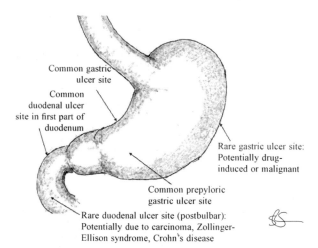

Figure 3.2: Locations for peptic ulcer disease.

Investigations

Blood tests:

- FBC: to check for a drop in Hb.
- U&E: an isolated raised urea is indicative of the 'protein meal' in cases of bleeding associated with the ulcer.
- Clotting screen.
- Cross-match.
- Serum gastrin and calcium: to exclude rarer causes such as

Zollinger-Ellison syndrome and hyperparathyroidism, the serum gastrin and calcium could be considered if clinically indicated.

Upper GI endoscopy:

- Peptic ulcers are most common on the gastric lesser curve and in the first part of the duodenum.
- Gastric carcinomas characteristically have a rolled edge, and tend to affect the greater curvature and antrum.
- A biopsy must be taken to confirm the nature of the lesion.

There are a number of ways to test for H. *Pylori*. These include

- A urea breath test: H. pylori has a high content of the enzyme urease which breaks down urea to release carbon dioxide and ammonia. The test involves ingestion of ^{14}C-labelled urea and measuring the amount of $^{14}CO_2$ in the breath after. This test can only be performed 2 weeks after PPIs have been stopped.
- A stool antigen test: tissue cultures from a biopsy sample can test for the presence of H. *pylori*, as well as establish antibiotic sensitivities.
- IgG antibodies: a blood serology test can detect IgG antibodies against H *pylori*. This is preferred in uncomplicated patients in primary care and those patients who are under the age of 45 years. The serology remains positive after eradication so cannot be used to detect successful treatment.
- Gastric antral biopsy and Campylobacter-like organism (CLO) test at Oesophagogastroduodenoscopy (OGD): the biopsy sample is placed on a test gel containing urea and if H. *pylori* is present it will convert the urea to ammonia, changing the colour from yellow to red if a positive result.

Management

➤ Triple therapy for H. *pylori* eradication. This should be taken for 10–14 days:

Regimen 1	Regimen 2
Omeprazole 20 mg or Lansoprazole 30 mg BD	
Clarithromycin 500 mg BD	
Amoxicillin 1g BD	Metronidazole 400 mg BD
More than 80% of patients are cured with this combination of treatment and the relapse rate is less than 5%.	

Table 3.4: The common regimens of triple therapy.

➤ Patients should be advised to avoid NSAIDs and aspirin, and to stop smoking, lose weight, reduce alcohol intake.

➤ Proton pump inhibitors significantly reduce gastric acid secretion by irreversibly inhibiting the pump on the apical membrane which is the final common pathway for acid secretion.

  o They are more effective at ulcer healing, however, are more expensive.

  o They should be taken for at least 4–8 weeks.

➤ H$_2$-receptor antagonists inhibit the production of gastric acid.

   o Continuous treatment with this can help to prevent ulcer recurrence and haemorrhage if there is a history of bleeding associated with a duodenal ulcer.

➤ Antacids mostly have a role in symptomatic relief

➤ Surgical management is indicated where:

   o There is persistent bleeding or ulcer perforation

   o No response to maximal medical therapy

   o A malignant gastric ulcer has been diagnosed

Prognosis:

➤ Patients confirmed to have a gastric ulcer require a repeat OGD in 6–8 weeks to re-assess the ulcer, check for healing and to repeat biopsies and cytology to exclude the diagnosis of gastric carcinoma. This is performed even if the patient is asymptomatic with initial treatment.

➤ The annual recurrence rate is now as low as 2% since the introduction of H. *pylori* eradication therapy.

Inflammatory bowel disease

The term IBD encompasses two chronic disease processes: Ulcerative colitis (UC) and Crohn's disease (CD) which will be considered separately.

Ulcerative Colitis

Epidemiology

Primarily a disease of the developed world, where approximately 70 per 100,000 people are affected with an incidence of 10 per 100,000 per year. Most people present between the ages of 20 to 40 years.

Females are affected more than males and the incidence in higher in the white population, in particular Ashkenazi Jews. In Europe more northern populations are affected more frequently than those in the south.

Aetiology

Although not proven, the disease process is thought to result from an abnormal inflammatory response of the body to food products or bacteria which are present within the bowel lumen, which is determined by both genetic and environmental factors.

Other factors which have been implicated include infection, abnormalities in the immune response, defective mucous production, psychological and social factors. Interestingly smoking cigarettes has a protective role!

Regardless of what the initial stimulating factor is, the leucocytes of the colonic mucosa are activated to produce a large amount of cytokines such as interleukin-1 and tumour necrosis factor alpha which encourage inflammation.

In genetic studies there is a 10% concordance rate in monozygotic twins and some associations with the HLA region chromosome 6 have been found.

Pathophysiology

UC starts in the rectum and spreads proximally. A disease primarily of the mucosa which initially becomes inflamed and oedematous. As the disease progresses granuloma formation, bleeding, pus production and eventually ulceration of the epithelial layer is seen. Healing is by granulation of the mucosa and this results in the formation of pseudopolyps.

Microscopic features:

• Crypt abscesses form as the inflammatory cells penetrate the lamina propria.

• Reduction in the number of mucous-producing goblet cells.

Long-standing colitis may result in:

• Muscular changes resulting in shortening and narrowing of the colon, i.e. the 'hosepipe' colon.

• Pseudo-polyp formation.

• Epithelial dysplastic changes predisposing to the development of carcinoma.

Key features in the history/examination

• Symptoms tend to be of gradual onset but can present acutely. They vary with disease extent and severity.

• The disease runs a chronic course with episodes of relapse and remission over a period of several years, where patients may be symptom-free in between episodes of disease relapse.

• The precipitating factors for relapse include psychological stress, coincidental infection, gastroenteritis, antibiotic therapy and use of other drugs such as NSAIDs.

The symptoms depend on how extensive the disease is in its active stage:

Type	Features
Proctitis	Mainly features of bleeding and mucous per rectum, anal pruritus and tenesmus (feeling of incomplete evacuation). The stool is well formed and the patient tends to be systemically well with a normal examination.
Procto-sigmoiditis	There is bleeding and mucous per rectum associated with diarrhoea, abdominal pain and the urgency to defaecate. The patient may report lethargy however, the overall examination is usually normal (less than 6 episodes per 24 hours).
Extensive colitis	This involves persistent and frequent episodes of diarrhoea associated with blood and mucous (more than 6 episodes per 24 hours). The patient is systemically unwell with a fever, lethargy, reduced appetite, weight loss and may have other extra-intestinal features as well. Signs on examination include a thin appearance, tachycardia, pallor, and signs of dehydration.

Table 3.5: The different forms of UC and presentations.

On acute admission with a flare of UC an assessment needs to be made of the disease severity, which will govern management. Truelove and Witt's criteria are widely used to identify acute severe disease:

Truelove and Witts criteria:
More than 6 episodes bloody diarrhoea/24 hrs
Pulse > 90
Fever
Hb < 10.5
Elevated inflammatory markers

Table 3.6: Truelove and Witts criteria.

Gastrointestinal complications of UC:

- Haemorrhage: chronic minimal blood loss is common and results in iron deficiency anaemia. Massive haemorrhage is an indication for emergency surgery, but is rare.
- Toxic megacolon: a rare occurrence in patients with extensive colitis. The patient can quickly deteriorate with features such as tachycardia, hypotension and fever. The abdomen becomes painful and distended, and there is an absence of bowel sounds.
  - A plain abdominal X-ray will confirm the diagnosis and will show lack of faecal shadows, mucosal thickening, dilated loops of colon (toxic dilatation is more than 6 cm).

- Colonic perforation: may or may not be preceded by toxic megacolon and usually occurs where there is active and extensive colitis. Peritonitis may result.
- Carcinoma: in patients who have suffered from extensive UC for more than 10 years there is an increased risk of development of colonic carcinoma. Those also at risk are patients with disease onset in childhood, frequent relapses and the presence of primary sclerosing cholangitis.

Systemic complications of UC:

- General: weight loss, lethargy, growth retardation.
- Blood: increased risk of venous and arterial thrombosis.
- Eyes: episcleritis and uveitis.
- Liver and biliary tree: fatty changes in the liver, primary sclerosing cholangitis and carcinoma of the bile duct.
- Skin: erythema nodosum, pyoderma gangrenosum.
- Musculoskeletal: arthritis (peripheral and axial) with an identical picture to ankylosing spondylitis and sacroiliitis. Clubbing.

Investigations

Blood tests:

- FBC: anaemia and increased WBC is usual.
- Inflammatory markers: ESR and CRP are raised.

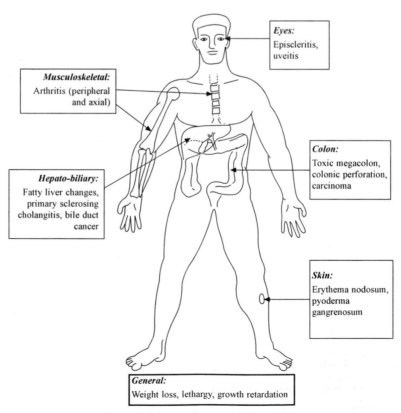

Figure 3.3: Systemic complications of UC.

- Biochemistry: albumin may be low.
- Cross-match.

Imaging:

- Erect chest x-ray if perforation suspected.
- Abdominal X-ray shows dilatation of large bowel loops, toxic megacolon, mucosal oedema, and proximal faecal loading where the disease is limited to proctitis.

Sigmoidoscopy/colonoscopy:

- Inflammation of the colonic mucosa, oedema, ulceration, active bleeding and occasionally pseudopolyps.
- Colonoscopy should never be performed in acute flare ups of UC as there is a significant risk of perforation due to the friable nature of the mucosa. It can help to define the extent of disease and differentiate UC from Crohn's disease as well as screen for any evidence of dysplasia.

Histology:

- Biopsy confirms diagnosis and determines the extent of disease activity.

Other:

- Stool microscopy and culture to exclude an infective cause of the diarrhoea.

Management

The mainstay of treatment is to induce and maintain remission.

➢ It is essential to provide the patient and their family with a full explanation of the disease and the effects it can potentially have upon their lifestyle.

➢ Patient support groups are often helpful such as the National Association for Colitis and Crohn's disease.

➢ Dietician referral for advice and support as they can often have nutritional deficiencies. Iron and folate supplements may be required.

➢ They should be under a Gastroenterologist for long term follow-up and monitoring of their disease.

➢ Referral to a clinical psychologist may be helpful.

➢ There is some evidence for the use of pre-biotics, especially in pouchitis, but research is ongoing in this area.

During an acute flare
➢ A to E assessment and initial resuscitation if required.
➢ The need for emergency surgery must be considered.
➢ In severe relapses of UC, but with only mild to moderate rectal bleeding, prophylactic clexane is given to reduce the risk of thromboembolism.
➢ With toxic megacolon, nasogastric tube insertion is required with regular suctioning with prophylactic wide spectrum antibiotic therapy and surgical review. With colonic perforation ensure antibiotics are given.
➢ Many Trusts will have local guidelines.

Table 3.7: Management during an acute flare up

Pharmacological measures:

1. Corticosteroids:
   ➢ Very effective for inducing remission.
   ➢ There are 3 modes of administration usually used including topical (enema, foam, or suppository), oral or intravenous, and they can be given up to a few weeks during and after an acute flare-up of symptoms.
     o Mode of treatment used is somewhat dependent upon the site of disease activity.
     o Usually given for 4 weeks in a mild relapse (< 4 stools per day), for example Prednisolone at 20 mg/day orally.
     o In moderate relapse (4–6 stools per day), Prednisolone is started at 40 mg per day for a week, then reduced to 30 mg per day for a week, then 20 mg per day for a further 4 weeks. Twice daily steroid enemas can be given as well.
   ➢ In a severe relapse, the patient may require IV Hydrocortisone at 100 mg 6 hourly. This can be changed to oral Prednisolone at 40 mg per day if the patient shows signs of improvement after 5 days.
   ➢ Adverse effects with long term use include an increased risk of diabetes, hypertension, osteoporosis and myopathy. It can also cause hypokalaemia.
     o Long term use is avoided if possible, especially in patients with pre-existing hypertension or diabetes.
     o Regular monitoring of BP, blood glucose and bone mineral density is indicated in patients on long-term therapy.
     o It may be necessary to treat with calcium/vitamin D3 supplementation and bisphosphonates.

2. 5-Aminosalicylates (Mesalazine or Sulphasalazine):
   ➢ First line therapy in inducing and maintaining remission in mild/moderate disease, reducing the rate of relapse from 80% to 20% per year.
   ➢ Can be administered orally, as an enema, as a suppository or in combination.
   ➢ Their action is thought to be by reducing the production of inflammatory mediators.
   ➢ Adverse effects include rash, headache, acid reflux, diarrhoea and rarely blood dyscrasias which may be potentially life threatening.
     o Due to the side-effects and need to apply treatments predominantly to the left side of the colon, slower release preparations have been formulated such as Asacol and Pentasa which rely on colonic bacteria for breakdown and release of the active component.

3. Azathioprine:
   ➢ Has a role in prevention of relapses and also has a steroid-sparing effect. It is usually continued for several months.
   ➢ Administered orally, and has an immunosuppressive effect.
   ➢ Adverse effects include nausea, rash, headache, bone marrow suppression and hepatitis.

o Hence it is essential to monitor the patient's FBC and liver function tests (LFTs) regularly.

➢ Due to its adverse effects, its use is not recommended in patients who are septic.

4. Ciclosporin:

➢ Used in conjunction with other steroid therapy in patients with an acute severe episode of relapse which is not responding to therapy within 5 days.

➢ Acts as an immunosuppressive agent by inhibiting T lymphocyte function. It is very effective in inducing remission in severe UC and helps reduce the need for urgent surgical intervention.

➢ Adverse effects are potentially serious such as electrolyte abnormalities, renal dysfunction, hypertension, seizures, and opportunistic infections.

o Regular measurement of the ciclosporin level is essential.

5. Infliximab:

➢ Useful as rescue therapy for acute severe colitis, however clinical trials are ongoing to define its effectiveness compared to ciclosporin.

Surgical management:

➢ Elective: indicated in those patients with chronic UC which is not responsive to maximal medical therapy, if there is carcinoma or in order to prevent its development, and in children where the aim is to prevent adverse effects upon their growth.

➢ Urgent: colonic perforation or massive haemorrhage, toxic megacolon and failure of medical therapy.

➢ Operative procedures used are:

o Total colectomy with end ileostomy (also for emergency surgery).

o Proctocolectomy with ileo-rectal anastomosis.

o Proctocolectomy with formation of ileo-anal pouch.

Malignancy:

➢ Increased risk of colorectal carcinoma which is dependent on disease length and severity.

➢ Patients who have extensive (pan-colic) UC for longer than 8–10 years should be enrolled in a surveillance colonoscopy programme with biopsies every 1–3 years to monitor for any dysplastic changes and reduce the risk of cancer development.

➢ If there is evidence of severe dysplasia, a colectomy is indicated.

Prognosis:

➢ The majority of patients with UC suffer from recurrent relapses, however their overall mortality is comparable to the general population.

➢ The main causes of morbidity and mortality are recurrent severe flare-ups of colitis which are unresponsive to therapy and the development of colon cancer in patients who have long-standing disease.

➢ After surgery and pouch formation there remains a 40% 10 year risk of inflammation called 'pouchitis', which carries a small risk of pouch failure and further surgery.

Crohn's Disease

Epidemiology

Less common than UC, Crohn's disease is more common in Europe and North America with a prevalence of 50 in 100,000 and an incidence of around 5 per 100,000 per year. Patients present in early adulthood but there is a second peak in the seventh decade. Small bowel disease is more common in the younger population (teens and early 20s): where as older individuals tend to have more colonic features of disease. There is a female preponderance and again an increased risk in Ashkenazi Jews and in Northern Europeans.

Aetiology

Genetic factors are thought to have a larger role than in UC.

The first-degree relatives of affected individuals have an increased risk of disease (>10%). In genetic studies a 40% concordance has been found in monozygotic twins.

Mutations have been discovered in the CARD 15 gene and anomalies in the anti-BPI antibodies. Smoking increases the risk of disease by 4-fold and worsens disease progression. Other factors are ill-defined but include gut infections, diet and abnormal immune responses.

Pathophysiology

Crohn's can affect any part of the gastrointestinal system from mouth to anus.

It most commonly affects the terminal ileum and ileo-caecal regions. 'Skip lesions' are seen where the disease affects segments of the gut in a discontinuous pattern.

Initially there are superficial aphthous ulcers, which develop into deep serpinginous fissuring ulcers with features such as 'cobblestoning', oedema, fibrosis and finally formation of strictures, adhesions and fistulas. The strictures may result in obstruction.

Microscopic features include a transmural inflammation and a characteristic feature is non-caseating epithelioid granuloma formation.

Key features in the history/examination

• The main features are of diarrhoea, abdominal pain, weight loss, malaise, anorexia, rectal bleeding and occasionally fever.

• Symptoms are variable depending on extent and location of GI involvement.

• Those with primarily small bowel disease may have steatorrhoea.

• Increased rectal bleeding in large bowel disease.

• On examination, the patient may appear thin and have features of malabsorption such as abdominal distension, pallor, oedema, bruising, and mouth ulcers.

- Perianal features such as skin tags, fissures, fistulae and abscesses are common.
- As the disease commonly involves the ileo-caecal region, a mass in the right iliac fossa may be palpable.
- Clubbing in patients with long-standing disease.

Gastrointestinal complications of Crohn's disease:

- Strictures: may result in obstruction.
- Perforation: usually contained locally and may result in abscess formation.
- Abscess and fistula: abscesses tend to form around inflamed bowel and hence discharge via fistulae into areas such as the colon, bladder (recurrent UTI, haematuria), skin and vagina (faeculent discharge or flatus per vagina). Patients may have:
- Anal fissures, abscesses and fistulae.
- Haemorrhage: that is usually mild and long-standing resulting in anaemia.
- Toxic megacolon is very uncommon.
- Carcinoma: there is a slightly higher incidence of bowel cancer in Crohn's patients comp ared to the general population.

Systemic complications of Crohn's disease:

- General: weight loss, fever, short stature in children.
- Eyes: episcleritis and uveitis.
- Oral: mouth ulcers.

- Blood: vascular thrombosis, autoimmune haemolytic anaemia.
- Kidneys: uric acid calculi and/or oxalate calculi.
- Liver and biliary tree: gallstones, bile duct carcinoma, fatty changes, sclerosing cholangitis (more commonly in UC).
- Gastrointestinal: diarrhoea, abdominal pain, rectal bleeding, steatorrhoea, peri-anal features.
- Skin: erythema nodosum, pyoderma gangrenosum.
- Musculoskeletal: arthritis (peripheral and axial) with an identical picture to ankylosing spondylitis and sacroiliitis. Clubbing.

Investigations

Blood tests:

- FBC: anaemia due to iron, vitamin B12 or folate deficiency, reactive thrombocytosis.
- Inflammatory markers: increased ESR, CRP and WCC.
- Biochemistry: reduced albumin, which can be a marker of malabsorption/malnutrition and reduced calcium.

Microbiology:

- Stool culture to exclude an infective cause for the diarrhoea.

Imaging:

- Sinogram necessary where there is an enterocutaneous fistulae to map out the fistula tract prior to surgery.

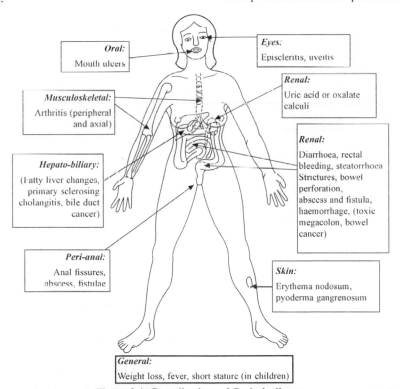

Figure 3.4: Complications of Crohn's disease.

- Ultrasound and CT scan required if an intra-abdominal abscess or mass is suspected.
- MRI is the first choice for complicated peri-anal disease.

Sigmoidoscopy/colonoscopy:

- Help to determine the extent of the disease and may illustrate features such as a thickened bowel wall, patchy inflammation and cobblestoning.
- Capsule endoscopy may be helpful in purely small bowel disease.

Histology:

- Biopsy from the rectum or large bowel is required for accurate diagnosis.

Other:

- Barium follow-through/small bowel enema will illustrate features such as strictures, fistulae, abscesses, 'rose thorn' ulcers and polyps.

Management

The main aim of treatment is to induce and maintain a period of remission.

- It is essential to provide the patient and their family with a full explanation of the disease and the effects it can potentially have upon their lifestyle.
- Patient support groups are often helpful such as the National Association for Colitis and Crohn's disease.
- Dietician referral for advice and support as they can often have nutritional deficiencies.
  - Iron and folate supplements may be required.
  - With patients with small bowel strictures it is especially important to avoid high-residue foods such as sweetcorn, uncooked vegetables and nuts as they can act as food boluses and result in obstruction.
  - In-patients with severe relapses may require enteral feeds or total parenteral nutrition.
- They should be under a Gastroenterologist for long term follow-up and monitoring of their disease.
- Referral to a clinical psychologist may be helpful.
- Loperamide or codeine phosphate can sometimes be used to reduce diarrhoea.
- Prophylactic clexane is given to reduce the risk of vascular thrombosis during an acute illness.

During an acute flare
➤ A to E assessment and initial resuscitation if required.
➤ The need for emergency surgery must be considered (see below).
➤ IV fluids with electrolyte replacement.
➤ With toxic megacolon, nasogastric tube insertion is required with regular suctioning with prophylactic wide spectrum antibiotic therapy and surgical review.
o With colonic perforation ensure antibiotics are given.

Table 3.8: Management during an acute flare up.

Pharmacological measures:

1. Corticosteroids:
   - Proven efficacy for use in the treatment of relapses of Crohn's disease, however they are not helpful in maintaining long-term remission
     - In mild attacks, 30 mg per day are given for 1 week followed by 20 mg per day for a month. They are gradually reduced by 5mg every 2–4 weeks.
     - In severe attacks, IV hydrocortisone is required at 100 mg per day, which can be changed to oral prednisolone at 40 mg per day if the patient improves after 5 days. Rectal steroids can also be given for proctitis.
   - Oral budesonide is preferred for use in patients with ileo-caecal involvement as the formulation releases the drug in the ileum so reducing systemic side effects.
2. 5-Aminosalicylates:
   - Sulfasalazine is more effective in Crohn's colitis compared to small bowel disease and is primarily a maintenance treatment.
   - A slow release preparation of mesalazine such as Pentasa is primarily active in the small bowel and is used in the treatment of active disease as well as maintenance.
3. Azathioprine:
   - An immunosuppressive agent, and has a role as a steroid-sparing agent as in UC.
   - Indicated in refractory Crohn's.
4. Methotrexate:
   - An immunosuppressive agent administered either orally or as a once weekly intramuscular injection, can be used instead of azathioprine in patients who do not tolerate this drug.
   - Indicated in refractory Crohn's.
   - Adverse effects include bone marrow suppression, hepatic fibrosis and pneumonitis.
   - Hence patients require full blood count and liver function tests at least once a month.
5. Antibiotics:
   - Metronidazole and ciprofloxacin are usually used in active Crohn's, especially, when patients have perianal involvement.
6. Infliximab:
   - A chimeric monoclonal antibody to TNF which can induce remission in patients with severe Crohn's which is unresponsive to maximal medical therapy.
   - Administered by intravenous infusion which can be repeated.
   - Adverse effects include infection, infusion reaction, and rarely B cell lymphoma.

Dietary Management:

- Elemental diets can be as effective as steroid therapy. It improves nutritional status and is of low residue and hence does not contain the usual food antigens which may trigger relapse.

➢ It is expensive with an unpleasant taste, and patients relapse more rapidly than those treated with steroid therapy.

Surgical Management:

➢ Up to 80% of Crohn's patients with long-standing relapses require surgical treatment.

  o Due to the risk of recurrence, up to half of these patients may require a further operation within 10 years.

  o Strictures are managed with minimal resection or a strictureplasty.

  o Surgical resection depends on the location of disease. The most common procedure is excision of the caecum and terminal ileum with side-to-side anastomosis.

  o Intra-abdominal abscesses are drained, often under radiological guidance and enteric fistulae are usually resected. Antibiotics are also used.

Prognosis:

➢ Mortality is twice that of the general population but this may be decreasing with better medical management and the trend to a more conservative surgical management.

➢ There is an increased risk of both colorectal and small bowel adenocarcinoma.

Irritable bowel syndrome (IBS)

Epidemiology

Irritable Bowel Syndrome (IBS) is the most common complaint in gastroenterology clinics. 1 in 10 adults have episodic symptoms of IBS. The Female-to-male ratio is 3:1. Peak incidence is between 20 and 30 years of age.

Aetiology

No organic cause has been found for the condition. There is an association with abnormal intestinal motility, and may be influenced by abnormal communication between the enteric nervous system and the central nervous system.

There is an association with anxiety, depressed mental state or suffering from food intolerances. It may at times result after an episode of acute infective gastroenteritis.

Key features in the history/examination

The diagnosis is clinical with no diagnostic tests. There is an international agreed set of diagnostic criteria for IBS known as ROME II:

At least 3 months in 1 year of abdominal discomfort (central/ lower) that has at least 2 or the following features starting with the pain:
Relief on defaecation
Change in bowel frequency
Change in the appearance and consistency of stool

Table 3.9: ROME II criteria.

Other supporting symptoms include:

• Frequency of <3/week and >3/day (alternating constipation and diarrhoea).

• Straining at stool.

• Hard/lumpy or loose/watery stool.

• Urgency to defaecate.

• Tenesmus.

• Passage of mucous per rectum.

• Abdominal bloating.

➢ Other gastrointestinal features may be seen, but are non-diagnostic:

  o Nausea and vomiting.

  o Dyspepsia and heartburn.

  o Dysphagia.

  o Anal pain due to muscle spasm of levator ani.

➢ There is a strong association between IBS and psychiatric disorders as well as symptoms in other organ systems:

  o Anxiety, stress, depression and obsession with bowel habit.

  o History of adverse life events.

  o Higher rates of reported sexual and physical abuse.

  o Gynaecological symptoms such as dyspareunia, dysmenorrhoea, and the bowel symptoms tend to occur around the same time as menstruation.

  o Urinary symptoms such as frequency and urgency.

  o General symptoms including headaches, and lethargy.

Remembering that IBS is largely a diagnosis of exclusion, the following features in the history should cause 'alarm' and require further investigation:

Alarm symptoms requiring further investigation
Weight loss
Rectal bleeding
Anorexia
Patients over 40 years
Nocturnal abdominal pain or diarrhoea
Mouth ulcers

Table 3.10: Alarm symptoms that require further investigations.

• On examination the patient is generally normal.

• Patient may be anxious, with diffuse or localised abdominal tenderness.

• Occasionally, the descending colon may be palpable and tender.

Investigations

The diagnosis is primarily clinical and investigations are primarily to exclude another cause.

Blood tests:

- FBC
- U&Es
- LFTs
- Inflammatory markers: CRP and ESR usually normal.
- Thyroid function tests and anti-tissue transglutaminase antibodies to exclude thyrotoxicosis and coeliac disease.

Sigmoidoscopy/colonoscopy:

- Rectal biopsy and barium enema can be performed if there is uncertainty regarding the diagnosis.

Other:

- Stool microscopy culture and sensitivity (MC&S).

Management

- ➢ Ensure an organic cause for the symptoms have been excluded.
- ➢ Reassurance is key in this condition in order to reduce the patient's anxiety regarding their symptoms.
- ➢ Anxiety not dispelled may require treatment with relaxation classes, cognitive-behavioural therapy or hypnosis.
- ➢ If the patient has persistent psychiatric symptoms, a psychiatric referral may be appropriate.

Pharmacological measures:

Drug therapy is tailored towards symptom control:

- ➢ Mostly pain: antispasmodics such as mebeverine, calcium channel blockers and peppermint oil are commonly used as well as tricyclic anti-depressants such as amitriptyline and selective serotonin reuptake inhibitors such as paroxetine.
  - o Dietary triggers such as wheat can be avoided by patients for example, cereal, dairy and fructose products.
  - o Antispasmodics such as buscopan can be effective when taken before meals.
- ➢ Mostly diarrhoea: loperamide or codeine can reduce the frequency of bowel motions and improve the stool consistency.
- ➢ Mostly constipation: a high-fiber diet and/or bulking agents such as fybogel can be effective in symptom relief. Ensure that overflow diarrhoea is excluded if the usual symptom is predominantly constipation.

Prognosis:

- ➢ Most patients are symptom-free after 5 years with the symptoms.

Urinary tract infection and pyelonephritis

UTI is the presence of $>10^5$ bacteria/ml in a freshly voided sample of urine.

Pyelonephritis is an infection of the renal parenchyma, usually following ascending infection from the bladder.

Epidemiology

UTI is a very common condition worldwide, accounting for 2% of GP consultations in the UK. It is significantly more common in women. 35% of women will experience symptomatic UTI at some time. It is more common in the elderly and very much more common in those living in care homes.

Pyelonephritis has an incidence of approximately 10/10,000 per year in women and 2/10,000 per year in males. Pyelonephritis is more common in younger women.

Aetiology

Infection most commonly is caused by bacteria entering the bladder via the urethra but blood borne infection is also seen. The most common infecting organisms are part of the normal gut flora, in particular *Escherichia coli* (70–80%). Staphylococcus, streptococcus, pseudomonas, klebsiella and proteus are also common infecting organisms. Common causes of sterile pyuria include partially treated bacterial infection, tuberculosis or inflammation from a non-infective cause.

Pathophysiology

There are various risk factors which lead to UTIs:

- **Females** have a shorter urethra allowing easier access for organisms to the bladder. During micturition, there may be backflow of urine in the shorter female urethra, which does not usually occur in the longer male urethra.
- **Sexual activity** can predispose to infection in females especially with a change in partner. It is advised for females to empty their bladder prior to and following sexual intercourse.
- **Urinary retention and incomplete emptying of the bladder** in patients results in the static urine within the bladder increasing the likelihood of infection.
- **Chronic prostate disease** in males.
- **Urinary catheterisation** can introduce bacteria into the urinary tract and hence a sterile technique is essential. Indwelling catheters in particular create a potential for infection, with colonisation of the biofilm within days of insertion.
- **Immunosuppressed or diabetic** patients are at an increased risk of infection.
- **Pregnancy** increases progesterone level which causes dilatation and relaxation of the ureters. This enables reflux of urine into the ureters increasing the risk of more serious upper tract infection.

Key features in the history/examination

- Can vary from asymptomatic UTI to acute pyelonephritis with severe sepsis.
- Ask about risk factors:

Risk factors
Diabetes
Previous history of UTI/pyelonephritis
Renal or kidney stones
Abnormalities within the renal tract
Ask about childhood UTIs and the possibility of reflux nephropathy
Any cause to be immunosuppressed

Table 3.11: Risk factors for UTI or pyelonephritis.

Lower tract infection (cystitis)	Upper tract infection (pyelonephritis)
<ul><li>Dysuria</li><li>Increased frequency and urgency</li><li>Offensive smelling urine</li><li>Urine has a cloudy appearance (pyuria)</li><li>Haematuria</li><li>Suprapubic pain</li><li>Confusion, especially in the elderly</li></ul>	<ul><li>Loin pain</li><li>Flank tenderness</li><li>Pyuria</li><li>Rigors, fever, vomiting</li></ul>

Table 3.12: The clinical features of cystitis and pyelonephritis.

UTI may reveal few examination findings:
- Look for signs of sepsis.
- Suprapubic tenderness.
- Palpable bladder if acute retention has developed.

Pyelonephritis will reveal more signs on examination:
- Clearer signs of sepsis, i.e. fever, tachycardia, hypotension
- Rigors may be seen.
- Loin/renal angle tenderness.

Investigations

Investigations for both UTI and pyelonephritis are the same.

Urine dipstick:
- Nitrites positive, produced from bacterial conversion of urinary nitrates.
- Leucocytes positive confirms pyuria.
- A trace of protein or blood may be present.
- The dipstick does not positively diagnose an infection nor firmly exclude one.

Mid-stream urine (MSU) for microscopy and culture:
- Organisms may be present and identified along with antibiotic susceptibility.
- White cells suggest infection and white cell casts indicate involvement of the upper tract as the casts are formed in the renal tubules.

- A UTI is diagnosed if there are $>10^5$ bacteria per ml of urine.
- Send a morning first-pass urine sample from the first micturition of the day for patients suspected of having mycobacterial infection.

Blood tests:
- FBC: An increased white cell count (neutrophilia).
- U&E: Increased urea and creatinine in dehydration or if there is outflow tract obstruction.
- Increased inflammatory markers such as CRP.
- Glucose to exclude diabetes.
- Blood cultures.

In children and men, patients with recurrent UTIs and all pyelonephritis further investigations are required. These include:

- Abdominal X-ray to exclude calculi (see figure 3.5).
- Ultrasound kidneys-ureter-bladder (KUB).
- Further tests as indicated: intravenous urogram (IVU), isotope scans such as DMSA (Dimercaptosuccinic acid), cystoscopy.

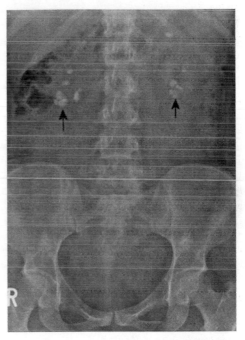

Figure 3.5: KUB X-Ray showing bilateral multiple renal calculi (arrows).

Management
- Analgesia.
- Increased fluid intake. Oral if possible but pyelonephritis may require IV fluids due to more profound dehydration and associated nausea and vomiting.

➤ Antibiotics:

○ Empirical antibiotics should be commenced if symptomatic with a positive urine dip.

○ Antibiotics should be prescribed according to local policy and changed if necessary when further microbiology advice is available.

○ A 3-day course of trimethoprim is the usual first choice for an uncomplicated UTI.

○ For pyelonephritis IV antibiotics are often required initially and should be based on local guidelines.

○ An asymptomatic positive dipstick does not require treatment except in pregnant women.

➤ Indwelling catheters should be changed.

➤ In both males and females a cause should be sought in recurrent infection.

➤ A urine dip can be performed following treatment of the UTI to ensure resolution.

➤ Complications of recurrent UTIs include renal scarring and chronic renal impairment.

Prevention of recurrent UTIs:

➤ Avoid constipation as this can prevent complete bladder emptying.

➤ Avoid bubble baths and soapy irritants in bath water.

➤ Double voiding on mictruition, which involves attempting to completely empty the bladder initially and then voiding again after 5 minutes.

➤ If UTI is associated with sexual intercourse, encourage micturition afterwards.

➤ Drinking plenty of fluid and in particular cranberry juice which has been shown reduce the incidence of bacteriuria.

➤ Good catheter care and early removal of unnecessary catheters.

➤ Prophylaxis with a low-dose of antibiotic daily but this should only be instigated on specialist advice.

Further reading and references

➤ British Society of Gastroenterology (2007). *Guidelines for osteoporosis in inflammatory bowel disease and coeliac disease.*

British Society of Gastroenterology (2004). *Guidelines for the management of inflammatory bowel disease in adults.*

➤ National Centre for Health and Clinical Excellence (2008). *Irritable bowel syndrome (CG061).*

➤ Scottish Intercollegiate Guidelines Network (2006). *Management of suspected bacterial urinary tract infection in adults.*

➤ Vakil N, van Zanten SV, Kahrilas P, Dent J, Jones R. The Montreal definition and Classification of gastroesophageal reflux disease: a global evidence-based consensus. *Am J Gastroenterol* 2006; 101: 1900–20.

➤ Warren JR, Marshall BJ (1986). Unidentified curved bacilli on gastric epithelium in active chronic gastritis, *Lancet* 1: 1273–5.

ACUTE BACK PAIN

Differential diagnosis

System/Organ	Disease
Mechanical back pain	**Back pain** Sciatica
Degenerative	**Osteoarthritis**
Traumatic	**Osteoporosis (vertebral fracture)**
Inflammatory	**Ankylosing Spondylitis** Discitis
Infective	Osteomyelitis Tuberculosis (Pott's disease)
Tumours	**Tumours of the bone** Primary (malignant and benign) Metastases

Back Pain

Epidemiology

A very common complaint; around 80% adults experience back pain at some time in their lifetime. It carries a significant level of morbidity, accounts for about 5% of GP consultations and is responsible for approximately 50 million lost working days per year in the UK.

It is mostly self-limiting, settling within 2 months, however there are a number of more serious causes which must be considered and the 'red flag' symptoms sought. The history should include the 'yellow flag' symptoms for chronicity. These are outlined in Table 3.13.

Red Flag Symptoms	Yellow Flag Symptoms
• Age under 20 or over 55 • Non-mechanical pain which is worsening • Pyrexia of unknown origin • Pain in the thoracic region of the spine • Focal neurological features • Major trauma (or more minor trauma if there is a diagnosis of osteoporosis) • Cancer • Systemic features such as weight loss • Immunosuppression • Use of steroids • New structural deformity • New bladder dysfunction • New faecal incontinence • Saddle anaesthesia	• Belief that the pain is harmful and disabling • Avoidance behaviour • Reduced activity levels • Low mood/depression • Social withdrawal • Problems at work • Lack of social/family support

Table 3.13: Key red and yellow flag features to elicit in patients with back pain.

Mechanical back pain is most common in those aged 15–30 years. Degenerative joint disease and osteoporosis are most common in those over the age of 50 years. In middle aged individuals (30–50 years) causes such as malignancy and a prolapsed intervertebral disc must be considered.

Aetiology

The following Table 3.14 outlines the various causes of back pain, relevant differentials to consider as well as ways in which to determine the cause by the clinical findings on history and examination.

Risk factors:

- Abnormal posture
- Insufficient back support
- Wearing high-heeled shoes
- Unequal leg length
- Heavy manual labour
- Anxiety/depression
- Pregnancy
- Ageing

3. Medicine

Causes	Differentials	Characteristics to differentiate the causes of back pain
Simple/ mechanical	- Intervertebral disc prolapse (can compress the nerve root resulting in sciatica) - Injury to facet joints, spinal ligaments or muscle - Degenerative changes including osteoarthritis - Fractures - Spondylolisthesis is when there is anterior displacement of one vertebra relative to the one below. - Spondylolysis is a stress fracture of the pars interarticularis (most commonly of L5), common in gymnasts and is a cause of Spondylolisthesis - Spinal stenosis	- Tends to be of sudden onset - Often unilateral pain affecting the leg and buttock - Pain mostly in evenings - No morning stiffness - Pain is worse on movement in particular after exercise - Relief with rest
Inflammatory/ infective	- Ankylosing spondylitis - Mycobacterium tuberculosis - Salmonella - Brucella	- More gradual onset - Often bilateral pain - Pain is constant and is at its worst in the mornings - Associated with morning stiffness - Exercise tends to relieve symptoms
Sinister cause	- Metastatic carcinoma (from carcinoma of breast, lung, kidney, thyroid, and prostate) - Myeloma - Bacterial/Tuberculosis/Osteomyelitis - Cauda equina syndrome - Cord compression	- A constant pain with no relieving factors - Systemic symptoms usually present such as fever, weight loss, night sweats, anorexia - Localised bony tenderness - Neurological signs involving more than one spinal root level - Signs present in both lower limbs - Altered bowel, bladder, sexual function
Metabolic	- Osteomalacia - Osteoporosis - Wilson's disease - Haemochromatosis - Paget's disease	
Referred pain	- Pelvic disease - Vasculature for example an aortic aneurysm - Genitourinary (bladder, prostate) - Gastrointestinal disease such as pancreatitis - Retroperitoneal structures such as the uterus and kidneys	

Table 3.14: Causes of back pain, differential diagnosis and key clinical features.

Pathophysiology

Pathophysiology is dependent on aetiology.

Key features in the history/examination

- Age, sex, and occupation.
- History of trauma or injury to the back or other precipitating factors such as falls, heavy lifting or a new strenuous activity.
- Any previous back conditions or surgery.
- Onset of symptoms and duration.
- Character of pain e.g. sharp, dull, shooting.
- Radiation of pain.
- Exacerbating or relieving factors.
- Paraesthesia.
- Weakness in leg(s).
- Bowel or bladder dysfunction.
- Early morning stiffness (and duration).
- Relevant medical conditions such as rheumatoid arthritis, osteoporosis, osteoarthritis.
- Check for any contraindications to using NSAIDs.
- Any stress at work or at home.

Examine for signs of medical emergencies as follows:

Cauda equina syndrome:
- Nerve root pain in both lower limbs
- Sacral paresthesia a saddle distribution
- Flaccid paralysis of the lower limbs
- Bladder or bowel dysfunction

Acute cord compression:
- Usually bilateral
- Lower motor neuron deficit at the level of cord compression with upper motor neuron features below this level
- Disturbance of sphincter function

Perforated aneurysm:
- Pulsatile mass in the abdomen
- Signs of peritonism
- Evidence of shock
- Radio-femoral delay

Also examine carefully for the following features:
- Scars or obvious deformity in the back, e.g. due to scoliosis or kyphosis.
- Observe the gait for any abnormal posture or limping.
- Palpate the spine in order to elicit any vertebral body or para-spinal tenderness.
- Check movements such as flexion, extension, lateral flexion, rotation, and also push the iliac crests together in order to elicit any restriction of movement at the sacroiliac joints.

- Look for any clubbing, muscle wasting, signs of weight loss such as cachexia, and anaemia.
- Feel for any masses in the abdomen.
- Assess the presence of peripheral pulses and degree of peripheral perfusion.
- A full neurological examination.
- Straight leg raise.
- A digital rectal exam to assess anal tone.
- Always check the perineal and perianal sensation.

Investigations

Blood tests:
- Full blood count (FBC): anaemia or raised white cell count (WCC) may be present.
- Inflammatory markers: may be raised such as C-reactive protein (CRP) and erythrocyte sedimentation rate (ESR).
- Bone profile: levels of calcium, phosphate and alkaline phosphatise (ALP) An increased level of calcium and ALP may be suggestive of bony metastases. Calcium is increased and ALP remains normal in myeloma. The ALP is increased and the calcium remains normal in metabolic bone disease.
- Prostate specific antigen (PSA) must be measured in men in whom prostate disease is suspected.

Microbiology:
- Blood cultures: Including acid fast bacillus (AFB) if spinal infection is suspected.

Imaging:
- X-rays:
  ○ History of trauma, especially in those over the age of 55 years.
  ○ Degenerative changes in osteoarthritis.
  ○ Signal alignment abnormalities such as in kyphosis and scoliosis.
  ○ Destruction of vertebral bodies by presence of infection or malignancy.
  ○ Pathological fractures.
  ○ Spondylolisthesis (most commonly at L5/S1 where there is forward subluxation of one vertebral body on the one below it).
- Computer tomography (CT):
  ○ Will allow imaging of the spinal canal in order to elicit any specific pathology.
- Magnetic resonance imaging (MRI):
  ○ Indicated if any of the surgical emergencies are suspected.
  ○ Especially useful for detecting any intervertebral disc abnormalities.
  ○ The best investigation to demonstrate cord compression.

3. Medicine

o Will show intra-spinal tumours, as well as any cysts or abscesses.

- Bone scan: 'Hot' spots will indicate areas of infection, malignant lesions or fractures as well as degenerative disease.

Management

➤ The more sinister causes of pain must be excluded and managed accordingly before using treatments for non-specific back pain.

➤ Empower the patient to help manage their pain.

➤ Provide education about lower back pain and the usual course.

➤ Explore patient concerns and expectations.

➤ Encourage physical activity and avoid total bed rest as this will worsen symptoms. However more strenuous activities should be moderated.

➤ Initial medical treatment includes Paracetamol, non-steroidal anti-inflammatory drugs and weak opioids.

➤ Adjuncts may include muscle relaxants such as Diazepam, and low-dose antidepressants such as Amitriptylline.

➤ Strong opioids can be used but consider referral to a pain clinic.

➤ In addition to pharmacological treatments, National Institute for Health and Clinical Excellence (NICE) recommends offering the following (taking patient choice into consideration):

o Physiotherapy/exercise programme: helps to strengthen the core muscles and adopt an improved posture.

o Manual therapy: includes spinal manipulation, spinal mobilisation and massage.

o Acupuncture.

➤ Surgical management such as spinal fusion may be considered for non-specific back pain and is indicated for significant ongoing pain which is not responsive to medical treatment.

Prognosis

➤ Most patients (more than 90%) with acute back pain will be symptom-free after six weeks.

➤ A number of patients develop chronic back pain which can result in significant morbidity.

Osteoarthritis

Osteoarthritis is a group of conditions affecting synovial joints characterised by loss of articular cartilage, resulting in pain, deformity and loss of function. Although previously thought of as a normal consequence of ageing associated with 'wear and tear' it is now known that it is caused by localised inflammation.

Epidemiology

Incidence and prevalence increase with age. It is the commonest cause of arthritis in the elderly, the commonest cause of hip and knee joint replacements and one of the commonest causes of GP consultations.

Aetiology

A multifactorial condition which can be primary or secondary.

Risk factors include:

- Increasing age
- Obesity
- Gender: males are affected more than females under the age of 45 years but above 45 years females are more effected
- Smoking
- Occupation
- Joint trauma
- Abnormal joint loading
- Genetic: polygenetic inheritance

Pathophysiology

There are three main disease mechanisms:

1. Loss of cartilage: the chondrocytes produce an increased amount of the enzymes which are responsible for the degradation of cartilage.

2. Remodelling of bone: increased bone turn-over results in subchondral bone sclerosis with the formation of cysts and proliferation of new bone and osteophyte formation. The joint contour changes as a result of these.

3. Inflammation of the synovium: there is an increase in the amount of synovial fluid.

Key features in the history/examination

When taking the history from the patient, enquire into the following areas in particular:

- Joint pain:
  o particular joints which are involved.
  o severity and nature of pain.
  o impact on activities of daily living.

- Joint stiffness: after inactivity, which is usually more problematic first thing in the morning, lasting less than 30 minutes.

- Hand: what daily tasks are becoming difficult.

- Hip: pain in the groin, buttock or anterior thigh.

- Knee: pain on kneeling, climbing stairs and getting in and out of cars.

- Spine: pain on movement. The cervical and lumbar regions are more commonly affected.

When examining the patient, bear in mind that joint deformities lead to a reduced range of movement in the affected joints.

- Hands:
  o Heberden's nodes (swelling at the distal interphalangeal joints).
  o Bouchard's node (swelling at the proximal interphalangeal joints).

- Hip:
  - o Check for pain on internal rotation as this is usually the first sign of osteoarthritis of the hip.
  - o Mobilise and look at gait.
- Knee:
  - o Deformity often obvious on examination.
  - o Reduced usage of the knee joints may result in wasting of the quadriceps.
  - o Knee pain may represent referred pain from the hip, so always examine the hip joint as well.
- Spine:
  - o Palpate the bony prominences of the spine for localised pain.
  - o Perform a neurological examination to look for signs indicative of nerve entrapment.

Investigations

Mainly a clinical diagnosis with confirmation on imaging.

Imaging:

- X-rays: of affected joints
  - o Loss of joint space
  - o Osteophytes
  - o Subchondral sclerosis
  - o Subchondral cysts
  - o Joint subluxation
  - o Soft-tissue swelling
- CT/MRI scan of the spine:
  - o Vertebral disc pathology
  - o Spinal canal stenosis

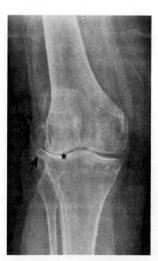

Figure 3.6: Plain X-Ray of right knee showing decreased joint space in the lateral compartment (star) with osteophyte formation (arrow) in keeping with osteoarthritis.

- o Cord compression
- o Facet joint arthritis
- o Square appearance of the hand (subluxation of the base of the thumb).
- o The wrist and metacarpophalangeal (MCP) joints are usually not affected which can help to differentiate the disease from rheumatoid arthritis.

Management

The treatment priorities are symptom relief, maintenance of function and quality of life. It should be patient centred and take a holistic approach as advocated by NICE. See further reading and references. The following are also key considerations:

- ➤ Patient education and empowerment.
- ➤ Formulate a plan in conjunction with the patient, family and carers.
- ➤ Weight loss and management.
- ➤ Physiotherapy, which can aid pain reduction, increase joint mobility and strengthen the supporting muscles such as the quadriceps for the knee.
- ➤ Occupational therapy.
- ➤ Other non-pharmacological treatments include orthotic aids, walking aids, appropriate footwear, heat/cold treatment, TENS and hydrotherapy.
- ➤ Analgesia:
  - o Oral (use World Health Organisation (WHO) analgesic ladder).
  - o Topical (including non-steroidal anti-inflammatory drugs (NSAIDs), Capsaicin).
- ➤ Intra-articular corticosteroid injections when pain is moderate to severe.
- ➤ Surgery:
  - o Mainly for the purpose of pain relief, or to increase the degree of movement in those with a severe disability.
  - o Arthroscopy and debridement.
  - o Arthrodesis.
  - o Osteotomy.
  - o Joint replacement, typically of the hip or knee.

Prognosis:

- A slowly progressive disease with significant degree of morbidity.

Osteoporosis

A systemic condition resulting from a reduction in the bone mass and quality, resulting in thin and fragile bones which have increased susceptibility to fractures.

Epidemiology

Osteoporosis is seen most commonly in white post-menopausal

women and more than 70% of osteoporotic fractures are in females. The incidence increases with age. It is more common in the developed countries.

The lifetime risk of fragility fracture is 40% for a white woman and 13% for a white man. There are over 300,000 fragility fractures per year in the UK.

Hip fractures are seen with an incidence of 4.3 per 100,000 females aged 45–64 years and 90.1 per 100,000 females aged 65–85 years per year.

Vertebral fractures occur in around 1–2% of females aged 44–54 years, increasing to more than 10% in those aged over 65 years.

Aetiology

The following risk factors are implicated in the development of osteoporosis:

- Female sex
- Family history fragility fracture
- Inflammatory bowel disease and coeliac disease
- Post-menopausal
- Low body mass index (BMI)
- Smoking
- Caucasian
- Glucocorticoid excess
- Excessive alcohol use
- Older age
- Hyperthyroidism
- Low dietary calcium
- Past history of fracture

Pathophysiology

Osteoporosis may result from a reduced peak bone mass. Peak bone mass is achieved in the early 20s, and is governed by both genetic and environmental factors.

More usually, osteoporosis results from bone loss seen with the ageing process. This loss occurs at about 1% per year except in post-menopausal women where the reduction in oestrogen causes a more rapid deterioration. There is usually an increase in bone resorption and a reduction in bone formation. Both factors contribute to thin and fragile bones which are more susceptible to fractures from low-impact trauma. Mostly fractures involve the hips, wrists and vertebral bodies.

Key features in the history/examination

Ensure enquiries are made into the following when taking a history:

- Pain: onset, location and any deformity.
- History of trauma (including low-impact trauma).
- Family history of osteoporosis and fragility fracture.
- Menstrual history.
- Corticosteroid use.

- Smoking and alcohol history.
- Medical history of diabetes, Cushing's syndrome, multiple myeloma.
- Any reduction in height.
- History of falls.

On examination, the following should be considered:

- Location of pain.
- Deformity, especially kyphosis.
- Features of steroid excess: moon facies, buffalo hump, bruising, straiae.
- Examine gait for any abnormalities.

Investigations

Blood tests:

- FBC.
- Urea & electrolytes (U&Es): this is usually normal.
- Thyroid function tests (TFT).
- Calcium: may be high in hyperparathyroidism and low in vitamin D deficiency.
- ALP: levels will be raised if there has been a recent fracture.
- Further tests will depend on clinical suspicion of an underlying cause, e.g. parathyroid hormone and vitamin D level, myeloma screen, cortisol levels.

Imaging:

- X-ray: confirm the presence of a fracture.
- Spinal X-rays: may show vertebral body compression fractures.
- Bones may appear osteopenic (osteoporosis cannot be diagnosed on plain X-rays).

T-score	Interpretation
–1.0 or above	Normal
–2.5 to –1.0	Osteopenia
–2.5 or below	Osteoporosis

Table 3.15: Diagnostic T-score score levels set by WHO.

- Isotope bone scan: this will help determine whether a vertebral body collapsed secondary to osteoporosis or if there is a more sinister cause such as malignancy.
- Dual energy X-ray absorptiometry (DEXA) scan: measure the bone mineral density at the proximal femur and lumbar spine (most common areas).
  - o Considered the 'gold standard' diagnostic test.
  - o A 'T-score' is obtained which compares the tested bone mineral density to a reference population of healthy young adults, and is expressed as the number of standard deviations below this reference population, as shown below in Table 3.15.

When an osteoporotic fracture has occurred, the diagnosis is 'established osteoporosis'.

Management

Acute management of non-vertebral fractures will be dictated by the orthopaedic surgeons.

Acute spinal cord compression from vertebral fracture is a medical emergency. (See section on weakness and paralysis).

➢ In acute cases of vertebral fracture and collapse, the mainstay of treatment is analgesia, followed by early mobilisation and physiotherapy.

➢ A multidisciplinary approach will facilitate rehabilitation.

➢ Prevention is necessary, both primary and secondary. Current guidelines do not completely agree so knowledge of local practice is necessary.

➢ Options include:

  o Lifestyle changes such as more exercise, smoking cessation, reducing alcohol.

  o Hormone replacement therapy.

  o Calcium (1–1.5 g) and Vitamin D (400–800 units) daily.

  o Bisphosphonates. Work by inhibiting osteoclast activity and therefore reduce bone resorption. The major side effects are gastro-intestinal. They must be taken at least 30 minutes before food, with the patient sat upright for that period.

  o Other therapies include Strontium ranelate, Raloxifine (a selective estrogen receptor modulator) and Teriparatide (a recombinant parathyroid hormone)

  o Aim to reduce steroid therapies if possible.

➢ If falls have been a problem, a referral to the falls service may help prevent future fractures.

Prognosis:

➢ There is a high mortality in those who suffer from a hip fracture, i.e. 10% within 1 month and 30% within 1 year.

➢ A further 30% may require institutional support following a hip fracture as it causes them to lose their independence and their level of mobility is reduced.

➢ Osteoporotic compression fracture of the spine causes a considerable morbidity with pain and loss of independence.

Ankylosing spondylitis

Ankylosing spondylitis is a chronic inflammatory disease. It is one of the spondylarthropathies, and is characterised by sacroiliitis, peripheral arthropathy, rheumatoid factor negativity, a familial tendency and involvement of other tissues, in particular the heart, lungs, skin and eyes.

The two widely-used diagnostic criteria are as shown below:

New York Criteria (1968)	European spondylarthropathy study group
• Limited movement of the lumbar spine in 3 planes • Pain in lumbar spine • Chest expansion <2.5 centimetres • Radiologically unilateral sacroiliitis grade III-IV or bilateral grade II	• Inflammatory spinal pain or synovitis along with at least one of: positive family history, psoriasis, inflammatory bowel disease, buttock pain, enthesopathy, sacroiliitis.

Table 3.16: Diagnostic criteria for ankylosing spondylitis.

Epidemiology

Prevalence is 0.1 to 0.5% of the population, with a male preponderance. Onset is typically in the second or third decades. The disease is rare in Japanese and Black African individuals but very common in North American Pima Indians. There is a 5:2 male to female ratio.

Aetiology

There is a combination of genetic and environmental influences. An association with the human leukocyte antigen-B27 (HLA-B27) gene on chromosome 6 has been suggested. This is present in about 10% of the Caucasian population but in over 95% of those with the disease. Multiple other loci on other genes have also been identified which confer additional susceptibility. The specific role of all of these genes is unclear. In monozygotic twins with HLA-B27 positivity, concordance is over 70% but it is only about 20% for dizygotic twins. It is hypothesised that infective agents within the environment are involved in triggering ankylosing spondylitis, and these are unknown.

Pathophysiology

Affected joints become infiltrated with lymphoid and plasma cells causing bony erosions and cartilage destruction. Eventually, there is fibrosis and hence joint stiffness and immobility, which is known as ankylosis.

Key features in the history/examination

The key features are pain, stiffness and fatigue which have been present for at least three months. The stiffness is worse in the morning and improves with exercise.

Skeletal symptoms:

• Back pain, stiffness and a progressive reduction in the range of movement at the spine.

• Worse in the morning and after prolonged periods of immobility and relieved by activity.

• A 'question mark' spine is classical and due to the combination increased thoracic kyphosis and loss of lumbar lordosis. This posture can result in reduced chest expansion and problems with mobility if severe.

- Symptoms are persistent with intermittent worsening and result in deformities which develop over a period of 10 or more years.
- Peripheral arthropathy, especially in the lower limbs.
- Enthesopthies giving tenderness on the chest wall from the intercostal muscle insertions and the sternocostal joints. Also plantar fasciitis and Achilles tendinitis.
- Osteoporosis.

Extra-articular manifestations:

- Anterior uveitis.
- Apical lung fibrosis.
- Cardiac involvement, i.e. aortic valve incompetence and AV nodal conduction defects.
- Association with inflammatory bowel disease.
- Amyloidosis.

When examining the patient, the following should be performed:

- Ask the patient to look from side to side; they will need to turn the whole body to achieve this.
- The Schober test: make two marks over the spine with the patient standing, the first at the level of the posterior superior iliac spine and the second 10 cm above that. Ask the patient to bend forward as far as possible and measure the distance between the marks. This should increase to more than 15 cm.
- Ask the patient to stand with their heels and back flush to the wall; their occiput will not be able to touch the wall at the same time.

Investigations

Blood tests:

- FBC: a chronic anaemia is usual.
- Inflammatory markers: CRP and ESR will be increased.
- Serum IgA levels: May be raised.
- Rheumatoid factor: Will be negative.
- HLA-B27 testing: This is not usually routinely performed.

Imaging:

Early disease may provide no radiological changes.

- X-ray pelvis: At the sacroiliac joints, there may be blurring of the joint margins as well sclerosis and loss of joint space indicating sacroiliitis.
- X-ray spine: With disease progression, there is squaring of the vertebral bodies, syndesmophyte formation and bridging of the bones with fusion of the vertebrae giving the 'bamboo spine' appearance (see Figure 3.7).
- Chest X-ray: may reveal apical fibrosis.

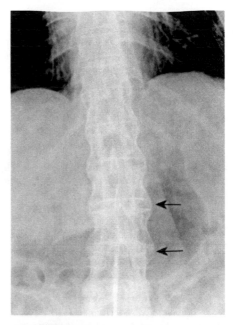

Figure 3.7: A bamboo spine: a plain frontal X-ray of the thoracolumbar spine showing flowing osteophytes in keeping with ankylosing spondylitis.

Other:

- Pulmonary function tests: Usually reveal a restrictive abnormality.
- ECG: Excludes cardiac involvement.
- Echocardiography: Excludes cardiac involvement.

Management

The mainstay of treatment is to relieve pain, prevent the formation of spinal deformity and to enhance mobility. The following features should be considered:

- Patient education and provision of information.
- Awareness of the National Ankylosing Spondylitis Society (www.nass.co.uk).
- Genetic counselling may be required.
- Physiotherapy to teach exercises to maintain posture and mobility and to encourage general fitness. Swimming is especially beneficial.
- Analgesia, especially NSAIDs, are effective in reducing symptoms of pain as well as morning stiffness.
- Disease modifying agents such as Sulfasalazine and Methotrexate can help to improve any peripheral joint symptoms but have little effects on the spine.
- Bisphosphonates.
- Newer biological therapies such as Infliximab are showing promise.
- Surgical intervention is rare, but hip replacement is the commonest operation performed for severe hip arthritis.

3. Medicine

Prognosis:

➤ With appropriate anti-inflammatory drug therapy, disease-modifying agents, and physiotherapy there is a good chance that the patient can lead a normal life with a normal life expectancy. More than 75% of sufferers remain in full-time employment.

Tumours of the bone

Epidemiology

Primary malignant tumours affecting the bone are rare. It makes up 0.2% of all neoplasms and approximately 400 cases are diagnosed each year in the UK.

Aetiology

Tissue	Benign	Malignant
Bone	Osteoma	Osteosarcoma
		Ewing's sarcoma
Cartilage	Chondroma	Chondrosarcoma
Bone marrow	–	Lymphoma
		Myeloma
Synovium	–	Synovial sarcoma

Table 3.17: Primary tumours of the bone.

Secondary malignant tumours are significantly more frequent and are most commonly from the breast, prostate, thyroid, kidney, lung and bowel (in descending order of frequency). The vertebrae are the commonest site affected by metastatic disease, but only 10% are symptomatic.

Pathophysiology

Pathophysiology is dependent on the aetiology.

Key features in the history/examination

- Local pain, swelling, and signs of a pathological fracture.
- Neurological symptoms from nerve root or spinal cord compression (progressive lower limb motor weakness, altered bladder and bowel function and saddle anaesthesia).
- Non-specific features of weight loss, lethargy and reduced appetite.
- Any symptoms from a non-bone primary neoplasm.

Investigations

Blood tests:

- FBC
- U&Es
- Liver function tests (LFT)
- Bone profile
- Inflammatory markers: CRP and ESR
- Protein electrophoresis (paired serum and urine)

Imaging:

- X-ray spine: To check the spine for any abnormal features.
- CXR: Look for primary tumours in the chest.
- CT/MRI:
  o Look for signs of cord compromise.
  o Can also define local spread (see Figure 3.8)

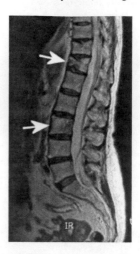

Figure 3.8: Sagittal MRI image of the lumbar spine showing multiple regions of abnormal signal intensity in keeping with bony metastases (arrows).

Others:

- Bone biopsy

Management

The management of primary bone neoplasms should be dictated by a multidisciplinary team at a specialist bone unit. It will depend on tumour type and stage and may include chemotherapy, radiotherapy, and surgical resection.

The priorities when treating secondary metastatic deposits are to control pain, prevent fractures and maintain function and mobility.

➤ Adequate analgesia. Use the WHO analgesic ladder, but often strong opiates are required as well as adjunctive therapy for neuropathic pain.

➤ Bisphosphonates inhibit osteoclastic activity and can help reduce pain.

➤ Some types of chemotherapy help e.g. Tamoxifen may be indicated in breast cancer.

➤ Radiotherapy can be useful in reducing pain and by shrinking tumours can relieve spinal cord compression.

➤ Surgery may be helpful in stabilising an unstable spine.

Prognosis:

➤ This varies according to the type of neoplasm and stage. Secondary metastatic deposits carry a poor prognosis.

Further reading and references

➤ British Orthopaedic Association (2007). *The care of patients with fragility fracture.*

➤ National Ankylosing Spondylitis Society www.nass.co.uk

➤ National Institute for Health and Clinical Excellence (2008). *Alendronate, etidronate, risedronate, raloxifene, strontium ranelate and teriparatide for the secondary prevention of osteoporotic fragility fractures in postmenopausal women (TA161).*

➤ National Institute for Health and Clinical Excellence (2008). *Alendronate, etidronate, risedronate, raloxifene and strontium ranelate for the primary prevention of osteoporotic fragility fractures in postmenopausal women (TA160).*

➤ National Institute for Health and Clinical Excellence (2009). *Low Back Pain (CG088).*

➤ National Institute for Health and Clinical Excellence (2008). *Osteoarthritis (CG059).*

➤ National Osteoporosis Guideline Group (2008). *Guideline for the diagnosis and management of osteoporosis in postmenopausal women and men from the age of 50 years in the UK.*

ACUTE CONFUSION

Differential Diagnosis

System/Organ	Disease
Central nervous system (CNS)	**Delirium (Acute confusional state/Toxic confusional state)**
Alcohol-related	**Alcohol withdrawal and Wernicke's encephalopathy**
Infection	**Cerebral abscess** Sepsis (UTI, chest infection, septicaemia) Encephalitis
Liver disease	**Acute hepatic failure and encephalopathy**
Drugs	Intoxication or side effects
Metabolic	Hyponatraemia Hypercalcaemia
Others	Hypoxia Post-ictal period in epileptics Intracranial bleed Stroke Post-head injury Constipation

In the elderly, acute on chronic confusion is most likely where there is some underlying dementia with the acute worsening usually secondary to an inter-current illness such as infection.

Metabolic causes – Please refer to the section on metabolic disturbances.

Delirium (Acute confusional state/Toxic confusional state)

A state in which there is impairment of level of consciousness as well as a disturbance in the patient's behaviour, cognition and their interaction with others. Although the state of hyperactive delirium is well recognised, patients may also suffer from a hypoactive subtype or a mixed subtype.

Epidemiology

Seen in 10–15% of patients admitted to hospital. Mostly occurs at the extremes of ages, especially the elderly population who have a 40% chance of developing it as an in-patient. Its presence is associated with a worse prognosis in the acute phase of the illness.

Aetiology

There are multiple potential causes of acute confusion as shown in Table 3.18.

Non-CNS infection	Especially urinary sepsis and chest sepsis.
Alcohol withdrawal	Known as delirium tremens, this occurs in patients with alcohol dependency and cannot have their regular intake due to hospital admission.
Drugs	In the younger population the use of recreational drugs must be excluded. In the elderly population it is common for drug interactions to cause symptoms of confusion. Opiates. Benzodiazepines.
Stroke or intracranial bleed	Must be excluded in patients who present with a very sudden onset of confusion, usually, but not necessarily associated with focal neurological signs.
Metabolic and Endocrine abnormalities	Hypernatraemia/Hyponatraemia. Hypercalcaemia. Hypoglycaemia/hyperglycaemia. Thiamine deficiency (Wernicke's encephalopathy) can occur in alcoholics, dietary deficiency, and in patients with excessive periods of vomiting such as hyperemesis in pregnancy. Adrenal crisis. Hypothyroidism.
Epilepsy	Patients who are immediately post-ictal may be confused and disoriented.
CNS infection	Meningitis, encephalitis, and cerebral abscess.
Others	Hypoxia. Pain. Post head injury. Post-operative. Hepatic encephalopathy. Renal failure. Myocardial infarction. Acute urinary retention.

Table 3.18: Causes of acute confusion.

Pathophysiology

The precise pathophysiology is unclear to date. It most likely involves a combination of disordered neurotransmission, toxins and abnormal cytokine activity.

Key features in the history/examination

- Confusion tends to be of rapid onset ranging from a few hours to a few days.
- Symptoms run a fluctuating course.
- Classically, levels of confusion are increased at night.
- Hallucinations are common, most often visual in nature and can be frightening for the patient.
- Obtain a collateral history from a third party e.g. relative or carer.
- Circumstances of this episode.
- Past history of dementia - this does not cause an acute confusional state but increases the risk of having one.
- Past history of co-morbid conditions which may contribute to the delirium.
- Drug history including over-the-counter medications.
- Alcohol history.
- It is important to remember that when assessing patients who are disorientated, restless, aggressive or agitated and having visual hallucinations that these symptoms are more likely to be due to an underlying medical disorder rather than a psychiatric disorder.
- In a patient presenting with dysphasia and 'appearing acutely confused', an underlying stroke or space occupying lesion must be excluded before diagnosing an acute confusional state.
- A CNS infection or intracranial bleed is suggested by meningism - neck stiffness, positive Kernig's sign and photophobia.
- If focal neurological signs or papilloedema are present it is suggestive of an intracranial lesion.
- There are usually no focal neurological signs in a toxic confusional state.
- Cognitive testing may reveal deficits in orientation, registration, immediate recall and attention.
- The abbreviated mental test score must be performed in any patient who presents with acute confusion and is outlined in Table 3.19.

Abbreviated mental test score (AMTS):

1.	Age
2.	Date of birth
3.	State an address such as 42 West Street and ask the patient to recall and repeat this after a few minutes
4.	Year
5.	Time (morning, afternoon, evening)
6.	Place (name of hospital or department)
7.	Recognise 2 people, for example, a doctor and a nurse
8.	Recall the dates of World War 1
9.	Count backwards from 20 to 1
10.	Monarch

Table 3.19: Abbreviated mental test score.

Investigations

Blood tests:

- Full blood Count (FBC): may reveal a haematological disorder, vitamin deficiencies, and evidence of infection.
- Erythrocyte sedimentation rate (ESR) and C-reactive protein (CRP): will be raised in inflammatory disorders.
- Urea and Electrolytes (U&Es), blood glucose, liver function test (LFTs), thyroid function test (TFTs) and calcium should be measured as an imbalance may be responsible for acute confusion.
- Arterial blood gas (ABG): required to exclude hypoxia and show acid/base status.

Microbiology:

- Blood cultures: are essential, especially when there is pyrexia.
- Urine dipstick and Mid-Stream Urine (MSU).
- Other samples as appropriate e.g. sputum, cerebrospinal fluid (CSF), pleural fluid, ascites.

Imaging:

- Chest X-ray: forms part of the septic screen and can reveal an unsuspected pneumonia or malignancy.

Other:

- ECG
- EEG if seizures suspected

Management

The aim is to identify and treat the cause of the confusion.

- ➤ All patients should be nursed in a calm, well-lit environment under close supervision to ensure safety of the confused patient, other patients and staff.
- ➤ Treat any sepsis found.
- ➤ Treat any metabolic or endocrine abnormality found.
- ➤ Ensure good hydration.
- ➤ Ensure patient is free from pain.
- ➤ The patient's medications should be reviewed and any potential contributors to the confusion should be discontinued.
- ➤ Sedation should be avoided if at all possible, but may become necessary if they are agitated, frightened and putting themselves or others in danger. Take care with the dosage of sedatives in the elderly as drug metabolism tends to slow in the presence of infection.
- ➤ IV thiamine should be given if there is suggestion of Wernicke's encephalopathy.

Prognosis:

- ➤ Usually considered rapidly reversible with appropriate treatment tailored to the cause however more recent evidence points to a prolonged recovery over months.

> There is a high level of morbidity with prolonged hospital length of stay and complications.

> There is at least a doubling of mortality rates in the acutely confused.

> Wernicke's encephalopathy can be potentially fatal without treatment and there may be little clinical improvement despite appropriate medical therapy.

Alcohol withdrawal and Wernicke's encephalopathy

Epidemiology

Around 20% of women and 33% of men in the UK regularly consume quantities of alcohol which exceed the recommended limits. There is an increase in morbidity and mortality due to alcohol in the UK. Binge drinking is particularly problematic in the late teens and early twenties.

Wernicke's encephalopathy is most common in patients with alcohol dependence, with a prevalence of is approximately 10%.

Aetiology

Alcohol withdrawal is group of symptoms and signs seen on cessation of drinking alcohol in patients with excessive alcohol consumption and alcohol dependency. Alcohol dependence results from a combination of factors which may be physical, psychological or social in nature. For example, the feeling of intoxication may help to 'numb' painful feelings experienced by the patient. Those who lack social contact are particularly susceptible.

Wernicke's encephalopathy is a severely confused state usually resulting from chronic alcohol abuse.

Pathophysiology

The precise pathophysiology of withdrawal is unclear. There are chronic changes in neurotransmission especially in the GABAergic, serotinergic and dopaminergic neurones. These chronic changes are responsible for the phenomena of dependence, addiction and withdrawal.

Wernicke's encephalopathy results from thiamine deficiency, which can result from poor nutritional status secondary to alcohol but can also result from chronic vomiting, cancer and chronic haemodialysis.

Key features in the history/examination

It is important to make an estimate of the patient's weekly alcohol intake in order to gauge the severity of their dependence. One unit is equivalent to a glass of wine, one measure of spirits, or one half of a pint of beer.

The **CAGE** screening tool is used in suspected alcohol dependence:

- Have you ever thought about **Cutting** down your alcohol intake?
- Do you feel **Annoyed** if people criticise your intake of alcohol?
- Have you ever felt **Guilty** regarding your drinking habits?
- Do you ever need to have a drink first thing in the morning to relieve symptoms of a hangover? (**Eye-opener**)

Table 3.20: CAGE criteria.

Alcohol dependence:
- Patient is aware of their compulsion to consume alcohol.
- Developed a tolerance to the effects of the alcohol.
- Have withdrawal symptoms in the absence of consumption.
- They consume alcohol in order to relieve or avoid the symptoms of withdrawal.
- Alcohol use takes precedence over other activities in their life.
- Rapid return to consumption after a period of abstinence.

Alcohol withdrawal syndrome:
- Features begin to present around 12 hours after the most recent intake of alcohol with sweating, nausea, insomnia, anxiety.

Seizures:
- Can occur as early as 12 hours after the last drink and peak around 48 hours.
- Patients with a background of epilepsy or previous withdrawal seizures are at an increased risk.

Delirium Tremens (DTs):
- Usually occurs around 72 hours after the last drink.
- Features include confusion, tremor, agitation, restlessness, fright, sweating, nausea, fever, tachycardia and dehydration.
- Hallucinations are a classical feature, both visual (e.g. seeing insects crawling on the body) and tactile (e.g. feeling insects crawling on the body).
- Those with higher alcohol consumption are at an increased risk, as are those with a long-standing history of alcohol dependence, an increased age and features of severe withdrawal on presentation.

Wernicke's encephalopathy:
- The classic triad of signs are: confusion, gait ataxia and nystagmus/opthalmoplegia (but all three are seen in less than 25%).
- Peripheral neuropathy may also be a feature.
- There is a high risk of irreversible brain damage with this condition.

A sequalae may be ***Korsakoff's psychosis***. However this can also result from persistent vomiting such as in pregnant women with hyperemesis.

- There are degenerative changes within the areas of the brain which are responsible for forming memories as well as the recall of short and long term memory, for example, the hippocampus.
- Patients are fully alert and conscious but with impairment of their intermediate memory and short-term recall of information.
- Usually, they are oriented and can register and recall new information temporarily.
- There is both antegrade and retrograde amnesia.
- Often patients confabulate as they are unable to recall actual information. However this can also be a feature of dementia.
- Treatment with thiamine may cause an improvement in symptoms.
- Neurorehabilitation can help the patient to optimise their abilities in order to allow for independent living as much as possible. However, this is rarely undertaken.
- Improvement is unlikely; however, it is thought that if the patient remains abstinent from alcohol there may be resolution of symptoms to some extent.

Investigations:

There are no specific diagnostic tests for alcohol withdrawal.

Blood tests:

- FBC: usually shows a macrocytosis (raised MCV) with the absence of anaemia.
- LFTs: will reveal an increased gamma-glutamyl transferase level.
- Clotting screen: an indicator of the synthetic function of the liver and may reveal a derangement secondary to alcohol use.
- Glucose: hypoglycaemia may feature.
- Magnesium: hypomagnesaemia may be found.

Imaging:

- Chest X-ray.
- CT or MRI brain is indicated in Wernicke's encephalopathy.

Others:

- ECG.

Management

1. Withdrawal symptoms:

➤ Benzodiazepines are first line treatment.
➤ A reducing regime of Chlordiazepoxide is required to reduce the severity of withdrawal symptoms and also acts to prevent progression to seizures.
➤ Usually tapered over 6 days.
➤ Ensure PRN doses are charted.

➤ An alternative is to use a symptom-triggered approach with the Chlordiazepoxide administered on the basis of symptomatology rather than using a purely a fixed-time approach.

2. Withdrawal seizures:

➤ Usually self-resolving.
➤ If required, 2mg of IV Lorazepam is effective at terminating prolonged seizures.

3. Psychosis:

➤ Haloperidol may be given as well as Chlordiazepoxide, up to a maximum of 5 mg TDS.

4. Vitamin/mineral replacement:

➤ In those at low risk of Wernicke's encephalopathy, oral supplements are sufficient with Thiamine 100–200 mg per day, Vitamin B complex strong 30 mg OD and Folate 5 mg per day.
➤ For higher risk or showing actual signs of Wernicke's encephalopathy, institute Pabrinex (vials 1 & 2) three times per day for up to 3 days. (Pabrinex contains Vitamins B1, B2, B6 and Nicotinamide)
➤ Multivitamin supplements.
➤ Supplement glucose if necessary, but beware of acutely precipitating Wernicke's encephalopathy.
➤ Replace magnesium if necessary.

5. Follow-up:

➤ Nutritional advice and dietician referral.
➤ If the patient has a strong social support network, no history of epilepsy or withdrawal seizures, and is otherwise well, the detoxification schedule can be performed as an out-patient.
➤ Oral vitamin supplements should be continued as an out-patient.
➤ A specialist alcohol team would be responsible for managing the patient in the community in terms of counselling or group therapy.
➤ There are voluntary organisations such as Alcoholics Anonymous which provide support in the community.

Prognosis:

➤ Usually, around 30–40% maintain their abstinence from alcohol or have controlled their drinking with a view to cutting down.
➤ Mortality is up to 3 times higher in patients who are alcohol dependent compared to the general population.
➤ Delirium tremens is fatal in 15% if left untreated.

Cerebral Abscess

Epidemiology

Occurs in 1 per 100,000 patients per year.

Aetiology

Most cerebral abscesses contain polymicrobial infection, the most common causative organism being *Streptococcus*. If the infection arises from neighbouring structures such as the frontal, mastoid, or maxillary sinuses, or ear as a result of chronic otitis media, then the organisms found will be those responsible for the primary infection such as *Pneumococcus, Haemophilus, Moraxella catarrhalis, beta-haemolytic Streptococci* and *Streptococcus pyogenes*. They can also form following a compound skull fracture or if there is a penetrating head injury with a foreign body which is contaminated with infection.

Chronic lung sepsis in the form of bronchiectasis is a common source of infection. They affect all lobes of the brain. Anaerobic organisms include; *Bacteroides* spp, *Porphyromonas* spp, and anaerobic cocci. Aerobic organisms include; *Strep milleri, Staph aureus and Proteus* spp.

Immunocompromised individuals show a novel range of infections e.g. toxoplasmosis, Cryptococcus, *Aspergillus* and tuberculosis. Multiple abscesses are common in these patients.

Patients with miliary tuberculosis are at risk of forming multiple small tuberculomas within the brain.

Pathophysiology

Cerebral abscesses arise either from the spread of infection from other sites in the body or directly from infection around or near the meninges. There is a localised area of bacterial infection in the cerebral substance which is associated with production of pus. A mass lesion may form which can expand and act as a intracranial space-occupying lesion.

Key features in the history/examination

- Symptoms may in fact be progressive over a number of days or weeks.
- Abscesses in the cerebellum tend to develop more acutely and can produce hydrocephalus.
- Headache, fever, nausea, vomiting and malaise are classical.
- There may be signs of meningism with neck stiffness and photophobia.
- Focal neurological deficits may occur such as hemiparesis, aphasia, hemianopia.
- Patients tend to be drowsy, confused and disorientated with a deteriorating level of consciousness.
- Tachycardia is common as well as signs of an intracerebral space-occupying lesion such as papilloedema (present in less than half of patients).
- Thorough examination of the head, ears, sinuses, lungs and abdomen is essential.
- Always look for features which may indicate the source of infection or an increased susceptibility to infection, for example congenital heart disease, tuberculosis, AIDS, endocarditis, bronchiectasis, infected sinuses, ears or the mastoid bone, and chronic dental infections.

- Occasionally, they may be no systemic features associated with the abscess.

Investigations

Blood tests:
- FBC: may show a leucocytosis.
- CRP and ESR: will most likely be raised.

Microbiology:
- Blood cultures.
- If the abscess is drained, pus should be sent for microscopy and culture in order to determine the responsible organisms. This must be done quickly as anaerobic organisms will be killed by atmospheric oxygen and are often key in diagnosis.

Imaging:
- CT or MRI brain scan: ring-enhancing lesion(s) may be seen.

Other:
- Lumbar puncture: This is more dangerous as the presence of a space-occupying lesion poses an increased risk of coning. A CT brain is mandatory prior to the procedure.

Management

Surgery has a key role in both diagnosis and management.
- Aspiration or open drainage of the abscess – a decision to be made by neurosurgeons.
- Surgical decompression of the abscess may be required if there is an inadequate response to antibiotic therapy.

Antibiotics are given based on clinical suspicion of the causative organisms and their degree of penetrance across the blood-brain barrier.
- May need to be changed according to culture results from the pus sample obtained at surgery.
- Mostly, antibiotics are given to cover infection with anaerobes such as Metronidazole.
- *Streptococci, Staphylococci*, and gram-negative anaerobes are covered with Cefotaxime.
- Flucloxacillin or chloramphenicol may be administered in addition in suspected *Haemophilus* infection.

Prognosis:
- Risk of mortality is 30% despite appropriate management.
- Of the survivors, there is a 30% risk of subsequent epilepsy and often, all surviving patients are given anti-epileptic medication upon discharge.

Acute hepatic failure and encephalopathy

Epidemiology

The actual incidence of hepatic encephalopathy is not clearly known.

Aetiology

The main causes of acute liver failure in the UK are:

- Paracetamol overdose (45%)
- Viral hepatitis A, B, C (55%)
- Drug induced (e.g. halothane), Wilson's disease, sepsis, pregnancy, malignancy (combined account for (<5%)

Table 3.21: Main causes of acute liver failure.

The aetiology of encephalopathy is thought to be due to an excess of ammonium. This is unlikely to be the whole story as there is only a poor correlation between encephalopathy and ammonium levels. The factors implicated in the development of encephalopathy include:

- Sepsis (gram negative sepsis as well as spontaneous bacterial peritonitis).
- Drugs (such as sedatives or narcotics).
- Acute alcoholic intoxication.
- Hepatic or portal vein thrombosis.
- Gastrointestinal bleeding which produces an excess of protein in the bowel.
- Electrolyte abnormalities (potassium or sodium depletion which can result from diuretics which are used to treat oedema or ascites).
- Constipation.
- Trauma (includes both minor and major surgical procedures as well as paracentesis).

Pathophysiology

When liver failure is associated with encephalopathy, it is known as fulminant hepatic failure. Defined as symptoms of encephalopathy (a spectrum of neuropsychiatric symptoms and signs) in a patient within 8 weeks of the onset of symptoms of liver failure, prior to which the individual had a normal liver. It is essential to recognise the symptoms early as the risk of mortality is high.

Encephalopathy is poorly understood, however, is thought to result from the failure of the liver to eliminate the toxic substances from the blood. There is absorption of nitrogen from the bowel, and a stimulation of the GABA (Benzodiazepine) receptors in the brain.

Key features in the history/examination

On examination, there may be many of the peripheral stigmata of chronic liver disease:

- Clubbing
- Koilonychia
- Leuconychia
- Asterixis
- Palmar erythema
- Jaundice

- Excoriation
- Purpura
- Parotid hypertrophy
- Spider naevi
- Gynaecomastia
- Dilated cardiomyopathy
- Splenomegaly
- Ascites
- Caput medusae
- With fatty liver there may be hepatomegaly with a palpable liver edge but as cirrhosis progresses, gradually it shrinks and is no longer palpable.
- Constructional apraxia may be illustrated by asking the patient to draw or copy a star.
- Hypoglycaemia is a late sign as the production of glucose from the liver tails off.
- At the later stages of the condition, there may be multi-system failure with:
  - Cerebral oedema
  - Renal failure
  - Adult respiratory distress syndrome
  - Vasomotor disturbances
  - Sepsis
- Encephalopathic patients may initially demonstrate subtle features of mild sleep disturbance and difficulty in performing basic daily tasks such as dressing and tying shoelaces. They will become increasingly irritable, confused and drowsy and may have reducing Glasgow Coma Scale.

There are 4 grades of hepatic encephalopathy:

1. Mild or intermittent drowsiness, with altered mood and behaviour, impaired concentration; however, patients remain coherent and rousable.
2. Patient becomes increasingly drowsy, confused and disorientated, with slurring of the speech. They remain rousable and participate in conversation.
3. Increasingly drowsy, disorientated, confused, aggressive, with incoherent speech, however, they do respond to simple and basic commands.
4. Coma, where patients only respond to painful stimuli (4a) or none (4b).

Table 3.22: Grading of hepatic encephalopathy.

Investigations

Blood tests:

- FBC: may show a low haemoglobin with a high MCV in an alcoholic patient presenting with encephalopathy.
- Clotting: may be deranged with raised INR.
- LFTs: indicate severe hepatitis with levels of transaminases above 5000 IU/l.

- U&Es
- Glucose

Microbiology:

- Urine dip and MSU
- Blood cultures

Imaging:

- Chest X-ray
- Hepatic ultrasound
- CT brain to exclude acute subdural haematoma

Other:

- EEG: Delta waves and a triphasic pattern are common features (patients with hypoglycaemia and carbon monoxide retention may also have this feature).

Management

➤ Support of a hepatologist will be urgently required.

➤ Early input from intensive care unit (ICU) should be considered.

➤ Specialist management from a tertiary centre may be required and in some cases a transplant may be appropriate. Such patients should be transferred to the appropriate facility as soon as possible. It is important to clarify the time of onset of symptoms of acute hepatic failure prior to the development of encephalopathy. The shorter the time period the better the prognosis. This can range from hyperacute (2 weeks) to subacute (8–26 weeks).

➤ It is essential to identify and correct precipitating causes.

➤ Patients require supportive therapy and close monitoring.

➤ Correct any electrolyte imbalance.

➤ Early treatment of hypoglycaemia and sepsis is essential in management.

   o Prophylactic antibiotic therapy can be given as patients are at high risk of infection (to cover bacteria and fungi).

   o For example Neomycin can reduce the risk of spontaneous bacterial peritonitis.

➤ Lactulose to reduce nitrogen load in the gut.

➤ If there is active bleeding any clotting abnormalities will need urgent correction.

➤ Avoid fluid overload as this will precipitate cerebral oedema, which is recognised, and should be treated rapidly.

➤ Ascitic tap with large volume paracentesis if required (tense ascites causing discomfort or diaphragmatic splinting).

➤ Supportive management for any renal or cardiovascular symptoms.

   o Dialysis needs to be considered for severe renal impairment.

   o Prone to hypotension and so central line insertion must be considered.

   o Inotropic support may be indicated if the patient is unable to sustain their blood pressure despite supportive management.

   o Respiratory support with ventilation is indicated in order to maintain their PaO_2.

   o Oral potassium replacement is sufficient to treat hypokalaemia.

➤ A proton pump inhibitor or H_2 receptor blocker is given to minimise the risk of developing gastric erosions and upper gastrointestinal bleeding.

➤ Early nutritional support with dietician assessment and advice is important.

   o Nasogastric tube insertion.

   o A low-protein diet (40 g per day) and Lactulose may alleviate symptoms as it produces an osmotic diarrhoea which removes both protein and any blood from the bowel and prevents the increase in ammonia-producing organisms.

   o IV Pabrinex as thiamine deficiency is common in alcoholics.

➤ In patients where a Paracetamol overdose is evident or suspected, the antidote N-acetylcysteine should be administered either with the blood Paracetamol level (if in the toxic range) or promptly in cases of doubt. (See Poisoning chapter later).

➤ If the patient shows features of severe disease (more than grade 2 encephalopathy), or persistently low blood pressure (less than 100 mmHg systolic), hyponatraemia or thrombocytopenia, INR >3 or factor 5 <20%, consider early transfer to dedicated liver unit for ongoing treatment and consideration of transplantation.

Prognosis:

➤ Generally poor, but influenced by the underlying cause and degree of liver damage.

➤ Mortality rates are as high as 90% if there is grade 4 encephalopathy with no transplantation possible.

➤ Most common causes of death include:

   o Cerebral oedema

   o Sepsis (can be bacterial or fungal)

   o Cardiovascular instability

Further reading and references

➤ www.alcoholics-anonymous.org.uk

➤ British Geriatrics Society (2006). *Guidelines for the Prevention, Diagnosis and Management of Delirium in Older People in Hospital.*

➤ Scottish Intercollegiate Guideline Network (2004). *The management of harmful drinking and alcohol dependence in primary care (Guideline 74).*

➤ Thomson, A.D., Cook, C.C.H., Touquet, R., et al. (2002). The Royal College of Physicians Report on Alcohol: Guidelines for Managing Wernicke's Encephalopathy in the Accident and Emergency Department. *Alcohol & Alcoholism* Vol. 37, No. 6, pp. 513–521.

3. Medicine

BREATHLESSNESS

Differential Diagnosis

System/Causes	Disease
Respiratory	**Pneumothorax**
	Pulmonary oedema
	Pulmonary embolism (PE)
	Lower respiratory tract infection/pneumonia
	Asthma
	Chronic obstructive pulmonary disease (COPD)
	Aspiration pneumonia
	Fibrosing alveolitis
	Cystic fibrosis
Other	Anaemia
	Anaphylaxis
	Anxiety
	Aortic Stenosis
	Metabolic Acidosis
	Neuromuscular Disorders
	Trauma

Pneumothorax

Epidemiology

The incidence is 24 in 100,000 for males and overall, 10 in 100,000 per year in the UK. Mostly occurs in young adults or in elderly individuals with pre-existing respiratory disease.

Aetiology

Primary spontaneous pneumothorax occurs where there is no underlying lung condition. Typically affects tall, young thin males and is attributable to the rupture of small sub-pleural blebs at the lung apex. The risk is increased by:

- Smoking
- Marfans syndrome
- Homocystinuria
- Family history

Secondary spontaneous pneumothorax occurs as a complication of underlying respiratory disease, for example:

- Asthma and bullous emphysema.
- Positive pressure ventilation in an intensive care setting.
- Infections such as tuberculosis or pneumonia especially *Pneumocystis jerovici.*
- Genetic disorders with lung involvement such as cystic fibrosis.

Trauma can also lead to a pneumothorax. Penetrating chest wall injury such as a stab wound and blunt chest wall injuries such as a road traffic accident are common traumas. Pneumothorax can result following a therapeutic procedure such as insertion of a central line into the subclavian vein or following pleural aspiration or biopsy.

Tension pneumothorax can occur with any of these types. It is a medical emergency where prompt recognition is essential to management. However it is rare.

Pathophysiology

The alveolar pressure is greater than intrapleural pressure. If there is a break in the integrity of the alveoli, the pleura or the chest wall then the air will follow the pressure gradient and accumulate in the intrapleural space. The flow will continue until the pressure gradient is equalised or the break in integrity has been sealed.

Tension pneumothorax occurs when a one-way valve develops that causes an accumulation of air during inspiration without allowing release during expiration. The volume of air and therefore the pressure within the pleural space increases. Results in severe breathlessness, mediastinal shift, hypoxaemia, with progression to shock as a result of reduced venous return to the heart.

Key features in the history/examination

Important points to consider when taking the history are as follows:

- Should always be considered as a differential in patients with known lung disease who present with an acute onset of shortness of breath.
- Sudden onset of sharp pleuritic chest pain associated with shortness of breath.
- Hypoxia
- Tachycardia
- Tachypnoea
- Presence of risk factors.

Essential features on examination are as follows:

- On examination, there will be reduced chest wall movement on the affected side of the chest.
- The percussion note will be normal or hyper-resonant on the affected side.
- Breath sounds are absent or diminished over the pneumothorax.
- Reduced vocal resonance and tactile vocal fremitus on the affected side.
- If it is large, there will be mediastinal shift away from the affected side with deviation of the trachea.
- Other late signs include hypotension and distension of the neck veins.

Investigations

The diagnosis of tension pneumothorax is a clinical diagnosis, no initial investigations are required.

Blood tests:

- ABG which will give a typical picture of hyperventilation with a respiratory alkalosis.

Imaging:

- Chest X-ray: inspiratory and expiratory films may be needed in cases of a small pneumothorax (See Figure 3.9).
- CT scan may be required to further evaluate the chest and any suspected underlying pathology.

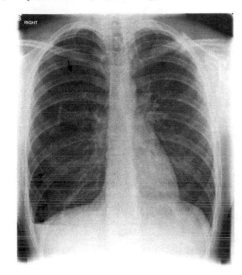

Figure 3.9: Chest X-Ray showing a large right pneumothorax. Note the absence of lung markings in the periphery and the edge of the collapsed lung (arrows).

Management

All patients should have a referral made to the respiratory team.

Primary spontaneous pneumothorax:

- ➤ If less than 2 cm rim visible between the lung and chest wall – observation and high flow oxygen. High flow oxygen has been shown to quadruple the rate of resorption.
- ➤ If 2 cm or more rim visible between the lung margin and the chest wall – needle aspiration (see relevant section in DOPS) and high flow oxygen.
- ➤ If needle aspiration fails a repeat attempt should be considered and if still unsuccessful, a chest drain should be inserted.

Secondary spontaneous pneumothorax:

- ➤ If the pneumothorax has a 2 cm or more rim of air visible, the patient is symptomatically breathless or is older than 50 years, then chest drain insertion and high flow oxygen is required (caution if the patient is known to have COPD with a hypoxic drive).
- ➤ If small (<2 cm) pneumothorax and the patient is clinically stable then attempt aspiration and manage with high flow oxygen and observation for at least 24 hours.

- ➤ If needle aspiration fails a repeat should not be attempted but a chest drain should be inserted.
- ➤ If very small (<1 cm) and asymptomatic, admission for observation is the management of choice.

Traumatic pneumothorax:

- ➤ The management for traumatic pneumothorax is similar to that of secondary spontaneous pneumothorax.
- ➤ If the patient continues to deteriorate they may require a thoracotomy.

Tension pneumothorax:

- ➤ Immediate decompression by insertion of 14G or 16G cannula into the second intercostal space, mid-clavicular line followed by insertion of chest drain.

Chest drain insertion:

- ➤ Complications of chest drain insertion include:
  - o Penetration of internal organ e.g. lung, heart, great vessel, liver or spleen.
  - o Infection.
  - o Surgical emphysema.
- ➤ A repeat chest X-ray must be performed post-procedure to ensure resolution or reduction in size of the pneumothorax.
- ➤ Recurrent pneumothoracies can be treated with pleurodesis or by surgery on the advice of a respiratory specialist.
- ➤ Patients should be advised:
  - o Avoid flying until resolution confirmed.
  - o Not to dive.

Prognosis:

- ➤ Around 1 in 5 patients who present with a primary spontaneous pneumothorax will have a recurrence on the same side.
- ➤ The risk of recurrence increases up to 80% with each subsequent pneumothorax.
- ➤ Patients with secondary spontaneous pneumothoraces are at greater risk of recurrence.

Pulmonary oedema

Epidemiology

A common occurrence affecting over 1 in a 100 individuals over the age of 65 years and a potentially life-threatening emergency.

Aetiology

A variety of different mechanisms can cause pulmonary oedema, as shown in Table 3.23 below:

Pathophysiology

The most common causative mechanism is a raised capillary pressure. When there is a rise in the pulmonary capillary pressure

3. Medicine

Mechanism	Feature
Raised capillary pressure	Cardiogenic causes
	Myocardial infarction (MI)
	Ventricular septal rupture
	Aortic valve regurgitation or stenosis
	Mitral valve regurgitation or stenosis
	Severe uncontrolled hypertension
	Arrhythmia
	Myocarditis
	Atrial myxoma
	Tamponade
	Aortic dissection
	Cardiomyopathy
Renal	Acute and chronic renal failure
	Renal artery stenosis
Increased pulmonary capillary permeability	Liver failure
	Fat embolism
	Amniotic embolism
	Acute respiratory distress syndrome
	High altitude
	Inhaled/aspirated toxin
Severe brain insult	–
High output heart failure	Septicaemia
	Anaemia
	Thyrotoxic crisis
Lymphatic obstruction	–
Acute or chronic upper airway obstruction	–

Table 3.23: Causes of pulmonary oedema.

(usually more than 24 mmHg), there is a leakage of fluid in to the interstitial space of the lungs. With further increases in pressure, the fluid enters in to the alveoli as well. If there is co-existing hypoalbuminaemia, then pulmonary oedema will result at a lower pulmonary capillary pressure. An acute increase in the left atrial pressure results in a rise in the pulmonary capillary pressure.

Key features in history/examination

Elicit the following from the patients history:

- Dyspnoea with orthopnoea and paroxysmal nocturnal dyspnoea.
- Cough (dry or productive) – classically pink frothy sputum.
- Pedal oedema.
- Rapid or insidious onset.
- Past medical history.
- Drug history and concordance with therapy.
- Ask about chest pain because oedema can be precipitated by MI.

The main features which may be present on examination are as follows:

- Pale
- Sweaty
- Cyanosis
- Raised jugular venous pressure (JVP)
- Tachycardia
- Pulsus alterans
- Gallop rhythm
- Tachypnoea
- Bibasal crackles on auscultation
- Pitting oedema
- Valvular murmurs
- Cardiogenic shock
- Hypotension
- Low cardiac output
- Oliguria
- Signs of right heart failure: peripheral oedema and hepatomegaly
- In long-standing cases, cardiac cachexia may be seen

Investigations

Blood tests:

- FBC
- U&Es
- TFT
- LFTs: low albumin in liver failure and nephrotic syndrome.
- Troponin: to exclude an acute MI.
- ABG: shows hypoxaemia with an initial fall in $PaCO_2$ due to tachypnoea followed by an increase due to impairment of gas exchange.
- Brain-type natriuretic peptide (BNP) if available.

Imaging:

- Chest X-ray: may show an enlarged heart, upper lobe diversion, bilateral perihilar shadowing with a typical 'bat's wing' distribution. Kerley B lines and fluid in the horizontal fissure indicate interstitial oedema. (See Figure 3.10 below).

Others:

- Echocardiogram
- ECG: may reveal an arrhythmia or myocardial infarction.

Management

➢ A to E assessment.
➢ Sit patient upright.
➢ Oxygen.
➢ Intravenous nitrates (e.g. a Glyceryl trinitrate infusion):

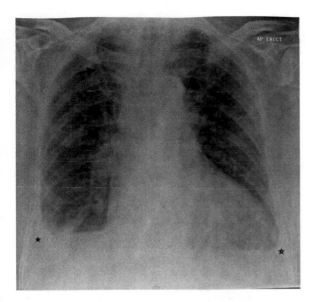

Figure 3.10: Chest X-Ray showing a big heart with bilateral small pleural effusions and blunting of costo phrenic angle (stars). Also note the prominent upper lobe pulmonary vessels in keeping with upper lobe blood diversion (arrow).

Class	Sign	Hospital mortality (%)
I	No signs of left ventricular dysfunction	6
II	S3 gallop with mild/moderate pulmonary congestions	20
III	Severe pulmonary oedema	40
IV	Cardiogenic shock	80–90

Table 3.24: Killip classification for pulmonary oedema.

Pulmonary embolism (PE)

Epidemiology

PE is one of the most common cardiovascular diseases with 28,600 cases reported in the UK between 2006 and 2007. There is equal distribution across age groups and sex. The prevalence is not accurately known as many are missed or undiagnosed; however, it is estimated at 1 in 500.

Aetiology

PE can have three different methods of causation, which is known as Virchow's triad, as shown in Table 3.25:

Pathophysiology

PE occurs when a thrombus lodges in the pulmonary vasculature, most commonly within the lower lung lobes. It is mostly caused by thrombi embolising from a pre-existing venous thrombus commonly in the pelvic or femoral veins (70 to 80%). However thrombi which occur in the veins below the knee very rarely result in a PE.

The composition of the emboli can range from a clot from a deep vein thrombosis (DVT) to a tumour or even material which has been injected intravenously. The thrombus obstructs the vasculature and leads to increased pulmonary vascular resistance, increasing the workload of the right ventricle. The heart rate increases in an attempt to compensate. If the vascular resistance continues to increase the compensation fails and causes right ventricle distension, decreases right ventricular cardiac output and increases end-diastolic pressures.

There is a decreased right ventricular output which results in a reduced left ventricular preload, and a decreased left ventricular preload results in a reduced left ventricular filling and cardiac output followed by a drop in mean arterial pressure. A drop in mean arterial pressure can lead to hypotension and cardiogenic shock can occur with 50% occlusion in a previous healthy individual. Ventilation-perfusion mismatch occurs as there is vascular occlusion despite normal ventilation.

There are 3 different types of PE:

- **Acute PE**
- **Acute massive PE:** the impairment to the pulmonary circulation is so great as to cause circulatory collapse.
- **Chronic thromboembolic disease:** very rarely occurs when

○ Vasodilation.

○ Reduce preload.

○ Caution should be used. Titrate infusion to keep systolic blood pressure > 90 mmHg.

➤ Intravenous diuretics such as Furosemide will cause an immediate vasodilatation. The subsequent diuresis reduces the filling pressures of the heart and results in symptomatic relief.

➤ Intravenous opiates, commonly Diamorphine 2.5–5.0 mg.

○ Reduces anxiety and causes vasodilatation.

○ Reduces vasomotor tone and so there is a reduction in the filling pressures of the heart resulting in symptomatic relief as well as a reduction in the systolic blood pressure.

○ Large doses must be avoided as they can cause respiratory depression.

➤ Catheterisation and measurement of urine output.

➤ CPAP may be required if there is a failure of other measures to support respiration.

➤ May require intensive care review for consideration of intubation, ventilation, inotropes and intra-aortic balloon pumping.

Prognosis:

➤ Prognosis of cardiogenic pulmonary oedema is generally poor.

➤ Killip classification can be used in those whose oedema is caused by acute MI as outlined in Table 3.24:

3. Medicine

Type of cause	Features
Vessel wall damage	<ul><li>Trauma</li><li>Surgery</li><li>Previous thrombosis</li><li>Central venous cannulation</li><li>Intravenous drug use</li></ul>
Venous stasis	Venous stasis and reduced blood flow increases the chance for emboli to form. Venous stasis is linked to:<ul><li>Increasing age</li><li>Immobility: caused by general anaesthesia, paralysis, previous stroke, spinal cord injury.</li><li>MI</li><li>Varicose veins</li><li>COPD</li></ul>
Hypercoagulability	Inherited conditions:<ul><li>Factor V Leiden mutation</li><li>Prothrombin gene mutation</li><li>Protein C and S deficiency</li><li>Antithrombin III deficiency</li><li>Antiphospholipid antibody syndrome</li></ul>Acquired conditions:<ul><li>Cancer</li><li>Inflammatory bowel disease</li><li>Nephrotic syndrome</li></ul>Other:<ul><li>Sepsis</li><li>Blood transfusion</li><li>High-oestrogen states (obesity, late pregnancy and hormone replacement)</li></ul>

Table 3.25: Virchow's triad in PE.

multiple small emboli cause a gradual occlusion of the pulmonary vascular tree over a period of a few months or years resulting in pulmonary hypertension.

Key features in history/examination

The presenting symptoms and signs may be very non-specific, so a high degree of clinical suspicion is required. Some of the following symptoms may be elicited in the history.

- Dyspnoea is the commonest symptom.
- Pleuritic chest pain as a result of pulmonary infarction which involves the pleural surface.
- Cough.
- Haemoptysis.
- Presence of risk factors.

The following features are common on examination:

- Tachypnoea.
- Tachycardia.
- Fever: low grade fever present in about 50% of patients.
- Crackles or a pleural rub.
- Symptoms of cor pulmonale in chronic PE i.e. elevated JVP, parasternal heave, loud pulmonary S2.
- Unilateral limb swelling may be present: only one in five patients will have evidence of a DVT on examination.

Massive PE:

As well as the findings similar to PE patients will present with:

- Signs of shock i.e. hypotension, cyanosis and reduced level of consciousness.
- Engorged neck veins.
- Syncope may result from reduced cardiac output associated with right heart obstruction.

Investigations

Complete the Wells score to determine clinical probability of PE:

Factor	Score
Clinically suspected DVT	3.0
Alternative diagnosis less likely than PE	3.0
Tachycardia	1.5
Immobilisation/surgery in last 4 weeks	1.5
History of DVT/PE	1.5
Haemoptysis	1.0
Malignancy	1.0

Table 3.26: The Wells score.

Interpretation of Wells score:

Probability	Score
High probability	≥ 7.0
Intermediate probability	2.0–6.0
Low Probability	0–1

Table 3.27: Interpretation of the Wells score.

Blood tests:

Most Trusts have policies to govern investigations and you should be familiar with these. The tests commonly used are:

- FBC: to exclude infection.
- U&Es: to get a baseline levels.
- Coagulation screen.
- D-dimer: most useful if Wells score suggests a low probability of PE.
  - A negative D-Dimer excludes PE in low probability patients.

o A negative D-Dimer does not exclude a PE in intermediate and high probability patients and hence D-Dimer is not indicated in these patients – imaging should be requested as the first-line investigation.

o False positive D-dimers are seen in a number of conditions including sepsis, DIC, post-operative state, malignancy and pregnancy.

- ABG: when there is an acute and massive PE.

- Thrombophilia screen: to be considered especially if the patient is young with no obvious risk factors. If necessary it should be done before anticoagulation is commenced.

Imaging:

- Chest X-ray: the classical finding is a wedge-shaped shadow representing an area of infarct. In acute massive PE there may be an area of pulmonary oligaemia as a result of pulmonary artery obstruction.

- VQ scan: only appropriate with a normal chest X-ray and no other concurrent cardio-respiratory disease.

- CT pulmonary angiogram (CTPA).

Others:

- ECG: wide range of changes may be present. Classically S1 Q3 T3 is seen whereby a deep S waves in lead 1, with Q waves and inverted T waves in lead 3 appears. Features of right heart strain are found in those with chronic disease.

- Pregnancy test: if female of child-bearing age.

- Echocardiography: may be a useful bedside test to rapidly confirm the diagnosis of massive PE.

Management

PE:

➤ Oxygen if saturations less than 92%.

➤ Analgesia

➤ Anticoagulation: usually low-molecular-weight heparin (LMWH). However different Trusts may use different types of LMWH. This should be commenced whilst awaiting definitive imaging.

➤ Ongoing anticoagulation with warfarin with concurrent LMWH until the INR is therapeutic and referral to anticoagulation clinic.

➤ Inferior vena cava filter occasionally indicated for failed anticoagulation.

Massive PE:

➤ An A to E assessment

➤ Oxygen

➤ Haemodynamic support with fluid resuscitation and inotropes.

➤ Thrombolysis

➤ Surgical embolectomy.

➤ Anticoagulation post intervention with LMWH. Ongoing anticoagulation with warfarin (with concurrent LMWH until the INR is therapeutic) and referral to anticoagulation clinic.

Prognosis:

➤ Second commonest cause of unexpected death in all age groups.

➤ Untreated mortality rate 30%.

➤ May contribute to 15–20% of acute hospital deaths.

➤ Massive PE has a mortality rate of between 16–57% with best results seen in specialist centres.

Asthma

Epidemiology

10–15% of all individuals will be affected by symptoms of asthma at some point in their lives with 4–7% of people worldwide having asthma. There are over 2000 deaths per year as a result of asthma.

The peak hospital attendances in the UK are between September and October and currently 5.4 million people are receiving treatment for asthma in the UK.

Aetiology

A chronic condition where there is inflammation of the lung airways resulting in partial obstruction. There are three main features:

1. Reversible limitation of airflow in the airways.

2. Hyper-responsiveness of the airways to variable stimuli within the environment.

3. Inflammatory changes within the bronchi.

The changes associated with asthma are caused by a complex interaction of atopy and genetic factors.

Atopy:

Asthmatics readily form IgE antibodies to normal environmental antigens and tend to have an exaggerated response to these. These antibodies bind to mast cells within the lumen and mucosa of the bronchi which degranulate and release histamine. This results in an inflammatory reaction within the bronchi increasing their responsiveness. The normal environmental antigens comprise of:

- Allergens: house dust mite, pollen, cat hair and spores from fungi such as *aspergillus*.

- Occupational allergens and drugs: non-steroidal anti-inflammatory drugs and Aspirin.

- Viral infections: *rhinovirus, influenza* virus, *respiratory syncytial* virus.

- Bacterial infections: *Mycoplasma pneumonia, Chlamydia pneumonia.*

- Other non-specific bronchial stimuli: cold air, exercise, stress and pollution.

Genetic factors:

Many genes are implemented in asthma, including:

- ADAM 33
- Dipentidyl peptidase 10
- PHD finger protein 11
- Prostanoid DP1 receptor
- Chromosome 12q
- Polymorphisms in tumour necrosis factor (TNF)

It is thought that asthma may be caused by abnormalities in calcium ion exchange across the cell membranes resulting in increased smooth muscle contraction and mast cell degranulation.

Risk factors for developing asthma include:

- Family history
- Obesity
- Parental smoking
- Atopic history of eczema or rhinitis
- Nasal polyps
- Prematurity or low birth rate
- Socioeconomic deprivation
- Smoking
- Early exposure to broad spectrum antibiotics
- Viral infections in early childhood

Pathophysiology

The main abnormality is airway narrowing as a result of:

- Smooth muscle contraction.
- Thickening of the airway wall due to inflammatory changes.
- Increased secretions within the bronchial lumen.

The inflammatory changes involve eosinophils, macrophages, mast cell and T-lymphocytes. These cells move to the airways causing changes to the airway epithelium and the airway tone which is under autonomic neural control. Increased mucus secretion, ciliary dysfunction and an increased smooth muscle response are also caused by the inflammatory cells.

Macrophages are thought to have a role in the uptake and presentation of environmental allergens to the T-lymphocytes. They release cytokines which have a role in the activation of mast cells and eosinophils. There is also production of IgE molecules which attach to the mast cells causing release of histamine, which acts on the smooth muscle and small blood vessels.

Over time there is remodelling of the airways. The smooth muscle of the airway undergoes changes such as hypertrophy and hyperplasia causing a larger proportion of the airway diameter to be composed of smooth muscle. Damage to the airway epithelium with destruction of the cilia on the surface of columnar cells within the lumen also occurs. The metaplasia of the epithelium results in an increase in the proportion of mucous-secreting goblet cells.

A small group of individuals have severe asthma. This is potentially life-threatening as it may occur either acutely as a sudden deterioration of chronic stable asthma or at the end-stage of chronic but progressively deteriorating asthma. A small number of patients have brittle asthma where they quickly develop acute and life-threatening asthma attacks despite being normally well controlled with treatment.

Key features in history/examination

Main features in the history are:

- Dyspnoea
- Expiratory wheeze
- Chest tightness
- Cough
- Presence of risk factors
- Past medical history and family history
- Recent history of upper respiratory infection
- More frequent/worse symptoms during the night and early morning
- Exercise induced asthma

During an acute asthma attack, on examination, there will be:

- Reduced chest expansion
- Prolonged expiratory phase
- Polyphonic expiratory wheeze
- Associated crepitations if there is an infective precipitant

Identification of acute severe asthma or life-threatening asthma as illustrated in Table 3.28:

Acute severe asthma	Life-threatening
<ul><li>Peak expiratory flow rate (PEFR): 33–50% of best or predicted</li><li>Respiratory rate > 25</li><li>Pulse rate > 110</li><li>Inability to complete full sentences in a single breath</li></ul>	<ul><li>PEFR < 33% of best or predicted</li><li>Oxygen saturations < 92%</li><li>$PaO_2 < 8$ kPa</li><li>$PaCO_2$ normal or raised</li><li>Exhaustion</li><li>Altered consciousness level</li><li>Poor respiratory effort</li><li>Silent chest</li><li>Cyanosis</li><li>Arrhythmia: bradycardia is a late sign</li></ul>

Table 3.28: Cardinal features of acute and life threatening asthma.

Investigations

Mostly a clinical diagnosis based on history and reversibility of symptoms in response to bronchodilator therapy.

Blood tests:

- FBC: may show eosinphilia.
- Serology: may show IgE to the antigen.

Imaging:

- Chest X-ray may reveal a hyperinflated chest.

Others:

- Lung function tests.
- Spirometry: FEV_1 less than 80% of predicted.
- Peak expiratory flow meter: measured early morning, once during the day, and then before sleeping. This gives an indication as to the range of airflow limitation of the patient. Asthmatics usually show a diurnal variation in their peak flow with a typical 'morning dip'.
- There will be an improvement in the patient's FEV_1 or peak expiratory flow rate of more than 15% after treatment with a bronchodilator.
- Skin prick testing: will identify allergens to which the patient is most sensitive.

Management

General measures include:

➤ Patient education.

➤ Written personalised asthma plan.

➤ Avoid precipitants:

○ Patients should be actively discouraged from smoking.

○ Reduction in house dust mite allergens, which can be achieved by regular cleaning of the household and using bedding covers.

○ Avoid any occupational allergens where relevant.

○ Avoid contact with household pets if they seem to precipitate symptoms.

➤ Use of the British Thoracic Society guidelines for the stepwise management of chronic asthma. (See Figure 3.11).

Prognosis:

➤ The mortality rate is significant in acute severe asthma.

➤ There is a good prognosis in those with asthma who are treated adequately.

➤ Occasionally, where there is onset of asthma in the middle ages, there is a slow progressive deterioration of symptoms despite optimal treatment.

Chronic obstructive pulmonary disease

Chronic obstructive pulmonary disease (COPD) is characterised by progressive airways obstruction which is poorly reversible. It does not change markedly over several months

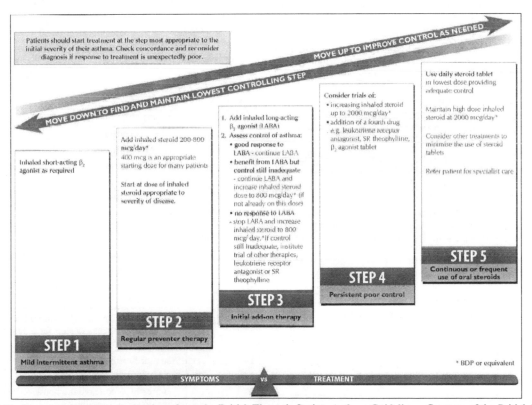

Figure 3.11: Stepwise management of asthma from the British Thoracic Society Asthma Guidelines. *Courtesy of the British Thoracic Society. Reproduced with permission*

Epidemiology

One million people in the UK have COPD with an additional undiagnosed burden of disease. Around 18% of males and 14% of females who are smokers are affected and around 5–10% of people over the age of 50 years are affected. Symptoms develop over a prolonged period of many years and will rarely present with symptoms before the age of 50 years. It is the fifth most common cause of death in the UK.

Aetiology

The main causes include cigarette smoking, pollution in the atmosphere and infection of the respiratory tract.

Smoking (and passive smoking): is the primary causative agent. Smoking activates the macrophages and epithelial cells in the respiratory tract. There is a release of neutrophils resulting in the release of proteases which break down the connective tissue within the lungs. The result being destruction of the alveolar wall and mucus hyper-secretion.

Pollution: plays a small role in the development of COPD compared to smoking.

Alpha-1 antitrypsin deficiency: is a rare cause (<1% cases) and should be considered in patients with an early onset of symptoms. The enzyme is a protease inhibitor (encoded on chromosome 14) and a lack of it permits unopposed protease activity and

therefore chronic lung damage occurs. It mainly affects lower lung lobes.

Pathophysiology

Chronic inflammation affecting the central and peripheral airways, lung parenchyma and pulmonary vasculature. The main changes are:

- Narrowing and remodelling of airways.
- Enlargement of mucus-secreting glands and increased goblet cells in the central airways.
- Subsequent vascular bed changes.

These changes cause increased airway resistance which results in expiratory flow limitation which leads to hyperinflation. Hyperinflation and destruction of lung parenchyma causes hypoxia which worsens on exertion. Progressive hypoxia causes vascular smooth muscle thickening which leads to pulmonary hypertension. Pulmonary hypertension has a poor prognosis. Classically there is a clinical distinction in place between those with mostly emphysematous symptoms, known as 'pink puffers,' and those with mostly bronchitis are known as 'blue bloaters'.

Key features in history/examination

- Presence of risk factors in particular smoking history. Try to calculate the number of pack-years smoked (1 pack-year is defined as the equivalent of smoking 20 cigarettes per day for 1 year).
- Cough: initially morning cough which then becomes constant as disease progresses. It is usually productive.
- Shortness of breath: initially on exertion which then becomes more constant as disease progresses. They may be unable to speak in sentences.
- Wheeze.
- Headache: due to vasodilation caused by hypercapnia.
- Fatigue: due to sleep disturbance.
- Home oxygen and/or nebulisers.
- History of exacerbations: frequency, severity and ICU admissions.

Assess disability using Medical Research Council (MRC) dyspnoea scale as shown below in Table 3.30:

Pathology	Features
Chronic bronchitis	• Narrowing of the airways and limitation of airflow due to hypertrophy and hyperplasia of the mucus-producing glands within the bronchial tree and hence an increased mucus production. The excess mucus is expelled by coughing. • Inflammation of the bronchial wall as well as mucosal oedema causing cillia dysfunction. • There may be ulceration of the epithelial cell layer and as these heal, squamous epithelium will replace columnar epithelium. • Diagnosed clinically where there is a cough productive of sputum on most days for at least 3 months within a year for at least 2 years in a row.
Emphysema	• A loss of elastic recoil which usually enables the airways to stay open during expiration. • Airflow limitation with expiration. • Air trapping within the alveoli. • A pathological diagnosis and involves dilatation and destruction of the lung tissue which lies distal to the terminal bronchioles.

Table 3.29: Pathological features of chronic bronchitis and emphysema.

MRC Grade	Description
I	Not troubled by breathlessness except on strenuous exercise
II	Short of breath when hurrying or walking up slight incline
III	Walks slower than contemporaries because of breathlessness or has to stop for breath when walking at own pace.
IV	Stops for breath after walking 100 m or for a few minutes on level ground
V	Too breathless to leave the house or breathless when dressing or undressing

Table 3.30: The Medical Research Council (MRC) dyspnoea scale.

On examination, the following features should be sought:

- Barrel chest secondary to hyperinflation and air trapping
- Pursed lip breathing to increase own positive end pressure ventilation to counteract air trapping
- Hyper-resonance to percussion
- Poor air movement with distant breath sounds
- Wheeze audible particularly during exacerbations
- Hypoxia
- Confusion caused by hypoxia
- Tachypnoea with use of accessory muscles
- Asterixis
- Cyanosis
- If cor pulmonale present, there may be:
  - o Distended neck veins
  - o Lower-extremity swelling
  - o Loud P2
  - o Hepatosplenomegaly

Assess disease severity using the National Institute for Health and Clinical Excellence (NICE) guidelines. It defines the severity of airflow obstruction as:

Severity	FEV$_1$/FEC ratio
Mild	50–80%
Moderate	30–49%
Severe	< 30%

Table 3.31: Assessment of disease severity according to NICE guidelines.

Investigations

Blood tests:

- FBC: may reveal a raised haematocrit. Differential white cells in cases of infective exacerbation could be done although it may be of little use.
- ABG: may be normal but it may show PaCO$_2$ > 50 mmHg +/– PaO$_2$ < 60 mmHg.
- Alpha-1 antitrypsin level: indicated if the patient is young or there is a family history.
- Blood cultures: if infective exacerbation is suspected.

Microbiology:

Sputum cultures: if infective exacerbation suspected. Purulent sputum should be treated empirically.

Imaging:

Chest X-ray: may show hyperinflation, flattened hemidiaphragms, increased intercostal spacing and complications of COPD. (See Figure 3.12).

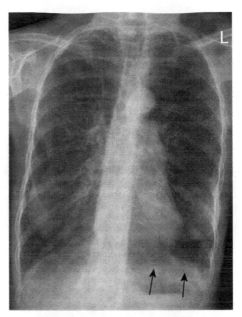

Figure 3.12: Chest X-ray showing hyperinflated lungs with flattening of the diaphragm (arrows) with long narrow cardiac silhouette.

- CT: of the chest may show location and type of tissue damage.

Others:

- ECG: co-morbidity of ischaemic heart disease.
- Pulse oximetry.
- Spirometry: may show airflow obstruction:
  - o FEV$_1$ < 80% of normal.
  - o FEV$_1$/FEC ratio < 70%.
  - o Evidence of reversibility with a bronchodilator is not required for a diagnosis of COPD.
- Exercise testing.
- Respiratory muscle function: patients with poor nutrition and steroid-induced muscle wasting.

Management

General measures

- ➤ Patient education and empowerment with written information.
- ➤ Advice about exercise.
- ➤ Influenza vaccination yearly.
- ➤ Pneumococcal vaccination 5 yearly.
- ➤ Smoking cessation.
- ➤ Assessment of osteoporosis risk.
- ➤ Assessment of inhaler technique.
- ➤ A stepwise approach is taken to improve breathlessness:

3. Medicine

o Short-acting bronchodilator PRN (beta2 agonist or anticholinergic).

o Combined therapy with short-acting beta2 agonist and short-acting anticholinergic.

o Add inhaled corticosteroids.

o Consider Theophylline.

Advanced therapies

Long term oxygen therapy:

➢ Has been shown to reduce mortality when used for at least 19 hours daily at a flow rate of 1–3 L per minute via nasal cannulae in order to maintain oxygen saturation levels above 90%.

➢ Should be used for more than 15 hours per day.

➢ Criteria for ambulatory oxygen:

o $PaO_2 \leq 7.3$ kPa or $SaO_2 \leq 88\%$ with or without hypercapnia.

o PaO_2 between 7.3 kPa and 8.0 kPa or SaO_2 of 88% if pulmonary hypertension, congestive cardiac failure or polycythaemia (haematocrit > 55%).

Surgical interventions:

➢ Most common are bullectomy or lung volume reduction therapy.

➢ Lung transplantation can improve functional capacity and quality of life but does not appear to increase survival.

➢ Criteria for consideration:

o FEV_1 25% predicted or less (without reversibility).

o +/– $PaCO_2$ > 7.3 Kpa.

o +/– elevated $PaCO_2$ with progressive deterioration requiring long term oxygen therapy.

o Or elevated pulmonary artery pressure with progressive deterioration.

Other therapies:

➢ Mucolytic: if ongoing productive cough.

➢ Pulmonary rehabilitation: MRC 3 or greater.

➢ Physiotherapy: teach active cycle of breathing techniques.

➢ Dietician: if low or reducing BMI.

➢ Occupational therapy: if COPD limits performance of ADLs.

➢ Assessment of depression and anxiety may require a psychiatric referral.

➢ Palliative care if required.

Prognosis:

➢ COPD has an indeterminate course and variable prognosis.

➢ Poor prognosis is indicated by frequent exacerbations or FEV_1 < 50% predicted (mortality of 5–10% per year).

➢ There is a 50% mortality in patients with severe breathlessness and a PaO_2 of less than 8 kPa or a $PaCO_2$ of more than 7 kPa as a result of severely impaired gas exchange.

Further reading and references

➢ Anderson D.R., Ginsberg J.S., Kearon C., et al. (2000). Derivation of a simple clinical model to categorize patients probability of pulmonary embolism: increasing the models utility with the SimpliRED d-dimer. *Thromb Haemost* 83: 416–20.

➢ Arnold T., Harvey J., Henry M. on behalf of the BTS Pleural Disease Group, a subgroup of the BTS Standards of Care Committee (2003). BTS guidelines for the management of spontaneous pneumothorax. *Thorax* 58 (Supplement 2): ii39–ii52.

➢ British Thoracic Society Standards of Care Committee Pulmonary Embolism Guideline Development Group (2003). British Thoracic Society guidelines for the management of suspected acute pulmonary embolism. *Thorax* 58: 470–483.

➢ British Thoracic Society and the Scottish Intercollegiate Guidelines Network (2008). *British Guideline on the Management of asthma.*

➢ National Institute for Health and Clinical Excellence (2004). *Chronic Obstructive Pulmonary Disease (CG12).*

CHEST PAIN

Differential diagnosis

System	Disease
Cardiovascular	**Acute coronary syndrome (ACS)**
	Aortic stenosis (AS)
	Aortic dissection
	Pulmonary embolus (PE)
	Pericarditis
	Hypertrophic cardiomyopathy (HCM)
	Myocarditis
	Takotsubo cardiomyopathy
Respiratory	Pneumonia
	Pneumothorax
Gut	Gastro-oesophageal reflux disease (GORD)
	Oesophagitis
	Peptic ulcer disease
Musculoskeletal	**Musculoskeletal chest pain**

Acute coronary syndrome (ACS)

ACS is a clinical syndrome characterised by symptoms and signs suggestive of potential or actual myocardial infarction (MI). It consists of three possible underlying diagnoses:

1. *ST Elevation Myocardial Infarction (STEMI):* ST elevation on electrocardiogram (ECG) accompanied by Troponin rise

2. **Non-ST Elevation Myocardial Infarction (NSTEMI):** No ST elevation seen on ECG but 12-hour Troponin rise detected

3. **Unstable angina (UA):** No ST elevation and normal 12-hour Troponin

Epidemiology

MI in the UK: 275,000 per year (DH NSF for Coronary Heart Disease).

Aetiology

- Smoking
- Hypertension
- Hypercholesterolaemia
- Diabetes
- Increasing age
- Male sex
- Family history
- Ethnicity
- Obesity

Pathophysiology

The majority of ACS is caused by coronary artery atherosclerosis. This is a dynamic process, but the following stages are identified:

1. Fatty streak formation: macrophages and oxidised cholesterol (foam cells) form a thin layer underneath the endothelium.

2. Endothelial damage stimulates platelet deposition and macrophage activation leading to localised release of inflammatory mediators.

3. Inflammatory mediators stimulate smooth muscle and fibroblast proliferation leading to the formation of an atherosclerotic plaque (lipid core with fibrous cap).

Stable angina (not an ACS) results from a fixed reduction in coronary blood flow due to arterial narrowing causing ischaemia and predictable chest pain on exertion.

The lipid core of atherosclerotic plaque is highly thrombogenic and as the atherosclerotic plaque increases in size, it is prone to rupture. Plaque rupture causes thrombus formation which may embolise and block the affected coronary artery distally. This results in an acute reduction or total loss of blood flow to the affected myocardium which initially becomes ischaemic and eventually may become infarcted resulting in an ACS.

Key features in the history/examination

- Chest pain: Central, severe tight or squeezing pain across chest. May be confused for "indigestion" pain. May radiate to neck, jaw, shoulders or arms. Onset typically occurs over a period of minutes to maximum severity and may last for minutes to hours.

- Other associated symptoms: Dyspnoea, nausea, vomiting, sweating, palpitations (related to increased sympathetic drive)

- Beware atypical presentations:
  - Silent MI: no chest pain experienced during MI. May occur in diabetic patients due to sensory neuropathy.
  - Epigastric pain: the patient admitted on the surgical take with an "acute abdomen" secondary to an inferior MI. Always do an ECG!

- General observation: Patient in distress, possibly a tachycardia (or bradycardia from heart block e.g. following inferior MI), tachypnoea, blood pressure (BP) may be normal, raised or low, sweating and pallor.

- Levine's sign: patient clenches fist over chest indicating area of pain.

- Systemic examination: often little to find but may include signs of heart failure (raised JVP, S3, basal lung crepitations, peripheral oedema), heart murmur due to existing valvular heart disease or papillary muscle infarction/rupture or a pericardial friction rub.

Investigations

Blood tests:

- Full blood count (FBC): anaemia may precipitate MI due to reduced oxygen carrying capacity.

- White cell count (WCC): may be raised due to inflammatory response secondary to MI or demargination due to an acute stress response.

- Platelets: monitor for thrombocytopenia following low molecular weight heparin use.

- Renal function: impaired renal function increases the risk of intravenous (IV) contrast induced nephropathy following coronary angiography.

- Lipid profile: deranged in hypercholesterolaemia and hypertriglyceridaemia

- Glucose: if raised, consider insulin sliding scale. Subsequent fasting blood glucose to check for diabetes (if no prior diagnosis).

- Cardiac enzymes: creatine kinase (CK), creatine kinase muscle/brain type (CK-MB), aspartate aminotransferase (AST), lactate dehydrogenase (LDH) and troponin T or I.

Cardiac troponin assays are sensitive and specific for myocardial damage. In the presence of a suggestive history and/or ECG changes, a raised troponin is indicative of irreversible myocardial damage following MI. The peak of the troponin rise occurs 12–24 hours following MI so the level must be tested at least 12 hours following initial onset of symptoms. Note that troponin levels may be raised in other conditions including heart failure, chronic renal failure, pulmonary embolus, pericarditis and cardiomyopathy. A negative 12-hour troponin rules out the possibility of MI in ACS.

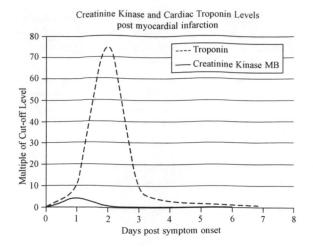

Figure 3.13: Graph of plasma levels of troponin and CK-MB following MI.

Area of infarct	Vessel occluded
Anterior MI ($V_2 - V_4$)	Left anterior descending (LAD) artery
Inferior MI (II/III/aVF)	Right coronary artery (RCA)
Septal (V_1/V_2)	Left anterior descending (LAD) artery
Lateral MI(I/aVL/V_5/V_6)	Circumflex (Cx) artery

Table 3.32: ECG changes that indicate the area of infarction.

Imaging:

- Chest X-ray (CXR): signs of heart failure, consolidation and mediastinal widening.

Management

Initial management:

➢ ABCDE and resuscitate if necessary

➢ Cardiac monitor

➢ High flow oxygen and establish IV access

➢ Aspirin 300 mg per oral (PO)

➢ Clopidogrel 300–600 mg PO

➢ Low molecular weight heparin (e.g. Enoxaparin 1 mg/Kg)

➢ Sublingual glyceryl trinitrate (GTN)

➢ Morphine 2.5–5 mg IV (and anti-emetic)

➢ Beta-blocker (e.g. Metoprolol 5 mg IV) unless contraindicated due to asthma/chronic obstructive pulmonary disease (COPD), bradycardia or hypotension.

➢ For STEMI urgent primary percutaneous coronary intervention (PCI). This may require transfer to a tertiary centre. If unavailable, consider thrombolysis.

ECG:

- STEMI: ST segment elevation in at least two consecutive leads of at least 1 mm in the limb leads or 2 mm in the chest leads. Reciprocal ST segment depression may be present and a posterior MI will have ST depression in the septal leads and a dominant R wave in V1. New left bundle branch block (LBBB) with a history of ischaemic chest pain should be treated as STEMI.

- NSTEMI/UA: T wave flattening or inversion, ST depression. May also be normal.

The area of the heart infarcted is indicated by the pattern of ECG changes in the different leads:

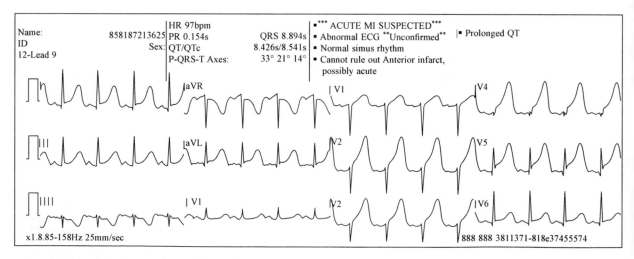

Figure 3.14: Anterior-lateral MI with ST elevation.

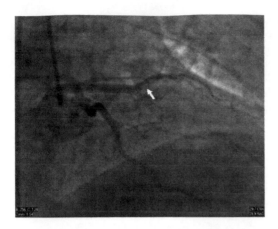

Figure 3.15: Angiogram of the occluded LAD (white arrow).

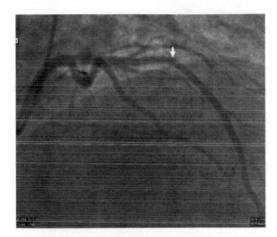

Figure 3.16: Angiogram of the LAD post stent deployment (white arrow) shows patent artery.

➢ As it takes 12 hours from the onset of symptoms to determine whether a patient without ST elevation has sustained MI (by measuring cardiac troponin levels), all patients who present with symptoms consistent with ACS are initially treated on the assumption that they have had an MI until the 12-hour troponin measurement proves otherwise.

Ongoing management for UA/NSTEMI:

➢ Angiotensin converting enzyme (ACE) inhibitor or Angiotensin receptor blocker (e.g. Ramipril 1.25 mg OD titrated up as tolerated).

➢ Statin (e.g. Simvastatin 40 mg OD)

➢ Consider converting to long acting beta blocker (e.g. Bisoprolol 1.25 mg OD titrated up as tolerated) or calcium channel blocker if this is contraindicated (e.g. Verapamil or Diltiazem).

Risk stratification:

Risk stratification will be governed by advice from the cardiology team, but may include:

➢ Echocardiography: regional wall motion abnormality, left ventricular (LV) function, valvular disease.

➢ Exercise tolerance test/stress echocardiography/myocardial perfusion scan/CMR perfusion scan.

➢ Angiography and PCI.

➢ Coronary artery bypass grafting (CABG) may be indicated.

➢ Clopidogrel should be continued for at least 12 months (CURE Trial, Yusuf et al. 2001).

➢ Cardiac rehabilitation.

➢ Ongoing aggressive risk factor reduction: smoking cessation, dietary modification, exercise, weight reduction, good glycaemic and BP control, cholesterol reduction and patient education.

Prognosis:

➢ Depends on TIMI risk score:

Risk factor (1 point for each of the following)		
Age > 65		
More than three of the following risk factors: family history, smoking, hypertension, diabetes, hyperlipidaemia		
Elevated cardiac markers: CK-MB or troponin		
Known coronary artery disease: coronary angiography > 50%		
Aspirin use in the last 7 days		
Severe angina: more than two episodes of chest pain in 24 hours		
ST deviation on ECG: horizontal ST depression or transient ST elevation > 1 mm		
Total Score	**Rate of death or MI in 14 days (%)**	**Rate of death or MI or urgent revascularisation (%)**
0–1	3	4.75
2	3	8.3
3	5	13.2
4	7	19.9
5	12	26.2
6–7	19	40.9

Table 3.33: Table of TIMI risk score and 14 day event rate for UA and NSTEMI. (Antman E et al., JAMA 2000)

Aortic stenosis

Aortic stenosis (AS) is defined as being 'an obstruction to the outflow of blood from the LV at the level of the aortic valve'.

Epidemiology

It is the most common single valve lesion, with a higher frequency in Caucasian males. However, in the developed world, 2–3% of the general population aged 70 years or more will have a degree of AS. Given the ageing population, the prevalence of AS is increasing.

Aetiology

There are three main causes of valvular AS.

Degenerative:

This is the most common cause of AS in the developed world. With increasing age there are arteriosclerotic changes involving the valve leading to calcification and degeneration of the valve with subsequent loss of function. It is common above the age of 70 though most will not have severe stenosis.

Congenital bicuspid aortic valve:

Stenosis gradually results from a turbulent blood flow through the congenitally deformed aortic valve. The bicuspid valve eventually becomes calcified. This form of AS usually occurs in males and the mean age of symptom onset is 40 to 50 years.

Rheumatic fever:

This is the most common cause of AS worldwide. It involves a gradual thickening and calcification resulting in the fusion of an apparently healthy three-cusped aortic valve. The mitral valve is involved most frequently, followed by the aortic valve. Additionally, co-existent aortic incompetence is common.

Miscellaneous:

There are other causes of LV obstruction which prevent adequate emptying, and can mimic the symptoms and signs of AS:

- Hypertrophic obstructive cardiomyopathy (HCM) is when there is hypertrophy of the muscle of the ventricular septum, causing obstruction of the outflow of the LV.
- Supravalvular obstruction occurs in Williams syndrome, where there is a congenital fibrous tissue mass located above the aortic valve causing obstruction. The syndrome also includes features such as mental retardation and hypercalcaemia.
- Subvalvular AS is a congenital condition which manifests as:
  o Congenital obstruction of the LV outflow tract affecting approximately 3–10% of individuals with congenital heart disease.
  o A discrete subaortic membrane which accounts for 8–10% of all cases of LV outflow tract obstruction in children.
- The subaortic membrane presents as a membranous or fibromuscular ring below the aortic valve, either in isolation or in association with other congenital anomalies such as a ventricular septal defect, patent ductus arteriosus, coarctation of the aorta, bicuspid aortic valve, abnormal LV papillary muscle, atrioventricular septal defect, and persistent superior left vena cava. The jet from the narrowed subaortic tract can damage the aortic cusps and cause regurgitation.

Pathophysiology

When there is an obstruction to emptying from the LV, this causes an increase in pressure within the LV and hence there is LV hypertrophy as a result of the persistently elevated pressure. This results in an increase in the diastolic pressure, which causes a decrease in the trans-coronary pressure gradient. This leads to an increase in the left atrial pressure as well as the pulmonary venous pressure. LV myocardial ischaemia and hence symptoms of angina follows.

Symptoms are worsened upon exercising as the LV obstruction becomes more severe. In normal circumstances, upon exercise, the cardiac output is very much increased; however, where there is this narrowing of the aortic valve (fixed outflow obstruction), the increase in cardiac output is restricted. Hence, there is a fall in the systemic BP, with worsening of ischaemia in the coronary arteries. Thus, heart failure ensues and there is an increased tendency to develop ventricular arrhythmias.

Key features in the history/examination

- Usually asymptomatic until the degree of stenosis is significant, for example, when the aortic cavity is reduced down to one third of its normal size.
- The three main symptoms include:
  o Exercise-induced syncope and dizziness
  o Symptoms of dyspnoea
  o Angina
- History of gastrointestinal (GI) bleeding or iron deficiency anaemia:
  o Gastrointestinal angiodysplasia is thought to arise from chronically raised pressures within the submucosal mesenteric venous system due to AS
  o Heyde's syndrome:
    ■ The high shear stress across the stenotic valve leads to increased consumption of multimeric von Willebrand factor and may increase platelet clearance, therefore increasing susceptibility to GI bleeding
- Low volume and slow-rising carotid pulse (*pulsus parvus et tardus*).
- Ejection systolic thrill felt maximally at the right sternal edge in the aortic region.
- A heaving apex beat results from LV hypertrophy. The apex tends not to be displaced as hypertrophy will not cause cardiomegaly.
- A harsh or rasping, low pitched ejection systolic murmur is audible at the left sternal edge and aortic region with radiation into the carotid arteries.
  o The intensity of the murmur is actually reduced as the cardiac output decreases.
  o In very severe AS, the murmur may be inaudible.
- Where there is congenital disease, an ejection click may be heard as a result of the presence of a bicuspid valve.
- Once the valve leaflets become calcified and hence immobile, this will cause a softening of the second heart sound.
- There may also be splitting of second heart sound on expiration as well as a prominent fourth heart sound.

Investigations

Imaging:

- CXR:
  - Typically will reveal a small heart with a prominent enlarged ascending aorta as well as the LV border of the heart.
  - The enlargement (post-stenotic dilatation) results from turbulent blood flow above the region of aortic valve stenosis.
  - Calcified regions of the aortic valve may also be present.
  - Signs of heart failure should also be sought including any cardiac enlargement.

ECG:

- There are signs of LV hypertrophy and left axis deviation as a result of the increase in ventricular pressure.
- Changes such as ST depression and T wave inversion in leads I, AVL, V5 and V6 are indicative of LV strain especially in severe disease.
- Atrioventricular conduction disease is relatively common in degenerative AS due to the proximity of the AV node to the aortic valve, wherein the same disease process can affect both the aortic valve and AV node.
- Left bundle branch block may also occur due to the same mechanism.
- Any ventricular arrhythmias may be revealed.

Echocardiogram:

- Demonstrates the thickened, calcified and immobile cups of the aortic valve.
- Degree of LV hypertrophy.
- Estimation of the gradient across the valve may also be made using Doppler.
- With a normal ventricular function, a gradient of up to 30 mmHg indicates a mild degree of AS, a gradient of 30–70 mmHg is moderate and with a gradient above 70 mmHg the stenosis is severe.
- However, where there is impairment of the LV function with a poor cardiac output, the gradient values are less for each of these degrees of stenosis.
- A dobutamine stress echocardiogram may be required to differentiate between a pseudoaortic stenosis due to a low cardiac output state and true AS.

Cardiac catheterisation:

- This aids confirmation of the diagnosis and also allows an assessment of the integrity of the coronary circulation (which will be required prior to aortic valve intervention).
- Also the pressure gradient between the aorta and the LV can be recorded.
- When it is above 50 mmHg, this is usually indicative of the need for surgical intervention.

Management

- Patients should be advised to avoid strenuous activity such as intense sporting activities.
- Beta blockers are indicated for the treatment of symptoms of angina.
- Nitrates, such as GTN spray or isosorbide mononitrate, must be avoided as these may precipitate symptoms of exertional syncope.
- ACE inhibitors are contraindicated and use is only indicated when prescribed by a cardiologist.
- The mainstay of treatment is an aortic valve replacement with either a tissue or mechanical prosthetic valve. Cardiopulmonary bypass is required in order to perform a valve replacement.
- In childhood, there is an alternative treatment where a open or closed valvotomy may be performed in order to split the valve cusps. This gives short-term relief from the obstruction, however, an aortic valve replacement is commonly required in adulthood.
- Percutaneous balloon valvuloplasty:
  - Usually a bridging measure for patients who are too unwell for surgery (cardiac or non-cardiac).
  - High AS recurrence rate.
- Percutaneous tissue aortic valve replacement:
  - Relatively new technique, for patients who are deemed to be unsuitable candidates for conventional aortic valve surgery.
  - Prosthetic aortic valve can be delivered via the femoral artery (retrograde) or via a small incision in the left lateral chest wall to access the LV apex and deliver the aortic valve via a transapical incision (antegrade).
- Prevention of bacterial endocarditis:
  - Current evidence fails to show any benefit from prophylactic antibiotics before dental surgery in at-risk patients.
  - General dental hygiene appears to be important in those at risk and general background bacteraemia from activites such as cleaning teeth appears to be a greater risk than dental surgery.
  - In 2006 the Working Party of the British Society for Antimicrobial Chemotherapy recommended that the indication for antibiotic prophylaxis for dental treatment should be restricted to patients who have a history of previous endocarditis, or who have had cardiac valve replacement surgery, or those with a surgically constructed systemic or pulmonary shunt or conduit.

Prognosis:

- Overall, adults with AS have a mortality rate of 9% per year.
- Sudden death occurs in 3 to 5% of patients with AS.
- When symptoms of angina, syncope or heart failure develop, sudden death rises to 15 to 20% per year.
- The approximate interval from the onset of symptoms to death is:

3. Medicine

- o   2 years for heart failure
- o   3 years for syncope
- o   5 years for angina.
- Even in the absence of significant obstruction, aortic sclerosis in the elderly is associated with a 50% increase in the risk of death from MI.
- The prognosis in even mild or moderate stenosis should not be underestimated as the outcome is rather poor.

Aortic dissection

Epidemiology

0.5–3 per 100,000 per year. It most commonly occurs in the sixth and seventh decades.

Aetiology

- Hypertension
- Atherosclerosis
- Bicuspid aortic valve
- Connective tissue disorders including Marfan's syndrome and Ehlers Danlos syndrome
- Turner's syndrome
- Vascular inflammation (giant cell arteritis)
- Deceleration trauma
- Pregnancy (most common in third trimester)
- Iatrogenic (during endovascular interventions or aortic surgery)

Pathophysiology

A tear in the intima results in the generation of a false lumen within the medial layer of the aortic wall, which is separated from the true lumen by a dissection flap. The intraluminal pressure drives blood into the tear, progressively dissecting the wall. This may progress in both retrograde and antegrade directions. The dissection may cause occlusion of the aortic branch arteries, including the coronary arteries and can cause acute aortic valvular incompetence. If the dissection flap breaches the full thickness of the vessel wall then haemothorax or haemopericardium may occur.

There are two common classification systems for aortic dissection; De Bakey and Stanford. The Stanford is simpler and classes Type A as all dissections involving the ascending aorta and Type B as all dissections not involving the ascending aorta.

Key features in the history/examination

- The commonest presenting symptom is of sudden onset severe 'tearing' chest pain, radiating to the back, typically to the inter-scapular area. This may migrate as the dissection progresses.
- Clinical findings depend on the extent of the dissection and any occlusion of branch arteries.
- The classical pulse and BP discrepancy between arms may

be found. If the dissection progresses proximally towards the heart it may affect the coronary arteries leading to MI as well as affecting the aortic valve leading to acute aortic regurgitation and signs and symptoms of cardiac failure.

- Patients may also show paraplegia (spinal artery involvement), stroke (carotid artery), abdominal pain (superior mesenteric artery) and/or acute renal failure (renal arteries).
- If bleeding into the pericardium or thorax has occurred, the patient may present in hypovolaemic shock and signs of cardiac tamponade may be found.

Investigations

Blood tests:

- FBC
- Coagulation screen
- Renal function
- Group and save

Imaging:

- CXR: Widened mediastinum (but may be normal)
- Computer tomography (CT) angiography: this will demonstrate the intimal flap within a dissected aorta and determines whether the dissection is Stanford class A or B. This is currently the gold-standard for diagnosis.
- Magnetic resonance imaging (MRI): excellent imaging of ascending and descending aorta but not widely available.

Others:

- ECG: look for evidence of myocardial ischaemia or infarction.
- Transoesophageal echocardiography (TOE): where available, a useful imaging modality for patients who cannot tolerate IV contrast due to renal impairment. Will also demonstrate aortic regurgitation if the aortic valve is affected. TOE cannot reliably demonstrate dissection which only affects the distal descending aorta.

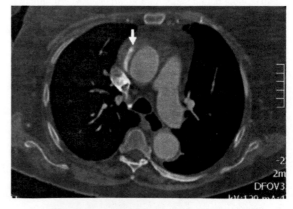

Figure 3.17: CT scan showing an aortic dissection (white arrow).

Management

➢ ABCDE and resuscitate if necessary

➢ Adequate analgesia

➢ Urgent CT angiogram to determine whether Stanford class A or B

➢ If Stanford class A: urgent referral to cardiothoracic centre for consideration of surgical repair. This may be open repair or by endovascular stenting.

➢ If Stanford class B: medical management aimed at controlling BP (aim for systolic BP approximately 100 mmHg). This may require IV nitrates or Labetalol. Surgery may be necessary to restore end-organ perfusion by stenting of occluded branch arteries.

Pericarditis

Epidemiology

1 in 1,000 hospital admissions

Aetiology

- Idiopathic is the most common in the developed world.
- Viral: Coxsackie virus, Echovirus, Epstein-Barr virus (EBV) cytomegalovirus (CMV).
- Bacterial: *Pneumococcus*, *Staphylococcus*, *Streptococcus* and *Neisseria* spp.
- TB.
- Other infections: fungal, toxoplasmosis, Lyme disease.
- Autoimmune: associated with systemic lupus erythematous (SLE) or rheumatoid arthritis.
- Post MI/cardiac surgery.
- Uraemia.
- Neoplastic.

Pathophysiology

Inflammatory response in the pericardium associated with fibrin deposition and occasionally pericardial effusion. Pericardial inflammation irritates the underlying myocardium as well as causing a systemic inflammatory response. Large pericardial effusion can lead to cardiac tamponade.

Key features in the history/examination

- Chest pain, usually pleuritic in nature, which may sometimes be relieved by sitting forward.
- Often associated with dyspnoea and fever.
- Pericardial friction rub.
- In the presence of a pericardial effusion causing tamponade, Beck's triad will be present: hypotension, raised jugular venous pressure (JVP) and muffled heart sounds.
- A high level of clinical suspicion is often required to make the diagnosis.

Investigations

Blood tests:

- FBC.
- Renal function.
- Inflammatory markers: C-reactive protein (CRP).
- Viral serology.
- Antinuclear antibodies (ANA) and rheumatoid factor.

Microbiology:

- Blood cultures

Imaging:

- CXR: enlarged cardiac silhouette may indicate pericardial effusion.
- CT/MRI: may further characterise the nature of a pericardial effusion (e.g. contrast enhancement indicates haemopericardium as opposed to an infective/inflammatory effusion) or the presence of pericardial thickening (e.g. with TB).

Others:

- ECG: saddle-shaped ST segment elevation across several leads (not confined to conventional coronary artery anatomy as for MI) leading to T wave flattening and inversion.
- Echocardiography: readily detects pericardial effusion and provides an indication of whether cardiac haemodynamics are affected.

Management

- ABCDE and resuscitate if necessary.
- Non-steroidal anti-inflammatory drugs (NSAIDs).
- Treat underlying cause where identified.
- Pericardiocentesis may be required to tap or drain a pericardial effusion if tamponade or empyema suspected.
- Recurrent, haemodynamically significant pericardial effusions will require surgical intervention with a pericardial window.

Myocarditis

Epidemiology

The mean age of presentation is approximately 40 years. The actual prevalence of the disease is unknown as many cases are asymptomatic. Myocarditis accounts for 8–12% of sudden cardiac death in young adults.

Aetiology

- Viral: Most common cause in the developed world, e.g. Coxsackie virus, Echovirus, EBV, CMV and human immunodeficiency virus (HIV).
- Bacterial: *Diphtheria, Staphylococcus, Streptococcus.*

- Spirochaete: Borrelia burgdorferi (Lyme disease).
- Protozoa: *Trypanosoma cruzi* (Chagas disease).
- Drugs: Clozapine, Penicillin, Hydrochlorothiazide, Methyldopa, Sulfonamides, Lithium, Doxorubicin, cocaine, Paracetamol, Zidovudine.
- Environmental: Lead, arsenic and carbon monoxide.
- Wasp, scorpion, and spider stings.
- Radiation therapy.
- Autoimmune: SLE, rheumatoid arthritis or dermatomyositis.
- Idiopathic inflammatory and infiltrative disorders: Kawasaki disease, sarcoidosis and giant cell arteritis.

Pathophysiology

Viral myocarditis can produce variable degrees of illness, ranging from focal disease to diffuse pancarditis involving myocardium, pericardium, and valve structures. Viral myocarditis is usually a self-limited, acute-to-subacute disease of the heart muscle that most often leads to the dilated type of cardiomyopathy.

The exact mechanism for myocardial injury in viral cardiomyopathy is controversial. Several mechanisms have been proposed. Viruses affect cardiac myocytes by direct cytotoxic effects and by cell-mediated (T-helper cells) destruction of myofibers. Other mechanisms include disturbances in cellular metabolism, vascular supply of myocytes, and other immunological mechanisms.

Key features in the history/examination

- Symptoms include chest pain which can mimic an ACS, and symptoms similar to those of congestive cardiac failure (CCF). Often these are subclinical.
- Many patients experience a flu-like prodrome (viral myocarditis).
- Confirming the diagnosis can be difficult because symptoms of heart failure can occur several months after the initial infection.
- If there is additional pericardial involvement (myopericarditis) then there may be a pericardial rub and/or any other clinical features of pericarditis (see Pericarditis section).

Investigations

Myocarditis is almost always a clinically presumed diagnosis because it is not associated with any pathognomonic sign or specific acute diagnostic laboratory test result. The diagnosis of myocarditis is mainly indicated by a compatible history and the absence of other potential aetiologies, particularly if it can be confirmed with acute or convalescent sera.

Blood tests:

- Serum markers: The initial diagnostic strategies should be to evaluate serum markers for myocardial necrosis. Raised troponin I or T, CK or CK-MB in the absence of MI and the proper clinical setting confirm acute myocarditis.

Imaging:

- Cardiac Magnetic Resonance imaging can be used as a means of highlighting inflammation due to myocarditis from early gadolinium enhancement.

Histology:

- Biopsy: Evidence suggests no advantage for immunosuppressive therapy in biopsy-proven myocarditis, so myocardial biopsy is not routinely performed.

Others:

- ECG: demonstrates varying degrees of ST-T wave changes reflecting myocarditis and, sometimes, varying degrees of conduction disturbances.
- Echocardiography: this is a crucial aid in classifying this disease process, which manifests mostly as a dilated type of cardiomyopathy.

Management

➢ The immunological mechanism of myocyte destruction has led to several trials having investigated the use of immunomodulatory medications. The Myocarditis Treatment Trial demonstrated no survival benefit with Prednisolone plus Cyclosporin or Azathioprine in patients with viral (lymphocytic) myocarditis.

➢ Randomised trials are underway to evaluate IV immunoglobulin as treatment for viral myocarditis.

➢ If there is impairment of ventricular function, treatment is with standard heart failure therapy, including ACE-inhibitors and Beta-blockers.

➢ Targeted therapy:
  o Removal of the offending agent e.g. drugs or environmental causes.
  o Treatment of the underlying condition e.g. bacterial, protozoal or spirochaetal infections, autoimmune or inflammatory diseases.

Prognosis:

➢ Viral myocarditis may resolve over several months during the treatment of LV systolic dysfunction.

➢ The main issue in recovery is ventricular size.

➢ Reduction of ventricular size is associated with long-term improvement; otherwise, the course of the disease is characterised by progressive dilatation and development of a dilated cardiomyopathy.

Musculoskeletal chest pain

Epidemiology

Common, particularly in young patients with minimal cardiac risk factors.

Aetiology

May occur spontaneously or as a result of trauma

Pathophysiology

Strain or injury to chest wall structures results in costochondritis and inflammation of connective tissue structures within the chest wall. Direct trauma may result in a fractured rib.

Key features in the history/examination

➢ Sharp, stabbing pain localised to a particular area of the chest wall

➢ No radiation of pain to surrounding structures

➢ No associated autonomic symptoms

➢ Pain usually lasts a short duration and may be pleuritic in nature and worse on movement.

➢ Palpation of the site of pain may reveal chest wall tenderness (but note this does not exclude other diagnoses).

Investigations

Blood tests:

• 12 hour troponin: normal

ECG:

• No evidence of ST segment or T wave changes

Imaging:

• CXR: no evidence of cardiac or pulmonary pathology. Fractured ribs are not always identifiable.

Management

➢ This is often a diagnosis made after exclusion of more serious pathologies. Simple analgesics, advice on breathing exercises and reassurance should be given.

Further reading and references

➢ Antman E, Cohen M, Bernink P, et al. (2000) The TIMI Risk Score for Unstable Angina/Non-ST Elevation MI. A Method for Prognostication and Therapeutic Decision Making *JAMA*. 284(7): 835–842

➢ Gould FK, Elliott TS J, Foweraker J, et al. (2006) Guidelines for the prevention of endocarditis. Report of the Working Party of the British Society for Antimicrobial Chemotherapy. *J Antimicrob Chemother*. 57(6): 1035–42.

➢ Mason JW, O'Connell JB, Herskowitz A, Rose NR, McManus BM, Billingham ME. A clinical trial of immunosuppressive therapy for myocarditis. The Myocarditis Treatment Trial Investigators. *NEJM*. Aug 3 1995; 333(5): 269–75.

➢ Otto CM, Lind BK, Kitzman DW, et al. (1999) Association of aortic-valve sclerosis with cardiovascular mortality and morbidity in the elderly. *NEJM* 15; 341(3): 142–7.

➢ Yusuf S, Zhao F, Mehta S R, et al. (2001). Effects of clopidogrel

in addition to aspirin in patients with acute coronary syndromes without ST-segment elevation. *NEJM* 345: 494–502.

COUGH

Differential Diagnosis

System	Disease
Respiratory	**Lower respiratory tract infection**
	Pneumonia
	Comunity acquired pneumonia
	Hospital acquired pneumonia
	Aspiration pneumonia
	Pneumonia in the immunocompromised
	Exacerbation of asthma
	Exacerbation of chronic obstructive pulmonary disease
	Bronchial carcinoma
	Upper respiratory tract infection
	Pulmonary tuberculosis
	Bronchiectasis
	Pulmonary oedema
	Pulmonary embolus
Other	Drugs such as ACE inhibitors
	Foreign body ingestion
	Gastro-oesophageal reflux disease
	Post nasal drip

Lower respiratory tract infection

Epidemiology

Mostly occurs in the winter period.

Aetiology

Most cases of lower respiratory infection are viral in nature but occasionally bacterial infections arise. Those with pre-existing lung disease are at an increased risk, for example, those with chronic bronchitis. Table 3.34 below shows the main causative organisms:

Viral infections	Bacterial infections
• *Adenovirus*	• *Streptococcus pneumoniae*
• *Influenza*	• *Haemophilus influenzae*
• *Respiratory syncytial virus*	

Table 3.34: Principal causes of lower respiratory infections.

Key features in history/examination

• Typically presents with a dry and tickly cough as well as retrosternal discomfort.

• Bronchospasm may be an associated feature.

- Bacterial infection is associated with the production of purulent sputum.

Investigations

Microbiology:

- Sputum culture to exclude a bacterial cause.

Management

➢ Usually self-resolving.

➢ Potential risk of development in to bronchopneumonia.

➢ Antibiotic therapy is usually continued for 5 to 7 days which mostly results in resolution of infection.

Pneumonia

There is an acute lung inflammation with filling of the alveoli with inflammatory cells due to infiltration by micro-organisms. Infection is either confined to a lung lobe or occurs in a patchy distribution within the lung fields (bronchopneumonia). Causative organisms vary according to how and where the infection was acquired as well as host factors.

- Community acquired pneumonia.
- Hospital acquired pneumonia.
- Aspiration pneumonia.
- Pneumonia in the immunocompromised.

Community acquired pneumonia

Epidemiology

Has an incidence of 5–10 per 1,000 adults per year. It is responsible for over 1 million hospital admissions per year in the UK.

Aetiology

Transmission is via the respiratory route with droplet inhalation. Ciliary function is impaired in those who smoke cigarettes and consume alcohol predisposing them to infection. The organisms overwhelm the body's lung defence mechanisms resulting in consolidation. The phagocytic response of the lungs is reduced by the use of steroids as well.

Pathophysiology

Lobar pneumonia involves consolidation of the alveoli with fibrin and red blood cells. There is inflammation of the overlying pleural surface which may eventually result in the formation of a pleural effusion. The red cells are subsequently re-absorbed and the alveoli are infiltrated by leucocytes.

Bronchopneumonia involves a patchy consolidation with pus leaking in to the bronchi.

The main causative organisms are:

- **Streptococcus pneumoniae:** responsible for the majority of cases in all ages. It is a normal commensal of the upper respiratory tract.

- **Mycoplasma pneumoniae:** common around the autumn period with epidemics every 3 to 4 years.
- **Haemophilus influenzae:** commonly found to cause pneumonia in chronic obstructive pulmonary disease patients.
- **Legionella pneumophila:** is classically found in poorly maintained air-conditioning systems. It occurs in previously fit individuals who have been exposed to the agent in the aerosols of infected water such as in a communal gym. Those who are elderly or immunocompromised are particularly at risk. Mostly occurs in men and in the winter periods.
- **Viruses:** are rarer cause of pneumonia in those who are immunocompetent. *Influenza, Parainfluenza,* and the *Adenoviruses* more commonly cause pneumonia in the extremes of the age range.
- **Psittacosis:** is transmitted by birds and hence can occur in those who work in close proximity with them.
- **Coxiella burnetti:** can result in Q fever which is carried by cattle and sheep. Farmers and abattoir workers are mostly affected.
- **Staphylococcus aureus:** pneumonia is rare and tends to occur as a complication of viral pneumonia.

Key features in history/examination

- Cough.
- Increased respiratory rate.
- Worsening shortness of breath (SOB) with increased oxygen requirement.
- Increase in purulence and or volume of sputum.
- Fever.

Certain features are said to be indicative of the underlying causative organism:

- *Streptococcus pneumoniae* classically presents in winter or spring with pleuritic type chest pain often following an URTI. It has a rapid onset with high fever and a non-productive cough. Tachypnoea and cyanosis are late signs when there is extensive consolidation. A rusty coloured sputum is produced after a few days of the illness.
- *Mycoplasma pneumoniae* should be suspected in young and fit patients with an insidious onset occurring over many days. Look for other features such as rash, polyarthritis, myocarditis, pericarditis and meningoencephalitis.
- *Haemophilus influenzae* is more common in those with chronic underlying lung conditions or immunocompromised (especially alcoholics).
- *Legionella pneumophila* infection is more common in those who have travelled from abroad, are confused, very pyrexial (above 39 degrees), with deranged liver function tests, hyponatraemia, and hypoalbuminaemia. It has an incubation period of up to 10 days. Systemic features of headache, lethargy, myalgia, gastrointestinal symptoms and confusion are seen.
- *Staphylococcus aureus* initially gives mild features of 'flu', however tends to rapidly worsen with the development of a productive cough. Subsequently it causes high fever with shortness of breath. The infection may spread to other organs with abscess formation particularly in intravenous drug users.

- *Coxiella burnetti* follows a prolonged course with fever, lethargy and headaches and myalgia being the most common features.
- *Psittacosis* has a gradual onset up to several weeks. It occurs in patients with close contact with infected birds. Malaise and a low-grade fever are usual features.
- 'Cavitating' organisms – *Staphylococcus aureus, Klebsiella* spp, anaerobes and *Tuberculosis*.

Investigations

Blood tests:

- FBC
- U&E's
- LFTs
- ABG
- Paired serology: for atypical organisms is rarely helpful.
- CRP

Urine:

- Pneumococcal antigen may be present.
- Legionella antigen if severe symptoms or clinical suspicion.

Microbiology:

- Sputum sample: for microscopy, culture and sensitivity including gram stain.
- Blood cultures.
- Pleural aspiration: is considered if there is a pleural effusion especially if there is a suspicion of an empyema.

Imaging:

- Chest X-ray (CXR): Look for consolidation, air bronchograms, effusions and cavitating lesions (See Figure 3.18).

CXR features will vary according to the causative organism as shown below in Table 3.35:

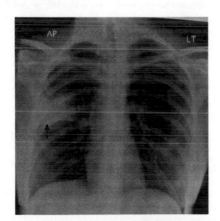

Figure 3.18: Plain X-ray showing consolidation (arrow) in the right upper lobe in keeping with pneumonia.

Causative organism	Features
Streptococcus pneumonia	Results in patchy changes within the lung field as well as lobar consolidation and occasionally a pleural effusion.
Mycoplasma pneumonia	Usually causes a lobar consolidation or patchy areas of shadowing.
Haemophilus influenza	Can cause extensive shadowing as well as scattered consolidation of the alveoli.
Legionella pneumophila	Legionnaire's disease results in a pneumonia which progressively spreads within the lung.
Psittacosis	May cause a diffuse pattern of infection.
Coxiella burnetti	Results in patchy changes within the lung fields.
Staphylococcus aureus	Results in spreading infection, associated with patchy changes, consolidation and abscesses. Frequently results in complication such as pneumothorax, pleural effusion and empyema.

Table 3.35: CXR features associated with various causative organisms of pneumonia.

CURB-65 score

The severity of the pneumonia should be assessed using the CURB-65 scoring system outlined below.

C: New onset confusion (Abbreviated Mental Test 8 or less)
U: Urea >7 mMol/l
R: Respiratory rate >30
B: Blood pressure <90 systolic or <60 diastolic
65: Age over 65

Table 3.36: The CURB 65 score for assessment of severity of pneumonia.

A score of 2 or greater predicts a high risk of death, so all scoring this should be admitted to hospital and treated as severe pneumonia. For all with 4 or 5 consider ICU/HDU referral.

Other factors should be considered whilst assessing severity, including multi-lobar or bilateral involvement and patient co-morbidities.

Management

➢ Oxygen therapy.

➢ Antibiotic therapy should be directed by local policy.

➢ A broad spectrum antibiotic such as Amoxicillin is commonly used.

➢ A macrolide may be added if an atypical organism is suspected.

➤ *Staphylococcus* infection requires addition of intravenous Flucloxacillin.

➤ In cases of deterioration with ongoing hypoxia, review by a respiratory specialist or the intensive care unit may be appropriate.

➤ May require invasive ventilation if severe hypoxia and signs of respiratory failure.

Complications:

➤ Lung abscess: a swinging fever is typical and intravenous antibiotic therapy must be given. Surgical drainage may be required.

➤ Pneumothorax formation is particularly common in *Staphylococcus aureus* infection and requires aspiration or chest drain insertion (see BTS guidelines).

➤ An empyema will also require chest drain insertion and intravenous antibiotic therapy. Again, surgical drainage may be required.

➤ Repeat CXR at 4–6 weeks post discharge to ensure resolution of changes.

➤ In the case of slow or no resolution, consider:

    o Incorrect diagnosis e.g. malignancy or cryptogenic organising pneumonia.

    o Incorrect or unexpected pathogen.

    o Antibiotic resistance.

    o Complications.

Prognosis:

➤ Severe pneumonia requires prompt and effective management especially if it results in severe sepsis.

➤ Carries approximately 5–10% mortality if hospitalised, especially in the elderly.

Hospital acquired pneumonia

When a new pneumonia develops after 48 hours as a hospital in-patient.

Epidemiology

Occurs in around 5% of in-patients.

Aetiology

Risk factors include:

• Extremes of age.

• Immunocompromise.

• Pre-existing lung disease.

• Recent major surgery.

• Mechanical ventilation.

• Supine position.

• Antacid therapy.

• Poor hand hygiene in healthcare workers.

• There may be reduced host defence mechanisms in hospitalised patients due to prior infection or illness.

Pathophysiology

Usually caused by gram negative bacteria (more than 50%) such as *E. coli* and *Proteus. Pseudomonas* is common in ventilated patients in the intensive care unit, and in those with bronchiectasis and cystic fibrosis. *Klebsiella pneumoniae* affects the elderly and those with a background of lung disease and has a high mortality rate.

Key features in history/examination

• Features of pneumonia as above, however symptoms tend to be more severe than in community-acquired pneumonia.

• *Klebsiella* typically causes an acute onset of symptoms of a severe pneumonia which tends to be confined to a single lobe. Patients are very unwell and produce copious amounts of purulent and blood-stained sputum. It may even result in lobe destruction when infection is very serious.

Investigations

• As for community acquired pneumonia.

• If an effusion is seen an aspiration should be performed to exclude complicated effusion and empyema.

Management

➤ Empirical antibiotics must be initiated even if sensitivities are not available and should be based on local guidelines and microbiology advice.

➤ Usually a broad spectrum antibiotic is used.

➤ Chest physiotherapy is an important part of management.

➤ Aspiration pneumonia will respond to treatment with a third generation cephalosporin such as Cefotaxime and Metronidazole which will cover anaerobes.

➤ Multiresistant strains of *Staphylococcus aureus* are increasing and therapy is very difficult. Flucloxacillin is usually used.

➤ Pseudomonas infection will respond to Gentamicin or a Quinolone such as Ciprofloxacin.

Prevention:

➤ Patients are encouraged not to smoke pre-operatively.

➤ Early mobilisation and chest physiotherapy are very important.

➤ High-risk individuals should be closely monitored.

Aspiration Pneumonia

Bacteria usually commensal to the oropharynx enter the lower respiratory tract and cause infection. Aspiration itself is very common in healthy people, especially at night. However the bronchial defences and small volume involved means that infection does not occur.

3. Medicine

It is usually caused by anaerobic bacteria and the right lower lobe is often involved due to the structure of the bronchial tree. Risk factors for aspiration include dental caries and poor mouth hygiene, oropharyngeal sepsis, reduced level of consciousness, stroke and other neurological conditions causing bulbar weakness, cognitive impairment, a hiatus hernia and binge drinking.

As with other infections, aspiration pneumonia should be treated along local policy guidelines. Metronidazole is commonly used.

Pneumonia in the immunocompromised

Epidemiology

Pneumonia has a high mortality rate in the immunocompromised. The diagnosis tends to be more difficult in the elderly as they produce fewer clinical features than in younger individuals. The risk of pneumonia in patients with HIV is up to 100 times greater. Overall there is a 14% risk of mortality, especially in those at the extremes of age. There is a greater incidence in males compared to females.

Aetiology

Immunocompromised individuals are more susceptible not only to the usual range of respiratory tract pathogens but also to a wide range of opportunistic organisms. These patients can be infected by more than one organism at any one time and the symptoms and signs of infection may be 'atypical'. Invasive procedures such as bronchoscopy are often required to obtain samples for microbiological investigations.

Most common organisms include *Pneumocystis jiroveci* (causing PCP and formerly known as *Pneumocystis carinii*), *Mycobacterium tuberculosis*, *Candida albicans* and *Cytomegalovirus*.

Pathophysiology

Immunocompromised patients tend to be susceptible to pneumonia as they carry defects within the neutrophils, immunoglobulins or in the T-cells, rendering the immune defences dysfunctional.

Key features in history/examination

- Clinical features are dependent upon the causative organism.
- Commonly there is an insidious onset of a non-productive cough, difficulty in breathing and fever.
- Pyrexia and scattered crackles on auscultation of the chest are common on examination.
- Around 70% of patients may have no features on examination especially if they are neutropenic where often the only presenting feature is fever.

Investigations

Blood tests:

- FBC: Individuals with HIV will have a lymphopenia (in particular a low CD4 count).

- ABG: classical findings in PCP include unexpectedly severe hypoxaemia and exercise induced oxygen desaturation.

Imaging:

- Chest X-ray: a PCP infection will typically show symmetrical peri-hilar alveolar shadowing in a butterfly distribution – classically 'ground-glass'. This may be very subtle and the CXR is normal in over 20% cases.

Microbiology:

- A sputum sample is required for definitive diagnosis. Pneumocysts will be visible on examination of the sputum.

Bronchoscopy:

- When PCP is suspected, a bronchoscopy must be considered. Bronchio-alveolar lavage can obtain samples to look for pneumocysts and a transbronchial bopsy will confirm the diagnosis in almost 95% of patients.

Management

- ➤ For PCP oral or intravenous Co-trimoxazole is first-line treatment.
- ➤ Steroids may be added as well as Pentamidine.
- ➤ CMV infection requires intravenous Ganciclovir and occasionally hyperimmune gammaglobulin.
- ➤ Mycobacterium tuberculosis responds to anti-tuberculous therapy.
- ➤ Candiasis is treated with Fluconazole or Amphotericin. It is important to change any indwelling medical devices.

Prognosis:

- ➤ Around 80% of patients will respond to treatment with their first episode of pneumonia unless there are complications with very severe infection where ventilation may be required.
- ➤ Overall mortality rate is 15 to 20%.

Exacerbation of asthma

Epidemiology

Asthma is a common chronic condition characterised by airways hyperresponsiveness and reversible airflow limitation. Around 7% of the population are affected. The bronchospasm and inflammation can be induced by a variety of stimulants, including infection, allergens, air pollution, exercise and emotions.

There is a significant mortality attached to acute asthma exacerbations, but this can be minimised by early interventions by the patient, seeking help early and by effective management by healthcare professionals.

Aetiology

Refer to section on Asthma.

Pathophysiology

Refer to section on Asthma.

Key features in history/examination

If there are one or more of the following features, it is suggestive of an acute exacerbation of asthma:

- Tachypnoea: a respiratory rate of more than 30 per minute.
- Tachycardia of more than 100 beats per minute.
- Inability to speak in full sentences.
- Peak flow less than 40% of the patient's predicted best normal value according to their height and age.

Investigations

Refer to section on Asthma.

Management

Chronic asthma should be managed using the stepwise approach advocated by the British Thoraic Society (BTS). Patients should all have a personalised treatment plan in writing with instructions about what to do in the event of an exacerbation.

All patients should be assessed starting with ABC:

> Airway
>
> Breathing
>
> Circulation

Prior to hospital admission:

- Self administration of inhaled salbutamol, preferably via a spacer.
- Early administration of salbutamol nebulisers (5 mg) and ipratropium bromide nebulisers (0.5 mg) by the ambulance crews.
- High flow oxygen.
- Oral steroids if available.

In hospital:

- Urgent assessment using the A to E approach.
  - PEFR < 33%
  - ABG if sats <92% or features of severe asthma.
  - CXR to exclude pneumothorax and infection if indicated.
- Use the BTS guidelines to aid correct investigations and management.

The signs of acute life-threatening asthma are shown in Table 3.28 in the chapter on Asthma.

Standard treatment for severe and life-threatening asthma is:

- Regular nebulised beta agonists and Ipratropium bromide.
- Steroid therapy.

- Magnesium sulphate (2 g IV) if the patient is unresponsive to maximal therapy with steroids and bronchodilators.

Further management:

- If there is little or no improvement with the above therapy then an intravenous beta agonist or Theophylline is required. Caution is needed when patients have already been on oral Theophylline as toxic serum levels may result.
- Intravenous antibiotics are administered if there is clinical suspicion or radiological evidence of a chest infection causing the exacerbation, which is unusual in asthma.
- Intravenous fluids.
- Electrolyte correction is occasionally required as there may be hypokalaemia due to beta agonist therapy.
- Indicators for referral to the intensive care unit:
  - Hypoxia with PaO_2 < 8 kPa despite high flow oxygen therapy.
  - Continued or worsening hypercapnia.
  - Worsening acidosis.
  - Exhaustion.
  - Bradycardia.
  - Hypotension.
  - Confusion and drowsiness.
  - Loss of consciousness.
  - Respiratory depression.

Overall, the prognosis of acute severe asthma is improved if it is recognised and treated promptly and adequately.

Exacerbation of COPD

Epidemiology

As defined by the Global initiative for chronic obstructive lung disease, COPD is a 'preventable and treatable disease. Its pulmonary component is characterised by airflow limitation which is not fully reversible. The airflow limitation is usually progressive.' The WHO has defined an exacerbation as '…a change in the patient's dyspnoea, cough and/or sputum that is beyond normal day-to-day variations, is acute in onset and may warrant a change in regular medication.'

Exacerbations of COPD are usually triggered by viral or bacterial infection and account for about 15% of all hospital admissions. There is a significant mortality and exacerbations can cause a marked reduction in quality of life.

Aetiology

Refer to section on COPD.

Pathophysiology

Refer to section on COPD.

Key features in history/examination

- Patients with an acute exacerbation present with symptoms of shortness of breath, increasing cough and increased volume or purulence of sputum.

- Chest tightness, confusion and a reduced exercise tolerance are associated features.

- On examination, such patients typically have tachypnoea with wheeze, poor air entry, pursed lip breathing and possibly cyanosis.

- They will give a history of reduced exercise tolerance and a marked reduction in their ability to conduct the normal activities of daily living.

Investigations

Refer to section on COPD.

Management

➢ Check for local Trust guidelines.

➢ Full A to E assessment.

➢ NICE guidelines for exacerbation of COPD (see Figure 3.19).

Permission granted from NICE

➢ A chest X-ray should always be performed to exclude a pneumothorax or confirm evidence of infection. In COPD the chest X-ray will usually have a hyperexpanded appearance with flattened hemi-diaphragms. (See Figure 3.20).

➢ Patients should be sat up and given oxygen according to the BTS guidelines (BTS 2008).

    ○ If hypercapnia is thought to be a problem commence with 28% oxygen via a venturi mask whilst awaiting the ABG results, aiming for sats of between 88–92%.

    ○ After ABG, if the $PaCO_2$ is normal then the target should be adjusted upwards to 94–98%.

    ○ The oxygenation must be carefully monitored and adjusted dependent on the clinical situation and the ABG results.

➢ Salbutamol (2.5–5 mg) and Atrovent (0.5 mg) nebulisers are given as well as Prednisolone (30–40 mg) or intravenous Hydrocortisone (200 mg) if unable to tolerate oral medications.

➢ It is usual to give antibiotics.

➢ If patients are unresponsive to the above treatment IV Aminophylline or Salbutamol can be administered.

➢ Non-invasive ventilation (NIV) – commonly referred to as BIPAP – is considered when patients are clinically worsening despite maximal medical therapy.

    ○ Uses a machine which aids patient's ventilation via a tightly fitting mask.

    ○ Indicated in type 2 respiratory failure due to exacerbation of COPD (i.e. PaO_2 less than 8 kPa)

    ○ Most commonly used when patients have a pH of 7.25–7.35 and $PaCO_2$ of more than 6.0 kPa.

    ○ It should only be commenced under senior guidance and only with a documented escalation plan in the event of treatment failure.

    ○ The patient must be conscious and able to co-operate with the therapy and protect their airway. Other contraindications include pneumothorax, severe agitation, vomiting, facial trauma and focal consolidation on the CXR.

Bronchial carcinoma

Epidemiology

The leading type of cancer causing death in men and the second leading cause in women. It accounts for over 30,000 deaths per year. Individuals aged 60 to 70 years are mostly affected. There is a strong correlation between socioeconomic deprivation and the incidence of lung cancer. The incidence is falling in males but rising in females, reflecting trends in smoking patterns.

Aetiology

Cigarette smoking is the main risk factor (accounts for over 90% of cases). Factors such as the duration of smoking and the number smoked are important. The number of pack years should be calculated (number smoked per day divided by 20 then multiplied by years smoked).

Family history is also an important risk factor. A first degree relative more than doubles the risk, especially if the relative was aged under 60 years.

Other risk factors include:

- Passive smoking, cigar and pipe smoking.

- Occupation exposure – asbestos, radon gas and uranium mining.

- COPD and interstitial lung disease.

Pathophysiology

Traditionally grouped as small-cell lung cancer (SCLC) and non-small-cell lung cancer (NSCLC). The main types of bronchial carcinoma are shown in Table 3.37 below.

Key features in history/examination

Local:

- The early stages of lung cancer are mostly asymptomatic, with the cancer being incidentally detected.

- Persistent cough.

- Haemoptysis.

- Fatigue and lethargy.

- Weight loss.

- A pneumonia which is slow to resolve or recurrent pneumonias.

- Chest pain due to involvement of the pleura or chest wall.

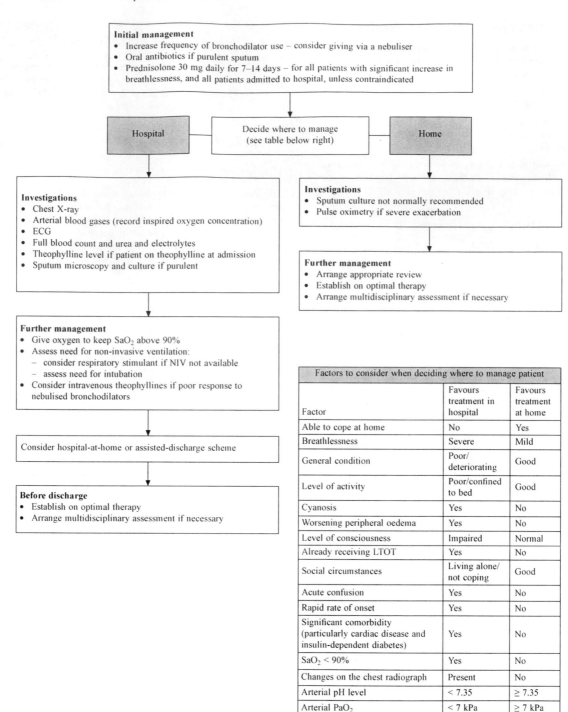

Initial management
- Increase frequency of bronchodilator use – consider giving via a nebuliser
- Oral antibiotics if purulent sputum
- Prednisolone 30 mg daily for 7–14 days – for all patients with significant increase in breathlessness, and all patients admitted to hospital, unless contraindicated

Hospital

Decide where to manage (see table below right)

Home

Investigations
- Chest X-ray
- Arterial blood gases (record inspired oxygen concentration)
- ECG
- Full blood count and urea and electrolytes
- Theophylline level if patient on theophylline at admission
- Sputum microscopy and culture if purulent

Investigations
- Sputum culture not normally recommended
- Pulse oximetry if severe exacerbation

Further management
- Arrange appropriate review
- Establish on optimal therapy
- Arrange multidisciplinary assessment if necessary

Further management
- Give oxygen to keep SaO_2 above 90%
- Assess need for non-invasive ventilation:
  - consider respiratory stimulant if NIV not available
  - assess need for intubation
- Consider intravenous theophyllines if poor response to nebulised bronchodilators

Consider hospital-at-home or assisted-discharge scheme

Before discharge
- Establish on optimal therapy
- Arrange multidisciplinary assessment if necessary

Factors to consider when deciding where to manage patient		
Factor	Favours treatment in hospital	Favours treatment at home
Able to cope at home	No	Yes
Breathlessness	Severe	Mild
General condition	Poor/deteriorating	Good
Level of activity	Poor/confined to bed	Good
Cyanosis	Yes	No
Worsening peripheral oedema	Yes	No
Level of consciousness	Impaired	Normal
Already receiving LTOT	Yes	No
Social circumstances	Living alone/not coping	Good
Acute confusion	Yes	No
Rapid rate of onset	Yes	No
Significant comorbidity (particularly cardiac disease and insulin-dependent diabetes)	Yes	No
SaO_2 < 90%	Yes	No
Changes on the chest radiograph	Present	No
Arterial pH level	< 7.35	≥ 7.35
Arterial PaO_2	< 7 kPa	≥ 7 kPa

Figure 3.19: NICE guidelines on managing exacerbations of COPD.

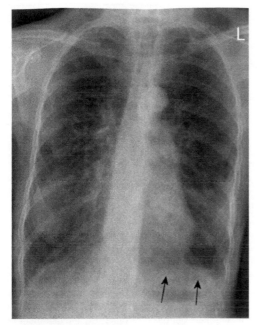

Figure 3.20: Chest X-ray showing hyper inflated lungs with flattening of the diaphragm (black arrow) with long narrow cardiac silhouette.

Type of cancer	Features
Small cell (Oat cell)	Accounts for about 20% of cases. Usually found in the large airways. Very rapidly dividing. Metastasises early (at least 75% have metastases at the time of diagnosis).
Squamous cell	Accounts for about 45% of cases. Usually only locally invasive and may form cavitating lesions.
Adenocarcinoma	Accounts for about 30% of cases. A relatively slow growing tumour which metastasises late. The tumour is often peripheral. Less strong association with smoking.
Large cell	Features are common to both squamous and small cell carcinoma.
Others	Alveolar cell carcinoma.

Table 3.37: Different types of bronchial carcinoma.

- Shortness of breath from lung or lobar collapse or pleural effusion or phrenic nerve palsy.
- A tumour occurring at the left hilar region may involve the left recurrent laryngeal nerve resulting in a hoarse voice and harsh cough.
- A tumour causing compression on the trachea or main bronchus will cause stridor or wheeze which may be acute or progressive in nature.

- Tumour invading the mediastinum can cause obstruction of the superior vena cava and the subsequent features such as swelling of the face, neck and upper limbs and venous engorgement in the upper chest wall.
- Invasion of the pericardium may result in arrythmias such as atrial fibrillation.
- An apical 'Pancoast's' tumour can potentially invade the brachial plexus and hence result in arm and shoulder pain as well as involving the lower cervical sympathetic chain giving the classical Horner's syndrome with features of ptosis, meiosis, enophthalmos, and anhydrosis.

Metastases:

- Around 15% of patients may present with features of metastases.
- Brain, which can cause headache, epilepsy, and confusion.
- Bone, which can cause pain, pathological fractures and can also give features of cord compression.
- Liver, which can cause jaundice, hepatomegaly and hepatic capsular pain.
- Feel for supraclavicular lymph nodes.

Non-metastatic (paraneoplastic) features:

Paraneoplastic syndromes are found in 15% of patients.

Endocrine:

- Hypercalcaemia, secondary to excess production of parathyroid hormone-like peptide or from bone metastases. (Most commonly from squamous cell).
- Hyponatraemia from the syndrome of inappropriate antidiuretic hormone secretion (SIADH).
- The tumour itself may secrete adrenocorticotrophic hormone (ACTH), resulting in hypokalaemia.
- Eaton-Lambert Syndrome.

Skin:

- Clubbing of the digits.
- Hypertrophic pulmonary osteoarthropathy.
- Dermatomyositis.

Haematological:

- Persistent anaemia or disseminated intravascular coagulation.

Investigations

Blood tests:

- FBC
- U&Es
- LFTs
- Bone Profile as a minimum.

3. Medicine

Imaging:

- Chest X-ray: must be performed in all patients presenting with haemoptysis, and has been shown to illustrate over 90% of bronchial tumours on presentation. (See Figure 3.21). Lesions which tend to be missed are those which are less than 15 mm in size and in the central lung areas.
- CT: more useful in identifying smaller lesions, will also demonstrate any local and metastatic spread. It is an essential part of staging and will be required before any surgical intervention.

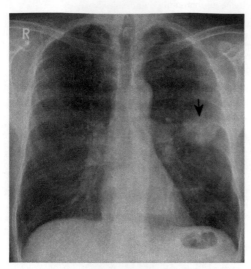

Figure 3.21: Plain X-ray demonstrating a soft tissue mass (arrow) in the left mid zone in keeping with malignancy.

Cytology:

- Sputum: 3 separate samples are required.
- Aspiration of any pleural effusion.

Histology:

- Peripheral lesions: percutanous needle biopsy under CT or ultrasound guidance.
- More central lesions: bronchoscopy and transbronchial needle aspiration.
- Biopsy of metastases or peripheral lymph nodes.

Other:

- Spirometry: this is especially important if surgery is being contemplated. Spirometry alone is sufficient if the post-bronchodilator FEV1 is >1.5 litres for a lobectomy or >2.0 litres for a pneumonectomy, provided that there is no evidence of interstitial lung disease.
- Pulmonary Function Tests: are required if the patient does not fulfil the operative criteria on spirometry.
- Assessment of performance status (PS): the PS will influence treatment decisions as a PS of more than 2 indicates a poor outcome with chemotherapy and radiotherapy.

0:	Fully fit
1:	Symptomatic but capable of light work eg housework
2:	Up and about more than 50% of waking hours (able to live at home with some assistance)
3:	Confined to chair or bed more than 50% of waking hours (unable to care for self)
4:	Confined to chair or bed

Table 3.38: The WHO performance status (PS) scale.

As governed by specialist advice:

- Positron Emission Tomography (PET).
- Thoracoscopy.
- Surgical biopsy.

Management

All suspected or diagnosed lung cancer patients should be referred to the Lung MDT. They will determine further investigations, confirm the diagnosis, determine the 'stage' of the neoplasm and decide on treatment options. The diagnosis and treatment options must be sensitively communicated to the patient. NSCLC uses the TNM staging classification, whereas SCLC use a system of 'limited or extensive' disease.

Surgery:

- Only 1 in 5 patients will be suitable for surgery depending on their state of health and the staging of the tumour as well as time of presentation.
- A lobectomy or pneumonectomy can be curative.
- Those with a peripheral lung tumour tend to fare better.
- It is essential for the patient to have pre-operative investigations in order to establish the nature and presence of any metastases.
- Tests of cardiovascular and respiratory function are required to ensure the patient will have a good chance of recovery from the surgery.

Chemotherapy:

- Multi-drug platinum-based chemotherapy is the primary treatment for SCLC.
- Usually used in the higher-stage NSCLC and also as adjunctive therapy.
- However, it is associated with many side-effects and is usually not curative.
- Neutropenic sepsis must always be considered in a patient presenting 7–10 days post chemotherapy.
- The mean survival after presentation is around 1 year.

Radiotherapy:

- Effective as palliative therapy in particular for bone pain and superior vena cava obstruction.

> Radical radiotherapy is offered in the form of Continuous Hyperfractionated Accelerated Radiotherapy (CHART).

Palliative care:

> End of life care should be facilitated by a specialist MDT, exploring the patient's wishes, involving the family if the patient wants and commencing advanced care planning at an early stage.
> The aim is to maintain symptomatic relief. This may include:
>   o Medical therapies especially analgesia.
>   o Surgical therapies such as tumour de-bulking.
>   o Bronchial stenting which provides symptomatic relief in those with localised tumours which are obstructing the main airways.
>   o Radiotherapy.
>   o Pleurodesis.
> Hospice care may be of benefit to some patients.

Prognosis:

> Poor due to late presentation and high frequency of metastatic disease at the time of presentation.
> The 5-year survival rate is less than 5%.

Upper respiratory tract infection

Although cough is a feature in the presentation of upper respiratory tract infection, it is not commonly the predominant feature. The main categories of upper respiratory tract are outlined below.

One of the major causes of chronic cough (cough lasting longer than 8 weeks) in a patient with a normal chest x-ray and no 'red-flag' symptoms is rhinitis and post-nasal drip. There is no specific definition for post-nasal drip, but it may be suspected if the patient describes a dripping sensation down the back of the throat or a frequent impulse to clear their throat. A trial of treatment with nasal steroids, decongestants or antihistamines is useful.

Common cold

- Commonly caused by *Rhinoviruses* and *Coronaviruses*, but also *Parainfluenzae*, *Echo-* and *Adeno-* *viruses* and *Respiratory syncytial virus*.
- Very infectious, spread via the aerosol route.
- Symptoms develop over a number of hours.
- Sneezing and rhinorrhoea are common features with swelling of the mucosal passages causing a blocked sensation.
- There may be secondary bacterial infection which will result in sinusitis.
- No investigations are required.
- Symptomatic management is all that is needed, with resolution in a few days.

Pharyngitis

- Infection of the pharynx, including tonsils and adenoids.

- Mostly viral in nature caused by *Coxsackie, Adeno-* and *Echo-viruses* but *Haemolytic streptococci* may also be a causative agent.
- Mainly causes a sore throat and systemic features including fever.
- The tonsils may appear enlarged with visible pus. Complications include a peritonsillar abscess (quinsy) which will require surgical drainage.
- The *Coxsackie* virus will cause a very painful dysphagia.
- Throat swabs and *anti-streptolysin-O* (ASO) titres should be taken.
- Antibiotics are only given in bacterial infections.
- Symptoms will resolve within a week if they are caused by a virus.

Sinusitis

- Inflammation of the nasal sinuses.
- Commonly causes headache, facial pain and a blocked nose.
- Imaging of the sinuses is rarely required.
- If there is bacterial infection, antibiotics will be required.
- Chronic sinusitis if very hard to treat and may require frequent surgical washouts of the sinuses.

Laryngitis

- The larynx is infected.
- Mostly viral in nature caused by *Influenza, Para-influenza,* or *Respiratory syncytial virus*, but may be bacterial such as *Streptococcus pneumoniae* or *Haemophilus influenza*.
- Common symptoms are hoarseness of the voice, malaise and fever.
- Since there is a natural narrowing of the airway at the larynx, any tissue swelling can potentially affect breathing and this is particularly troublesome in children.
- Throat swabs should be taken.
- Antibiotics are required only if a bacterial cause is identified.
- Symptoms will resolve with treatment.

Pulmonary tuberculosis

Tuberculosis (TB) most commonly affects the lungs, however, it can affect any body part (e.g. the spine in Pott's disease). It is caused by *Mycobacterium tuberculosis.*

Epidemiology

TB is the commonest cause of death from a treatable infection worldwide with 3 million deaths per year. Approximately 10 million individuals are affected. The worst affected areas are sub-Saharan Africa and Eastern Europe/Russia. The incidence has increased with the rise of HIV worldwide with widespread co-infection. It is relatively uncommon in the UK with an incidence of 1–2 per 1,000 per year. The incidence is rising but this is due to the influx of migrants from areas of high TB prevalence.

Aetiology

There is an increased risk of infection in the immunocompromised e.g. people with HIV, diabetes, lymphoma, patients on steroids or chemotherapy, the elderly and malnourished individuals.

Transmission is via the airbourne route and so the greatest risk is living with infected persons with TB in their sputum.

Pathophysiology

Primary pulmonary tuberculosis:

Transmission via inhalation. A small amount of the bacillus mycobacterium tuberculosis is required for infection and it tends to reside in the poorly perfused but well-ventilated regions of the lung field (mostly the upper lobes).

The primary inflammatory response involves a leucocytosis. Macrophages are released which engulf the tubercle bacilli and self-destruct leaving a lesion which eventually develops into a granuloma. Granulomata usually have a central area of necrotic tissue which is composed of caseous material and is surrounded by Langerhans' giant cells which together form the Ghon focus. This eventually fibroses and calcifies. There is lymph node enlargement related to the area of involved lung field. Both of these in combination form the 'primary complex'.

It can take up to 2 months for the development of the primary complex following primary infection with TB but it usually heals fully. The tubercle bacilli may, in rare cases, overwhelm the host defence system and hence result in the development of tuberculous pneumonia and pleural effusion. Spread of the bacilli throughout the body can result in serious consequences such as tuberculous meningitis. Miliary tuberculosis occurs when host defences are particularly poor and hence the bacilli spread throughout the blood, which can be potentially fatal.

Post-primary tuberculosis:

This occurs when the Ghon focus does not heal fully or if there is re-activation of the primary infection.

Key features in history/examination

Primary pulmonary tuberculosis:

- Development of the primary complex tends to be early on and may sometimes be associated with a mild fever and erythema nodosum.
- There will usually be no signs on examination however a minor pleural effusion may be present and compression of the bronchus by significant hilar lymphadenopathy can cause wheeze and signs of lung collapse.

Post-primary pulmonary tuberculosis:

- Features develop over several months and includes:

  - Cough, usually chronic, may be dry or purulent
  - Weight loss and anorexia
  - Fever
  - Night sweats
  - Malaise
  - Haemoptysis
  - Breathlessness
  - Chest pain

- The diagnosis of TB should be considered in any cough lasting longer than 3 weeks, particularly if courses of antibiotics have had no effect.
- On examination there may be few signs. Commonly there may be signs of a pneumonia or pleural effusion, more rarely finger clubbing or cervical lymphadenopathy are seen.

Miliary tuberculosis:

- A persistent fever associated with malaise and weight loss is characteristic.
- There may be hepatosplenomegaly on examination as well as tubercles visible within the retina.

Investigations

Blood tests:

- FBC: anaemia may be the only feature.
- U&Es and bone profile: there may be hyponatraemia and potentially hypercalcaemia.

Immunology:

- Mantoux tests: are mostly used. Strongly positive in those with post-primary pulmonary tuberculosis. Negative if there is miliary tuberculosis or if the patient is immunocompromised, such as those with HIV.

Microbiology:

- Sputum smear microscopy (Ziehl Neelsen stain): is the most important diagnostic test. It is rapid, cheap and identifies 80% cases with 1 sample. 3 early morning samples should be sent to the laboratory on 3 consecutive days.
- Sputum sample culture: can take up to 6 weeks as the tubercle bacilli are slow growing.
- It may be necessary to obtain samples by inducing sputum using hypertonic saline or by bronchial lavage on bronchoscopy.
- If TB is suspected from another site, samples should be sent of relevant tissue/fluids, clearly marked with the suspicion of TB.

Imaging:

- Chest X-ray: may show consolidation and a cavitating lesion, especially in the upper zones. (See Figure 3.22).

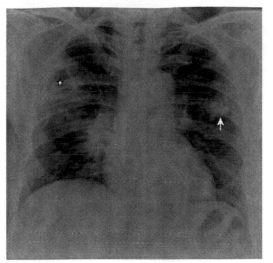

Figure 3.22: Cavitating mass in the RUL in keeping with a TB cavity (star) also note further focal consolidation in left lung (arrow).

- Miliary tuberculosis gives a distinctive pattern of many tiny nodules (up to 2 mm in size) distributed throughout the lung fields with the appearance of millet seeds (hence 'miliary' TB) which can be easily missed. (See Figure 3.23). However there is a time lag between disease and X-ray changes so up to 30% have a normal CXR.

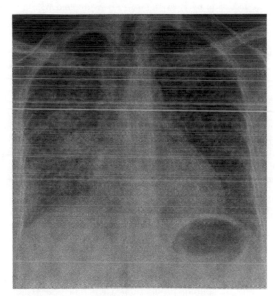

Figure 3.23: CXR showing numerous well defined tiny nodules throughout the lung in keeping with miliary spread of TB.

Histology:

- Pleural effusion sample: if there is a significant pleural effusion it may be aspirated to obtain a sample, which usually contains granulomata.

- Tissue biopsy: from either the lung or the liver obtained via bronchoscopy, will provide definitive diagnosis of miliary tuberculosis in up to 70% of patients.

Management

➢ Any patient with suspected pulmonary TB should be isolated in a negative pressure side-room. For TB elsewhere in the body, isolation need not be as strict. Patients should be managed at home if at all possible.

➢ Masks should be worn by staff within the side-room until the patient is considered non-infectious.

➢ Children and those not immunised against TB should not have contact until the patient is considered non-infectious.

➢ HIV testing should be encouraged.

➢ Isolation would normally be discontinued after 14 days in an uncomplicated case of TB.

Medication:

➢ The treatment of pulmonary TB should be supervised by a respiratory or infectious disease consultant and should involve a multidisciplinary team to support the patient and encourage concordance.

➢ A combination of drugs is used in order to minimise the risk of multi-drug resistant strains developing. The standard first line therapy is Isoniazid, Rifampicin, Ethambutol and Pyrazinamide for 2 months. The Isoniazid and Rifampicin are continued for a further 4 months. Pyridoxine is given with Isoniazid to reduce the incidence of neuropathy.

➢ All anti-tuberculous drugs have side-effects and these should be monitored for:

   o Rifampicin: turns secretions red and induces the cytochrome p 450 enzyme complex. Warn about avoiding contact lenses and reduced effectiveness of the oral contraceptive pill.

   o Isoniazid: idiosyncratic hepatitis and peripheral neuropathy.

   o Pyrazinamide: hepatitis, arthritis and gout.

   o Ethambutol: optic neuritis. Monitor with the ishihara test.

➢ For complicated cases such as drug resistance and extra-pulmonary involvement, other antibiotic choices may be needed and the treatment must be longer, for example for 18 months if there is any bone involvement.

➢ Increasing drug concordance:

   o Health education stressing the importance of the medication regime with the provision of written information.

   o Provision of a single point of contact to obtain help and support e.g. a respiratory specialist nurse.

   o Home visits.

   o Patient diary.

   o Random urine tests and other monitoring (for example, pill counts).

   o Information about help with paying for prescriptions where relevant.

   o Directly observed therapy (DOT).

Prevention:

➤ The BCG vaccination consists of a non-virulent strain of bovine tuberculosis and results in the development of immunity and a 70% risk reduction for the development of infection.

➤ Usually given to school children aged 12 to 13 years and also offered to infants at high-risk such as those born in endemic areas.

➤ Only those with a negative mantoux test will be vaccinated.

Contact tracing:

➤ If an affected individual has sputum positive TB any close contacts must be screened and treated if necessary. The risk is proportionate to the closeness of the contact, ranging from 1:3 for a partner to 1:100 for work colleagues.

➤ The algorithms in the NICE guidelines should be used. The principle test is the mantoux. If this is positive, an interferon gamma test should be performed to reduce the number of false-positives given by the mantoux. If this is also positive and a CXR/clinical examination reveals evidence of TB then treatment for latent TB should be instigated.

➤ Standard treatment is 3 months of rifampicin and isoniazid or 6 months of isoniazid.

➤ It is a notifiable disease.

Prognosis:

➤ A good prognosis unless the patient is immuno-compromised or the TB strain shows resistance to anti-tuberculous treatments.

Multi-drug resistant TB (MDRTB) and extremely drug resistant TB (XDRTB):

➤ Single drug resistance, commonly to Isoniazid is relatively common (<10% in the UK) but is associated with an increased mortality (5%).

➤ MDRTB shows resistance to Rifampicin and Isoniazid. Although the prevalence is still low, it is increasing. It is harder to treat than sensitive TB and carries a greater mortality (>30%).

➤ XDRTB shows resistance to Rifampicin and Isoniazid as well as a Fluoroquinolone and an injectable treatment (e.g. Amikacin). There have been case reports in the UK. There has been much interest in XDRTB, especially in South Africa where it is especially prevalent. The majority of cases have HIV co-infection and the mortality is high (>50%).

➤ These should be suspected in patients with a past history of poor concordance with TB treatment, HIV co-infection, failure to respond to standard treatment after 2 months and birth in, or travel to, an area where these strains are endemic (e.g. Eastern Europe and Southern Africa).

Bronchiectasis

Bronchiectasis is an irreversible dilatation of bronchi characterised by chronic inflammation, chronic cough and sputum production

Epidemiology

Bronchiectasis effects around 1 in 1,000 individuals. It usually starts from childhood but may present at any age. Those with pre-existing lung disease are more commonly affected, for example cystic fibrosis. The diagnosis is increasing in part due to increased availability of high resolution CT scanning. There is a higher incidence in the developing countries.

Aetiology

Bronchiectasis is the resultant end-point of a number of pathologies. Cystic fibrosis is the most well known cause (with over 7,000 sufferers in the UK) but bronchiectasis in association with COPD is increasingly being recognised. Other causes include:

• Post-infectious: bacterial pneumonia, whooping cough, tuberculosis, aspergillosis.

• Distal to bronchial obstruction e.g. foreign body, malignancy.

• Secondary to connective tissue disorder e.g. rheumatoid arthritis, SLE, systemic sclerosis.

• Primary cilliary dyskinesia.

• Immunodeficiency: hypogammaglobulinaemia, HIV.

• Other: idiopathic, ulcerative colitis-associated, post radiation therapy, alpha-1 antitrypsin deficiency and yellow nail syndrome.

Infective exacerbations are commonly caused by *Staphylococcus, Pneumococcus, H. influenzae* and *Pseudomonas aeroginosa*. Chronic infection by *P. aeroginosua* is associated with a worse prognosis.

Pathophysiology

There is damage to the elastic and muscular layers of the bronchial wall, leading to dilatation and inflammation of the bronchial walls. The normal transport of mucous through the airways via the ciliary transport mechanism is damaged which allowing accumulation of bronchial secretions. The damage predisposes to bacterial infections, resulting in a vicious cycle of further damage to the bronchial wall and ciliary system and further accumulation of secretions. Bacterial colonisation of the airways is the result.

Key features in history and examination

• Chronic cough with purulent sputum.

• Offensive smelling breath is common as well as wheeze, breathlessness, fatigue and chronic rhinosinusitis.

• Infective exacerbations of bronchiectasis result in increased volume of sputum production. There may be associated haemoptysis and chest pain.

• Crackles heard on examination of the chest on inspiration and expiration.

• There may be associated wheezing in particular with certain causative agents such as aspergillosis.

• Finger clubbing, right sided cardiac failure and delayed resolution of infection are all associated features.

Investigations

Blood tests:

- FBC: those with severe disease will have a low haemoglobin.
- May point to an underlying cause and are useful during an exacerbation.

Immunology:

- Bronchiectasis is more common in those who have an immunoglobin deficiency.

Microbiology:

- Microscopy and culture of the sputum, including acid fast bacilli.

Imaging:

- CXR: may show thickening of the bronchial wall as well as areas of cystic changes, but only in approximately 50%.
- CT: High resolution scanning will show the 'tramline' appearance of thickened airways, the 'signet-ring' sign of a dilated bronchi viewed end-on next to an artery and mucous plugging of airways. This is the diagnostic investigation of choice.

Histopathology:

- The bronchi have a deranged appearance and there is evidence of pulmonary fibrosis.

Management

The aim is to reduce disease progression by reducing ongoing lung damage. Patients will need to be managed by a multidisciplinary team which should include the doctor, specialist nurse and physiotherapist and should have a self-management plan which includes instructions on how to manage the disease on a daily basis and what to do in the event of an exacerbation.

General management:

- ➢ Treatment of any underlying conditions, and smoking cessation.
- ➢ Immunisation against *Pneumococcus* and *Influenza*.
- ➢ Dietician review to optimise nutrition.

Physiotherapy:

- ➢ Postural drainage – the patient is put in to certain positions and affected lung areas are percussed in order to encourage drainage.
- ➢ Active cycle of breathing techniques.
- ➢ Cough augmentation.
- ➢ General physical exercise.

Medications:

Antibiotics:

- ➢ Especially important in order to break the ongoing cycle of lung damage and recurrent infections. Care should be taken to give these promptly.
- ➢ The exact choice will depend on the results of sputum cultures and local guidelines. Microbiology advice must be sought. If there is no *Pseudomonas* present, it is usual to use a long course of a β-lactam or macrolide, but in cases of pseudomonal infection the usual choice is Ciprofloxacin. Nebulised Colomycin is also used.
- ➢ Long-term antibiotics may be required where patients have frequent exacerbations but should only be instituted on specialist advice.

Bronchodilators:

- ➢ Effectively used in patients with airflow obstruction and recurrent symptoms of wheeze.

Corticosteroids:

- ➢ Required in exacerbations and ongoing therapy in bronchiectasis associated with COPD and asthma.

Surgical treatment

- ➢ Lobectomy is sometimes performed for localised disease.
- ➢ Surgery may also be required for life-threatening haemoptysis.

Further reading and references

- ➢ The British Thoracic Society and Scottish Intercollegiate Guidelines Network (2008). *British Guideline on the Management of Asthma.*
- ➢ British Thoracic Society Cough Guideline Group; a sub-committee of the Standards of Care Committee of the British Thoracic Society (2006). Recommendations for the Management of Cough in Adults. *Thorax*, 61 (Suppl 1) i1–i24.
- ➢ British Thoracic Society Pleural Disease Group, a subgroup of the British Thoracic Society Standards of Care Committee (2003). British Thoracic Society Guidelines for the Management of Spontaneous Pneumothorax. *Thorax*. 58 (Suppl II): ii39–ii52.
- ➢ British Thoracic Society Pneumonia Guidelines Committee (2001). British Thoracic Society Guidelines for the Management of Community Acquired Pneumonia in Adults. *Thorax* 56: (suppl IV).
- ➢ National Institute for Health and Clinical Excellence (2004). *Chronic Obstructive Pulmonary Disease (CG12).*
- ➢ National Institute for Health and Clinical Excellence (2006). *Clinical diagnosis and management of tuberculosis, and measures for its prevention and control. (CG033).*
- ➢ National Institute for Clinical Excellence (2005). *The diagnosis and treatment of lung cancer (CG024).*

DIARRHOEA

Differential Diagnosis

System/Organ	Disease
Intestinal	Inflammatory (ulcerative colitis and Crohn's disease)
	Coeliac disease
	Colonic carcinoma
	Diverticular disease
	Gastroenteritis
	Irritable bowel disease
	Faecal impaction (overflow diarrhoea)
Infective	**Campylobacter jejuni**
	Salmonella spp
	Escherichia coli
	Yersinia enterocolitica
	Clostridium difficile
Pancreatic	**Chronic pancreatitis**
	Pancreatic cancer
	Cystic fibrosis
Other	Thyrotoxicosis
	Carcinoid syndrome
	Drugs such as antibiotics and laxatives
	Artificial enteral feeding

Coeliac disease

Epidemiology

The main cause of malabsorption involving the small intestine in the developed world. Affects 1 in 100 to 1 in 300 of the population in the UK and is slightly more common in the Irish population. The disease can remain subclinical for many years, so although the most common presentation is in early childhood it can present at any time from weaning to old age.

Aetiology

Also known as gluten-induced enteropathy, a malabsorption disorder in which there is damage to the enterocytes of the small intestine as a result of intolerance to dietary gluten.

Abnormalities develop within the proximal small bowel mucosa, which are reversible with the withdrawal of gluten from the patient's diet.

Genetics plays an important role and there is a 10–20% risk of disease development in first degree relatives. 85% of coeliac sufferers possess the HLA B8 antigen, which is present in only 20% of the general population. In those who are genetically susceptible, there is a specific immune reaction to a breakdown product of gluten, triggered by the ingestion of relevant foods. The specific genes involved in coeliac disease have not yet been identified, however, certain MHC class II gene alleles have been found to have a strong association: DR3/DQW 2 and DR7/DQW.

Patients with Down's and Turner's syndromes are at increased risk of developing coeliac disease.

Pathophysiology

Gluten refers to a number of water-insoluble proteins contained in cereal grains. Gliadin is the alcohol-insoluble fraction of this protein in wheat which is responsible for the toxicity and damage caused within the small intestine (the equivalent in rye is secalin and in barley is hardein).

An immunological basis is likely since there is an increased incidence of certain HLA haplotypes. The strong association with HLA-B8 is also seen with dermatitis herpetiformis; a skin disease found in up to 20% of coeliac patients.

There are four main processes thought to be responsible for the underlying pathology of coeliac disease:

Process 1	Direct toxic effect of the breakdown products of gluten upon enterocytes in genetically susceptible individuals.
Process 2	A possible enzyme defect within the enterocytes: also genetically associated, which results in reduced production of peptidase and therefore impaired breakdown of gluten resulting in potentially toxic products available to cause damage to enterocytes.
Process 3	An immune mediated response of mucosa exposed to gluten. There may be deficient IgA production and hence reduced antibody coverage which permits potentially toxic products of gluten to have access to the mucosa. Therefore, patients with hyposplenism and related impairments within the immune system are more susceptible to development of coeliac disease.
Process 4	There may be an association with human adenovirus type 12. Onset of disease may be preceded by an episode of gastroenteritis in susceptible individuals. This accounts for the unpredictable age of onset of disease and newly diagnosed cases in middle aged and even elderly individuals.

Table 3.39: The four main pathological processes involved in coeliac disease.

The pathological changes in coeliac disease can be classified by the Marsh Classification:

Marsh stage 0: Normal mucosa
Marsh stage 1: Increased intra-epithelial lymphocytes
Marsh stage 2: Crypt hypertrophy
Marsh stage 3: Partial or complete villous atrophy
Marsh stage 4: Hypoplasia of the small bowel architecture

Table 3.40: Marsh Classification for coeliac disease.

The proximal small bowel mucosa (duodenum and proximal jejunum) is predominantly involved with progressive reduction in severity towards the ileum. The result is malabsorption, particularly in the proximal small intestine:

- Sugars, fatty acids, monoglycerides and amino acids.
- Iron and calcium absorption are particularly affected since their absorption is predominantly in the proximal small intestine.
- Folic acid, vitamin C and B12 are mainly absorbed in the jejunum and ileum and so their absorption is only affected in advanced disease.

Production of hormones from the small intestine may be deficient and hence there is a decrease in pancreatic secretion and bile flow, which accounts for the malabsorption of fat.

There is an increased risk of lymphoma (100 fold) or carcinoma, greatest in those who are non-compliant or present late in life, in particular small bowel T-cell lymphoma (very rare in non-coeliac patients). Metabolic bone disease (osteomalacia and osteoporosis) is found in up to 25% of patients. Calcium malabsorption results in increased parathyroid hormone secretion, causing an increase in bone turnover and cortical bone loss.

Key features in history/examination

- May be asymptomatic.
- Diarrhoea – ask specifically about steatorrhoea (how easy is the stool to flush away?).
- Abdominal discomfort/pain.
- Flatulence and bloating.
- Weight loss.
- Look for dermatitis herpetiformis, which is a highly pruritic subepidermal bullous eruption typically affecting the extensors such as the elbow and the buttocks.
- Menstrual disturbances.
- In children may see features of failure to thrive.
- May present with symptoms of anaemia – either iron deficiency or folate deficiency (fatigue, pallor, glossitis, aphthous ulceration).
- Rarely vitamin D deficiency may cause fractures.
- Past or family history of atopy or autoimmune conditions such as thyroid disease, type 1 diabetes, Sjögren syndrome and primary biliary cirrhosis.
- Family history of coeliac disease.
- Neurological symptoms are rare and include seizures, ataxia and peripheral neuropathy.

On examination:

- Oedema
- Bruising
- Evidence of weight loss.
- Abdominal examination reveals pain and distension as well as bloating.
- Neurological examination reveals peripheral neuropathy and ataxia.
- Looking for dermatitis herpetiformis – a highly pruritic subepidermal bullous eruption typically affecting the extensors, such as the elbow, and the buttocks.

Investigations

Blood tests:

- Full blood count (FBC) and blood film: May show anaemia. Iron deficiency is a result of malabsorption of iron and gives a low MCV. Folate deficiency is more likely and results in an increased MCV. The blood film may show a dimorphic picture, plus hypersegmented polymorphonuclear leucocytes, all indicative of anaemia.
- Prothrombin time: may be prolonged with vitamin K deficiency, however, this is uncommon.
- Biochemistry: calcium and phosphate may be low and alkaline phosphatase levels may be raised, indicative of osteomalacia. Hypoalbuminaemia from protein malabsorption. Low folate and vitamin B12.
- Tissue transglutaminase (tTGA): this is the primary diagnostic blood test for coeliac disease. It has a 90% sensitivity and 97% specificity. There is a false negative result with IgA deficiency, so IgA levels must be measured concurrently.
- Endomyseal antibodies (IgA): a high specificity (about 100%) and sensitivity (90%) for the diagnosis of untreated coeliac disease. Used if the tTGA test is equivocal.

Endoscopy:

- Lesions are diagnostic and can range from an increased number of intra-epithelial lymphocytes to total villous atrophy.
- To confirm the mucosal lesion is gluten-induced, three biopsies may sometimes be required, i.e. before treatment, after gluten withdrawal, and after re-challenge with gluten.

Imaging:

- Small bowel barium follow-through: this may show evidence of dilatation of bowel loops as well as changes in the intestinal mucosa, such as coarsening. It is useful in terms of excluding other causes of malabsorption for instance terminal ileum Crohn's disease. It is also helpful to detect the development of any complications such as bowel strictures.
- DEXA scan: If osteoporosis is suspected.

Other:

- Absorption tests: these are rarely performed. Fat malabsorption can be confirmed by measuring the fat content of the patient's stools over a 3-day period whilst they are on a diet consisting of 100 g of fat daily. Less than 6 g of fat is normal and hence a higher content is indicative of malabsorption.

Management

➤ Patients require a detailed explanation of their diagnosis and its implications. This includes the implications for family members of a positive test.

➤ Patients should also be given information regarding support groups such as the Coeliac Society.

3. Medicine

➤ The mainstay of management is adherence to a strict gluten-free diet (see below), which must be emphasised to patients. This results in rapid improvement in clinical features (within days/weeks) and intestinal morphology (3–12 months).

➤ A dietician should be involved in advising and supporting dietary requirements.

➤ Non-compliance is the main cause of treatment failure.

Gluten-free diet:

➤ Patients need to permanently remove gluten-containing foods from their diet. Gluten is not a constituent of rice and maize, which are therefore permitted.

➤ This results in complete remission and protects against the potential complications of coeliac disease.

Other:

➤ Dermatitis herpetiformis usually resolves upon withdrawal of gluten from the diet.

    o   If there is no clinical improvement, treatment with Dapsone (50–200 mg daily) or sulphonamides may be commenced – this treats the skin symptoms and not the bowel.

    o   Dapsone carries a risk of liver damage, methaemoglobinaemia and aplastic anaemia, and so regular blood monitoring is required.

➤ Small bowel T cell lymphoma. Treatment is usually with surgery and resection, followed by chemotherapy and radiotherapy.

'Unresponsive' coeliac disease:

➤ Occurs in some patients where, despite compliance with a strict diet, there is no clinical improvement.

➤ Treatment with corticosteroids or immunosuppressants may induce remission.

➤ A small bowel biopsy is required after 3 months to confirm improvement.

Prognosis:

➤ In most patients prognosis is excellent with compliance to a strict gluten-free diet and patients can therefore lead a predominantly normal life.

➤ Lymphoma significantly increases the mortality.

Chronic Pancreatitis

A chronic inflammatory condition of the pancreas associated with irreversible destruction of the structure and function of the pancreas.

Epidemiology

Estimated that around 0.04% of the UK population are affected. There is a strong male predominance.

Aetiology

Most common causes are as follows:

Excess alcohol usage (60%)	• Usually presents after an average of 18 years of alcohol use in men and 11 years in women with a consumption of over 150 g per day. • The risk is also increased in those who smoke, have raised lipids and have chronic renal failure.
Idiopathic causes (30%)	• Two distinct population groups: younger – aged 15 to 30 years – and older – aged 50 to 70 years.
Gallstones	• Associated with the consumption of a high fat and high protein diet. • May enhance the damaging effects of alcohol.
Others	• Malnutrition • Cystic fibrosis • Hyperparathyroidism and hypercalcaemia. • Hereditary (autosomal dominant). • Autoimmune • Recurrent acute pancreatitis. • Ischaemic

Table 3.41: The principal causes of chronic pancreatitis.

Pathophysiology

A number of processes are proposed, each of which leads on to the chronic disease:

• Protein plugs deposit within the ducts of the pancreas.

• Mechanical obstruction by intra-ductal stones.

• Toxins or recurrent episodes of acute pancreatitis causing inflammation and fibrosis.

There is resultant duct dilatation and atrophy of the acinar cells. Widespread fibrosis increases and surrounds the pancreatic ducts and eventually, there are only few functioning acinar and islet cells. The pancreatic ducts are significantly dilated. The protein plugs become calcified and there is resultant formation of calculi.

Complications of chronic pancreatitis result from this inflammatory process and destruction of pancreatic function, and include:

• Chronic abdominal pain.

• Malabsorption.

• Diabetes mellitus.

• Pseudocyst formation.

• Stricture of the common bile duct.

• Bowel obstruction.

• Ascites.

• Aneurysm of the arteries which surround the pancreas.

• Thrombosis of the splenic vein causing portal hypertension.

Key features in the history/examination

- Most common presentation is with recurrent epigastric pain which radiates to the back, is often severe and described as 'deep'.
- Occasionally it can present with obstructive jaundice or diabetes.
- Bloating.
- Anorexia and weight loss.
- Steatorrhoea (results when the pancreatic lipase production is reduced by more than 90%).
- Past history of acute pancreatitis, gallstones or autoimmune diseases.
- Alcohol consumption.

On examination:

- There may be no specific signs.
- Epigastric or general abdominal tenderness.
- The patient may appear thin and wasted.
- Look for signs of anaemia and jaundice.

Investigations

Blood tests:

- Protein and albumin levels: may be reduced indicating ongoing malabsorption.
- Serum amylase: is normal or only modestly raised.
- LFTs may reveal a pattern of obstructive jaundice.
- Check calcium (and PTH if indicated).
- Fasting glucose or glucose tolerance test may be indicated if diabetes is suspected.
- IgG levels: if autoimmune suspected (will be raised).

Imaging:

- Abdominal X-ray: may reveal calcification of the pancreas.
- CT abdomen: will illustrate an irregular, calcified and fibrosed gland. May show complications e.g. pseudocyst.

Other:

- Level of fat in faeces test: this is rarely performed. It gives indication of the pancreatic function. If the fat content in the faeces is higher than 6 g in a 72 hour period it implies there is true steatorrhoea.
- Endoscopic retrograde cholangio-pancreatography (ERCP) or magnetic retrograde cholangio-pancreatography (MRCP): Outlines the pancreatic ducts and may show dilatation and strictures as well as pancreatic duct stones.
- Endoscopic ultrasound: the best way to visualise the pancreas in skilled hands.

Management

No curative treatment – usually supportive management only.

- Patients are advised to avoid the consumption of alcohol. This needs to be in conjunction with a multidisciplinary approach to assist with abstinence.
- Pain control tends to be very difficult in these patients.
  - Use the WHO pain ladder.
  - May require referral to a specialist pain team.
  - Pancreatic duct stenting or coeliac-plexus block may help with symptom management.
  - In those who are very severe, surgery may be required for partial or complete resection of the pancreas.
- Complications are managed conservatively with the aim of optimising symptom control.

Complications:

- Pancreatic pseudocysts are most common – occur in around 10% of patients.
  - Only requires treatment if large in size.
  - Tends to cause an increase in pain and associated nausea and vomiting.
  - Can be managed conservatively with aspiration and follow-up with ultrasound examination or definitive treatment with surgical resection may be indicated.
- Pancreatic ascites or pleural effusions.
  - Disruption of the pancreatic duct causes a communication between the pancreatic duct and peritoneal cavity.
  - The fluid will have a high level of amylase.
- Pancreatic enzyme replacements such as Creon or Pancrex V will aid in control of the symptoms which result from the inadequate exocrine function of the pancreas.
- Dietician to advise on diet and supplementation:
  - A low-fat diet (limit fat intake to 45 g per day).
  - High protein and calorie intake.
  - Fat soluble vitamin supplements.
- Patients who develop diabetes will require treatment usually with insulin and review by diabetic specialist.
- Gallstone removal is indicated if it is recognised as the causative factor.
- Surgical treatment is indicated to treat obstruction of the duodenum or biliary tree or to remove pseudocysts.
- Future therapies include pancreatic transplantation.

Prognosis:

- Improved in those who abstain from alcohol, but overall there is a 30% 10-year mortality.

Carcinoid syndrome

Epidemiology

Around 2 in 100,000 individuals are affected by a carcinoid tumour. Around 10% of small bowel carcinoid tumours result in carcinoid syndrome. It usually affects individuals from middle age onwards, with the median onset in the 6th decade.

Aetiology

The precise aetiology of carcinoid tumours is unknown. It can form a part of multiple endocrine neoplasia type 1, an autosomal dominant condition which results in the tendency to form tumours involving the endocrine organs.

Pathophysiology

Carcinoid tumours are derived from the enterochromaffin (APUD) cells in the bowel. The most common sites are the distal small bowel and the appendix. The next most common site for carcinoid tumours is the bronchus, but less than 5% of bronchial carcinomas are carcinoid.

Only 2% bronchial carcinoid tumours result in the carcinoid syndrome. The cells of the carcinoid tumour produce serotonin (5-hydroxytryptamine (5 HT)), bradykinin, histamine and tachykinins in addition to prostaglandins. Serotonin is responsible for the symptoms of diarrhoea and the cardiac abnormalities. Bradykinin is responsible for the skin flushing as it causes vasodilatation, bronchospasm and increased bowel motility.

These agents, when released from the primary tumour in the bowel, are inactivated by first pass metabolism in the liver. The symptoms of carcinoid syndrome only become apparent when this metabolism is compromised, for example when a carcinoid tumour metastasises to the liver.

Key features in history/examination

It is often asymptomatic, found incidentally in an excised appendix. The following are the most frequently encountered features:

- Flushing is the most frequent symptom. It is caused by a transient vasodilation causing reddening predominantly of the face, head and neck. Initially it lasts only a few minutes but can last significantly longer as the disease progresses. It can be precipitated by exertion, excitement or alcohol. If this occurs chronically then telangectasia can form in the affected areas.
- Most patients have recurrent abdominal pain and watery diarrhoea.
- Bronchospasm results in symptoms of dyspnoea and wheezing.
- May occasionally present with a complication such as intestinal obstruction, perforation or haemorrhage.
- Other common signs are palpitations, hypotension, fever, fatigue, dizziness and nausea and vomiting.
- Weight loss is usual in these patients.
- Symptoms can be associated with the primary tumour, such as recurrent haemoptysis or intermittent episodes of diarrhoea.
- 50% of patients have cardiac abnormalities involving the right side of the heart particularly tricuspid regurgitation. This may result in right ventricular hypertrophy and failure.
- Bronchial carcinoid affects the left side of the heart.
- There may be irregular hepatomegaly on examination of the abdomen.

Investigation

Blood tests:

- FBC
- U&Es
- LFTs
- clotting screen

Imaging:

- Ultrasound scan: will reveal any liver metastases.
- CXR and/or CT scan of the abdomen/thorax: can help to reveal the primary tumour.

Histopathology:

- Biopsy of the primary tumour may be possible.
- A liver biopsy to confirm the presence of metastases if necessary.

Other:

- ECG and echocardiogram may be useful to reveal involvement of the heart.
- Barium studies: can sometimes be useful to delineate the tumour.
- Radioisotope scanning with radio-labelled Octreotide can localise carcinoid tumours.
- Urine: the metabolism of serotonin results in the production of 5-hydroxyindoleacetic acid (5 HIAA), which is present in a significant amount in the urine. It is measured over a 24-hour period whilst the patient is kept on a low serotonin diet (exclusion of tomatoes, bananas and walnuts from the diet). The normal range should be 2 mg to 10 mg in a 24-hour period.

Management

Medical management:

➢ IV fluid resuscitation if necessary for severe diarrhoea.
➢ Octreotide is an octapeptide somatostatin analogue which prevents the production of a number of hormones from the bowel.
   o Given subcutaneously at 200 micrograms three times per day.
   o Relieves symptoms of flushing and diarrhoea.
   o Occasionally may inhibit tumour growth as well.
➢ Methysergide is a serotonin antagonist and is given at 1 mg to 2 mg four times a day.
➢ Anti-diarrhoeal agents can provide effective symptomatic relief.
➢ Methyldopa and corticosteroids can provide relief of symptoms such as flushing.
➢ Chemotherapy has a limited role in management – usually advanced disease.

Surgical management:

➢ Surgical resection of a localised carcinoid tumour is occasionally performed. This is only an option if the tumour is detected prior to the development of the syndrome.

➢ Resection of hepatic metastases may also be of benefit.

Prognosis:

➢ Carcinoid tumours tend to be slow-growing.

➢ Despite having metastases in carcinoid syndrome, the 5-year survival is estimated at 40% and the 10-year survival is 15%.

Gastroenteritis

Epidemiology

Gastroenteritis is a common condition affecting 20% of the population in the UK. Groups at increased risk include the immunocompromised, those at the extremes of age, as well as travellers. Infective diarrhoea is a major cause of mortality in the developing world with an estimated 2–3 million deaths per year in the under 5s.

Aetiology

Bacteria and viruses account for the majority of cases. See Table 3.42. Infection is commonly through contaminated food (such as meat, milk or egg) and water. Alternatively ingestion of organic or inorganic toxins can also cause symptoms of gastroenteritis.

Pathophysiology

The effects of infection within the gut depend largely on the following factors:

• The extent of adherence of organisms to surface enterocytes

• Production of enterotoxins – these activate secretion of water

Organism	Source	Incubation period	Symptoms	Diagnosis	Recovery time
Clostridium difficile	Release of spores from the bacteria found on contaminated toilets and floor – person to person spread or via hands of healthcare workers	1–10 days	Bloating, constipation, severe diarrhoea and abdominal pain	Stool culture for the c.diff toxin	Up to 30 days
Norovirus	Spread by aerosol route, person to person, or faecally contaminated food/water	24–48 hours	Nausea, vomiting, diarrhoea and abdominal pain. Lethragy, weakness, myalgia and headache may occur	Norovirus RNA in stool	Up to 60 hours
Staphylococcus aureus	Contaminated food, e.g. meat	2–6 hrs	Abdominal pain, diarrhoea, vomiting, dehydration	Culture the organism in stool or food	Usually a few hours
Bacillus cereus spores	Found in food e.g. rice	1–6 hrs	Diarrhoea, vomiting, dehydration	Culture the organism in stool or food	Usually rapid
E. coli	Uncooked beef and raw cow's milk	12–48 hrs	Watery diarrhoea, +/– haemorrhagic colitis, haemolytic uraemic syndrome	Stool culture	10–12 days
Salmonella	Found in meat, eggs, poultry	12–24 hrs	Abrupt onset of diarrhoea, vomiting, fever, septicaemia	Stool culture	From 2–14 days
Campylobacter jejuni	Found in milk, poultry, & water	2–5 days	Bloody diarrhoea, abdominal pain, malaise and fever	Stool culture	3–5 days
Shigella	Found in contaminated food	2–3 days	Sudden onset of watery, bloody diarrhoea	Stool culture	3–4 days
Rotavirus	Found in food or water	1–7 days	Diarrhoea, vomiting, fever, malaise	Stool culture	3–5 days
Clostridium perfringens spores	Found in food & survive boiling	8–22 hrs	Watery diarrhoea and cramping abdominal pain	Culture the organism in stool or food	2–3 days
Clostridium botulinum	Found in canned or bottled food & survive boiling	18–36 hrs	Brief episode of diarrhoea/ vomiting & paralysis due to neuromuscular blockade	Toxin found in food or faeces	10–14 days

Table 3.42: Causes of gastroenteritis and associated symptoms.

3. Medicine

and electrolytes from the small bowel resulting in watery diarrhoea.

- Once adhered, organisms can invade the intestinal mucosa and may cause bloody diarrhoea (dysentery).
- Organisms such as *clostridium difficile* and *shigella* multiply within the bowel lumen and directly invade the epithelial cells of the colon. Hence, they cause the production of cytotoxins which cause damage to the mucosa and cause inflammation.

Key features in the history/examination

- Symptoms tend to be of sudden onset, and can feature diarrhoea with or without vomiting as well as general malaise and cramping abdominal pain.
- Watery or bloody diarrhoea.
- The duration of symptoms, as well as the frequency and description of the vomitus and stool is important in diagnosis.
  o The Bristol stool chart can be used to record the types of stool the patient has and hence the progression of the illness and response to treatment (refer to Table 3.43).
- Note the recent food and fluid intake of the patient as well as how it was cooked, the time until onset of symptoms.
- Details of any medication they are taking can be important.
- Any other affected family members.
- Travel history and occupation.
- Any activities such as swimming, canoeing, diving etc are significant.
- Any systemic illnesses eg diabetes, hypothyroidism.

Bristol Stool Chart:

Type	Description
Type 1	Separate hard lumps shaped like pellets, difficult to pass stool
Type 2	Sausage shaped small lumps, some difficulty in passing stool
Type 3	Sausage shaped lumps which are hard with cracks on the surface
Type 4	Smooth, sausage shaped and long pieces of stool
Type 5	Small soft blobs which are well-defined and easy to pass
Type 6	Soft fluffy stool with irregular edges and mushy in nature
Type 7	Watery and liquid stool

Table 3.43: Bristol stool chart.

On examination one can expect:

- The patient may have fevers, sweating, and tenderness on examination of the abdomen.
- It is important to assess for the degree of dehydration and look for signs of shock.

Class 1 10–15% fluid loss 750 mls	Class 2 15–30% fluid loss 1500 mls	Class 3 30–40% fluid loss 2000 mls	Class 4 > 40% fluid loss > 2000 mls
Physiological compensation Thirst and dry mouth Reduced appetite Dry skin	Postural hypotension Flushed skin Concentrated urine Fatigue or weakness Rigors	Hypotension Tachycardia Tachypnoea Reduced sweating Reduced urine output Fever Increasing fatigue Muscle cramps Headache Nausea Reduced skin turgor Cool peripheries	Marked hypotension Vomiting Tachycardia Visual disturbance Confusion Difficulty in breathing Seizures Chest and abdominal pain Reduced level of consciousness

Table 3.44: Symptoms associated with varying degrees of shock.

Investigations

Blood tests:

- FBC, U&E, LFT, CRP, Amylase. There may be an increased white cell count and CRP, but this will not distinguish infective diarrhoea from an inflammatory cause. Reduced renal function will be seen if the patient is dehydrated.

Imaging:

- Abdominal X-ray

Other:

- Stool sample: microscopy and culture, *C. difficile* toxin and ova, cysts and parasites if indicated.
- If the patient is from an institution or day care or an outbreak is suspected the food source can be cultured to identify the causative organism.

Management:

➢ Supportive care is the mainstay as most cases resolve spontaneously within 1 to 6 days and is based around symptom control and ensuring adequate hydration.

➢ Isolation in a side room and barrier nursing to minimise risk of transmission to other patients and staff.

➢ Good hand hygiene should be emphasised.

➢ Small and frequent volumes of oral fluids (such as Dioralyte) should be encouraged if possible.

➢ IV fluids if the patient cannot tolerate oral intake or has significant dehydration.

➢ Anti-emetics.

> Antibiotics should only be prescribed as per hospital protocol or in discussion with the microbiologist. For example oral Metronidazole or Vancomycin for *C.difficile* and Ciprofloxacin (for travellers) with *campylobacter* and *shigella*.

> If the symptoms are persistent further differentials of diarrhoea must be considered

> Local notification procedures should be activated, with contact tracing and investigation of outbreaks.

Complications:

> Haemolytic-ureamic syndrome (HUS) after *enterohaemorrhagic E Coli*.

> Guillain-Barré syndrome after *campylobacter*.

> Aseptic arthritis after *salmonella*, *shigella* and *yersinia*.

> Irritable bowel syndrome is increasingly recognised post-infective complication.

Prevention:

> Typhoid and cholera vaccination if visiting endemic areas

> Good food and hand hygiene should be emphasised, especially when travelling abroad, avoiding unboiled or unbottled water, ice cubes and fresh salads.

Further reading and references

> Coeliac UK. www.coeliac.org.uk

> British Society of Gastroenterology (2007). *Guidelines for osteoporosis in inflammatory bowel disease and coeliac disease.*

> National Centre for Health and Clinical Excellence (2009). *Coeliac Disease (CG061).*

> Lewis SJ, Heaton KW (1997). Stool form scale as a useful guide to intestinal transit time. Scand. J. Gastroenterol. 32(9): 920–4.

FALLS

Differential diagnosis

System/Organ	Disease
Multisystem causes for falls	**Cardiac syncope**
	Neurally-mediated syncope
	Orthostatic (postural) hypotension
	Carotid sinus hypersensitivity
	Neurological
	Musculoskeletal
	Environmental
	Drugs
	Urinary incontinence
	Acute medical illness
	Accidental 'mechanical' fall

General principles of falls assessment

Falls are a very common occurrence, especially in the elderly population. They are one of the four 'geriatric giants' and require a careful and thoughtful assessment.

The definition of a fall, as used by National Institute for Health and Clinical Excellence (NICE), is 'an event whereby an individual comes to rest on the ground or another lower level with or without loss of consciousness.'

Falls often occur in hospital in-patients and FY doctors are likely to find that they are asked by nursing staff to review patients who have fallen. All patients deemed to be at risk of falling should have a falls risk assessment completed on admission. These should be reviewed regularly and updated should the patient's conditions alter. An example of a falls risk assessment tool is STRATIFY (Oliver et al, 1997), however there are other assessments that may be in use. As a FY doctor you should familiarise yourself with your Trust's risk assessment tool and the care that should be implemented to ensure patient safety. Once you have reviewed a patient who has fallen you should ensure that you document your findings in the medical notes and complete the necessary part of the Trust incident form.

Epidemiology

The incidence increases with age. Approximately 30% of the over-60 age group experience falls each year rising to 50% of the over-80s. Hospital inpatients and those living in institutional care are at increased risk compared to those living at home.

Falls have a number of consequences. The most common is physical injury directly relating to the falls. Around 40–60% of falls lead to an injury. The majority are only minor, but 5% of falls result in fractures (1% leading to hip fracture) and an additional 5% result in a non-fracture major injury.

Aetiology

There are a number of causes of falls, but it is common for there to be a multi-factorial aetiology with number of contributory causes, each of which needs to be identified and treated if possible.

Syncope:

- Cardiac Causes
  - Structural
  - Arrhythmic
- Orthostatic hypotension
- Neurally-mediated
- Carotid sinus hypersensitivity

Musculoskeletal:

- Arthritis
- Muscular deconditioning

Urinary incontinence

Neurological:

- Seizures
- Dementia or delirium
- Transient ischaemic attack (TIA) (focal neurological symptoms at the time of fall)
- Previous stroke with residual unilateral weakness
- Visual impairment (e.g. cataract, macular degeneration)
- Reduced vestibulo-ocular reflexes
- Vestibular dysfunction
- Peripheral neuropathy (e.g. diabetes)
- Normal pressure hydrocephalus

Environmental:

- Loose carpet/rugs
- Poor lighting
- Poor footwear
- Elderly and living alone

Accidental 'mechanical' fall

Drugs:

- Polypharmacy (4 or more medications)
- Psychoactive medications
- Alcohol

Acute medical illness:

- Sepsis
- Acute myocardial infarction (MI)
- Pulmonary embolus
- Aortic dissection

Pathophysiology

The pathophysiology is dependent on the aetiology.

Key features in the history/examination

- Circumstances leading up to the fall:
  - Where was the fall?
  - What was the patient doing at the time?
  - Was there any warning?
  - What preceding symptoms were felt?
  - Did the patient become pale?
- The fall:
  - Any loss of consciousness? If so for how long?
  - Any evidence of seizure activity?
  - Any injuries sustained?
- After the fall:
  - How were they after the fall?

- Where they confused/disorientated?
- Did they display signs of focal weakness?
- How long did these symptoms last?
- How long were they on the floor for?
- A witness account is invaluable
- Previous falls
- Previous cardiac history
- Past medical, drug and social history:
  - Ask specifically about night-time sedatives and number of episodes of nocturia as these are commonly overlooked as causes of nocturnal falls.
  - Any previous fractures or risk factors for fracture (e.g. steroid use).
  - Family history of sudden death, especially if the patient is young, should raise the suspicion of long QT syndrome.
- Mini mental state examination (MMSE) if evidence of cognitive impairment
- A full examination is required, but especially detailed cardiac, neurological (cranial and peripheral nerves) and musculoskeletal examinations are important.
  - Check for and document any pressure sores
- Correctly perform postural blood pressure (BP) measurement
  - Patient is relaxed and supine for at least 5 minutes
  - Measure BP
  - Stand patient
  - Measure BP at 1, 3 and 5 minutes after standing
  - Record any concurrent symptoms
- Level of consciousness
- Examine gait
- Timed Get up and Go Test: time the patient standing up from a chair, walking three meters (in a line), turning around, walking back to chair and sitting down. Less than ten seconds is considered normal and greater than 20 seconds is considered abnormal.

Investigation

Blood tests:

- FBC
- U&Es
- LFTs
- Bone profile
- TFT
- Clotting
- Creatinine kinase (CK): To exclude rhabdomyolysis if has been lying for a while
- Troponin: If MI suspected

Imaging:

- Chest X-ray (CXR)

Others:

- ECG

Further investigations will be determined by the history and examination findings, but may include:

Blood tests:

- Synacthen test: If Addison's disease likely

Imaging:

- CT brain – in the acute setting this may be required if a head injury has been sustained (eg after a fall downstairs). The NICE head injury guidelines should be adhered to.
- Dual energy X-ray absorptiometry (DEXA) scan

Other:

- 24 hour tape/7 day event recorder/Loop recorder: If arrhythmia considered likely
- EEG
- EMG
- Tilt test
- Carotid sinus massage
- Echocardiograph: if clinical evidence of valvular disease or signs of cardiac failure.

Management

- ➤ Acute management consists of identification and treatment of physical injuries.
- ➤ A to E assessment.
- ➤ Close attention should be paid to potential fractures, especially C-spine and neck of femur. All fractures should be reviewed by orthopaedic surgeons (with the exception of pubic ramus).
- ➤ Precise management will depend on the cause.
- ➤ Most acute NHS Trusts have a falls clinic, usually with referral criteria. Patients who meet the criteria should be referred to this clinic if they are being discharged home.
- ➤ Physiotherapy can help improve strength, mobility and balance.
- ➤ Occupational Therapy may be required if environmental risk factors are found.
- ➤ Consider need for primary or secondary osteoporosis prevention.
  - o Use FRAX, the World Health Organisation (WHO) fracture risk assessment tool (see references and further reading) which will give the ten-year risk for major osteoporotic and hip fractures.
  - o Use the linked National Osteoporosis Guideline Group tool to determine risk and therefore management:
    - ▪ **Low Risk** – lifestyle advice
    - ▪ **Medium Risk** – measure bone mineral density

- ▪ **High Risk** – Treat with bisphosphonate and calcium/vitamin D supplementation

Prognosis:

- ➤ The majority of falls do not cause significant immediate or long-term consequences. However there are a number of serious sequelae directly resulting from falls.
- ➤ Falls are the commonest cause of injury-related death in the elderly.
- ➤ Injuries can result in permanent reduction in mobility, which has a number of consequences:
  - o Loss of independence
  - o Social isolation with concomitant increase in loneliness and depression
  - o Increased risk of institutionalised care
  - o Anxiety and fear of falling

Syncope

Syncope is a symptom and not a diagnosis. It is a transient loss of consciousness, with a rapid onset and rapid recovery, due to transient cerebral hypoperfusion.

Epidemiology

Accounts for 3–5% of Accident & Emergency (A&E) attendances and incidence increases with age.

Aetiology

- Cardiac causes
  - o Structural
    - ▪ Valvular heart disease
    - ▪ Atrial myxoma
    - ▪ Cardiac tamponade
  - o Arrhythmic
    - ▪ Tachyarrhythmias
    - ▪ Bradyarrhythmias
    - ▪ Tachy-Brady or sick sinus syndrome
    - ▪ AV nodal conduction delay
    - ▪ Long QT interval
    - ▪ Pacemaker malfunction
- Orthostatic hypotension
- Neurally-mediated causes
  - o Vasovagal (faint)
  - o Situational – e.g. cough, micturition syncope
- Carotid sinus hypersensitivity

Pathophysiology

Cardiac causes for syncope are due to a reduction in cardiac output e.g. reduced rate in bradyarrhythmias and outflow obstruction in aortic stenosis. Neurally mediated causes lead to inappropriate vasodilatation.

Key features in the history/examination

- Classically a short prodrome with the patient becoming pale.
- Short period of loss of consciousness.
- Beware 'convulsive syncope' when a short burst of myoclonic jerks is witnessed. This is commonly mis-diagnosed as epilepsy.
- The elderly frequently have poor recall of events and may not remember a period of loss of consciousness. An eyewitness account should be sought if at all possible.
- See examination under 'general principles' section.

Investigations

See investigations under 'general principles' section. If the syncope remains unexplained after initial investigations, it is important to perform tilt table testing and carotid sinus massage.

Tilt test:

- Precise protocols vary.
  - The patient lies on the table and is strapped in place (to avoid injury)
  - The patient is attached to non-invasive monitoring of pulse and BP
  - Initially the patient lies horizontal for at least 10 minutes
  - A head-up tilt, usually of 60 degrees, is applied and the patient monitored for at least 20–40 minutes
  - Sublingual glyceryl trinitrate (GTN) may be given to try to stimulate symptoms
- A drop in pulse, BP (or both) associated with symptoms is considered a positive test

Carotid sinus massage:

- Used to diagnose carotid sinus hypersensitivity
- A firm massage of each side of the neck over the carotid sinus for five seconds.
- Performed supine and in the head-up tilt position
- Contra-indicated if a carotid bruit is heard or has had a recent stroke
- Cardioinhibitory response: More than three seconds of asystole
- Vasodepressor response: Drop of more than 50 mmHg BP
- A mixed response is also possible

Management

- Will depend on the cause
- Structural heart disease and arrhythmias may need cardiology referral

- A symptomatic three-second asystole on cardiac monitoring warrants referral for consideration of cardiac pacemaker insertion.
- Avoiding known triggers of vasovagal syncope.
- There are driving restrictions on patients with syncope and patients should be advised of these.

Orthostatic (postural) hypotension

Orthostatic (postural) hypotension is defined as drop of 20 mmHg or more in standing systolic BP or 10 mmHg or more in standing diastolic BP.

Epidemiology

Prevalence increases with age and is reported to be between 5 and 30% in the elderly. This wide variation reflects differences in evaluation methods, definitions and populations studied. One of the commonest causes of syncope in hospital practice, seen both as a presenting diagnosis but also developing during the admission. Must be considered as a cause of a fall on the ward. It is associated with an increased risk of falls and fractures.

Aetiology

Drug therapy:

This is the commonest cause of orthostatic hypotension. Drugs include:

- Anti-hypertensives: Beta-blockers, calcium-channel blockers ACE-inhibitors and alpha-blockers
- Diuretics
- Vasodilators: nitrates
- Antidepressants: tricyclic antidepressants, selective serotonin reuptake inhibitors (SSRIs)
- Anti-parkinsonian medication

Neurogenic causes:

- Primary autonomic failure: Parkinson's disease, Shy-Drager syndrome (combination of multisystem atrophy with autonomic failure).
- Secondary autonomic failure: Diabetes mellitus.
- Spinal cord lesions (syringobulbia, syringomyelia, cord transection, transverse myelitis, amyloid).

Volume depletion causes:

- Fluid loss: Acute haemorrhage, diarrhoea
- Sepsis
- Addison's disease

Pathophysiology

On standing there is rapid displacement of about 10% of the blood volume from the thorax to the lower body. The normal physiological response to maintain BP involves the neuroendocrine system, baroreflex function and beta-adrenergic responses. With increasing age these responses are decreased resulting in a fall in BP on standing.

Progressive orthostatic hypotension is characterised by a slow progressive decrease in systolic BP with a compensatory increase in heart rate on assuming the upright posture. Symptoms tend to occur after a few minutes of standing rather than immediately. It is mainly seen in the elderly and is associated with other co-morbidites and vasoactive drugs.

Key features in the history/examination

- Patients may be asymptomatic.
- Symptoms on, or soon after standing, including dizziness, visual disturbances and feeling light-headed.
- Unexplained falls.
- Drug history, especially those listed above and any recent changes.
- Correctly perform postural BP measurement:
  o Patient is relaxed and supine for at least 5 minutes
  o Measure BP
  o Stand patient
  o Measure BP at 1, 3 and 5 minutes after standing
  o Record any concurrent symptoms
- Postural changes are usually most marked in the morning.

Investigations

As for syncope.

- Tilt table testing is a useful tool if the diagnosis is unclear.

Management

- ➤ Stop any predisposing drugs if possible
- ➤ Ensure adequate hydration
- ➤ Drug therapy
  o Fludrocortisone (a mineralocorticoid). Fluid retention and hypertension are side effects.
  o Midrodine (an alpha agonist) has shown promising results in small studies but its use is limited by systemic vasoconstriction and hypertension.
  o Desmopressin (DDAVP) may be useful in patients with autonomic failure but hyponatraemia may limit its use.
- ➤ Non-pharmacological treatments
  o Encourage fluid intake
  o Encourage caffeine intake
  o Head-up tilt on the bed
  o Physiotherapy with balance classes
- ➤ Advise the patients to avoid
  o Suddenly standing up
  o Alcohol
  o Hot baths

Further reading and references

- ➤ Drivers Medical Group, DVLA, Swansea. For Medical Practitioners. (2009) *At a glance guide to the current medical standards of fitness to drive.*
- ➤ European Society of Cardiology (2004) Task Force Report. Guidelines on Management (Diagnosis and Treatment) of Syncope – Update 2004. Europace 6: 467–537
- ➤ National Institute for Health and Clinical Excellence (2004). *Falls: the assessment and prevention of falls in older people CG021.*
- ➤ National Institute for Health and Clinical Excellence. (2007) *Head injury: triage, assessment, investigation and early management of head injury in infants, children and adults: partial update of clinical guideline 4. CG056.*
- ➤ Oliver, D, Britton, M, Seed, P, et al. (1997) Development and evaluation of evidence-based risk assessment tool (STRATIFY) to predict which elderly patients will fall. *BMJ* 315: 1049–53
- ➤ World Health Organisation (2004). *WHO Scientific Group on the Assessment of Osteoporosis at Primary Health Care Level.*
- ➤ WHO Fracture Risk Assessment Tool http://www.shef.ac.uk/FRAX

FEVER

Differential diagnosis

Cause	Disease
Bacterial infection	Meningitis
	Pneumonia
	Urinary sepsis
	Infective endocarditis
	Staphylococcal toxic shock syndrome
Viral infection	Influenza
	Glandular fever
Fungal infection	**Aspergillosis**
	Candida albicans
	Cryptococcus neoformans
	Pneumocystis jiroveci
Immunocompromised	**Brucellosis**
	Cryptosporidium
	Toxoplasma gondii
Non-infective	Rheumatological diseases
	Malignancy (e.g. lymphoma)
	Transfusion reaction
	Rarer causes e.g. familial Mediterranean fever
Other	**Malaria**

A general approach to sepsis

Epidemiology

Sepsis is the body's response to infection and can range greatly in severity. Severe sepsis is still a leading cause of mortality,

3. Medicine

but good evidence shows that early goal-directed therapy can be instrumental in reducing this. In 1992 the Surviving Sepsis Campaign was launched to highlight this and many resources are available at www.survivingsepsis.org.

Sepsis is very common in in-patients and severe sepsis has an incidence of 1 in 200,000 per year. Mortality in severe sepsis varies widely (25–80%) with the greatest mortality in the elderly as well as those who are immunocompromised and have a chronic underlying disease.

Definitions:

Bacteraemia:

* A 'positive' blood culture.

Systemic inflammatory response syndrome (SIRS)

At least two of:

* Temp > 38 or < 36°C
* Heart rate (HR) > 90 beats per minute
* Respiratory rate (RR) > 20 or pCO_2 < 4.3 kPa
* White cell count (WCC) > 11×10^9/L or < 3.5×10^9/L

Sepsis:

* SIRS plus suspicion or evidence of microbial infection.

Severe sepsis:

* Sepsis plus organ dysfunction

Septic shock:

* Severe sepsis with hypotension despite adequate volume resuscitation.

Aetiology

The infecting organisms relates to the age and health of the patient. The most common organisms are:

* Gram-negative coliforms (40%)
* *Staphylococcus aureus* (12%)
* *Streptococcus pneumoniae* (10%)

Pathophysiology

Gram-negative organisms in particular, more commonly cause septic shock as they possess a lipopolysaccharide on their surface which triggers the release of tumour necrosis factor and interleukin-1 in to the circulation which potentiate the features of shock and tissue damage via the release of agents such as prostaglandins and nitrous oxide.

Key features in the history/examination

* Any recent illnesses or symptoms indicative of infection are significant, such as dysuria, diarrhoea, and a productive cough, all of which may indicate the cause of sepsis.
* History of recent surgery or procedures in particular involving the gastrointestinal or urinary tract.

* History of any implants or prosthetic devices.
* Establish any cause of immunosupression.
* Early features on examination include fever, rigors, nausea, confusion as well as signs such as tachycardia and warm peripheries.
* A later sign is hypotension with cold and clammy peripheries.
* Acute renal failure, metabolic acidosis and adult respiratory distress syndrome may ensue.
* Caution must be taken in the elderly as they are unable to generate some of the features of sepsis such as tachycardia and hence may present late in the illness.
* Sepsis in the immunosuppressed must be recognised early and treated aggressively as it may result in significant morbidity and mortality.
* Patients require a full examination in order to elicit any features which will help to identify the causative organism.
* Cardiovascular examination, especially listen for murmurs.
* Respiratory examination, especially listen for consolidation.
* Abdominal examination, especially look for signs of urinary tract or gastroenterological infections.
* Neurological, especially for any focal neurology, confusion or neck stiffness and photophobia which may indicate central nervous system (CNS) infection.
* Skin, looking for cellulitis, rash and other lesions such as erythema gangrenosum (a small (10 mm) erythematous lesion with a central necrotic region, specifically associated with gram negative infection).
* Musculoskeletal, especially for septic arthritis.
* Gynaecological (if female) to exclude a retained tampon if suspected.

Investigations

Blood tests:

* WCC: may be increased or decreased: this cannot be used in order to gauge the severity of infection as most patients with severe disease tend to have a reduced WCC
* U&Es
* LFTs
* Inflammatory markers
* ABG: will indicate any acidosis and establish the lactate level, both of which are important markers of severity
* Clotting screen: to exclude disseminated intravascular coagulation.

Microbiology:

Cultures must be taken of all possible sources of sepsis identified on history and examination. This may include:

* Blood cultures: Preferably three sets taken from different sites

at different times. If an indwelling central venous catheter is present blood should be sent from this. Preferably taken before antimicrobial treatment started.

- Sputum culture
- Urine culture
- Stool culture
- Effusions
- Ascites
- Cerebrospinal fluid (CSF)
- Wound/skin swabs
- If there are lines *in situ*, consider changing and sending the tips to microbiology

Imaging:

- CXR: this forms part of the septic screen. This may reveal a cause such as pneumonia, a pre-disposing illness such as bronchial carcinoma, as well as any complications such as adult respiratory distress syndrome.
- Other imaging will be directed by the clinical situation.

Management

➢ Each hospital has its own policy regarding antibiotic therapy in sepsis and this should be adhered to whenever possible.

➢ Antibiotics must be started promptly and can be directed towards the most likely suspected cause if known, for example, a recent urinary tract infection.

➢ In severe sepsis antibiotics should be commenced within 1 hour.

➢ If not able to ascertain a cause, broad spectrum antibiotics are given such as a broad spectrum Penicillin and an aminoglycoside such as Gentamicin, or a third-generation Cephalosporin.

➢ Patients who are immunocompromised or present with burns are at an increased risk of pseudomonas infection and hence this should be covered with antibiotic therapy such as Ceftazidime.

➢ If there is doubt or for complicated cases, the microbiology team should be contacted for advice.

➢ High flow oxygen should be given in the acute situation, and then titrated according to the patients requirement.

➢ Intravenous (IV) fluid resuscitation should be given as required.

➢ Urinary catheter may be required to monitor the urine output.

➢ If hypoadrenalism suspected IV Hydrocortisone should be given.

Prognosis:

➢ The risk of mortality is related to the general health of the patient.

➢ It is much higher (at least four times) in those with an underlying pre-existing illness.

➢ The overall mortality rate is as high as 20–50% which is why prompt recognition and treatment is essential.

Staphylococcal toxic shock syndrome

Epidemiology

It is a rare condition with up to 40 cases nationally per year; approximately 50% are related to a retained tampon. It occurs predominantly in younger adults.

Aetiology

Staphylococcal toxic shock syndrome is a serious infection resulting from the release of exotoxin from a localised staphylococcal infection commonly *staphyloccus aureus*. The most common exotoxins are toxic shock syndrome toxin-1 (75%) and staphylococcal enterotoxin B (20–25%). Staphylococcal toxic shock syndrome can follow burns, boils, insect bites, post operative infections and retained tampons.

Pathophysiology

Pathophysiology is dependent on the aetiology.

Key features in the history/examination

- Symptoms include fever, headache, abdominal pain, vomiting, myalgia and postural dizziness followed by profuse watery diarrhoea.
- Features include systemic upset, tachycardia and hypotension.
- There is an associated macular erythroderma which resembles sun burn.
- There will be evidence of multi-system failure.
- Characteristically causes a desquamation pattern of the hands and feet.

Investigations

Bloods tests:

- FBC will show an elevated white cell count.
- Inflammatory markers will be raised.
- Coagulation: elevated prothombin time
- U&Es: may give evidence of renal failure
- Bone profile: may give evidence of renal failure
- LFTs: hypoalbuminaemia is likely to be present (70%).

Microbiology:

- Blood cultures
- Urinalysis
- Swabs if indicated

Management

➢ The identification and decontamination of the site of the toxin production.
- o Drain abscesses
- o Debride lesions
- o Remove foreign material

➢ Aggressive fluid resuscitation: Up to 10 litres can be required in 24 hours.

➢ Anti-staphyloccocal antibiotics: currently with a semisynthetic Pencillin or Vancomycin, and for those with Pencillin allergies with Clindamycin or Gentamicin.

➢ If caused by methicillin-resistant *Staphylococcus aureus* (MRSA) need to use a suitable antibiotic as recommended by local microbiology protocols (often Vancomycin).

➢ Patients are often very unwell and are likely to require treatment in an intensive care setting for supportive management and treatment of multi-organ failure.

➢ Administration of pooled human immunoglobulin in refractory cases and cases with an undrainable or removable source of infection.

Prognosis:

➢ 2–3 people die per year.

➢ Mortality rate for menstrual cases is 2.5%, the incidence being 2–3 times higher for non-menstrual cases.

➢ Between 5–40% will be recurrent.

Pyrexia of unknown origin

Epidemiology

Pyrexia of unknown origin (PUO) is classified as:

- Classic: temperature of 38.3°C with no diagnosis reached with three outpatient visits, three days as an inpatient or one week of 'intelligent and invasive' ambulatory investigation.

- Nosocomial – at least 24 hours as an inpatient prior to onset of temperature of 38.3°C and no obvious source.

- Immune deficient (neutropenic): fever of 38.3°C, neutrophils of <1 with negative cultures and no diagnosis after three days.

- HIV related: fever of 38.3°C for four weeks as an outpatient or three days as an inpatient with no diagnosis after three days of investigation and at least two days for cultures to develop.

Aetiology

The causes tend to be unusual presentations of common diseases. There are five main categories of causes:

- Infections
- Neoplasms
- Connective tissue disease
- Miscellaneous i.e. alcoholic hepatitis

- Undiagnosed
- Between 50 and 80% of cases are attributable to infections and neoplasm. Around 10–20% are caused by autoimmune disorders. The diagnosis is one of exclusion.

The various causes of PUO are shown in Table 3.45:

Type	Disease
Bacterial	Abscesses
	TB
	Hepatobillary infection
	Osteomyelitis
	Brucellosis
	Borrelia
	Chlamydophila (Psittacosis)
Viral	Cytomegalovirus (CMV)
	Epstein-Barr Virus (EBV)
	HIV
Parasites	Toxoplasmosis
	Trypanosoma
	Leishmania
Neoplasms	Hodgkins and Non-Hodgkins Lymphoma
	Leukaemia
	Renal cell carcinoma
Collagen vascular and autoimmune disease	Juvenile rheumatoid arthritis (Still's disease)
	Polyarthritis nodosa
	Rheumatoid arthritis
Granulomatous disease	Sarcoidosis
	Crohn's disease
Vasculitides	Giant cell arteritis
	Polymyalgia rheumatica
	Behcet's disease
Inherited disease	Familial Mediterranean fever
Endocrine disorders	Hyperthyroidism
	Subacute thyroiditis
	Adrenal insufficiency
Drugs	Beta-lactam antibiotics
	Isoniazid

Table 3.45: Possible causes of PUO.

Pathophysiology

Pathophysiology is dependent on the aetiology.

Key features in history/examination

- Careful history taking is essential to elicit information that may inform and guide the identification of the source of the fever:

o History of travel and recreational activities.

o Contact with animals including pets such as dogs, cats and birds and any other relevant creatures.

o Sexual history and activity is important to enquire about.

o Occupation i.e. farmers, sewage workers, vets, doctors, nurses and foresters.

o Any meals consumed prepared outside of the home or ingestion of any unpasteurised milk or cheese or poorly cooked meat or eggs.

o Drug history can be important, both prescribed and non-prescribed medications. For example, certain antibiotics and phenytoin.

• A full physical examination on admission is required to identify any likely cause.

• Daily examination in order to reveal any features which have developed with progression of the fever.

o CNS: it is very difficult to detect intracranial abscesses clinically. Look for signs of raised intracranial pressure or focal neurological deficit on examination.

o Cardiovascular: murmurs, whether new or changing in nature, and any tenderness of the temporal arteries.

o Respiratory: any added sounds such as crepitations or crackles can be indicative of an early pneumonia.

o Focal abscesses can occur in respiratory conditions such as tuberculosis (TB) and bronchial carcinoma.

o Abdominal: any organomegaly must be identified. Inflammatory bowel disease in particular is associated with abscess formation.

o Musculoskeletal: any muscle stiffness or tenderness on examination.

o Examine all lymph glands for any enlargement.

o Examine the mouth for any evidence of abscesses.

o Inspect any lines or catheters which are in situ for signs of infection.

Investigations

Blood tests:

• Inflammatory markers such as WCC, and CRP – any neutrophilia or lymphocytosis associated with bacterial or viral infection respectively.

• A raised erythrocyte sedimentation rate (ESR) may be indicative of myeloma, temporal arteritis or even metastases.

• Liver function tests may reveal a derangement due to a primary tumour or metastases.

Microbiology:

• Urine dipstick can reveal microscopic haematuria which may accompany endocarditis and renal carcinoma.

• Sputum sample can be sent for microscopy and culture and to look for any organisms such as acid fast bacilli.

• 3 sets of blood cultures must be taken from separate sites at different times.

• Swabs should be taken from any suspected sources of infection such as lines or catheters, and send for microscopy and culture.

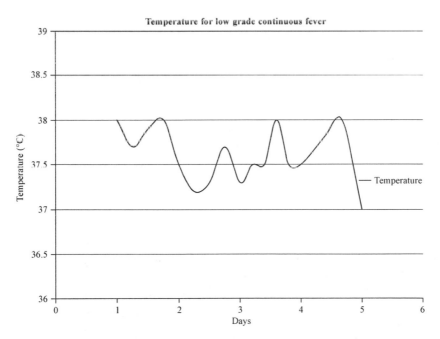

Figure 3.24: Temperature variation for a low grade continuous fever

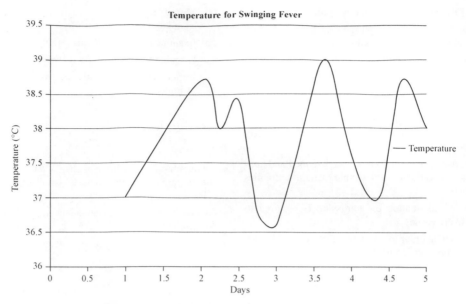

Figure 3.25: Temperature variation for a swinging fever.

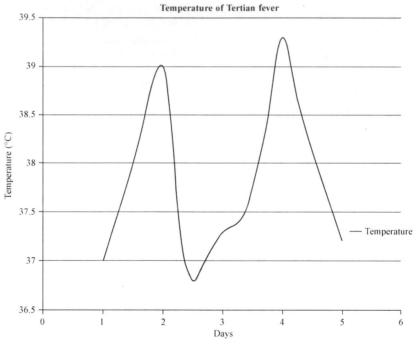

Figure 3.26: Temperature variation for a tertian fever.

- A lumbar puncture may be indicated if a CNS infection is suspected, however, a computer tomography (CT) scan may be needed prior to this procedure.

Imaging:

- CXR: may reveal either a primary lung tumour, metastases, an aspergilloma or another cause.

- Ultrasound (USS): to detect any un-identified lesions or masses within the abdomen or lymphadenopathy.

- CT: to detect any un-identified lesions or masses within the abdomen or lymphadenopathy.

- Magnetic resonance imaging (MRI): to detect any unidentified lesions or masses within the abdomen or lymphadenopathy.

Other:

- Further investigations should be chosen depending on history, examination findings and results of investigations.
- This may include:
  - Echocardiogram (to exclude vegetations as endocarditis may be a cause but not be clinically obvious)
  - Lymph node biopsy
  - Bone marrow aspiration

Management

➤ Immune deficient neutropenic cases should be treated aggressively with broad spectrum antibiotics immediately according to local microbiology guidelines. Cultures must be obtained, preferably prior to antibiotic administration
  - These patients should be closely monitored and reviewed by the microbiology team.
➤ Treat empirically if case suggestive of:
  - Culture negative endocarditis.
  - Cryptic disseminated tuberculosis (or other granulomatous infections).
  - Temporal arteritis (with vision loss).
➤ Otherwise treatment will be determined by achieving a definitive diagnosis.

Fungal infections

These must be considered in particular in those who are immunocompromised. Examples include:

Aspergillus fumigatus:

- Disseminated infection which typically occurs in advanced HIV disease.
- Symptoms of asthma such as chest tightness and wheezing as well as haemoptysis.
- Evidence of fungus ball on CXR.
- The main treatment is Amphotericin B.
- Ketoconazole has a limited role.
- Oral steroids may be effective in acute treatment.

Candida albicans:

- Oral features include white patches in the tongue and inner mouth as well as plaques in the oesophageal mucosa.
- Symptoms include dysphagia and retrosternal burning and pain.
- Vaginal infection will produce a white creamy discharge with surrounding erythema.
- Management depends on the location but includes Nystatin drops or lozenges, Clotrimazole pessary or cream as well as Fluconazole orally or amphotericin IV for severe infection.

Cryptococcus neoformans:

- Mostly causes symptoms of meningitis in the immunocompromised.

- Features include a progressive onset of headache associated with fever and nausea.
- Severe cases cause impairment in the level of consciousness.
- Lumbar puncture and CSF microscopy and culture with India ink staining.
- Requires IV Amphotericin B for at least 2 weeks and then high-dose Fluconazole.
- Treatment may be required long term in patients not on antiretroviral therapy.

Pneumocystis jiroveci (formally carinii) (PCP):

- Causes a severe pneumonia in human immunodeficiency virus (HIV) patients where the CD4 count has fallen to less than 200 cells/microlitre.
- Symptoms are of progressive onset and include a non-productive cough, fever, breathlessness, and malaise.
- Typically the CXR may be normal or reveal bilateral perihilar infiltrates which may further develop into diffuse shadowing throughout the lungs.
- Diagnosis is confirmed by revealing the organisms in samples obtained at bronchoscopy.
- Requires aggressive treatment with IV Co-trimoxazole, Pentamidine or Dapsone and Trimethoprim.
- Systemic steroid therapy is effective in reducing mortality where the lung gas exchange values are poor, for example, where the PaO_2 is less than 9.5 kPa.
- Prophylaxis is required in patients with a CD4 count of less than 200 cells per microlitre.

Infections to be considered in the immunocompromised

Brucellosis:

- Rare in the developed world.
- A zoonotic disease where the organism is transmitted to humans from livestock such as cows.
- Main features include fever, cough, myalgia, and splenomegaly.
- Arthralgia and meningoencephalitis are known complications.
- Diagnosis is by detection of antibodies on a standard agglutination test or enzyme-linked immunosorbent assay (ELISA).
- Blood cultures may also reveal the organism which is a small gram negative bacillus.
- Tetracycline or in addition to Streptomycin is effective, with Co-trimoxazole being an alternative.
- Occasionally where there are collections of pus, surgical drainage is indicated.

Cryptosporidium:

- Features are mainly severe chronic watery diarrhoea.

- Stool microscopy and culture as well as a small bowel biopsy samples obtained at endoscopy, will reveal typical cysts.
- Symptom management include anti-diarrhoeals and fluid and electrolyte replacement.

Toxoplasma gondii:

Mostly responsible for encephalitis and cerebral abscesses in acquired immune deficiency syndrome (AIDS) patients.

- Clinical features include focal neurological deficits, seizures, fever, headache and symptoms of confusion.
- Eye infection results in symptoms of chorioretinitis.
- Serological investigations will be positive for toxoplasmosis.
- MRI and CT scanning will reveal a number of ring-enhancing lesions when done with contrast enhancement.
- Treatment is mainly with Pyrimethamine, Sulfadiazine and Folinic acid (Leucovorin).
- Long term maintenance treatment may be indicated to prevent recurrence of infection.

Infectious mononucleosis (glandular fever)

Epidemiology

It has been found that more than half of all children have been exposed to the Epstein Barr Virus (EBV) and over three-quarters will have developed antibodies to the virus. The infection tends to be milder in children and may even be asymptomatic. Teenagers or young adults aged 15 to 20 years tend to be symptomatic with the virus.

Aetiology

The causative organism is EBV (*Human herpes virus 4*). The virus is present in saliva and is spread via close contact ('kissing disease').

Pathophysiology

EBV preferentially infects B lymphocytes.

Key features in history/examination

There are two types of presentation:

Anginose type:

- Production of exudate from the tonsils.
- Presence of petechiae on the hard palate.
- Oedema involving the tonsils and face.
- Splenomegaly may be a feature on examination.
- A change in voice making it more nasal in nature.
- Enlargement of the cervical lymph nodes.
- A macular-papular rash commonly occurs.

Juvenile type:

- Generalised lymphadenopathy and malaise.
- Mild sore-throat.
- Myalgia and arthralgia.
- Low-grade fever.
- Complications include dysphagia and threatened obstruction of the pharynx due to tonsillar enlargement.

Rarely there is secondary bacterial infection, splenic rupture, hepatitis or pancreatitis and meningoencephalitis.

Investigations

Blood test:

- FBC: reveals a lymphocytosis and usually a thrombocytopenia.
- Liver function tests are mildly deranged and inflammatory markers raised.
- Specific immunoglobulin M (IgM) antibodies indicate acute infection.
- The monospot (heterophil antibody) test.
- Blood film: atypical lymphocytes may be present.

Management

- ➢ Mostly symptomatic management.
- ➢ Bed rest, gargling with Aspirin for example, and anaesthetic lozenges.
- ➢ If there is impending obstruction of the airway due to enlarged tonsils, steroids are effective in reducing the oedema (Prednisolone given at 40mg per day for up to ten days).
- ➢ Ampicillin is occasionally given for the treatment of a sore throat, however, this should be avoided in patients with infectious mononucleosis as it results in a florid skin rash.

Prognosis:

- ➢ Generally good with the majority of patients make a full recovery.
- ➢ Complications are rare, but include chronic fatigue syndrome and Guillain-Barré syndrome.

Malaria

Epidemiology

A disease predominantly of the sub tropics, where more than 1.5 billion people are exposed to the risk of infection every year. It is endemic in Africa, Central and South America and Asia. Although malaria is no longer a problem in Europe and North America, there is a risk of imported cases with over 2,000 cases being reported per year in the UK. Individuals of all ages are at risk of the disease. It has been found that individuals who carry the sickle cell trait are at a reduced risk of disease, however those with sickle cell disease fare worse when infected.

Aetiology

Plasmodium falciparum, mostly found in Sub-Saharan Africa and Papua New Guinea, is particularly implicated in the imported cases, probably as a result of an increase in tourists travelling to Africa and the persistence of malaria in this region. *Plasmodium vivax* also commonly infects humans and is more common in South America and India. *Plasmodium ovale* is less common, found only in West Africa. *Plasmodium malariae* is much less common and occurs mainly in Africa. A number of factors influence the transmission of malaria such as:

- Environment
- Host:
  - Pregnant women and patients who have had a splenectomy will be affected more severely with the disease.
  - Children who are better nourished will in fact develop more severe disease when infected.
  - Sickle cell trait, alpha and beta thalassaemia trait, glucose-6-phosphate dehydrogenase (G6PD) deficiency and malnutrition all reduce the risk of disease and its severity if it is transmitted.
- Vector
- The female Anopheles mosquito

Pathophysiology

The malarial sporozoites enter the blood stream when a mosquito bites. They reach the hepatocytes and undergo multiple divisions over 1–2 weeks before the merozoite form re-emerges into the bloodstream. The merozoites enter the host erythrocytes, and a cycle of division within the erythrocyte, subsequent rupture with further merozoite release and infection of new red cells begins, resulting in a rapid increase in parasitaemia.

Incubation periods: P falciparum is about 1 month, but rarely presents up to 1 year after exposure. P vivax and P ovale are longer but additionally have a hypnozoite form which lies dormant in the liver, and can induce recurrence many months following the initial infection.

Key features in the history/examination

- Most commonly patients present with 'flu-like' symptoms – persistent fever, sweats, rigors, malaise, headache and myalgia following travel to an endemic area.
- A history of mosquito bites is not necessary to suspect the diagnosis; the patient may not have noticed.
- A history of good concordance with prophylaxis does not exclude infection.
- Diarrhoea, mild jaundice, confusion and seizures are also features.
- Hepatosplenomegaly and herpes of the labia are common on examination.
- More common in individuals who were non-compliant with their anti-malarial medication or did not take proper precautionary measures such as sleeping under mosquito nets.

- Recognition is the key as a delay in diagnosis is associated with an increased risk of mortality.
- The pattern of attacks of fever and rigors will indicate the diagnosis.
- Periods of fever indicate a rupture of the red cells infected with parasite.
- There may be a classical tertian (3-day) or quartan (4-day) cycle of fever.
- Tertian fever is where the fever peaks every other day and the quartan fever is where the fever peaks every third day.
- Usually more commonly occurs in patients who have some acquired immunity to the disease due to their origin from an endemic country.

Complications:

Complications are more common when there is a high parasite count and hence are more likely to occur in patients with no immunity, young children and travellers. They are more commonly seen in falciparum malaria.

- Hypovolaemic shock
- Cerebral malaria
- Pulmonary oedema: A frequent complication which can be prevented with careful monitoring of fluid balance.
- Renal failure
- Severe anaemia
- Blackwater fever:
  - There is haemoglobinuria due to severe haemolysis secondary to a high parasite count in the blood.
  - Use of quinine in patients with a G6PD deficiency can also result in this feature often described as 'coca-cola' coloured urine.
  - Where red cells infected with parasites obstruct the cerebral capillaries.
  - There is a reducing level of consciousness ranging from mildly drowsy to coma, seizures and psychosis.

Investigations

Blood tests:

- WCC: this is classically normal with a relative lymphopenia. A low platelet count is usual.
- Hyponatraemia, hypocalcaemia and hypoalbuminaemia are seen. An increased bilirubin may be secondary to haemolysis or associated with a general increase in LFTs.
- Glucose: may be low either from the infection or from quinine treatment.
- Antigens: may need to send malaria antigen.
- Blood film: Confirms the presence of parasites.
  - A parasite count is required. Parasitaemia of >2% is considered severe in patients with no immunocompromise.
  - At least three films are required and should be taken when the fever peaks and a short period afterwards.

Microbiology:
- Blood cultures: Look for supra-added bacterial infection.

Imaging:
- CXR: look for pneumonia and pulmonary oedema if suspected.

Others:
- Urine dipstick: look for haematuria.
- Pregnancy test: (in appropriate individuals) as pregnancy increases the risk associated with malaria.

Management

If the clinical suspicion of malaria is high after an initial negative blood film in the emergency department, admit for ongoing investigations. Cases should be notified to the local health protection agency.

Falciparum malaria:

➢ All cases should be admitted and assessed for severity and complications.
  - Parasitaemia greater than 2%
  - Acidosis (pH <7.3) or lactate >4.0
  - Shock
  - Reduced GCS
  - Hypoglycaemia (<2.2 mmol/L)
  - Fits
  - Renal impairment
  - Respiratory distress or pulmonary oedema
  - Haemoglobin less than 8.0 g/dL
  - Haemoglobinuria

➢ For mild to moderate, oral treatment with Quinine and then Fansidar is sufficient.
  - Quinine can cause renal impairment (which is more severe when the malaria infection also results in renal damage) and hypoglycaemia by increasing the production of insulin.

➢ Globally, artemesinin derivatives are now a key resource in combating falciparum malaria because there is very little resistance, they reduce parasitaemias faster than anything else, and they reduce gametocytaemia, thus impeding transmisssion back to the mosquito. To protect against the emergence of resistance, it is advocated that they should only ever be used as combination therapy.

➢ In the event of severe or complicated malaria immediately commence IV Quinine therapy and seek specialist advice.

➢ Consider intensive care unit (ICU)/high dependency unit (HDU) admission especially if there is renal or hepatic failure or signs of shock.

➢ Intravenous fluids must be given cautiously due to the risk of fluid retention and pulmonary oedema.

➢ In the event of shock, additionally treat for gram negative sepsis.

➢ Steroid therapy is avoided as it worsens the outcome.

➢ Exchange transfusion is indicated when patients are extremely ill and have a parasitaemia above 10%.

➢ Patients on treatment need review after four weeks to ensure a clinical improvement as well as reduction in parasitic load.

➢ Patients with splenomegaly must avoid contact sports and strenuous exercise as there is a considerable risk of splenic rupture.

Non-falciparum malaria:

➢ Usually appropriate for outpatient therapy with oral treatment.

➢ Chloroquine treatment is normally effective; however resistance is recognised in certain areas worldwide and hence it cannot always be relied upon.

➢ Liver parasites must subsequently be eradicated, so a course of Primaquine for 14 days follows.

➢ Patients with G6PD deficiency must be identified before treatment is initiated in order to avoid severe haemolysis with Primaquine.

Prevention:

➢ The mainstay is prevention of mosquito bites which mostly occur at night-time.

➢ Use bed-nets and chemical repellents.

➢ Prophylaxis with anti-malarials.
  - All those travelling to endemic areas should attend their GP or travel clinic for advice.
  - Treatment is started around one week prior to travel and continued for up to 6 weeks after their return.
  - There is no one set pattern of prophylaxis as the resistance of the organism is changing continually and varies geographically.
  - Common drugs used include Chloroquine, Mefloquine, Malarone and Doxycycline.

➢ Researchers are currently working towards the development of a vaccine against malaria, targeting the various stages of the mosquitoes' infection within the body.

Prognosis:

➢ Fatal infection is rare in healthy individuals.

➢ *Plasmodium falciparum* is an exception and potentially can result in a high risk of mortality in the immunocompromised.

Infective endocarditis

Epidemiology

Involves infection of the cardiac valves or the endocardium. It is commonly caused by streptococcal infections. Previously found to be more common in young individuals with rheumatic heart disease. It mostly affects those aged 50 or over with degenerative disease of the aortic and mitral valves. The prevalence is twice as high in men than women.

Aetiology

The usual causative organisms are as follows:

o *Streptococcus viridans* accounts for 50% of cases.

o *Staphylococcus aureus* (20% of cases) can result in rapid destruction of the cardiac valves.

o *Staphylococcus epidermis* is more common following valve replacement surgery.

o Gram-negative organisms will be found rarely in patients following heart valve surgery or in intravenous drug users.

o Fungal organisms (*candida, aspergillus*) are very rarely encountered.

Pathophysiology

The organisms generally arise from sources such as the teeth, tonsils, urinary tract, central venous catheterisation and the skin. Occasionally, it may be caused by a sexually transmitted disease (chlamydia *or* gonorrhoea). It usually involves abnormal heart valves, for example those involved in rheumatic heart disease at a younger age or those with congenital heart disease. Those with mitral valve prolapse or aortic stenosis are also at an increased risk.

Intravenous drug use has resulted in a higher incidence of right sided endocarditis, in particular involving the tricuspid valve, over the past few years. Patients with prosthetic heart valves are particularly at risk and once infection ensues, it is extremely difficult to resolve. Permanent pacemakers also increase the risk of endocarditis. The valve which is involved tends to form clusters of the infecting organism, with fibrin and platelets which aggregate together to form vegetations on the cusps of the valve. The valves usually get destroyed by this process and there is resultant regurgitation or stenosis and systemic embolisation may be a consequence. Hence, myocardial abscesses may develop.

Key features in the history/examination

- A low threshold of suspicion is required in patients who present with a new or different character to an existing heart murmur and a fluctuating fever ('swinging').

- Symptoms similar to influenza are common, as well as anaemia and weight loss.

- Extra-cardiovascular features result from systemic embolisation and deposition of immune complexes.

  o Emboli may result in splenic, gastrointestinal or renal infarction, myocardial infarction, ischaemic stroke, and loss of the peripheral pulses.

  o Deposition of immune complexes can result in vasculitis involving certain regions of the body. There may be small haemorrhages within the skin, mucosa, retina (Roth's spots) or nail beds (splinter haemorrhages).

  o Other associated features include small erythematous macules in the palms (Janeway lesions) and small, tender, subcutaneous swellings in the digits (Osler's nodes).

- Haematuria is a common feature and may be microscopic or macroscopic.

- Splenomegaly may occur as with any chronic infection, and splenic infarction will give symptoms of left sided abdominal pain.

- A late feature is finger clubbing.

- When there is right heart involvement, embolisation to the lungs can result in pleuritic-type chest pain with haemoptysis.

Investigations

Blood tests:

- FBC: raised WCC and a normochromic normocytic anaemia.

- Inflammatory markers: elevated ESR (present in 90% of cases) and CRP.

- U&Es: elevated

- LFTs: deranged

Microbiology:

- Blood cultures:

  o Must be taken over a 12 to 24 hour period and at least three sets are required from three different sites in the body.

  o They must be taken prior to the initiation of antibiotic therapy.

  o Around 80% are positive and the remaining 20% will be negative, usually in those individuals where antibiotics were started early on or where symptoms have been longstanding and the patient has developed high levels of antibodies.

  o Negative cultures have been shown to be associated with a poorer prognosis.

Imaging:

- CXR: may illustrate features of cardiac failure. If there is right-sided heart involvement, there may be evidence of a pulmonary emboli or lung abscess.

- CT: to check for myocardial abscesses.

- MRI: to check for myocardial abscesses.

Others:

- Echocardiogram:

  o An echocardiogram may confirm the presence of vegetations on the heart valves.

  o The absence of these does not exclude the diagnosis as they must be at least 2 mm in size to be visualised.

  o A transoesophageal echocardiogram has been shown to be more sensitive in identifying vegetations compared to a transthoracic echocardiogram.

- Urine dipstick: may be positive for both blood and protein.

- ECG: usually nothing to note on ECG, however, if the conducting tissue is involved, there may be a prolonged PR interval, which is indicative of severe infection.

3. Medicine

Management

> It is essential to identify the underlying source of infection for example, a tooth abscess may well be the cause which can be discovered using dental X-rays and may require prompt tooth extraction.

Pharmacological management:

> There will be local microbiology guidelines, however a common regime is IV Benzylpenicillin (Vancomycin if Penicillin allergy) and Gentamicin.

> The Gentamicin levels should be measured after the third dose and on alternate days thereafter.

> Antibiotic therapy can be altered when the blood culture and sensitivity results become available. The microbiologist will be involved in this decision.

> The minimal inhibitory concentration may be measured which is where the concentration of antibiotic required to inhibit the growth of the infective agent is measured.

> If the blood cultures are negative, broad spectrum antibiotics should be administered including Ampicillin instead of Penicillin.

> Since staphylococcal is extremely virulent, infection must be treated with three antibiotics such as Flucloxacillin, Fusidic acid, and Gentamicin.

> Intravenous antibiotic therapy is required for at least two weeks and then oral antibiotics for a further four weeks (unless complications arise).

Surgical management:

> 1 in 4 patients will require surgical intervention.
> The main indications for surgical management are:
>   o Worsening cardiac failure.
>   o Persistent infection with fever or worsening renal failure that is not responding to antibiotics or antifungals.
>   o Prosthetic heart valves – antibiotics are rarely effective in eradicating infection of prosthetic material.
>   o If there is evidence of myocardial abscesses which are suspected when there is a prolonged PR interval on ECG.
>   o If this is detected a temporary pacing wire is indicated as there is a high risk of complete heart block or even death.
>   o Regurgitation of heart valve.
> Types of surgical intervention:
>   o Valve repair
>   o Valve replacement
>   o Abscess drainage

Prognosis:

> The effectiveness of treatment is indicated when there is a reduction in the temperature, a decrease in the inflammatory markers and white cell count as well as a clinical improvement.

> The mortality rate is 20% mostly as a result of the increase in the number of prosthetic heart valve replacements, intravenous drug users and antibiotic resistance of the most virulent organisms.

> Without appropriate treatment, the mortality is as high as 95%.
> Usually from cardiac failure or valve destruction.

Prophylaxis:

Recent National Institute for Health and Clinical Excellence (NICE) guidance (NICE, 2008) recommends the administration of prophylactic antibiotics for patients with known valvular disease or a prosthetic heart valve, only when there is going to be a medical or surgical intervention at a site where there is a suspected infection in gullet, stomach, intestines, reproductive tract or urinary tract. Good oral and dental hygiene is imperative for those at risk.

Further reading and references

> British Infection Society (2007) Malaria – algorithm for initial assessment and management in adults.
> Dellinger RP, Mitchell LM, Carlet JM et al. (2008) Surviving Sepsis Campaign: International guidelines for management of severe sepsis and septic shock. *Intensive Care Med*: 34(1): 17–60, 2008.
> www.healthmap.org/promed – a useful website giving worldwide locations of disease outbreaks.
> National Institute for Health and Clinical Excellence (2008) *Prophylaxis against infective endocarditis (CG064).*
> Tidy H. (1952) Glandular Fever. *Br Med J* 2: 436–439.
> www.toxicshock.com

HAEMATEMESIS AND MELAENA

Differential diagnosis

System/Organ	Disease
Gastrointestinal	**Peptic ulcer disease**
	Oesophageal varices
	Mallory-Weiss tear
	Oesophagitis
	Dieulafoy lesion
	Upper gastrointestinal (GI) tract tumours
	Vascular malformations
	Angiodysplasia
	Hereditary haemorrhagic telangiectasia
	Aortoenteric fistula

Variceal bleeding

Epidemiology

Variceal bleeding is responsible for 50–60% of bleeding in patients with cirrhosis 5% of acute upper gastrointestinal bleeds in the UK. The risk of bleeding in patients rises to 15% per year with large varices.

Aetiology

Portal hypertension, and subsequent variceal formation, has a number of causes but the most common is cirrhosis caused by alcoholic liver disease. Other causes include:

- Primary biliary cirrhosis
- Budd-Chiari syndrome
- Sarcoidosis
- Schistosomiasis (important worldwide)
- Congenital hepatic fibrosis
- Idiopathic portal hypertension

Pathophysiology

Cirrhosis causes portal hypertension due to the distortion of hepatic architecture causing increased resistance to blood flow though the liver. In addition to the portal vein, the portal circulation also anastomoses with the systemic venous circulation at several other sites – the oesophagus, umbilicus and rectum.

In portal hypertension, increased flow at the sites of these anastomoses may lead to dilatation and the formation of dilated tortuous veins known as varices.

The formation of oesophageal varices is the most clinically important consequence of portal hypertension, and it is these varices which are most susceptible to rupture and bleeding.

Key features in the history/examination

- Haematemesis: ask about amount and frequency and any previous episodes. Copious fresh bleeding may raise the suspicion of a variceal source but does not rule out other causes.
- Melaena: loose, black, tar-like stool which is foul smelling. Ask about amount and frequency. When did it begin? Is there any associated bleeding per rectum (PR)?
- Alcohol: amount and frequency. Find out when last drank as a withdrawal regime may be necessary.
- Past medical history: known chronic liver disease and cirrhosis. Results of previous endoscopies. Exacerbating factors such as coagulopathies.
- Signs of hypovolaemic shock: tachycardia, tachypnoea, cool peripheries, prolonged capillary refill time, pallor, hypotension (or significant postural blood pressure (BP) drop).
- Signs of chronic anaemia: pale conjunctivae, pale palmar creases
- Signs of chronic liver disease: jaundice, encephalopathy, leuconychia, clubbing, palmar erythema, asterixis, spider naevi, gynaecomastia.
- Abdomen: tenderness, guarding, hepatomegaly, splenomegaly, ascites, epigastric mass.
- Rectal examination: blood or melaena.

Investigations

Blood tests:

- FBC: low haemoglobin (Hb), microcytic indices if chronic bleeding. Note, initial Hb may not be a true reflection of extent of blood loss and should be frequently rechecked. Platelets may be low in alcoholism and may be contributing to the bleeding.
- Renal function: note that urea may be disproportionately raised compared to creatinine owing to breakdown of haemoglobin in the upper GI tract.
- LFTs: may indicate chronic liver disease. If so, consider variceal bleeding as a possible cause of bleeding.
- Coagulation screen: PT may be prolonged in chronic liver disease.
- Cross-match.

Imaging:

- Erect chest X-ray (CXR) and abdominal X-ray (AXR): To look for free air under the diaphragm which may indicate perforation.

Urgent endoscopy:

- Oesophagogastroduodenoscopy (OGD), usually just referred to as 'endoscopy', is a diagnostic and therapeutic procedure which involves passing a flexible fibre-optic endoscope through the mouth and into the oesophagus, stomach and duodenum.

Management

Initial management:

➢ A to E assessment and urgent resuscitation
➢ High flow oxygen
➢ Consider early intensive care unit (ICU) review if haemodynamically compromised.
➢ Large-bore intravenous (IV) access. Initially two large-bore (16 gauge or above) but a central line may also become necessary.
➢ IV fluids
➢ Blood transfusion if Hb less than 10 g/dl
➢ Platelet transfusion if less than 50×10^9/L
➢ Reverse any coagulopathy: Vitamin K/fresh frozen plasma (FFP)
➢ Urinary catheter to monitor fluid balance
➢ Terlipressin (2 mg stat then 1–2 mg 6 hourly)
➢ Antibiotics: usually a cephalosporin
➢ Urgent referral to the endoscopist on-call (consider prompt surgical review if unavailable). All patients presenting with an acute upper GI bleed of suspected variceal origin should be considered for an urgent upper GI endoscopy (OGD). The usual treatment for varices found is by endoscopic banding. A special attachment on the end of the endoscope sucks up part of the varix allowing a small band to be placed around

the neck. This causes the varix to thrombose and can help control haemorrhage.

➤ Close monitoring of pulse, BP, urine output, stool chart, CVP (if central line *in situ*).

Ongoing management:

➤ If variceal bleeding not controlled at initial endoscopy, tamponade using a Sengstaken Blakemore tube should be considered. This is best performed by someone skilled in its use and under a general anaesthetic

➤ Continue Terlipressin

➤ Beta blocker (usually Propranolol)

➤ If still drinking give alcohol withdrawal regime – pabrinex/ benzodiazepine

➤ Enter a re-banding program until the varices are obliterated

➤ Tranjugular Intrahepatic Portosystemic Shunting (TIPSS): May be used to decrease the risk of rebleeding (or treat refractory bleeding) from varices. It is performed on the recommendation of a hepatologist. The procedure involves passing a catheter to the hepatic vein (via the jugular vein) and inserting a needle into the portal vein to create a shunt which is held open by deploying a metal stent. This helps to release pressure from the portal venous system thus reducing the pressure at sites of portosystemic anastomoses (including the oesophagus) to prevent further enlargement of varices.

Risk		Score
Age	< 60 years	0
	60–79 years	1
	≥ 80 years	2
Shock	None	0
	Pulse > 100, Systolic BP > 100	1
	Systolic BP < 100	2
Co-morbidity	None	0
	Cardiac failure, Ischaemic heart disease or any other major co-morbidity	2
	Renal /liver failure or disseminated malignancy	3

Table 3.46: Pre-endoscopy clinical Rockall score. Adapted from Rockall *et al.* 1996

Risk		Score
Diagnosis	No stigmata of recent haemorrhage	0
	Mallory-Weiss tear	0
	Malignancy	2
Major stigmata of haemorrhage	None or black spots	0
	Blood in lumen	2
	Clot	2
	Non-bleeding visible vessel	2
	Spurting haemorrhage	2

Table 3.47: Post-endoscopy clinical Rockall score. Adapted from Rockall *et al.* 1996

Prognosis:

➤ A variceal bleed has a high mortality rate – up to 30–50% in some series. See below for details of the Rockall scoring system.

➤ The Rockall score may be used to assess the severity of acute upper GI bleeding. There are two aspects of the score: pre-endoscopic assessment and post-endoscopic assessment. The scores are simply added together to yield a total score which indicates overall severity and prognosis and may be used to guide ongoing management.

Pre-endoscopy		Post-endoscopy		
Score	% death	Score	% death	% re-bleed
1	0	0–2	0	0–5.9
2	3	3	1.9	12
3	5.6	4	8	15
4	12	5	11	25
5	21	6	12	27
6	35	7	23	37
7	62	8+	40	37

Table 3.48: Rockall Score Interpretation. Adapted from Rockall *et al.* 1996

Non-Variceal bleeding

Epidemiology

The incidence of non-variceal bleeds ranges between 50 and 125 per 100,000 and causes 2,500 hospital admissions per year in the UK. Peptic ulcer disease is the most common, accounting for 50% of cases.

Aetiology

The commonest causes are:

• Peptic ulcer disease

• Oesophagitis/gastritis/duodenitis

• Mallory-Weiss tear

Pathophysiology

Peptic ulcer disease:

Peptic ulcers are the commonest cause of acute upper GI haemorrhage. They are caused by damage to the lining of the gastric or duodenal epithelium. The disease process is largely associated with inadequate protection of the mucosa to the effects of stomach acid although the underlying pathophysiology is multifactorial and may include *H. pylori* infection (which stimulates gastrin secretion and promotes parietal cell acid secretion), NSAID use (which inhibits prostaglandin production and mucus secretion) as well as steroid use, smoking and stress. As the ulcer erodes through the mucosa it may also erode into underlying blood vessels and cause haemorrhage.

Mallory-Weiss tear:

Caused by a small tear in the oesophageal mucosa which leads to bleeding in the upper GI tract. It is caused by forceful or repeated vomiting, retching or coughing, owing to the stress on the wall of the oesophagus caused by increased gastric pressure. Rarely, an oesophageal perforation may occur, if the force on the oesophagus is sufficiently great (Boerhaave syndrome).

Oesophagitis:

Gastro-oesophageal reflux disease (GORD) is the most common cause of oesophagitis (due to exposure of the oesophagus to stomach acid). Other causes include candidiasis, chemical corrosion and exposure to ionising radiation. Continued inflammation of the oesophagus may lead to localised bleeding.

Gastritis/duodenitis:

Gastritis and duodenitis disease is caused by damage to the epithelium with a similar pathophysiology to peptic ulcer disease above.

Key features in the history/examination

- Haematemesis: is defined as vomiting blood either fresh red or altered 'coffee ground'. Ask about amount and frequency and any previous episodes. Fresh bleeding may raise the suspicion of a variceal source but does not rule out other causes.

- Melaena: loose, black, tar-like stool which is foul smelling.

- Abdominal pain: epigastric pain may indicate underlying peptic ulcer disease or oesophagitis.

- Past medical history: known peptic ulcer disease or H. *pylori* infection, oesophagitis, hiatus hernia, chronic liver disease, renal failure, coagulopathies.

- Previous gastric surgery will help guide the endoscopist if there is aberrant anatomy (e.g. from previous gastrectomy).

- Drug history: Aspirin and non-steroidal anti-inflammatory drugs (NSAID) can contribute towards peptic ulcer disease and other anticoagulants (e.g. warfarin or heparin) may precipitate severe haemorrhage.

- Alcohol: heavy alcohol use is associated with peptic ulcer disease and may cause alcoholic liver cirrhosis which may lead to oesophageal varices.

- Neoplasm: history of weight loss, dysphagia, vomiting and early satiety may indicate an undiagnosed upper GI tumour.

- Signs of hypovolaemic shock: tachycardia, tachypnoea, cool peripheries, prolonged capillary refill time, pallor, hypotension (or significant postural BP drop).

- Signs of chronic anaemia: pale conjunctivae, pale palmar creases

- Signs of chronic liver disease: jaundice, encephalopathy, leuconychia, clubbing, palmar erythema, asterixis, spider naevi, gynaecomastia,

- Abdomen: tenderness, guarding, hepatomegaly, splenomegaly, ascites, epigastric mass

- Rectal examination: blood or melaena

Investigations

Blood tests:

- FBC: low Hb, microcytic indices if chronic bleeding. Note, initial Hb may not be a true reflection of extent of blood loss and should be frequently rechecked. Platelets may be low in alcoholism and may be contributing to the bleeding

- Renal function: note that urea may be disproportionately raised compared to creatinine owing to breakdown of haemoglobin in the upper GI tract

- LFTs: may indicate chronic liver disease. If so, consider variceal bleeding as a possible cause of bleeding

- Coagulation screen: PT may be prolonged in chronic liver disease

- Cross-match

Imaging:

- Erect CXR and AXR: to look for free air under the diaphragm which may indicate perforation.

Endoscopy:

➢ All patients presenting with an acute upper GI bleed should be considered for an OGD. The urgency will relate to the clinical picture – an acute bleed with haemodynamic compromise should be performed as soon as possible whereas a patient with a small bleed, stable Hb and haemodynamic markers may be able to have the endoscopy as an outpatient.

Management

Initial management:

➢ A to E assessment and urgent resuscitation

➢ High flow oxygen

➢ Consider early ICU review if haemodynamically compromised.

➢ Large bore IV access. Initially 2 large-bore (16 gauge or above) but a central line may also become necessary

➢ IV fluids

➢ Blood transfusion if Hb less than 10 g/dl

➢ Platelet transfusion if less than 50

➢ Reverse any coagulopathy: Vitamin K/FFP

➢ Urinary catheter to monitor fluid balance

➢ Consider ICU review if haemodynamically compromised or unable to maintain their own airway

➢ Consider prompt surgical review, especially if large, uncontrolled bleeding

➢ Close monitoring of pulse, BP, urine output, stool chart, CVP (if central line in situ)

➢ Upper GI endoscopy

    ○ In so doing, it is possible to directly visualise any gross pathology within the upper GI tract.

    ○ In addition to visualising the upper GI tract, instruments may also be passed down the endoscope to obtain mucosal biopsies and give treatment. For bleeding ulcers, adrenaline injection, electrocoagulation and sclerotherapy are used. Preferably using 2 treatments to reduce the risk of rebleed.

    ○ Prior to endoscopy, the patient must remain nil by mouth for at least 6 hours.

    ○ Topical anaesthetic is sprayed into the oropharynx and the patient may also be sedated during the procedure.

    ○ Risks of the procedure are few but may include bleeding and perforation.

Ongoing management:

➢ Effective management of a patient following acute upper GI haemorrhage does not end with endoscopy. It is vital to continue to monitor the patient's vital signs and to look for any signs of re-bleeding (haemodynamic compromise or further episodes of haematemesis or malaena).

➢ Stop predisposing drugs if possible.

➢ H. *pylori* testing and eradication: a biopsy for the CLO test is usually taken at the time of OGD.

➢ Proton pump inhibitor: these are given to patients following peptic ulcer bleeding to reduce the risk of further ulcer erosion and repeat bleed. PPIs work by inhibiting the H^+/ATPase transporter in gastric parietal cells reducing H^+ secretion into the lumen thus increasing pH and reducing the exposure of the gastric and duodenal mucosa to acid.

➢ For a significant non-variceal haemorrhage the regime is 80 mg omeprazole IV STAT followed by 8 mg per hour IV infusion for 72 hours.

➢ Ongoing oral PPI choice is as per local policy.

➢ Rebleed: the rate is 15% and most commonly occurs within the first 24 hours. The patient should have urgent surgical review. Treatment options include redo endoscopy, surgery or angiography and arterial embolisation.

Prognosis:

➢ The overall unselected mortality is 10%.

Further reading and references

➢ Rockall TA, Logan RF, Devlin HB, et al. (1996). Risk assessment after acute upper gastrointestinal haemorrhage. *Gut* 38 (3): 316–21.

➢ Scottish Intercollegiate Guidelines Network (2008) *Management of acute upper and lower gastrointestinal bleeding.*

HEADACHE

Differential diagnosis

System/Organ	Disease
Primary headache	**Migraine**
	Tension-type
	Cluster headache
	Hemicranias continua
	Benign exertional/sex headache
Secondary headaches	Infection
	Meningitis/encephalitis
	Sinusitis
	Dental abscess
	Vascular
	Subarachnoid haemorrhage (SAH)
Subdural haemorrhage (SDH)	Cerebral venous thrombosis
	Vasculitis
Vasculitis	**Temporal arteritis/Giant cell arteritis**
Other	Carbon monoxide poisoning
	Tumour
	Raised intracranial pressure (ICP)
	Primary angle-closure glaucoma

Headache is a very common medical condition that accounts for approximately 5% of General Practice (GP) consultations with nine out of ten people likely to suffer from headache at some point. Almost a third (30%) of neurology out-patient appointments are related to headache.

Primary headaches may carry a heavy morbidity but secondary headaches, i.e. those with an underlying pathological condition, have a significant mortality, which is a source of much litigation when incorrectly treated.

When investigating headaches taking an accurate history is important since many significant pathologies can result in few clinical signs and, especially in the case of meningitis and SAH, rapid diagnosis and treatment can have a beneficial impact on outcome. Investigations need to be directed and will be dictated by the history.

'Red flag' features need to be enquired about during the history:

• New onset/change in headache in the over 50-year-olds.

• Thunderclap onset, i.e. less than five minutes to peak severity.

• Focal neurological symptoms

• New cognitive impairment

• Headache changing with posture

• Headache precipitated by exertion or Valsalva manoeuvre

• Headache causes sufferer to awake from sleep

• Jaw claudication

- Neck stiffness or fever
- New onset with history of human immunodeficiency virus (HIV) infection or cancer.

Migraine

Epidemiology

Migraine is the commonest cause of a recurrent disabling headache and it accounts for 5–20% of those presenting to the emergency department (ED) with headache. There is a female preponderance with an annual prevalence of 15% in female and 6% in males. Attacks commonly start with the onset of puberty and there is often a family history of migraine.

Aetiology

Stress, missed sleep and strenuous exercise are well known trigger factors. 20% report a dietary trigger, commonly cheese, chocolate and alcohol. Women are more susceptible to migraines around the time of menses and there is an increased risk of stroke in women with migraine using the combined oral contraceptive pill (OCP) with relative risk of 8.7.

Pathophysiology

Aura/prodome is thought to be related to low levels of serotonin causing artery spasm and pain, i.e. headache caused by subsequent dilation of arteries. It is thought to be linked to hormone level fluctuation but the exact mechanism is unclear.

Key features in the history/examination

- Headache, usually with gradual onset, classically lasting 4–72 hours.
- Throbbing, usually unilateral.
- The sufferer finds they want to lie down and stay still.
- Nausea and vomiting are common.
- 50% of patients have a prodrome, feeling fatigued, irritable with neck stiffness.
- 15% of patients have an aura, which may include blurring of vision, transient loss of vision, photophobia, zigzag lights and parasthesia, particularly of the face and hands. This lasts up to an hour before the headache.
- The International Headache Society has formulated a diagnostic criteria for migraine without aura. (See Table 3.49).
- During a migraine the patient may have loss of vision and paresthesia.

Investigations

No specific investigations will aid the diagnosis of migraine, however in cases of diagnostic doubt a secondary cause for the headache may need excluding. Patient should be advised to keep a diary of attacks asking them to note what they were doing at the time and what they had consumed.

Diagnostic criteria for migraine without aura:

More than four headaches lasting 4–72 hours

With at least two of:

- Unilateral headache (but bilateral in 20%)
- Pulsating
- Moderate or severe
- Worsened by physical activity

And at least one of:

- Nausea/vomiting
- Photophobia
- Phonophobia

Table 3.49: International Headache Society has formulated a diagnostic criteria for migraine without aura.

Management

- If possible drug therapies during an attack should be combined with rest. Treatment should begin as soon as possible after the attack starts.
- Simple analgesia with anti-emetics. Paracetamol or Ibuprofen (400 mg) is recommended with a prokinetic anti-emetic such as metoclopramide if required.
- Sumatriptan, or other triptans (5-hydroxytryptamine type 1 ($5HT_1$) agonist) administered orally/subcutaneously/nasal/per rectum (PR). Sumitryptan injections relieve 80% of migraines within one hour. Caution is needed in uncontrolled hypertension and with concomitant cardiovascular disease.
- Opiates increase nausea and vomiting and should not be used to treat acute migraine.
- Prophylaxis includes avoidance of trigger factors.
- Preventative medication can be considered in the event of frequent attacks. These should be continued for six months and withdrawn slowly.
  - ○ Propranolol 160 mg BD or other beta-blocker
  - ○ Tricyclic antidepressants e.g. Amitriptyline 10–100 mg OD
  - ○ Anti-epileptics e.g. Valproate 300–1000 mg BD, Topiramate 50 mg BD
  - ○ Methylsergide 1–2 mg TDS

Tension-type headache

Epidemiology

Tension-type headaches are the most common type of headache. They affect 78% of the general population.

Aetiology

As with the other primary headache syndromes, the precise aetiology is uncertain. There is an association with stress and with musculoskeletal problems in the head or neck. Prolonged usage of analgesia in chronic tension-type headache may lead to medication overuse headache.

Pathophysiology

Pathophysiology is not fully understood but there is a possible link to muscle tension. Recent evidence suggests that could be linked to serotonin levels.

Chronic Tension-type headache occurs, by definition, on more than 14 days per month. This can be disabling and may not respond well to analgesics. The hyperexcitability of central nociceptive neurons in trigeminal spinal nucleus, thalamus, and cerebral cortex are believed to be involved. Possibly related to a dysfunction in the pain inhibitory systems.

Key features in the history/examination

- Bilateral, non-throbbing headache which is not as incapacitating as migraine.
- Classically described as a 'pressure' or 'band' around the head.
- May spread into the neck.
- Usually last a few hours.
- There is an association with hormone replacement therapy (HRT).
- Examination will be normal.

Investigations

No specific investigations will aid the diagnosis, however in cases of diagnostic doubt a secondary cause for the headache may need excluding. Patient should be advised to keep a headache diary which may help aid diagnosis.

Management

- Reassurance and explanation.
- Address stress and musculoskeletal triggers.
- Simple analgesia.
- Tricyclic antidepressants may be of benefit e.g. Amitriptyline titrated to 100–150 mg nocte.
- A trial of analgesic withdrawal may resolve medication overuse headache.
- Referral to pain clinics or for cognitive therapies.

Cluster headache

Epidemiology

Cluster headaches have a prevalence of 0.05%. It more commonly affects middle aged men and there is a male-to-female ratio of 6:1.

Aetiology

The aetiology is not known but a familial predisposition may exist. It has been linked to a history of head trauma, heavy cigarette smoking and heavy alcohol intake. Sleep apnoea is common in people with the disease, suggesting that hypoxia might trigger attacks, which often occur at night.

Pathophysiology

The pathophysiology is not well understood.

Key features in the history/examination

- Rapid onset of intense unilateral headache
- Lasting 45–90 minutes typically
- Several attacks per day, usually self-terminating within 2–3 weeks
- Sufferers feel agitated and find themselves pacing around
- Can experience migraine-type symptoms of photophobia, phonophobia, nausea and vomiting.
- Prominent ipsilateral autonomic features: conjunctival injection, lacrimation, nasal congestion, rhinorrhea, flushing, sweating.
- May result in a partial Horner's syndrome.

Investigations

No specific investigations will aid the diagnosis, however in cases of diagnostic doubt a secondary cause for the headache may need excluding. Patient should be advised to keep a headache diary which may help aid diagnosis.

Management

- Initially simple analgesia, but this rarely achieves adequate relief
- Subcutaneous Sumatriptan 6 mg can be very helpful in some.
- Explanation of the diagnosis
- Avoidance of alcohol during the period of the cluster
- Prophylactic drug treatment, starting as soon as possible after the start of a cluster
  - Verapamil 80 mg TDS, titrated upwards
  - Prednisolone 60–100 mg OD

Subarachnoid haemorrhage

Epidemiology

The incidence of SAH is 8–10 per 100,000 per year with peak incidence in the 6th decade. It accounts for approximately 3% attendances to ED with headache, but for 10–25% of those presenting with an acute headache.

Aetiology

Up to 75% spontaneous SAH are due to a ruptured berry aneurysm. Most commonly found on the anterior communicating artery, followed by the internal carotid artery, middle cerebral artery and finally the vertebrobasilar circulation. The risk is increased by smoking and hypertension. 20% have no identifiable cause but rarer causes are:

- Arteriovenous malformations of the brain or spine

- Arterial dissection
- Sympathomimetic drugs, including cocaine
- Tumours
- Connective tissue disorders and vasculitis

Pathophysiology

Blood in subarachnoid space causes chemical meningitis and subsequent increase in ICP leads to cerebral oedema.

Key features in the history/examination

- Acute severe headache, maximal immediately or within a few seconds (less than five minutes).
- Lasting longer than an hour and can continue for many days.
- Often described as 'thunderclap' and 'worst ever.'
- In 10% of cases of SAH headache is the only symptom.
- Symptoms of meningism: nausea, vomiting, photophobia and neck stiffness.
- Headaches prior to the SAH have been described apparently resulting from 'sentinel bleeds' but evidence suggests that these headaches have other causes, or perhaps are 'missed' SAH.
- Examination may be completely normal. Remember there is no such thing as 'too well for SAH'.
- Focal neurological symptoms including hemiparesis and cranial nerve palsies.
- Loss of consciousness which may be transient or persisting.
- Epileptic seizures in about 6% of cases.
- 10% of cases of spontaneous subarachnoid haemorrhage present with sudden death.
- Pain may be relieved by simple analgesia and sometimes from tripans which is a diagnostic pitfall.

Investigations

Blood tests:

- FBC
- U&Es
- Clotting
- Glucose

Imaging:

- Computer tomography (CT): of the brain is performed as soon as possible. (See Figure 3.27). Subarachnoid blood is rapidly reabsorbed.

  The sensitivity of CT rapidly decreases with time (almost 100% within 24 hours reducing to 50% at first week and almost 0% at third week). Interpretation should be by a neuroradiologist. Such scans will miss about 2% SAH at 12 hours, rising to 7% at 24 hours.

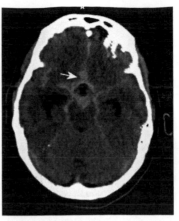

Figure 3.27: Non contrast enhanced CT brain showing increased density along the circle of Willis (arrow) in keeping with an acute subarachnoid haemorrhage.

- CT angiography: will also be necessary if presenting more than two weeks after a bleed. A normal CT and lumbar puncture (LP) in these circumstances will not exclude SAH.

Others:

- Electrocardiogram (ECG)
- LP: is mandatory with a history of acute headache and a negative CT brain. Ideally delay until 12 hours post headache onset (unless meningitis suspected). Measure opening pressure which will be raised in 60% SAH. One sample is sent to look for protein and glucose and another is sent to microscopy to look for red blood cells. Final sample is sent to look for xanthochromia hence do not place in vacuum transport system and ensure protected from light. (See Table 3.50). LP may be negative if performed too early (<6 hours) which is a diagnostic pitfall.

> CSF findings:
>
> Red blood cells leaking into the subarachnoid space lyse and the haemoglobin degrades first to oxyhaemoglobin and then bilirubin. It is this bilirubin which causes the yellowish colouration of xanthochromia detected in the laboratory by spectrophotometry. The presence of bilirubin is diagnostic of SAH as it is only produced in vivo. Oxyhaemoglobin may result from a traumatic LP (10–20% of LPs) or from agitation of red blood cells, for instance in vacuum transport tubes. Since light causes degradation of bilirubin the sample must be protected in transport.

Table 3.50: Laboratory findings in the CSF.

Management

- ➢ Adequate analgesia
- ➢ Deep vein thrombosis (DVT) prophylaxis
- ➢ Nimodipine 60 mg every four hours to reduce vasospasm
- ➢ Ongoing monitoring of neurological status using the Glasgow coma score (GCS).

➢ Monitoring for hyponatraemia caused by cerebral salt wasting or syndrome of inappropriate anti-diuretic hormone secretion (SIADH).

➢ Careful management to reduce secondary brain injury, i.e. avoid hypoxia and hypotension ensuring good hydration.

➢ Neurosurgical referral for endovascular coiling or open surgery to apply clips.

Prognosis:

➢ There is 50% mortality with about 25% mortality in the first 24 hours

➢ 20% survivors have long term dependency

➢ If left untreated up to 20% will re-bleed within the first two weeks with a long term re-bleeding risk of 3% per annum

➢ Re-bleeds have a greater mortality, so SAH is an important diagnosis to make

➢ Hydrocephalus is seen in 10–30% which sometimes requires ventriculo-peritoneal shunt placement

Cerebral venous thrombosis

Epidemiology

Estimated incidence 3–4 cases per million per year. It is most common in the third decade and 75% are female.

Aetiology

There are various risk factors for cerebral venous sinus thrombosis:

- Infections: meningitis, mastoiditis and sinusitis.
- Drugs: OCP, HRT, androgens, and anabolic steroids.
- Pregnancy and puerperium.
- Coagulopathies: factor V Leiden, protein C, protein S or antithrombin deficiency.
- Systemic diseases with pro-coagulant states: nephrotic syndrome, Polycythemia vera and Systemic lupus erythematosus (SLE).
- Head injury.
- Intracerebral space occupying lesions (SOL).

Pathophysiology

Thrombus formation within a venous sinus can create a partial or complete blockage leading to localised congestion within the venous system and the brain. Venous congestion causes increased ICP, massive ischaemia, and infarction of cerebral tissue. Haemorrhagic conversion can occur in larger infarctions. Frequently occluded venous sinuses are the superior sagittal and the left and right transverse sinuses.

Key features in the history/examination

- Headache (90%) This may be of gradual onset, but can also be 'thunderclap' in presentation

- Nausea and vomiting
- Past medical history of thrombophilia
- Drug history of sinusitis/mastoiditis
- Focal neurology mimicking a stroke
- Seizures
- Signs of raised ICP: papilloedema and reduced level of consciousness
- May have signs of nystagmus, dysphagia, hearing loss, and cerebellar incoordination

Investigations
Blood tests:

- Thrombophilia screen

Imaging:

- Contrast-enhanced CT: of the brain may show the empty delta sign in the superior sagittal sinus, i.e. enhancement of the collateral veins surrounding the less dense thrombosed sinus.
- Magnetic resonance venogram: is the investigation of choice.

Management

➢ Full A to E assessment

➢ Intravenous (IV) fluids

➢ Control any seizures

➢ Treat any underlying infection

➢ Stop oral contraceptive/hormone replacement therapy

➢ Anticoagulation: heparin in the first instance

Prognosis:

- Estimated mortality of 20%.
- However in survivors the frequency of long term neurological deficits and epilepsy is low.
- A recurrent thrombosis occurs in about 20% if no treatment is given.

Meningitis/encephalitis

Epidemiology

Bacterial have an incidence of 5 per 100,000 while viral encephalitis has an incidence of 5–10 per 100,000.

Aetiology

Risk of meningitis is increased when defences against infection are lowered, especially in any condition which results in immune deficiency. Organisms can enter by haematogenous spread or by direct invasion from infection in local tissues. The typical causative organism of bacterial meningitis varies according to age. (See Table 3.51).

Age	Pathogens
< 1 month	Group B Streptococcus, E. coli, Klebsiella, proteus spp, L. monocytogenes
1–3 months	Group B Streptococcus, E. coli, Klebsiella, proteus spp, L. monocytogenes, S. pneumonia, N. meningitides, H. influenzae type B
3 months-5 years	S. pneumonia, N. meningitides, H. influenzae type B
5–50 years	S. pneumonia, N. meningitides
> 50 years	S. pneumonia, N. meningitides, L. monocytogenes, gram negative bacilli

Table 3.51: Microbes usually found to cause meningitis in different age groups.

The causes of viral meningo-encephalitis are herpes simplex virus (HSV), enteroviruses, cytomegalovirus (CMV), Epstein-Barr Virus (EBV) and HIV.

Pathophysiology

Neutrophils are drawn into the CSF by bacterial surface components, complement, and inflammatory cytokines (e.g. tumour necrosis factor (TNF), interleukin-1). The neutrophils release metabolites that damage cell membranes including those of the vascular endothelium leading to vasculitis and thrombophlebitis, which can cause focal ischaemia or infarction, and oedema. Vasculitis also disrupts the blood-brain barrier, further increasing oedema. The purulent exudate in the CSF blocks CSF reabsorption by the arachnoid villi, causing hydrocephalus. Brain oedema and hydrocephalus increase ICP.

Key Features in the history/examination

- Headache, usually of subacute onset, but can be sudden.
- Photophobia.
- Neck stiffness (absent in 30%).
- Fever.

- Encephalitic symptoms, including abnormal behaviour, reduced level of consciousness, focal neurological signs and seizures.
- Neck stiffness (absent in 30%).
- Meningococcal meningitis and septicaemia give a non-blanching purpuric rash.

Investigations

Blood tests:

- FBC
- U&Es
- Inflammatory markers: C-reactive protein (CRP)
- Clotting screen

Microbiology:

- Blood cultures: ideally some should be taken before the antibiotics are given, but the antibiotics should not be delayed if they have not been.

Imaging:

- CT: if required. This may need discussion with the radiologist on call, but if the patient has GCS 15/15, normal neurological examination (including fundoscopy), no history of cancer or intracerebral SOL and no evidence of immunosupression then CT brain is not usually required prior to LP.

Others:

- LP: for analysis of CSF. See Table 3.52.

Management

➤ On clinical suspicion of meningitis do not delay in giving antibiotics. IV Ceftriaxone 2 g is usually given but see local hospital guideline to be sure.

➤ Steroids are sometimes given in meningitis but only on senior advice.

	WBC	Protein	Glucose	Gram Stain	Comments
Normal	< 5 cells/mm	0.15–0.45 g/L	> 2/3 plasma	–	Opening pressure 10–20 cmH$_2$O
Bacterial	> 1000 neutrophils	Increased (> 1.0 g/L)	Decreased (< 1/3 plasma)	Positive in 60–90%	–
Partially treated bacterial	100–1000 neutrophils or lymphocytes	Normal or increased	Normal or decreased	Positive in 40–60%	Listeria will also give this picture
Viral	10–100 lymphocytes	Normal or mild increase	Normal or decreased	Normal	HSV polymerase chain reaction (PCR)
Tuberculous	10–100 lymphocytes	Increased (> 1.0 g/L)	Decreased	Normal	AFB on Z-N stain and PCR
Fungal	10–100 lymphocytes	Increased	Increased	Normal	India Ink and Cryptococcal antigen

Table 3.52: Interpretation of CSF results.

Temporal arteritis/giant cell arteritis

Epidemiology

Prevalence of 18–22/100,000 of population. Predominantly in over 50's and more common in women than men (2.5 times more likely). Rare in Asian and Afro-Caribbeans.

Aetiology

The aetiology is not proven, but is felt to be a maladaptive autoimmune response to an environmental stimulus. These environmental stimuli are either infectious or non-infectious. Infectious causes include human para-influenza virus, parvovirus B19 and *Mycoplasma pneumoniae* while non-infectious causes include smoking.

Pathophysiology

Vasculitis primarily affecting the elastic lamina of medium and large arteries. Typically affects the temporal arteries. Transmural inflammation of the artery is seen with infiltration by multinucleated giant cells. The hyperplasia can result in arterial luminal narrowing, which may cause ischaemia distally. The major complication is irreversible blindness, and consequently is considered a medical and opthelmological emergency.

Key features in the history/examination

- Consider in any new headache in the over-50s age group
- Usually a unilateral headache, but can be bilateral (usually not localised to the temples)
- Associated with jaw claudication and visual disturbances
- Symptoms of polymyalgia rheumatica (PMR) may be present, including muscle aches and fatigue
- Enlarged, tender temporal arteries
- Scalp tenderness may be present

Investigations

Blood tests:

- Inflammatory markers: erythrocyte sedimentation rate (ESR) is usually raised to more than 50 mm/hr but sometimes normal. CRP, on the other hand, is always raised.

Others:

- Temporal artery biopsy

Management

➢ High dose steroids: 1 mg/kg Prednisolone.
➢ Steroids should be instituted on clinical grounds before temporal artery biopsy due to the risk of blindness.
➢ This will give a rapid improvement in symptoms.

Raised intracranial pressure

Epidemiology

Varies dependent on the causation.

Aetiology

Raised ICP is caused by a number of pathologies including tumour, abscesses, encephalitis, hydrocephalus and trauma. It can also be idiopathic in obese young women.

Pathophysiology

The pathophysiology is dependent on the aetiology.

Key features in the history/examination

- Diffuse headache
- Exacerbated by lying down, valsalva manoeuvre and exertion
- Neurological signs are usually present:
  o Localising: directly from the pathology
  o False: resulting from the raised ICP, classically a cranial nerve VI palsy
- Papilloedema: ensure fundoscopy performed
- As pressure rises, bradycardia and hypertension
- As 'coning' begins: unilateral then bilateral fixed dilated pupil, cranial nerve III palsy

Investigations

Imaging:

- CT: of the brain.

Others:

- LP: with particular emphasis on the opening pressure.

Management

➢ Pressure will be relieved by LP
➢ Acetazolamide
➢ Treatment of the underlying cause e.g. abscess drainage or tumour removal
➢ Neurosurgical referral for consideration of shunt placement

Trigeminal neuralgia

Epidemiology

There is an annual incidence of about 4–5 per 100,000. It most commonly occurs after the age of 40 and females are more affected.

Aetiology

Rarely it can be seen in association with multiple sclerosis (MS) (3%) or result from a tumour compressing the nerve root (6%). There may also be a genetic predisposition as there have been observations of familial clustering. Idiopathic cases exist too.

Pathophysiology

The underlying pathology can be due to compression of the trigeminal nerve or degeneration of the nerve.

Compression of blood vessels may press on the trigeminal nerve as it leaves the brainstem at the level of the pons. This is more likely as vessels become more ectatic with age. Compression of the nerve leads to demyelination. This results in spontaneous generation of electric impulses. This probably accounts for up to 90% of cases that were originally classified as idiopathic.

Some have postulated it to be part of the ageing process as with increasing age the brain atrophies leading to redundant arterial loops which can cause compression. Myelin sheath infiltration e.g. tumour or amyloidosis.

Key features in the history/examination

- Usually a disease of the over-50s and is more common in women
- Severe knife-like pain lasting a few seconds at a time
- There may be triggers to the pain, typically chewing, speaking and touching the affected area
- Previously called tic douloureux as there may be facial spasms associated with the pain
- Confined to the distribution of the trigeminal nerve (CN V) on 1 side, usually the maxillary or mandibular divisions

Investigations

Imaging:

- Magnetic resonance imaging (MRI): of the brain may be indicated to exclude multiple sclerosis (MS) or a tumour

There are no diagnostic investigations.

Management

➢ Most patients respond well to Carbamazepine or Gabapentin
➢ Surgical decompression is only indicated for the most intractable cases

Further reading and references

➢ Al-Shahi R., Davenport R.A., Lindsay K.W., et al. (2006). Subarachnoid haemorrhage. *BMJ* 333: 235–240.
➢ www.bash.org.uk
➢ www.britishinfectionsociety.org
➢ www.i-h-s.org

➢ Scottish Intercollegiate Guidelines Network (2008). *Guideline 107: Diagnosis and Management of Headache in Adults.*

JAUNDICE

Differential diagnosis

System/Organ	Disease
Pre-hepatic	Hereditary Spherocytosis
	Sickle cell disease
	Glucose-6-phosphate dehydrogenase (G6PD) deficiency
	Malaria
	Transfusion reaction
	Hypersplenism
Hepatic	Hepato-cellular carcinoma (refer to insidious onset)
	Viral hepatitis
	Fatty Liver
	Alcoholic hepatitis
	Drug induced hepatitis
	Autoimmune hepatitis
	Ischaemic hepatitis
	Infiltrative disease
	Cirrhosis (covered in medical section)
	Primary biliary cirrhosis (PBC)
	Haemochromatosis
	Wilson's disease
	Gilberts syndrome
	Crigler-Najjar syndrome
Post-hepatic	Acute cholecystitis
	Obstructive jaundice
	Ascending cholangitis (refer to acute abdominal pain)
	Sclerosing cholangitis
	Acute pancreatitis (refer to acute abdominal pain)
	Sclerosing cholangitis
	Biliary stricture
	Cholangiocarcinoma (refer to insidious onset)
	Gallbladder cancer (refer to insidious onset)
	Pancreatic carcinoma (refer to insidious onset)
	Pancreatic pseudocyst

Alcoholic liver disease

The incidence of alcoholic liver disease is increasing in the UK as individuals are starting to consume alcohol at a younger age. Traditionally it was men aged 40 to 50 years of age who were affected but this has changed along with the drinking patterns in the UK. Alcohol is the most common cause of liver disease. The risk of developing the disease depends upon the following:

- The amount of alcohol consumed. The safe limits are 14 units for females and 21 units for males, per week.
- Females are more susceptible than males.
- Obesity.
- Co-existing disease affecting the liver such as chronic hepatitic viral infection, alpha-1-antitrypsin deficiency and haemochromatosis.

The harmful effects of alcohol are mostly attributable to acetaldehyde, which is the primary product of metabolism of ethanol. Alcohol causes three different types of liver damage:

- Fatty liver
- Alcoholic hepatitis
- Alcoholic cirrhosis

Fatty liver

Epidemiology

The incidence of fatty liver is increasing due to increased alcohol consumption.

Aetiology

Fatty liver is caused by chronic excessive alcohol consumption.

Pathophysiology

Fatty liver is the most common finding in alcoholic individuals and also an early finding in excessive alcohol intake. Alcohol metabolism within the liver results in fat production and this accumulates in the liver cells. Fat will dissipate with alcohol withdrawal but continued consumption will result in progression to fibrosis and cirrhosis.

Key features in the history/examination

- History of increased alcohol intake over a prolonged period of time. However patients may not be fully accurate when detailing the amount of alcohol they drink.
- Risk factors for hepato-toxicity may be found in the past medical history and drug history to look for other.
- Patients may well be asymptomatic.
- Patients could smell of ethanol.
- Hepatomegaly is usual and jaundice is sometimes seen.
- May demonstrate signs suggestive of alcohol withdrawal e.g. profuse sweating, shaking, agitation.

Investigations

Blood tests:

- FBC: Macrocytosis without anaemia
- Liver biochemistry: Aspartate aminotransferase (AST) will be raised more than alanine aminotransferase (ALT). Gamma-glutamyl transferase (GGT) will also be raised.

Imaging:

- Ultrasound scan (USS): will reveal diffuse areas of high echogenicity within the liver.

Others:

- Liver biopsy: will show fatty infiltration of the liver cells with enlargement of the cells and the nuclei.

Management

- ➤ Targeted at the cause of disease and hence abstinence from alcohol and weight reduction is essential.
- ➤ Provide patients with information about alcohol related liver damage and the consequences of continuing alcohol consumption.
- ➤ Refer to or provide information about local alcohol support services.

Prognosis:

- ➤ Usually a very good prognosis, but only if alcohol consumption is curtailed.

Alcoholic hepatitis

Epidemiology

The incidence of alcoholic hepatitis is increasing due to increased alcohol consumption.

Aetiology

Alcoholic hepatitis is caused by too much alcohol consumption.

Pathophysiology

Alcoholic hepatitis involves necrosis of the hepatocytes and leucocyte infiltration. There is accumulation of dense cytoplasmic material within the liver cells known as Mallory bodies. Continued consumption of alcohol will lead to cirrhosis.

Key features in the history/examination

- Patients have a significant intake of alcohol per day.
- Other risk factors for hepato-toxicity may be present in the past medical history and drug history.
- There can be variable features ranging from mild and non-specific to very severe, progressive and potentially fatal.
- It commonly causes jaundice and right upper quadrant abdominal pain.
- On examination, milder cases may have no findings. However, more severe cases may have evidence of chronic liver disease and portal hypertension.
- It is often accompanied by fever.

Investigations

Blood tests:

- FBC: macrocytosis and a leucocytosis (mainly a neutrophilia). Thrombocytopenia is common.

- Liver biochemistry: The classical picture is of raised AST with normal or mildly raised ALT. Also seen is an increased serum bilirubin, a normal or mildly raised alkaline phosphatise (ALP), a markedly raised GGT (reflecting the alcohol intake).

- Liver function tests (LFTs): hypoalbuminaemia may be present. A prolonged prothrombin time is a late feature.

- Inflammatory markers.

Imaging:

- USS: of the liver will show enlargement with no focal lesions.

- Chest X-ray (CXR): to exclude concurrent sepsis.

Others:

- Urinalysis: to exclude concurrent sepsis.

- Liver biopsy: will reveal necrosis of the liver cells, infiltration with neutrophils, steatosis, as well as features of fibrosis. It is not always necessary to make the diagnosis but may be more useful if there is diagnostic doubt.

Management

➢ Management is mainly supportive and targeted at symptom control, especially during alcohol withdrawal.

➢ Abstinence from alcohol.

➢ Essential to maintain nutritional support and refer to the dietician. Vitamin B supplements as well as dietary supplements may be indicated.

➢ 10 mg if vitamin K for three days if there is a raised International Normalized Ratio (INR).

➢ Steroids such as Prednisolone 40–60 mg per day has been shown to reduce the risk of premature death. However it is not recommended for use in those with encephalopathy.

Prognosis:

➢ Prognosis is worse if individuals continue with excessive alcohol consumption.

➢ In severe disease, there is renal failure and increasing symptoms of jaundice due to worsening liver function as well as prolonged clotting times. Such features precede death.

Alcoholic cirrhosis

Epidemiology

The incidence of alcoholic cirrhosis is increasing due to increased alcohol consumption.

Aetiology

Alcoholic cirrhosis is caused by too much alcohol consumption.

Pathophysiology

Alcoholic cirrhosis is the final stage of alcoholic liver disease and an irreversible process. Chronic hepatic injury with regeneration results in fibrosis, nodule formation and distortion of the hepatic architecture. The intra-hepatic changes cause disruption of the sinusoids, increasing vascular resistance and therefore causing portal hypertension.

Key features in the history/examination

- Full alcohol history

- Other risk factors for hepato-toxicity may be present in the past medical history and drug history

- Main features include jaundice and ascites

- Look for all the features of chronic liver disease

- Variceal haemorrhage which is a complication of alcoholic cirrhosis. (See Haematemesis and Melaena section)

- Encephalopathy which is a complication of alcoholic cirrhosis. (See Confusion section)

- Ascites which is a complication of alcoholic cirrhosis:

  o Distension of the abdomen

  o Accumulation of fluid results in weight gain

  o Shifting dullness when the abdomen is percussed

Investigations

Blood tests:

- FBC: anaemia and thrombocytosis

- U&Es: hyponatraemia is common. Exclude renal failure seen in hepatorenal syndrome

- Liver biochemistry: raised transaminases predominate but raised bilirubin will also be seen

- LFTs: decreased albumin

- Coagulopathy

Imaging:

- CXR: to exclude sepsis as a cause for decompensation.

- USS of the liver: shows a small, nodular liver with dilation of the portal vein. Hepatocellular carcinoma can be identified.

Others:

- Liver biopsy: shows features including Mallory's hyaline, fibrosis, and fatty infiltration.

- Ascitic tap: it is positive if the neutrophil count is more than 250/ml.

- Endoscopy may be indicated, especially if variceal bleed suspected. May also show portal hypertensive gastropathy.

3. Medicine

Management

➤ Management is mainly supportive and targeted at symptom control, especially during alcohol withdrawal.

➤ Counselling and close support for alcohol abstinence.

➤ Avoidance of other hepatic insults, especially drugs.

➤ 10 mg of vitamin K for three days.

➤ Treatment of complications.

Varicies:

➤ Variceal banding programme

➤ Propranolol to reduce portal hypertension

Ascites:

➤ Dietary manipulation: low sodium diet

➤ Diuretics are first line treatment:

  o Spironolactone typically 200 mg per day

  o Furosemide if required

  o Monitoring of U&Es is required

Large volume paracentesis:

➤ This is performed in order to drain the ascites.

➤ May be required acutely for a decompensation with rapid accumulation.

➤ For diuretic resistant ascites a programme of planned paracentesis may be instigated.

➤ It is essential to administer intravenous (IV) salt-poor albumin. Check your local policy for precise regime.

➤ Indications for paracentesis include:

  o Splinting of diaphragm

  o Suspected infection

  o Tense, uncomfortable ascites

➤ There is a high risk of infection, so the drain must only be left in for 6–8 hours.

➤ There is also a high risk of physiological upset, especially hepato-renal syndrome, so only a maximum of ten litres should be drained.

Spontaneous bacterial peritonitis:

➤ Antibiotics

➤ Drainage of ascites

➤ Patients must be given prophylactic antibiotics in order to reduce the risk of bacterial infection and the associated mortality. Most commonly used antibiotics are:

  o Ciprofloxacin

  o Co-trimoxazole

  o Co-amoxiclav

Hepatorenal syndrome:

➤ Very difficult to manage, may require input from hepatologist, nephrologist and an intensivist.

➤ Fluid replacement with albumin.

➤ Close monitoring of fluid balance and regular clinical assessment.

➤ Central line may be required.

➤ Trans-jugular intra-hepatic portasystemic stent shunt (TIPSS) placement may help for problematic portal hypertension with recurrent variceal bleeding.

➤ Liver transplant may be considered but strict criteria apply for the six months of abstinence prior to transplantation.

Prognosis:

➤ The Child-Pugh score is used to assess prognosis:

Factor	1 point	2 points	3 points
Bilirubin (micromol/L)	<34	34–50	>50
Albumin (g/L)	>35	28–35	<28
INR	<1.7	1.7–2.2	>2.2
Ascites	None	Present	Refractory
Encephalopathy	None	Grade I-II	Grade III-IV
Child-Pugh Class	Score	1 year survival	
A	5–6	100%	
B	7–9	80%	
C	10–15	45%	

Table 3.53: The Child-Pugh score.

➤ Prognosis improved generally in those individuals who abstain from alcohol.

Acute viral hepatitis

Hepatitis is the inflammation of the liver cells with no features of fibrosis or nodule formation. It is a very common condition worldwide. Hepatitis is primarily caused by hepatitis virus A, B, C. Cytomegalovirus (CMV), Epstein-Barr virus (EBV), and adenovirus can also cause hepatitis.

Hepatitis A virus

Epidemiology

Hepatitis A virus (HAV) is responsible for 30–40% of acute hepatitis worldwide. It mainly affects children aged 5–14 years and young adults. Infection is much more likely where there is overcrowding and poor sanitary conditions. It is most commonly found in Africa, India and parts of South America.

Aetiology

HAV is an ribonucleic acid (RNA) virus that is transmitted via the faecal-oral route and contaminated water and food products. Epidemics result from water or food contamination. Shellfish have been shown to be an important source as they consume sewage products. Rarely it is transmitted via blood.

The use of contaminated needles in IV drug users and unprotected sexual intercourse are sources of transmission.

Pathophysiology

HAV has an average incubation period of 28 days and will be found in the faeces up until the stage where jaundice appears.

Key features in the history/examination

- Assessment of risk factors: travel to an endemic region or close personal contact with a known case.
- There is a pre-icteric prodrome for one week and the icterus peaks at two weeks.
- Causes the following clinical features:
  - Fever
  - Hepatomegaly and right upper quadrant pain
  - Nausea and vomiting
  - Diarrhoea
  - Anorexia
  - Headache
  - Malaise
  - Jaundice, accompanied by dark urine and pale stools.

Investigations

Blood tests:

- FBC
- U&Es
- Liver biochemistry: a high serum AST and ALT are characteristic of hepatitis.
- Clotting: a marker of disease progression and severity.

Serology:

- IgM antibodies to HAV: indicate infection within the last 4–6 months.
- IgG antibodies to HAV: indicate previous infection.

Imaging:

- USS: of the abdomen to exclude bile duct obstruction, cirrhosis and hepatocellular carcinoma which is very rare with HAV infection.

Management

- Supportive management with avoidance of excessive alcohol.
- Prevention is key and hence the public health measures of careful attention to hygiene and adequate sanitation are essential.

- A vaccination is available and should be administered to those who are due to travel to endemic regions.
- Post-exposure prophylaxis in the form of human immunoglobulin and vaccination can be given to individuals at risk of infection which includes those that had close contact with infected individuals. Prophylaxis is given in order to control an epidemic in institutions.
- The virus will be found in the stools up to two weeks prior to the appearance of jaundice and usually a week afterwards.

Prognosis:

- There is rarely any long term sequelae with less than 1% progressing to fulminant liver failure.
- It is associated with a higher mortality in older individuals.
- Liver function will return to normal within three months of infection.

Hepatitis B virus

Epidemiology

Hepatitis B virus (HBV) is responsible for 0.2% of acute hepatitis in the UK. Around 350 million chronic carriers of the virus exist worldwide. It is commonly in Africa, China and South East Asia. Less than 1% incidence of chronic carriage in the UK.

Aetiology

HBV is spread by blood and any blood products. However very occasionally it spreads by mouth-to-mouth contact too. It can be found in bodily excretions such as saliva, vaginal and menstrual discharges, and seminal fluid. Modes of spread include:

- Horizontal: person to person when there is inoculation of tiny amounts of the contaminated fluid via needles or sexually.
- Vertical: from mother to baby.

Those at higher risk of infection in the UK include immigrants from endemic regions, IV drug users and individuals with multiple sexual partners.

Pathophysiology

HBV is a deoxyribonucleic acid (DNA) virus of the hepadnavirus family. The incubation periods lasts up to six months. Important antigens are the surface antigen (HBsAg), the core antigen (HBcAg) and the pre-core or 'e' antigen (HBeAg). The precise function of (HBeAg) is unknown.

The majority of HBV infections are asymptomatic, with only about 30% having symptoms. Hence it progress to chronic disease in around 20% of patients. There is also a 15–30% chance of developing cirrhosis with chronic HBV carriage but the risk is greatest in those co-infected by hepatitis D virus (HDV) or human immunodeficiency virus (HIV).

Key features in the history/examination

- Assessment of risk factors: sexual history, in particular number of partners, sexual contact with an infected individual and men who have sex with men. Injection of drugs is another risk factor to look out for.

- 70% who are asymptomatic patients will be normal on examination.
- Clinical features in the symptomatic individuals will be broadly similar to those with HAV infection:
  o Fever
  o Hepatomegaly and right upper quadrant pain
  o Nausea and vomiting
  o Diarrhoea
  o Anorexia
  o Headache
  o Malaise
  o Jaundice, accompanied by dark urine and pale stools.

Investigations

Blood tests:

- FBC
- U&Es
- Liver biochemistry: a high serum AST and ALT are characteristic of hepatitis.
- HBV DNA: if present within the blood is diagnostic of infection. It can also be used to monitor progress of treatment.
- Clotting: a marker of disease progression and severity.

Serology:

- HBsAg: appears around six weeks after the initial acute infection and usually disappears by three months. Persistence longer than six months means chronic infection.
- HBcAg: is usually found only in the liver cells.
- HBeAg: is found early in the acute phase and usually undetectable after a few weeks. Positivity at three months indicates increased risk of chronicity. It is an indicator of high infectivity.
- Hepatitis B surface antibody (HBsAb): is detectable post-immunisation or post-infection, i.e. once infection has resolved.

Imaging:

- USS: of the abdomen to exclude bile duct obstruction, cirrhosis and hepatocellular carcinoma.

Others:

- Liver biopsy: may show evidence of cirrhosis. Ground glass cells are suggestive of HBV infection. Certain types of staining may illustrate the HBcAg and HBsAg in the liver cells.

Management

➢ Management is mostly supportive in the acute phase.
➢ Patients must be monitored in order to ensure clearance of the virus, i.e. through blood tests showing HBsAg negative results.

➢ If the HBsAg is found to persist for over a six month period, the diagnosis of chronic HBV infection is made.
➢ Chronic HBV is treated with agents such as pegylated interferon alpha and Lamivudine.
➢ Treatment goal is to render the patient HBeAg negative.
➢ Less than 5% of chronic HBV infection will become HBsAg negative.
➢ A vaccination is available and is given as an intramuscular (IM) injection at 0, 1 and 3 months.
  o Levels of anti-HBsAg must be monitored after vaccination at least every three years afterwards.
  o If levels are above 100 IU/ml this is indicative of a good level of immunity.
➢ Post-exposure prophylaxis in the form of human immunoglobulin and vaccination can be given to individuals at risk of infection:
  o Individuals who have a needle-stick injury
  o Sexual partners of infected individuals
  o Household contacts of infected individuals need only receive the vaccination
➢ Babies born to mothers with HBV require immunoglobulin and vaccination at birth.

Prognosis:

➢ Infection resolves completely for the majority of people.
➢ Around 20% of patients may go on to develop chronic infection.
➢ Cirrhotic patients should be monitored for complications including hepatocellulat carcinoma.

Hepatitis C virus

Epidemiology

HCV is responsible for 15–20% of acute hepatitis worldwide. Global prevalence of approaching 3%, but is closer to 0.5% in the UK. It is endemic in many parts of the world, especially in Southern Europe and Japan.

Aetiology

HCV is spread by exposure to contaminated blood, classically via blood transfusions prior to the introduction of screening. Sharing needles whilst injecting drugs is another mode of transmission. It can also be transmitted from mother to child during birth.

Pathophysiology

HCV is a single stranded RNA flavivirus and consists of six genotypes which all respond differently to therapy. The subtype 1b virus of the genotype 1 is the most virulent and the commonest genotypes in the UK the genotypes 1, 2 and 3. HCV is usually involved in post-transfusion hepatitis and there is a significantly higher risk of becoming chronically infected with HCV than with HBV.

Key features in history/examination

- Assessment of risk factors: IV drug use and previous blood transfusion.
- Patients may initially be asymptomatic but symptoms of mild jaundice follow.
- Later, features of chronic liver disease and cirrhosis may become evident.

Investigations

Blood tests:

- FBC
- U&Es
- Liver biochemistry: high serum AST and ALT are characteristic of hepatitis.
- Clotting: is marker of disease progression and severity.

Serology:

- HCV antibodies
- HCV RNA: done by using enzyme-linked immunosorbent assay (ELISA) or polymerase chain reaction (PCR), it is the most useful diagnostic test
- Viral genotyping: is useful in predicting response to treatment

Imaging:

- USS: of the abdomen to exclude bile duct obstruction, cirrhosis and hepatocellular carcinoma.

Others:

- Liver biopsy: In HBV or HCV it may show evidence of cirrhosis.

Management

- Acute infection is treated with interferon-alpha.
- The duration of the treatment required depends upon the specific viral genotype, for example, genotype 1 has a 50% six month cure rate, whereas those not of type 1 will respond well to six months of therapy.
- Treatment is associated with benefits such as reduction in the amount of fibrosis and a lower risk of developing hepatocellular carcinoma.
- Chronic carriers should be advised to abstain from alcohol, advised about safe sex especially to avoid co-infection with HIV, and should be offered HAV and HBV vaccination.
- Prevention involves awareness of the dangers of sharing needles and unprotected sexual intercourse. Needle exchange programmes have been shown to be successful.

- Advanced liver disease should be managed by a hepatologist and the possibility of liver transplantation should be considered.

Prognosis:

- The majority of affected individuals become chronic carriers and of those 20% will eventually develop cirrhosis over a 20-year period.
- Cirrhotic patients should be monitored for complications including hepatocellular carcinoma.
- Renal function should be monitored for the possibility of glomerulonephritis caused by cryoglobulinaemia.
- Older patients tend to have more aggressive symptoms.
- Very rarely there will be cases of acute liver failure.

Chronic hepatitis

Persistently deranged liver biochemistry for more than three months and evidence of necrosis of the liver cells on liver biopsy indicated chronic hepatitis. Causes of chronic hepatitis include:

- Autoimmune hepatitis
- Chronic HBV and HCV infection
- Wilson's disease
- Haemachromatosis
- Alpha-1-antitrypsin deficiency
- Certain drugs such as methyldopa

Eventually chronic liver disease will follow chronic hepatitis. Generally, the features of chronic liver disease are as follows, with the associated condition in brackets:

- Clubbing
- Palmar erythema
- Leukonychia (hypoalbuminaemia)
- Dupytren's contracture (alcohol dependence)
- Metabolic flap/asterixis (hepatic encephalopathy)
- Parotidomegaly (alcohol dependence)
- Keiser-Fleisher rings (Wilson's disease)
- Xanthelasmata (PBC)
- Excoriations
- Spider naevi
- Gynaecomastia
- Ascites (portal hypertension and hypoalbuminaemia)
- Small irregular shrunken liver (cirrhosis)
- Distended abdominal veins/caput madusae
- Testicular atrophy
- Reduction in body hair
- Anaemia
- Drowsiness (hepatic encephalopathy)

3. Medicine

- Hyperventilation (hepatic encephalopathy)
- Jaundice (excretory dysfunction)
- Peripheral oedema (hypoalbuminaemia)
- Bruising (coagulopathy)
- Peripheral neuropathy (alcohol and certain medications)
- Cerebellar signs (alcohol dependence and Wilson's disease)
- Hepatomegaly (alcohol dependence, non-alcoholic fatty liver disease (NAFLD), haemochromatosis)
- Increased pigmentation of the skin (haemochromatosis)
- Signs of right heart failure
- Tattoos (HCV infection)
- Signs of chronic obstructive pulmonary disease (COPD) (alpha-1 antitrypsin deficiency)

Autoimmune hepatitis

Epidemiology

Incidence approximately 1 per 100,000 per year. A bimodal distribution exists when considering age with peaks at ages 20–30 and 55–65 years. It is more common in females than males with a female to male ratio of 8:1.

Aetiology

The aetiology is unknown.

It is associated with human leukocyte antigen (HLA) phenotype B8, DR3 and DR4. Environmental triggers are unclear. There are four recognised subtypes of autoimmune hepatitis:

1. Positive for antinuclear antibodies (ANA) and smooth muscle antibodies (SMA) and raised IgG.
2. Positive for anti-liver/kidney/microsomal (anti-LKM) antibodies. This is typically found in female children and teenagers.
3. Positive for antibodies against soluble liver antigen (anti-SLA). This is clinically similar to group 1.
4. No auto-antibodies detected.

Pathophysiology

Autoimmune hepatitis is a chronic inflammatory disease characterised by autoimmune hepatocyte damage.

Key features in the history/examination

- Other auto-immune diseases such as hyperthyroidism, type 1 diabetes mellitus, ulcerative colitis (UC), coeliac disease and rheumatoid arthritis in the past medial history or family history.
- Presents with features of jaundice, pruritis, fatigue, nausea, anorexia, abdominal discomfort and arthralgia.
- Hepatomegaly is a common finding.
- Rarely presents with complications of liver disease such as ascites, splenomegaly, portal hypertension and encephalopathy.
- Always look for features of other undiagnosed autoimmune conditions.

Investigations

Blood tests:

- FBC
- U&Es
- Coagulation screen
- Liver biochemistry: transaminases are always moderately raised but ALP/GGT may be normal.

Serology:

- Auto-antibodies: look for ANA, SMA, anti-SLA and anti-LKM.
- Serum IgG is often found to be raised.

Others:

- Liver biopsy

Management

➢ Steroid regimen such as Prednisolone at 30–60 mg per day is the first-line treatment. The dose of steroids are reduced as the liver enzymes improve.
➢ Azathioprine can also be commenced as first-line or is added to therapy when the Prednisolone is reduced to 20 mg per day and if the LFTs have returned to normal.
➢ Life-long treatment with steroid or azathioprine is required and it can only be withdrawn successfully without relapse occasionally.
➢ Attention should be given to prevent osteoporosis with long term steroid use.
➢ Ciclosporin has also been shown to be effective.
➢ A liver transplant is indicated in patients who do not respond to treatment.

Prognosis:

➢ Over 80% of patients enter remission but this may take several years to achieve.
➢ There is a 50% 5-year survival rate without appropriate treatment.
➢ Treatment initiated before any features of cirrhosis results in a 90% 10-year survival, but it is considerably lower if cirrhosis is established.

Chronic HBV infection

This affects around 0.1% patients in the UK and up to 15% in the Far East and Africa. It is found to be more common in males than females.

Aetiology

Chronic HBV infection develops in up to 20% of patients with the acute infection.

Pathophysiology

Patients continue to be HBsAg positive and the persistence of this virus indicates a poor host immune response to the virus.

Key features in the history/examination

- The infection could be an incidental finding at a routine screening during pregnancy or at a genitourinary medicine (GUM) clinic.
- It can present with features such as jaundice, pruritus or complications associated with liver disease.

Investigations

Blood tests:

- FBC
- U&Es
- Liver biochemistry: can be normal or show subtle increases in the serum liver enzymes, ALP and bilirubin levels.
- Coagulation screen

Serology:

- HBV serology: is required in order to determine the management plan.

Others:

- Liver biopsy: may reveal minimal changes within the liver, ranging up to a chronic active hepatitis or cirrhosis. Ground glass liver cells are characteristic features.

Management

➢ Subcutaneous interferon-alpha therapy given regularly over a three-month period is effective in those who are HBV DNA positive.
➢ Lamivudine is effective in those with evidence of active viral replication.

Prognosis:

➢ Around 5% of patients will seroconvert by the first year compared to up to 50% of individuals who are treated.
➢ Without treatment the infection will progress to cirrhosis and eventually hepatocellular carcinoma with a much poorer prognosis.
➢ Those with low serum HBV DNA levels and high liver enzyme levels tend to have a better prognosis.
➢ Males tend to have a poorer prognosis.
➢ Those with established cirrhosis tend to have a poorer prognosis.

Chronic HCV infection

Chronic HCV infection is responsible for 50–70% of cases of what was previously known as cryptogenic cirrhosis.

Aetiology

Cause is HCV infection.

Pathophysiology

The disease can be rapidly progressive in older individuals and those with excessive alcohol consumption.

Key features in the history/examination

- There tends to be an insidious onset and patients tend to be asymptomatic until they develop symptoms.
- Symptoms of cirrhosis may be the presenting feature.
- Occasionally deranged liver biochemistry on a routine blood test may reveal the disease.

Investigations

Blood tests:

- FBC
- U&Es
- Coagulation screening
- Liver biochemistry: can be normal or show subtle increases in the serum liver enzymes, ALP, and bilirubin levels.

Serology:

- Antibodies to structural and non-structural viral proteins will be detected on serological testing. The presence of antibodies indicate active infection.

Others:

- Liver biopsy: will show features of mild hepatitis as well as fatty changes and aggregates of lymphoid cells.

Management

➢ Symptomatic treatment is important.
➢ Pegylated interferon-alpha and Ribavirin is required for at least 6–12 months tailored according to patient response to treatment.

Prognosis:

➢ Treatment response is confirmed with a reduction in the level of serum liver enzymes. This can be found in over 50% of patients.
➢ The rate of relapse is around 33%.
➢ At 20 years there is a 20% change of developing cirrhosis and of those with cirrhosis there is an annual 5% risk of developing liver failure or hepatocellular carcinoma.

Primary biliary cirrhosis

Primary biliary cirrhosis (PBC) is an autoimmune disease characterised by intra-hepatic duct inflammation, fibrosis and cirrhosis of the liver.

Epidemiology

It affects 1–2 in 5,000 women in Europe and rarely occurs in Africa and India. It mostly affects middle-aged individuals (40–60 years).

Aetiology

PBC has an autoimmune basis and hence may be associated with other autoimmune conditions such as:

- Sjögren syndrome
- Sicca syndrome
- Thyroid disease e.g. Grave's disease
- Vitiligo
- Coeliac disease
- Systemic sclerosis

Over 95% of patients are positive for AMA.

Pathophysiology

Progressive immune-mediated damage to the intra-hepatic bile ducts is seen with loss of ducts. Eventually this leads to cholestasis and the consequent damage to the liver itself results in cirrhosis.

Key features in the history/examination

- Autoimmune disease in the past medical history or family history.
- There are different presentations of this condition.
- The presentation may be asymptomatic and only an incidental finding.
- There may be progressive symptoms of pruritus, classically associated with PBC, followed by jaundice. Look for excoriation marks.
- The presentation may be with complications such as ascites, jaundice, and gastrointestinal (particularly variceal) bleeding. However these tend to represent advanced disease.
- Pale stools, dark urine and steatorrhoea.
- On examination, features such as hepatosplenomegaly are common early in the disease.
- Pigmentation and xanthomas in the periorbital region may be found.

Investigations

Blood tests:

- FBC: check for anaemia and platelet count
- U&Es
- Liver biochemistry: will initially reveal an increased ALP and GGT and as the disease progresses the serum bilirubin will rise.

- LFTs: as the disease progresses the prothrombin time will increase and albumin decrease.
- Clotting screen
- Alpha-fetoprotein

Serology:

- Serum immunoglobulins: will be increased in particular the level of IgM.
- Antimitochondrial antibodies: particularly the M2 subtype will be present.
- ANA: may be present as well but are less common.

Imaging:

- USS: of the liver is useful to exclude extra-hepatic biliary obstruction.

Others:

- Liver biopsy: will show infiltration of lymphocytes in and around the intra-hepatic bile ducts, followed by duct proliferation, fibrosis and eventually cirrhosis.

Management

- No treatment has been found to improve the prognosis in these patients.
- Ursodeoxycholic acid has been shown to improve the LFTs hence slowing the rate of deterioration.
- Cholestyramine is effective in reducing symptoms of pruritus as it binds the bile acids in the gut.
- Antihistamines such as Chlorpheniramine should be avoided as they are ineffective in cholestatic pruritis and may cause drowsiness.
- Fat-soluble vitamin supplements are required in these patients to prevent deficiencies.
- Patients with decompensated liver disease should be treated symptomatically for ascites, varicies and other complications. In addition they should be referred to a transplant centre for consideration of liver transplant since the 5-year survival rate is as much as 70%.

Prognosis:

- Follow-up should be done at least annually to screen for deteriorating hepatic function. This is achieved by monitoring bilirubin, albumin and prothrombin time. Monitor progression of portal hypertension and occurrence of hepatocellular carcinoma too.
- There is a variable survival rate which is inversely proportional to the bilirubin levels.

Further reading and references

- British Society of Gastroenterology (2003). *Guidance on the Treatment of Hepatitis C incorporating the Use of Pegylated Interferons.*

➤ British Society of Gastroenterology (2006). *Guidelines on the Management of Ascites in Cirrhosis.*

➤ Scottish Intercollegiate Guidelines Network (2008). *Management of acute upper and lower gastrointestinal bleeding.*

LIMB PAIN AND SWELLING

Differential Diagnosis

	Disease
Musculoskeletal (non-trauma)	Osteoarthritis
	Rheumatoid arthritis
	Gout
	Pseudogout
	Seronegative arthropathies
Trauma	Fracture
	Soft tissue injury (e.g. sprain)
	Compartment syndrome
Infections	Abscess
	Cellulitis
	Necrotising fasciitis
	Septic arthritis
Vascular	**Deep Vein Thrombosis**
	Venous insufficiency
Other	Lymphoedema
	Neuropathic pain
Bilateral Leg Swelling	Heart failure
	Cirrhosis
	Nephrotic syndrome
	Hypoalbuminaemia
	Hypothyroidism
	Dependent oedema
	Drug side-effects e.g. calcium channel blockers

In an acute mono-arthritis with a painful, red, hot, swollen joint, septic arthritis must be excluded.

Rheumatoid Arthritis

Rheumatoid arthritis (RA) is a chronic inflammatory condition which predominantly affects joints but also has significant multisystem involvement.

Epidemiology

RA affects approximately 1% of the population with a 2:1 female:male ratio.

The most common age of onset is in the 5th decade.

Aetiology

RA is an autoimmune disease of multi-factorial origin. There is evidence to suggest that some polymorphisms at the HLA loci on chromosome 6 can increase the chance of the disease. The environmental triggers are poorly understood.

Pathophysiology

The synovial tissue proliferates, eroding first the cartilage and then the underlying bone, resulting in joint deformity and joint destruction.

Key features in the history/examination

- The 1988 revised American College of Rheumatology criteria are used for diagnosis:

1. Morning stiffness lasting at least 1 hour
2. Arthritis of 3 or more joint areas simultaneously (the possible areas are left and right – proximal inter-phalangeal (PIP), metacarpophalangeal (MCP), wrist, elbow, knee, ankle and metatarsophalangeal)
3. Hand joint involvement
4. Symmetrical arthritis
5. Rheumatoid nodules (subcutaneous nodules, classically at the elbow)
6. Rheumatoid Factor positivity
7. Radiographic changes typical of RA on hand or wrist X-rays
If 4 of the 7 criteria are satisfied, then RA is diagnosed. The first 3 criteria must have been present for at least 6 weeks.

Table 3.54: American College of Rheumatology criteria.

- A full history of joint and extra-articular involvement.
- History/family history of other auto-immune diseases.
- Cardiovascular history.

Summary of features to expect on examination:

System	Feature
Rheumatoid hands	• Look for active synovitis, typically at the MCP and PIP joints (with sparing of the DIP joints) and the wrist
	• Ulnar deviation of the fingers at the MCP joints
	• Swan-neck and boutonnière deformities of the fingers and Z-thumbs
	• Dorsal subluxation of the ulna at the carpal joint
	• Wasting of the small muscles
	• Nail-fold infarcts
	• Palmar erythema
	• Carpal tunnel syndrome
	• A functional assessment should be made of the hands, including writing, combing hair and picking up coins.

Continued

3. Medicine

Lung	• Pleural effusions (exudates)
	• Fibrosis
	• Recurrent infections due to parenchymal lung damage and immunosuppression
Cardiac	• Pericardial rub
Neurological	• Mono-neuritis multiplex
	• Peripheral neuropathy
	• Cervical myelopathy caused by atlanto-axial subluxation
Skin	• Rheumatoid nodules
Ophthalmic	• Scleritis/episcleritis
	• Sjögren syndrome
Haematological (anaemia)	• Anaemia of chronic disease
	• NSAID – related gastrointestinal bleeding
	• Megaloblastic anaemia associated with pernicious anaemia/methotrexate therapy
	• Bone marrow suppression from DMARDs
	• Felty's Syndrome anaemia and splenomegaly

Table 3.55: Summary of features on examination in rheumatoid arthritis.

Investigations

Blood tests:

- FBC looking for anaemia, leucocytosis and thrombocytosis
- Raised ESR and CRP
- Rheumatoid Factor

Imaging:

- Joint X-rays: typical radiological features are: Joint space narrowing, joint erosions, juxta-articular osteoporosis, cysts, subluxation and deformation. Exclude other causes for the hot, inflamed joints.
- Chest X-ray: look for evidence of fibrosis, effusions, and rheumatoid nodules.
- CT: of chest if appropriate for confirmation or further clarification of X-rays. For example, bronchiolitis obliterans organising pneumonia (BOOP), which is identical to the idiopathic form.

Others:

- Joint aspiration: typically straw-coloured fluid with a slight neutrophilia. Check for crystals and send to microbiology to exclude infection.

Assessment of cardiovascular risk factors:

- Lipid profile

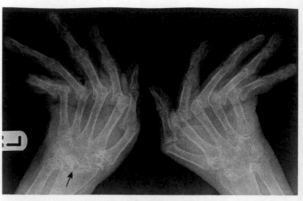

Figure 3.28: Plain X-ray of both hands showing multiple joint subluxations, periarticular cyst formation and erosions (arrow).

- Diabetes
- ECG

Management

➢ Analgesia, e.g. simple analgesia, Non steroidal anti-inflammatory drugs (NSAIDs)

➢ Corticosteroids

➢ Disease Modifying Anti-rheumatic Drugs (DMARDs), e.g. Hydroxychloroquine, Sulphasalazine, Methotrexate, Gold and Penicillamine

➢ Anti-cytokine agents e.g. Infliximab (anti-TNF-α)

➢ Physiotherapy

➢ Treatment of extra-articular features as required

➢ Reduce cardiovascular risks by advising lifestyle changes and prescribing Aspirin, anti-hypertensives and Statins

Gout

Epidemiology

Prevalence of approximately 1%.The prevalence is increasing. The reason for this is not clear but may be connected to increases in obesity and diuretic use. Gout is the commonest cause of crystal arthritis and much more common in men. Risk of gout increases with increasing uric acid levels.

Aetiology

Crystal arthropathy is caused by an inflammatory response to urate crystals in the joint space. Both genetic and environmental causes influence urate levels.

An acute attack may be precipitated by:

- Trauma
- Unusual physical exercise
- Severe systemic illness
- Dietary excess (diets containing high levels of red meat)

- Alcohol
- Surgery
- Drugs (cytotoxic drug therapy, diuretics, commencement of allopurinol, commencement of B12 for pernicious anaemia).

Pathophysiology

Uric acid is produced by purine metabolism. Purines may come from dietary intake or catabolism, especially of purine nucleotides.

Hyperuricaemia may result from reduced renal excretion of urate (90%) or increased urate production (about 10%):

Causes of reduced renal excretion	Causes of increased production
Diuretics (especially thiazide)	Glucose-6-phosphate deficiency
Aspirin	Lymphoproliferative disorders
Hypertension	Myeloproliferative disorders
Chronic kidney disease	Cytotoxic therapy
	Carcinomatosis
	Idiopathic

Table 3.56: Causes of hyperuricaemia

Key Features in the history/examination

- Usually presents as an acute mono-arthritis, typically in the first metatarsophalangeal joint.
- Polyarticular presentation in about 10% cases.
- May have previous episodes of arthritis.
- May have previous history of renal stones.
- Family history of gout.
- Sudden onset of hot, red, swollen and exquisitely tender joint(s).
- Chronic hyperuricaemia can result in renal impairment, renal calculi and gouty tophi, i.e. deposition of urate in the tissues especially in finger tendons and the pinnae.

Investigations

Blood tests:

- FBC: Raised WBC in acute gout
- U&E
- CRP
- Clotting
- Glucose
- Uric acid

Imaging:

- X-ray joint: any bony injury needs to be excluded. Look for

characteristic changes of punched out periarticular erosions, secondary degenerative change and soft tissue swelling.

Others:

- Joint aspiration: send for urgent microscopy to exclude septic arthritis, culture, sensitivity and polarised light microscopy. The presence of negatively birefringent (needle shaped) crystals confirms the diagnosis.

Management

- ➤ Analgesia: NSAIDs or colchicine 500 mcg TDS. Beware of diarrhoea with colchicine.
- ➤ Allopurinol should not be started during an attack because this can make matters worse or prolong the attack. It can be started after the attack has settled, usually with NSAID or colchicine cover.
- ➤ Consider injecting joint with long acting steroid if infection excluded.
- ➤ Physiotherapy.

Pseudogout

Epidemiology

Although chondrocalcinosis (soft tissue calcium deposition within the joint) is very common in the elderly population, attacks of pseudogout are relatively uncommon.

Aetiology

Crystal arthropathy caused by an inflammatory reaction to calcium pyrophosphate dehydrate (CPPD) in the joint. There may be no clear precipitating factor for an acute attack, but it may follow trauma or be triggered by an acute illness e.g. flu.

Pathophysiology

Risk factors include old age, osteoarthritis, hyperparathyroidism, haemochromatosis and hypothyroidism.

Key Features in the history/examination

- Usually presents as a mono-arthritis, typically the knee but also commonly the hip or wrist.
- It can be spontaneous but may be precipitated by illness or trauma.
- Hot, red, swollen and exquisitely tender joint(s).
- The joint may be stiff and painful to move due to the build-up of fluid.

Investigations

Blood tests:

- FBC
- U&E

3. Medicine

- CRP
- Clotting
- Glucose
- Uric acid

Imaging:

- X-ray joint: bony injury needs to be excluded. Chondrocalcinosis may be seen.

Other:

- Joint aspiration: Send for urgent microscopy to exclude septic arthritis, culture, sensitivity and polarised light microscopy. The presence of positively birefringent (rhomboid shaped) crystals confirms the diagnosis.

Management

➢ Usually self-limiting

➢ NSAID (or Colchicine if gastrointestinal or other contraindications)

➢ Consider injecting joint with long acting steroid (if infection excluded)

Cellulitis

Epidemiology

A common presentation on the medical on-call. It affects both sexes equally.

Aetiology

An acute dermal infection of the skin usually caused by gram positive bacteria, i.e. *Streptococci* and *Staphylococci*.

Risk factors:

- Trauma
- Surgery
- Obesity
- Peripheral Vascular Disease
- Ulcerated skin
- Concomitant skin disorder

Pathophysiology

Often caused by a break in the skin e.g. due to insect bite. In the hospital it may occur at a site of venepuncture or cannulation. Cellulitis may be a sign of reduced immunocompetence or the presence of diabetes. It is associated with a local inflammatory response with pain, oedema and warmth.

Key features in the history/examination

- Sudden onset
- History of break in skin integrity

- Past medical history or family history of diabetes or immunocompromise
- Fever may be present
- Affected site will demonstrate erythema, swelling and pain
- Characteristic 'peau d'orange' dimpling of skin
- Localised lymphadenopathy
- In the presence of abscess formation, there will be palpable defined edges

Investigations

Blood tests:

- FBC, CRP & ESR: elevated white cell count and inflammatory markers
- U&E
- LFT
- Glucose: to exclude a new diagnosis of diabetes mellitus.

Microbiology:

- Blood cultures, if there are signs of systemic illness.
- Wound swab, if wound is present.

Other:

- Mark extent of erythema to observe for signs of deterioration or improvement.

Management

➢ Antibiotics may be oral or intravenous depending on severity and causation

  ○ Typical regime is benzylpenicillin and flucloxacillin

➢ Surgical intervention if abscess present

➢ Elevation of affected limb

➢ Analgesia

Necrotising fasciitis

Epidemiology

An estimated 500 new cases per year with a mortality rate of 20%.

Aetiology

Progressive, rapidly spreading inflammatory infection of the deep fascia that causes necrosis of the subcutaneous tissue. Causative bacteria can be aerobic, anaerobic or mixed flora. The most common causative organism is *Streptococcus pyogenes*.

Necrotising fasciitis can occur after:

- Trauma
- Intramuscular or Intravenous injection

- Surgical procedures
- Insect bites
- Child birth

Peripheral vascular disease increases risk. The immunocompromised individuals are at more risk. There is a possible link to NSAID use during a varicella infection.

Causative Organisms	
Gram positive aerobic bacteria	Group A ß haemolytic streptoccoci
	Group B streptococci
	Enterococci
	Coagulase negative staphylococci
	Staphylococcus aureus
	Bacillus species
Gram negative aerobic bacteria	*Escherichia coli*
	Pseudomonas aeruginosa
	Proteus species
	Serratia species
	Anaerobic bacteria
	Bacteroides species
	Clostridium species
	Peptostreptococcus species
Fungi	Zygomycetes
	Aspergillus
	Candida
Other	*Vibrio* species

Table 3.57: Causative organisms of necrotising faciitis.

Pathophysiology

A rapidly spreading infection that causes the release of toxic substances leading to tissue hypoxia and death. The infective organisms release pyrogenic exotoxin A that stimulates the release of cytokines. Cytokines cause damage to the endothelium lining of vessels and alters the permeability of the cell membrane such that fluid leaks into the extravascular space. Subsequent reduced blood flow leads to tissue ischaemia and death. As vasculitis and thrombosis occurs damage to subcutaneous nerves occurs.

Key features in the history/examination

- History of trauma or recent surgery
- Sudden onset of pain and swelling at site
- Pain may be reported as intense
- Pain deteriorates into loss of sensation
- May report diarrhoea and vomiting
- Rapidly spreading erythema changing to a dusky pink colouration at site of insult
- Anaesthesia at site

- Signs of septic shock: Pyrexia, hypotension, tachycardia, confusion
- May have crepitations at the site of infection

Investigations

Diagnosis is clinical and treatment should not be delayed to wait for the results of any investigations.

Blood tests:

- FBC: raised WBC
- U&E: often elevation of urea and creatinine
- Glucose: often found to be raised
- ABG

Microbiology:

- Blood cultures
- Tissue biopsy and culture taken during surgical debridement to allow identification of pathogen

Imaging:

- X-ray can reveal presence of gas
- CT scan can identify the anatomical site and extent of necrosis
- MRI can identify the anatomical site and extent of necrosis

Management

➢ A to E assessment of patient
➢ IV fluid resuscitation
➢ Anti-pyretics such as Paracetamol
➢ Commence urgent broad spectrum antibiotics following local Trust policy (usually a combination of penicillin, gentamicin and either metronidazole or clindamycin) changing once sensitivities are known
➢ Amputation may be required to excise all the infected tissue
➢ Urgent aggressive surgical debridement and repeat debridement may be necessary
➢ May require intensive care to manage the septic shock

Prognosis:

➢ Very high mortality if not diagnosed and treated effectively.
➢ Even with good treatment mortality approaches 20%.

Deep Vein Thrombosis

Epidemiology

Deep Vein Thrombosis (DVT) is a common presentation to the medical on-call.

Aetiology

A DVT is a thrombus formed within the deep veins of the leg. It can occur anywhere from the deep veins of the calf to the ilio-femoral veins. In pregnancy most DVT are in the ilio-femoral region.

Pathophysiology

Virchow's triad tells us that thrombosis results from one or more of vascular wall injury, circulatory stasis and hypercoaguable state. A DVT will result from one of these.

Key features of history/examination

- Onset of pain and swelling.
- Presence of risk factors for DVT, e.g. cancer, immobility, trauma, surgery, pregnancy and the puerperium.
- Past history of DVT/pulmonary embolism (PE) or hypercoaguability (Antithrombin III, Protein C or S deficiency, antiphospholipid syndrome).
- Family history of DVT/PE.
- Oral contraceptive pill/hormone replacement therapy.
- Patients are often asymptomatic.
- The classical symptoms of DVT are limb pain, pitting oedema, erythema and dilation of the surface veins. However these are often not all present.
- Measure the calf circumference on both legs.
- Examination using Homans' test (dorsiflexion of foot giving pain in posterior calf) and Pratt's sign (squeezing of posterior calf gives pain) are unreliable diagnostically.
- Look for evidence of complications, principally pulmonary embolus.

Investigations

Many hospitals use a protocol for investigation of DVT. In many cases this will involve:

- Initial clinical examination and blood tests on presentation
- Dose of low molecular weight heparin (LMWH)
- Booking Duplex Doppler ultrasound
- Outpatient wait until Doppler if appropriate and required

Blood tests:

- FBC
- U&E
- CRP
- D-dimer

Duplex Doppler ultrasound:

- Which should identify a clot based on colour Doppler images

Venogram:

- The 'gold standard' test is a venogram, but this is rarely performed nowadays.

Calculate the Wells score:

Wells pre-test probability	
Clinical Feature	Score
Active Cancer	1
Paralysis/Plastered leg	1
Bedridden for 3 days in last 4 weeks	1
Localised tenderness along a deep vein	1
Entire leg swollen	1
Calf swollen >3 cm compared to normal	1
Pitting oedema	1
Superficial collateral veins	1
Alternative diagnosis more likely	−2
A score of <1 is low probability	
A score of 1–2 is medium probability	
A score of >2 is high probability	

Table 3.58: The Wells score.

Management

- For a confirmed DVT, the patient will require ongoing anticoagulation, usually with warfarin with additional LMWH until the INR (international normalised ratio) is within the therapeutic range.
- It may not be necessary to anticoagulate a below-knee DVT as the risk of embolisation is slight.
- If no clear cause for the DVT is found, this will need to be investigated. The precise investigations depend on the clinical scenario but may include:
  - Thrombophilia screen (taken before any anticoagulation is given).
  - Pelvic ultrasound.
  - Chest X-ray to look for lung cancer.
- Referral will need to be made to the anticoagulant clinic for stabilising the INR and warfarin dose.
- If DVT is not confirmed, an alternative diagnosis for the leg swelling must be sought.

Further reading and references

- Hasham, S, Matteucci, P., Stanley, P.R.W., Hart, N.B. (2005) Necrotising fasciitis *BMJ*; 330: 830–833
- National Institute for Health and Clinical Excellence (2009). *Rheumatoid Arthritis (CG079)*.
- National Institute for Health and Clinical Excellence (2007). *Rheumatoid arthritis - adalimumab, etanercept and infliximab (TA130)*.

METABOLIC AND ENDOCRINE

Differential Diagnosis

System	Disease
Endocrine abnormalities	Diabetic ketoacidosis
	Hyperosmolar Hyperglycaemic State (HHS)
	Hypoglycaemia
	Cushing's Disease/Syndrome
	Addison's Disease
	Conn's Syndrome
	Phaechromocytoma
	Hyperthyroidism
	Hypothyroidism
	Thyrotoxic crisis
	Myxoedema coma
	Acromegaly
Electrolyte disturbances	Hypernatraemia
	Hyponatraemia
	Hyperkalaemia
	Hypokalaemia
	Hypercalcaemia
	Hypocalcaemia
	Hypomagnesaemia

ENDOCRINE ABNORMALITIES

Diabetic ketoacidosis

Diabetic ketoacidosis (DKA) is a life threatening complication of diabetes. The diagnostic criteria are:

1. Raised serum glucose
2. Ketones of greater than 5 mmol/l, or more practically ketonuria on dipstick
3. Metabolic acidosis with serum bicarbonate < 15 mmol/l

Epidemiology

DKA is the most common acute hyperglycaemic diabetic emergency. Up to 5% of type 1 diabetics per year (although can occur in type 2 diabetics). Of these, 20% of cases are previously undiagnosed diabetics.

Aetiology

Infection is the most common precipitating cause. Other causes include inadequate insulin, newly diagnosed diabetes, myocardial infarction, stroke and drugs (e.g. sympathomimetics, beta-blockers, corticosteroids or diuretics).

Pathophysiology

Inadequate insulin level leads to insufficient cellular uptake of glucose and increased hepatic glucose release and consequently to hyperglycaemia. Catabolic hormones including catecholamines, cortisol and glucagon are released as part of the stress response. They increase peripheral insulin resistance and potentiate the hyperglycaemia.

The lack of intracellular glucose results in the body switching to the metabolism of fatty acids. The end result of fatty acid metabolism is the production of the ketone bodies 3-hydroxybutyrate and acetoacetate. The increased blood glucose acts as an osmotic diuretic leading to profound dehydration and therefore tissue hypoperfusion.

Lack of insulin also leads to extracellular hyperkalaemia and reduction in intracellular potassium stores as insulin promotes potassium uptake by cells.

Key features in the history/examination

- Polyuria and polydipsia
- Nausea and vomiting
- Weight loss (due to protein and fatty acid catabolism)
- Fatigue and weakness
- Abdominal pain
- Drowsiness and confusion
- In addition, it is important to ask about symptoms which may relate to precipitating factors such as fever, productive cough, dysuria, insulin dosing and injection sites, chest pain or recent changes in medication.
- Tachycardia
- Hypotension (or postural hypotension)
- Dyspnoea (which may lead to Kussmaul's breathing)
- Reduced level of consciousness
- Raised temperature (if septic)
- Ketone breath (characteristically smells like "pear drops")
- Signs of clinical dehydration: reduced skin turgor, dry mucous membranes, reduced urine output
- Evidence of infection may be present – localisation of source is important
- Neurological examination – focal neurological signs may be present due to the acute DKA, but there may be peripheral neuropathy caused by the diabetes

Investigations

Blood tests:

- FBC
- U&Es
- Inflammatory markers: CRP
- Osmolality
- Glucose
- ABG: shows metabolic acidosis
- Cardiac enzymes: to rule out silent MI

Microbiology:

- Blood cultures

Imaging:

- Chest X-ray: shows evidence of consolidation.

Others:

- ECG: may show ischaemic changes
- Urinalysis: ketones and glucose. May also show leucocytes and nitrites which may indicate UTI. If so, send urine sample for microscopy, culture and sensitivity

Management

General measures:

- A to E assessment
- Oxygen (high flow for the critically unwell)
- Close monitoring (initially hourly) with regular clinical review, careful monitoring of glucose and electrolytes and fluid status
- Urinary catheter to monitor fluid balance
- DVT prophylaxis
- Consider antibiotics if evidence of infection according to Trust microbiology policy
- Sodium bicarbonate is not recommended unless pH <6.9 and failing to improve despite other interventions
- Keep nil by mouth if vomiting or reduced GCS
- Consider ICU review if haemodynamically compromised or significantly reduced level of consciousness
- Diabetes specialist nurse/diabetologist referral

Specific therapies:

- Trusts have policies for treating DKA, and a number of differing styles are used. It is important to be aware of your local policy as DKA is frequently encountered on the acute medical on-call.

The principles behind management:

- Rapid fluid replacement
  - Patients often have a deficit of 4–6 litres.
  - 0.9% Saline is the usual choice

Suggested replacement with 0.9% saline:

- 1L in 30 mins, then
- 1L 1 hr
- 1L 2 hrs
- 1L 4 hrs
- 1L 6 hrs
- 1L 8 hrs
  - Careful monitoring of fluid balance with clinical

assessment will be required, especially if there are cardiac comorbidities

- Insulin replacement
  - Often using a sliding scale, but more common to use a 6 unit/hr infusion
  - Insulin infusion: aim to reduce plasma glucose by 3–5 mmol/l/hr
  - Continue until keto-acids are no longer detectable
  - If CBG low before this occurs, give concurrent glucose infusion

A specific example of insulin replacement is:

Give 10 units (U) actrapid IV stat (15 u intramuscular (IM) if IV access delayed).

Add 50 u actrapid to 50 ml 0.9% saline (giving a concentration of 1 unit per ml).

Initially infuse at 6 ml/hr until bicarbonate > 15 mmol/l

Then as per sliding scale:

Blood Glucose	Pump Setting
0–4.0 mmol/l	0.5 ml/hr
4.1–7.0 mmol/l	1.0 ml/hr
7.1–10.0 mmol/l	2.0 ml/hr
10.1–15.0 mmol/l	3.0 ml/hr
15.1–20.0 mmol/l	4.0 ml/hr
20.1–28.0 mmol/l	6.0 ml/hr
> 28.0 mmol/l	6.0 ml/hr + call doctor

Table 3.59: Sliding scale.

- Potassium replacement
  - Although initial potassium may be normal or high, there is a total body depletion
  - As acidosis improves and insulin given, potassium is driven intracellularly and plasma levels fall
  - Give potassium in the second and subsequent bags of IV fluid, with careful monitoring
  - Potassium should be measured every 2–4 hours for the first 24 hours

Prognosis:

- Has improved with better clinical care and mortality now stands at less than 5%.

Hyperglycaemic Hyperosmolar State (HHS) (formerly HONK)

Diagnostic criteria are:

1. Hyperglycaemia (usually 30–70 mmol/l)
2. High serum osmolality >350 mmol/kg
3. No or minimal ketones in the urine
4. No or minimal acidosis

Epidemiology

Incidence may be 10–20 per 100,000 per year.

Aetiology

The causes of HHS include:

- Infection
- Poor compliance with oral hypoglycaemics
- Myocardial infarction
- Stroke
- Pancreatitis
- Drugs (e.g. sympathomimetics, beta-blockers, corticosteroids or diuretics)

Pathophysiology

- Hyperglycaemia occurs due to relative insulin deficiency or insulin resistance.
- There is still sufficient insulin to prevent cellular metabolism switching to fatty acid catabolism therefore preventing ketoacidosis.
- Uncontrolled hyperglycaemia leads to osmotic diuresis and serum hyperosmolarity leading to profound dehydration and altered neurological states.
- Relative hyperviscosity due to dehydration increases the risk of venous thromboembolism.
- Untreated or poorly managed HHS can lead to disseminated intravascular coagulation (DIC).

Key features in the history/examination

- Drowsiness, confusion, generalised weakness
- Seizures
- Nausea and vomiting
- Symptoms relating to precipitating factors such as fever, productive cough and dysuria.
- Current hypoglycaemic therapy and compliance and any recent changes in medication
- Tachycardia
- Hypotension (or postural hypotension)
- Reduced level of consciousness
- Raised temperature (if septic)
- Signs of clinical dehydration: reduced skin turgor, dry mucous membranes, reduced urine output
- Signs of source of infection
- Neurological examination
- Symptoms of venous thromboembolism may be present

Investigations

Blood tests:

- FBC

- CRP
- U&Es: usually hypernatraemia but beware severe hyperglycaemia can cause pseudohyponatraemia
- Osmolality >350 mmol/Kg
- Glucose 30–70 mmol/L
- ABG: possible mild metabolic acidosis but may be normal
- Consider checking cardiac enzymes to rule out silent MI

Microbiology:

- Blood cultures

Imaging:

- CXR: shows evidence of consolidation

Others:

- ECG: may show ischaemic changes
- Urinalysis: glucose and possibly minimal ketones. May also show leucocytes and nitrites which may indicate UTI. If so, send urine sample for microscopy, culture and sensitivity.

Management

General measures:

➢ A to E assessment
➢ Close monitoring (initially hourly) with regular clinical review, careful monitoring of glucose and electrolytes and fluid status
➢ Urinary catheter to monitor fluid balance
➢ DVT prophylaxis: significantly greater risk of thrombosis compared to DKA so consider full anticoagulation with low molecular weight heparin
➢ Consider antibiotics if evidence of infection
➢ Keep nil by mouth if vomiting or reduced GCS
➢ Consider ITU review if haemodynamically compromised or significantly reduced level of consciousness
➢ Diabetes specialist nurse/diabetologist referral

Specific therapies:

➢ Trusts have policies for treating HHS, and a number of differing styles are used. It is important to be aware of your local policy as HHS is frequently encountered on the acute medical on-call.

The principles behind management:

➢ Fluid replacement
  o Patients are usually profoundly dehydrated
  o 0.9% Saline is the usual choice
  o Replacement should be less vigorous than with DKA

Suggested replacement with 0.9% saline:

- 1L 1 hr, then
- 1L 2 hrs
- 1L 2 hrs
- 1L 6–8 hrs thereafter
  - o Careful monitoring of fluid balance with clinical assessment will be required, especially if there are cardiac comorbidities
- ➤ Insulin replacement
  - o Often using a sliding scale
  - o Aim to reduce plasma glucose by 3–5 mmol/l/hr. Too fast will result in rapid osmolar shifts and could precipitate cerebral oedema
  - o If CBG low before this occurs, give concurrent glucose infusion
- ➤ A specific example of insulin replacement is:
  - o Add 50 u actrapid to 50 ml 0.9% saline (giving a concentration of 1 unit per ml).
  - o Initially infuse at 6 ml/hr until bicarbonate > 15 mmol/l
  - o Then as per sliding scale:

Blood Glucose	Pump Setting
0–4.0 mmol/l	0.5 ml/hr
4.1–7.0 mmol/l	1.0 ml/hr
7.1–10.0 mmol/l	2.0 ml/hr
10.1–15.0 mmol/l	3.0 ml/hr
15.1–20.0 mmol/l	4.0 ml/hr
20.1–28.0 mmol/l	6.0 ml/hr
> 28.0 mmol/l	6.0 ml/hr + call doctor

Table 3.60: Sliding scale.

- ➤ Potassium replacement
  - o Give potassium in the second and subsequent bags of IV fluid, with careful monitoring

Prognosis:
- ➤ Up to 15% mortality even with effective treatment
- ➤ Prognosis worse in the elderly

Hypoglycaemia

Diagnostic criterion is plasma glucose of <4 mmol/L.

Epidemiology

Most commonly occurs in patients being treated for diabetes mellitus with insulin or oral hypoglycaemics.

Aetiology

Causes of hypoglycaemia include:

- Overtreatment with insulin or oral hypoglycaemics (including deliberate overdose)
- Excess alcohol
- Inadequate carbohydrate intake
- Insulinoma
- Adrenal insufficiency

Pathophysiology

- Sympathetic symptoms typically start to appear when glucose concentrations fall below 3.0 mmol/L. They are due to increased secretion of glucagon, adrenaline, cortisol and growth hormone as the body tries to increase the plasma sugar levels. These may include sweating, anxiety, palpitations, nausea, hunger, and tremor.
- Neuroglycopenic symptoms are a result of cerebral hypoglycaemia. These include blurred vision, dizziness, confusion, lethargy and drowsiness. Focal neurological symptoms may be seen and in severe cases there may be seizures, coma and cardiac arrest.

Key features in the history/examination

- History of diabetes
- Treatment of diabetes including doses and what medications have actually been taken
- N.B. Metformin does not cause hypogylcaemia
- Time since last meal and nature of meal
- Awareness of 'hypo'
- Autonomic features: sweating, tremor, anxiety
- Palpitations
- Hunger
- Headache
- Alcohol history
- Neurological features: confusion, slurred speech, blurred vision, reduced level of consciousness, seizures
- Aggression or peculiar behaviour
- NB other potential causes of peculiar behaviour, reduced level of consciousness and seizures are stroke, subdural haematoma and alcohol intoxication, so these differentials should be borne in mind

Investigations

Blood tests:

- FBC
- U&Es and CRP
- LFTs
- Bone profile
- Glucose
- Hb$_{A1c}$: shows whether recent control has been too tight
- C-peptide: if insulinoma suspected

Management

➤ A to E assessment and resuscitate if necessary

➤ Patient conscious: oral glucose (e.g. Lucozade, dextrose tablet, hypostop)

➤ Patient unconscious: 25–50 ml 10% glucose IV, 0.5–1 mg glucagon IM

➤ Recheck glucose 10–15 mins later. If no improvement, give further oral or IV glucose until improvement obtained.

➤ Ensure either oral complex carbohydrate (eg a sandwich) or ongoing IV 5% glucose infusion given. With long acting insulins and sulphonylureas there is a danger of recurrence of hypoglycaemia

➤ Diabetic specialist nurse/diabetologist review

➤ Counsel about stopping driving and informing the DVLA if either having 'frequent hypoglycaemic episodes likely to impair driving' or 'impaired awareness of hypoglycaemia' (source: For Medical Practitioners. At a glance guide to the current medical standards of fitness to drive. DVLA February 2009).

Cushing's disease/syndrome

Cushing's syndrome results from prolonged exposure to excess glucocorticoids.

Cushing's disease results from a pituitary adenoma causing an ACTH dependent glucocorticoid excess.

Epidemiology

Incidence thought to be 1 in 250,000.

Aetiology

Cushing's syndrome can be ACTH dependent or non-ACTH dependent:

ACTH dependant	Non-ACTH dependant
• Pituitary adenoma (80% cases) • Ectopic ACTH secretion (particularly bronchial cancer)	• Benign adrenal adenoma • Adrenal carcinoma • Nodular adrenal hyperplasia • Exogenous glucocorticoid administration

Table 3.61: Aetiology of Cushing's syndrome

Pathophysiology

Glucocorticoid (cortisol) release from the adrenal cortex is stimulated from ACTH from the pituitary gland, which in turn is secreted in response to corticotrophin releasing hormone (CRH) from the pituitary. The hypothalamus-pituitary-adrenal axis is controlled physiologically with negative feedback. Pathologies affecting this axis can cause excess cortisol release.

Key features in the history/examination

• Easy bruising

• Psychiatric disturbances: typically depression or psychosis

• Unexplained fracture

• Recurrent infections

• Poor wound healing

• Drug history

• Diabetes

• Moon facies

• Buffalo hump

• Obesity

• Hypertension

• Abdominal striae

• Hirsutism

• Oligo/amenorrhoea

• Reduced libido

• Osteoporosis

• Proximal myopathy

• Pigmentation (with excess ACTH)

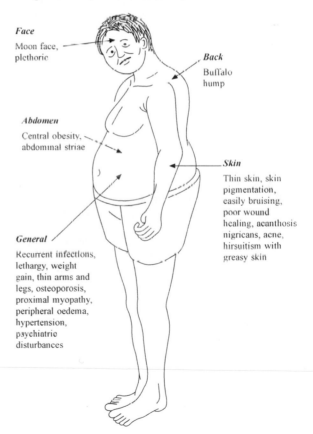

Face
Moon face, plethoric

Back
Buffalo hump

Abdomen
Central obesity, abdominal striae

Skin
Thin skin, skin pigmentation, easily bruising, poor wound healing, acanthosis nigricans, acne, hirsuitism with greasy skin

General
Recurrent infections, lethargy, weight gain, thin arms and legs, osteoporosis, proximal myopathy, peripheral oedema, hypertension, psychiatric disturbances

Figure 3.29: Clinical findings of a patient with Cushing's syndrome/disease.

Investigations

The diagnosis is in two stages:

Confirm the diagnosis:

- Three possible tests can be used
1. Low-dose dexamethasone suppression test (there are two possible ways of performing this):

Overnight test	48 hour test
1 mg dexamethasone given at 2300 and cortisol levels taken at 0900 the following day	0.5 mg dexamethasone given at 0900, 1500, 2100 and 0300 for 48 hours. Cortisol levels taken before and after the test.

Table 3.62: Difference between the overnight and 48 hour low does dexamethasone test.

For both tests a cortisol level of greater than 50 mmol/l is indicative of Cushing's syndrome

2. 24 hour urinary free cortisol
3. Midnight plasma cortisol: due to the loss of the normal circadian rhythm of cortisol levels, a midnight level of greater than 50 mmol/l is indicative

Localise the lesion and determine the cause:

- ACTH levels will distinguish ACTH and non-ACTH dependant causes
  - The sample must be taken immediately to the lab, preferably on ice, so it can be centrifuged and frozen immediately. It may be useful to call ahead before the sample is taken so the lab has some warming.
  - ACTH level of <5 pg/ml indicates an ACTH-independent cause, the commonest of which are an adrenal adenoma, adrenal carcinoma or exogenous corticosteroid administration.
  - ACTH level of >15 pg/ml indicates an ACTH-dependant cause, which are pituitary adenoma (Cushing's Disease) and ectopic ACTH release (commonest is from a bronchial neoplasm).
  - ACTH levels between 5–15 pg/ml are difficult to interpret, and the test should be repeated.
- High dose dexamethasone suppression test is used if an ACTH dependant cause is suspected. 2 mg dexamethasone is given 6 hourly for 48 hours and cortisol levels are measured at the beginning and the end. Suppression of cortisol levels to below 50% of the basal level is indicative of Cushing's disease as ectopic ACTH production will not be suppressed.

Blood tests:

- U&Es: shows hypokalaemia
- Glucose
- Corticotrophin Releasing Hormone level

Imaging:

This will depend on the results of the diagnostic tests:

- CXR: to exclude lung cancer
- MRI: of pituitary
- CT: of abdomen to visualise the adrenals

Others:

- Inferior petrosal sinus sampling

Management

➢ Pituitary disease: surgery, i.e. trans-sphenoidal adenomectomy and radiotherapy
➢ Adrenal disease: adrenalectomy (beware Nelson's syndrome if bilateral adrenalectomy performed)
➢ Excision of source of ectopic ACTH
➢ Metapyrone may be used in the short term to suppress cortisol synthesis
➢ Reduction in exogenous glucocorticoid therapy

Prognosis:

➢ Untreated has a high mortality (50% in five years).

Addison's disease

Primary adrenal insufficiency with reduced production of all of the adrenocortical hormones.

Epidemiology

Incidence is estimated to be 0.5/100,000 per year and females are predominantly effected. It may present with insidious onset or acutely with an adrenal crisis.

Aetiology and Pathophysiology

- Autoimmune (85–90% cases): can be seen as part of the polyglandular syndromes
- TB
- Metastases: predominantly lung, breast, lymphoma
- Haemorrhagic infarction (antiphospholipid syndrome)
- Fungal infection in immunocompromised individuals
- Congenital: congenital adrenal hyperplasia, enzyme deficiencies

Key features in the history/examination

- Many features are very non-specific
- Weight loss and anorexia
- Fatigue
- Myalgia and weakness
- Abdominal pain, diarrhoea and vomiting
- Reduced libido
- Depression

- Salt craving
- Past medical or family history of autoimmune diseases, especially type 1 diabetes
- Look for signs of dehydration (including postural hypotension)
- Hyperpigmentation
- Signs of other autoimmune disease e.g. goitre, vitiligo

Investigations

Blood tests:

- FBC: get baseline levels
- LFTs: get baseline levels
- U&Es: hyponatraemia and hyperkalaemia, with raised urea in dehydration
- Glucose
- TFTs
- Cortisol: will be low (preferably taken at 0900)
- ACTH: will be high

Confirm the diagnosis:

- Short synacthen test: 250 microgram synacthen (a synthetic ACTH) is given IM at 0900 and serum cortisol measured at 0, 30 and 60 minutes. A normal response is for the cortisol to rise to more than 550 nmol/L
- Adrenal autoantibodies

Others:

- Chest X-ray: look for TB, which may be the cause
- CT: of the abdomen may reveal metastases or a primary tumour, which may be the cause

Management

- ➢ Patient education and information
- ➢ Medic alert bracelet
- ➢ Provide written information and include the UK Addison's society
- ➢ Hormone replacement:
    - ○ Hydrocortisone: typically 10 mg, 5 mg and 5 mg
    - ○ Fludrocortisone: typically 50–100 microgram BD
- ➢ Ensure additional glucocorticoid is given during acute illness

Adrenal crisis:

- ➢ If an adrenal crisis is encountered:
    - ○ IV hydrocortisone
    - ○ Aggressive fluid replacement
    - ○ Correction of hypoglycaemia and any other electrolyte imbalances

Prognosis:

- ➢ With careful adherence to replacement therapy a normal life-expectancy is seen.

Conn's syndrome

Epidemiology

Conn's syndrome accounts for approximately 50% cases of primary hyperaldosteronism, but is rare. It is more common in women.

Aetiology

Conn's syndrome is a form of primary hyperaldosteronism resulting from a unilateral aldosterone-secreting adrenal adenoma.

Pathophysiology

Mineralocorticoid secretion from the zona glomerulosa of the adrenal cortex is governed by the renin-angiotensin system. Excess secretion can be due to a number of pathologies, which includes Conn's syndrome.

Key features in the history/examination

- Features of hypokalaemia including cramps, weakness and palpitations from tachydysrhythmias
- Hypertension, especially younger onset (below age 50)

Investigations

Blood tests:

- U&Es: classically hypernatraemia and hypokalaemia, but up to 40% of Conn's are normokalaemic
- Aldosterone
- Renin: a high/normal renin, in the absence of diuretic therapy, excludes the diagnosis
- ABG: shows metabolic alkalosis
- Adrenal venous sampling: in cases of diagnostic doubt

Imaging:

- Adrenal CT/MRI

Management

- ➢ Adrenalectomy with pre-operative spironolactone
- ➢ In non-surgical candidates, ongoing treatment with amiloride or spironolactone

Prognosis:

- ➢ If remains untreated, the patient faces all the risks induced by ongoing hypertension and in addition the risk of cardiac arrhythmias from hypokalaemia.

Phaeochromocytoma

Epidemiology

Rare condition which affects less than 1% of hypertensive patients. Prevalence is equal in males and females. There is a peak incidence between 30 and 50 years old.

Aetiology

The majority of phaeochromocytomas are tumours affecting chromaffin cells of the adrenal medulla. A small number will be extra-adrenal and affect the paraganglion cells in the ANS. There may be familial predisposition and approximately 24% are thought to be hereditary. However the majority are sporadic.

Hereditary tumours are associated with a number of other conditions:

- Multiple Endocrine Neoplasia (MEN) type 2
- Neurofibromatosis type 1
- Von Hippel-Lindau syndrome

10% rule describes the fact that 10% of phaeochromocytomas will be:

- Familial
- Bilateral
- Malignant
- Extra-adrenal

Pathophysiology

Phaeochromocytomas cause hyper-secretion of catecholamines (adrenaline, noradrenaline and rarely dopamine) and hence symptoms are related to increased stimulation of alpha and/or beta adrenergic receptors.

Malignant tumours are histologically similar to benign tumours however they either metastasise or have local invasion. Common sites of metastases are:

- Liver
- Lymph nodes
- Bone

Key features in the history/examination

- History of diabetes mellitus
- Familial history of phaeochromocytoma and endocrine disorders
- Headache
- Palpitations
- Panic attacks
- Hypertensive retinopathy
- Hypertension
- Pallor
- Tachyarrhythmias
- Diaphoresis
- Papilloedema: if untreated for prolonged period
- Tremor
- Occasionally an abdominal mass may be palpable

Investigations

Diagnosis is through 24 hour urine collection and measurement of urinary catecholamines.

Blood tests:

- FBC
- U&Es: if delayed treatment renal failure may be present
- Glucose: impaired glucose tolerance may be present due to affects of high levels of catecholamines
- Bone profile: Hypercalcaemia may be present in patients with primary hyperparathyroidism related to MEN 2 syndrome
- TFTs: elevated in MEN 2

Imaging:

- CT scan of the abdomen can detect adrenal phaeochromocytomas of 0.5 cm and extra-adrenal phaeochromocytomas of 1 cm diameter
- MRI: scan of localisation of tumour

Management

- ➢ Control of hypertension usually alpha blockers with the addition of beta blockers
- ➢ Surgical excision

Prognosis:

- ➢ Benign phaeochromocytoma
  - ○ Normal life expectancy if surgery is successful
  - ○ 95% 5-year survival rate
- ➢ Recurrence more likely in hereditary disease
- ➢ Malignant
  - ○ Untreated 50% 5-year survival rate
  - ○ Unpredictable: factors improving survival include early diagnosis and excision of primary tumour

Hyperthyroidism

Hyperthyroidism is an excessive quantity of thyroid hormones in the circulation. Thyrotoxicosis may occur without hyperthyroidism either when excessive amounts of hormone are released, e.g. in de Quervain's thyroiditis and post-partum thyroiditis, or with iatrogenic overdosing of Levothyroxine.

Epidemiology

This affects around 2% of females and 0.2% of males. Graves' disease is the most common form of hyperthyroidism and it usually affects individuals between the ages of 20 to 40 years.

Toxic multi-nodular goitre mostly affects those who are middle aged or over. There is an increased risk of disease in those with a positive family history.

Aetiology

The causes can be split into the following categories:

- Iatrogenic
- Secondary causes (rare)
- Toxic adenoma
- Toxic multi-nodular goitre
- Graves' disease

Pathophysiology

Graves' disease	• An autoimmune thyroid disease caused by thyroid-stimulating IgG antibodies which stimulate TSH receptors on the thyroid gland. Approximately 75% cases of hyperthyroidism
Toxic multi-nodular goitre	• Commonest cause of hyperthyroidism in the elderly
Toxic adenoma	• When there is a thyroid nodule which is over-productive of the thyroid hormones
Secondary causes (rare)	• TSH-secreting pituitary adenoma • Thyroid hormone resistance syndrome • Stimulation of the thyroid by human chorionic gonadotropin during pregnancy
Iatrogenic	• Amiodarone, glucocorticoids, levodopa, and iodine containing IV contrast agents

Table 3.63: Various pathophysiologies of hyperthyroidism.

Key features in history/examination

General features of hyperthyroidism:

- Weight loss despite a normal or increased appetite
- Sweating and heat intolerance
- Irritability, hyperactivity and insomnia
- Fine tremor of hands
- Brisk tendon reflexes
- Palpitations, tachycardia and AF
- Fatigue
- Muscle weakness, proximal myopathy
- Diarrhoea
- Oligomenorrhoea, decreased libido
- Lid lag
- Nervousness and psychosis
- Cardiac failure, particularly in the elderly

Dysthyroid eye disease:

- Dysthyroid eye disease is seen in any cause of hyperthyroidism.
- Lid lag: The increased levels of thyroid hormone causes an increase in catecholamine sensitivity which affects the levator palpebrae superioris muscle as it has some sympathetic innervation. The resultant muscle spasm causes upper eyelid retraction giving the typical 'staring' appearance.
- Patients tend to blink less frequently giving them a 'gritty' feeling within their eyes.

Graves' disease:

- Usually a painless diffuse goitre
- Ophthalmopathy:
  - Eye signs are seen in >60% of those with Graves' disease and are more severe in smokers.
  - Lymphocytic infiltration of the muscles and fatty tissues of the eye with oedema and later fibrosis, causing forward displacement of the eye.
  - CT/MRI shows fusiform enlargement of the extra-ocular muscles.
  - Proptosis (exophthalmos): examination will reveal prominent white sclera below the cornea as the patient looks straight ahead. Can be asymmetrical. It frequently causes corneal damage and keratitis as the patient is unable to close the eyelids fully. In severe cases there may be chemosis (oedema of the conjunctiva), an increase in the intraocular pressure, and papilloedema.
  - Complex ophthalmoplegia: may occur because of weakness in the extra-ocular muscles.
- Pretibial myxoedema
  - Affects 2% of Graves' disease sufferers
  - Painless thickening of the skin and subcutaneous tissue over the shin and foot causing nodule formation and showing characteristics similar to erythema nodosum.
- Thyroid acropachy
  - Rare (<1%)
  - Almost all have ophthalmopathy and pretibial myxoedema
  - A similar appearance to finger clubbing
  - X-rays may reveal some subperiosteal bone formation
- Other auto-immune diseases
  - Associated with type 1 diabetes, pernicious anaemia, vitiligo, myasthenia gravis and coeliac disease, either in the past medical history or family history.

Investigations

Blood tests:

- FBC: must be performed prior to commencing anti-thyroid drugs as they may cause agranulocytosis.
- Thyroid function tests: will reveal an increase in T3 and T4 In primary hyperthyroidism there will be a decreased TSH

level, in secondary there may be an increased TSH if the cause is hypothalamus-pituitary dysfunction.

- Serum antibodies against thyroglobulin and thyroid peroxidise: are found in 80% Graves' disease.

Imaging:

- Chest X-ray: look for retrosternal goitre
- Ultrasound
- Technetium-99 m or 131I scans aid in the differentiation between Graves' and toxic adenomas.

Others:

- ECG: To diagnose any rhythm abnormalities especially atrial fibrillation.
- Fine needle aspiration (FNA): This is the only non-surgical method used to differentiate between malignant and benign nodules. A needle is inserted into the nodule multiple times and cells are aspirated and collected in a syringe. The cells are then stained and examined on a slide. The nodule can be classified in to benign, suspicious or malignant in nature; if this is not possible it is classed as non-diagnostic.

Management

Medication:

- ➤ Anti-thyroid drug therapy is first-line for all patients.
- ➤ Carbimazole and Propylthiouracil:
  - ○ Reduces the production of thyroid hormone
  - ○ The 'titration' regime for carbimazole: initially treated with 40–60 mg per day for a period of 4–6 weeks and then reduced to 5–15 mg per day for maintenance. In Graves's disease this is continued for up to 2 years before stopping.
  - ○ The 'block-replace' regimen: Treatment of 40 mg (Carbimazole) continued and Levothyroxine given to prevent hypothyroidism
  - ○ The risk of relapse after treatment is higher in the first year and all patients should be carefully monitored with TFT checks
  - ○ Patients must be warned regarding the risk of agranulocytosis with Carbimazole (<0.1% of patients) and advised to seek medical attention if they develop fever or a sore throat.
  - ○ Other side effects include rash, arthralgia and nausea
  - ○ Propylthiouracil is used in pregnant patients as it is less teratogenic.
- ➤ Propranolol is useful in early stages of treatment and is effective in controlling symptoms such as palpitations and tremor.
- ➤ Radioactive iodine therapy
  - ○ Mostly offered to patients who are over the age of 40 years.
  - ○ I^{131} is administered by IV injection. This concentrates in the thyroid gland causing cell death.
  - ○ Patients must be made euthyroid with anti-thyroid medication prior to iodine administration, which must be stopped at least five days prior to therapy to enable the thyroid gland to take up the iodine.
  - ○ The treatment may need to be repeated several times in order to gain control of the symptoms.
  - ○ Hypothyroidism is the main complication with a 50% risk of developing hypothyroidism within a 10-year period, mostly occurring within the first two years.
  - ○ Regular TFTs are mandatory and treatment with Levothyroxine may be required.
  - ○ I^{131} is contraindicated in pregnancy and breastfeeding.

Surgery:

- ➤ Partial thyroidectomy is the most common procedure performed with the aim of normalising the patient's thyroid function.
- ➤ Useful in patients with a large or retrosternal goitre, a solitary toxic adenoma, those who cannot tolerate drug therapy or who have relapsed post therapy.
- ➤ Potassium iodide is used by some surgeons prior to surgery in order to reduce the vascularity of the gland and minimise the risks of haemorrhage.
- ➤ Specific complications include hypothyroidism, left recurrent laryngeal nerve damage, parathyroid gland damage, and haemorrhage into the neck with laryngeal oedema.
- ➤ The risk of hypothyroidism is 30% within a ten-year period.

Prognosis:

- ➤ A treatable disease.
- ➤ Graves' ophthalmopathy may not completely resolve on treatment
- ➤ There is increased mortality due to cardio- and cerebrovascular disease if left untreated
- ➤ Cardiac dysrhythmias, particularly atrial fibrillation
- ➤ Osteoporosis

Hypothyroidism

Hypothyroidism results from a deficiency of the thyroid hormones T4 and T3.

Epidemiology

Prevalence is around 10 in 1,000 women and 1 in 1,000 men. It can affect individuals of any age but is most common in middle-age or older patients. An association has been found with families who have a higher incidence of autoimmune disease. The incidence is higher in areas of the world where there is iodine deficiency, classically in mountainous regions in the developing world.

Aetiology

Hypothyroidism can be primary or secondary. Significant causes of secondary hypothyroidism include drugs, most commonly

Amiodarone and Lithium, and treatment of hyperthyroidism, which accounts for up to one in three cases of hypothyroidism in the developed world.

Iodine deficiency accounts for the majority of cases in the developing countries where as autoimmune disease is mostly responsible for cases in the developed world.

Pathophysiology

Hypothyroidism usually results from primary disease of the thyroid gland.

- Hashimoto's thyroiditis: An auto-immune disease presenting with a moderate sized diffuse painless goitre. Most commonly affects middle-aged and elderly women.

- Idiopathic atrophy: Likely to have an autoimmune cause (is associated with other autoimmune conditions). Again more common in middle-aged and elderly women.

Secondary hypothyroidism may rarely be due to dysfunction of the hypothalamus or pituitary gland resulting in lack of production of thyrotropin-releasing hormone or thyroid-stimulating hormone respectively.

Key features in history/examination

- Many symptoms are very non-specific and tend to be present for many months or even years prior to the development of signs of the disease
- Tiredness
- Weight gain
- Cold intolerance/cold peripheries
- Goitre
- Bradycardia
- Dry skin
- Slow relaxing reflexes
- Hyperlipidaemia
- Anaemia
- Angina
- Heart failure
- Pleural and pericardial effusions
- Carpal tunnel syndrome
- Cognitive impairment
- Peri-orbital swelling and Myxoedema
- Depression
- Constipation
- Oligomenorrhoea
- It is also important to enquire about symptoms and signs of other autoimmune conditions which may be seen in addition to hypothyroidism, especially vitiligo, pernicious anaemia, type 1 diabetes and Addison's disease.

Investigations

Blood tests:

- FBC: may show anaemia. It can be macrocytic, microcytic or normocytic patterns and also concurrent pernicious anaemia may also be seen.

- TFTs: confirm the diagnosis of primary hypothyroidism by revealing a low T4 level with an increased TSH level.

- Anti-thyroid antibodies (thyroglobulin or thyroid peroxidise): are strongly positive in Hashimoto's thyroiditis.

- Lipid profile

Imaging:

- Chest X-ray: to identify any pericardial or pleural effusions.

Others:

- ECG: There may be a sinus bradycardia with low voltage QRS complexes. Occasionally, ischaemic changes may be evident.

- A biopsy may reveal lymphocytic infiltration which is a typical feature.

Management

➢ Primary disease is managed with Levothyroxine.

    o Started at a dose of 25–50 micrograms once per day and can be increased up to 200 micrograms depending upon the patient's response to treatment and measurement of their TSH levels.

    o Take care in patients with ischaemic heart disease and the elderly. Start with a low dose and titrate slowly.

    o T4 has a long half life (1 week) so full clinical response and changes in TSH levels may take up to 6 weeks.

➢ 'Subclinical' hypothyroidism (normal T4 but TSH <10 mU/l) does not need pharmacological treatment, but TFTs should be monitored every 6 months.

➢ If secondary hypothyroidism is suspected, it is important not to start therapy with Levothyroxine.

    o Hypopituitary disease must be excluded as if there is a reduced reserve of ACTH, treatment with thyroxine replacement alone may cause an acute Addisonian crisis which can be very severe and associated with significant morbidity.

➢ Pregnancy may require a temporary increase in Levothyroxine dose.

Prognosis:

➢ Life expectancy is normal unless there is the presence of accelerated ischaemic heart disease.

Thyrotoxic crisis (Thyroid storm)

Epidemiology

This is an uncommon but life threatening medical emergency with a mortality approaching 50%.

Aetiology

Precipitating factors are: surgery, acute intercurrent illness particularly severe sepsis, radioiodine, iodine-based contrast media and withdrawal of anti-thyroid drugs. Prevention is the key.

Pathophysiology

The pathophysiology is dependent on the aetiology.

Key features in the history/examination

- Patients present with features of severe thyrotoxicosis and in addition fever, seizures, psychosis, coma and signs of heart failure may be present

Management

Treatment should be initiated promptly:

- ➤ A loading dose of Propylthiouracil or Carbimazole.
- ➤ Potassium iodide ('stable iodine') one hour later.
- ➤ Intravenous beta-blockers effectively reduce the symptoms of tachycardia and anxiety.
- ➤ Steroids, antipyretics and IV fluid therapy.
- ➤ Any specific treatments of precipitating causes.
- ➤ Thyroid function tests should be performed.

Prognosis:

- ➤ Prognosis is poor unless there is quick recognition and management of symptoms.

Myxoedema coma

Epidemiology

This is a rare medical emergency mostly affecting elderly individuals.

- 90% of individuals are females.
- Mostly in poor social communities and colder climates due to problems associated with non-compliance.

Aetiology

It is precipitated by exposure to cold weather, infections, or sedative treatment.

Pathophysiology

The pathophysiology is dependent on the aetiology.

Key features in the history/examination

- The principle presenting signs are hypothermia and reduced level of consciousness.
- Coma is not seen in everyone.
- Other features include hypotension, hypoventilation, hypoglycaemia and hyponatraemia.

Investigations

Blood tests:

- FBC
- U&Es
- TFTs
- Glucose and cortisol levels: to exclude Addison's disease

Management

- ➤ Thyroxine replacement is required, either T3 given intravenously, loading of 100 microgram then 20 microgram TDS, or T4 (via NG tube if necessary).
    - ○ Intravenous hydrocortisone should be administered (100 mg TDS). The adrenal glands are thought to function poorly in severe hypothyroidism.
- ➤ General supportive measures including IV fluids, slow re-warming, treatment of underlying infection and correction of electrolyte disturbances and hypoglycaemia.
- ➤ Associated with a poor prognosis especially in elderly individuals.

Acromegaly

Acromegaly is a chronic, progressive disease caused by excessive secretion of Growth Hormone (GH), usually from a pituitary adenoma.

Epidemiology

The prevalence is around 60 per 1,000,000 individuals. Males and females tend to be affected equally with an even distribution amongst all ethnic groups. Mostly diagnosed in individuals aged between 40–50 years, although the clinical features are often evident from the mid 20s.

Aetiology

Results from a growth hormone-producing pituitary tumour in the majority of cases (>98%). This may be seen as part of the MEN-1 syndrome. Excess growth hormone releasing hormone and ectopic production of growth hormone are very rare causes.

Pathophysiology

The chronic excessive circulating GH on the peripheral tissues via the stimulation of insulin-like growth factor 1 production cause the clinical features.

Key features in the history/examination

General features:

Ask about

- Change in facial appearance
  - Ask if there are any old photos to compare
- Changes in size of hands/feet – changes in glove or shoe size. Rings no longer fitting
- Increase in hat size (if known)
- Headache and visual disturbances (presenting feature in 25% patients)
- Carpal tunnel syndrome
- Oligo-amenorrhoea and galactorrhoea in females
- Reduced libido/impotence in males
- Deepening voice
- Breathlessness and peripheral oedema indicative of heart failure
- Arthropathy
- Excessive sweating
- Past history of diabetes/impaired glucose tolerance, hypertension and obstructive sleep apnoea. Ask specifically for colonic polyps and colonic cancer.

Examine for:

- Hands: large and moist from sweating. Classically described as 'spade-like' with a 'doughy' feel to the handshake.
- Axillae: skin tags and acanthosis nigricans
- Face: prominent supraorbital ridges, enlarged nose and lips. Thickened greasy skin
- Mouth: interdental separation and prognathism (protruded lower jaw) with malocclusion.
- Macroglossia: large tongue
- Eyes: test visual fields
- Neck: palpate for goitre, acanthosis nigricans
- Chest: gynaecomastia and galactorrhoea. Check for displaced apex beat.

Investigations

Blood tests:

- Growth hormone levels: GH release occurs as 'pulses' with low levels between pulses. Hence measurement is not always a useful test, however if levels are persistently below 0.4 ng/ml the diagnosis of acromegaly is very unlikely.
- Insulin-like growth factor 1 levels: these vary considerably, dependant on a number of factors. This makes interpreting levels difficult, so although levels are raised in acromegaly, this is not a useful diagnostic test.
- Oral glucose tolerance test (OGTT): considered the most

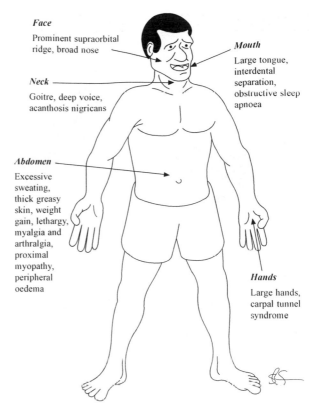

Face
Prominent supraorbital ridge, broad nose

Mouth
Large tongue, interdental separation, obstructive sleep apnoea

Neck
Goitre, deep voice, acanthosis nigricans

Abdomen
Excessive sweating, thick greasy skin, weight gain, lethargy, myalgia and arthralgia, proximal myopathy, peripheral oedema

Hands
Large hands, carpal tunnel syndrome

Figure 3.30: Clinical features of Acromegaly.

diagnostic test. An OGTT suppresses GH, and the standard 75 g is used. There is no complete consensus about precise levels, but those with acromegaly will typically fail to suppress the growth hormone level below 0.3 microgram/l (1 mU/L).

- In addition the OGTT will check for the presence of diabetes or impaired glucose tolerance.
- Other tests of pituitary function: Prolactin level (mid to moderate increase in around 30% of patients), TFT, 9:00 am cortisol, LH/FSH.

Imaging:

- MRI: of the pituitary gland is very sensitive for revealing the pituitary adenoma.
- Chest X-ray or CT chest and abdomen: may be required in the rare cases of ectopic GH production to locate the source.

Other:

- ECG
- Formal visual field perimetry

Management

➢ Treatment should be considered in all individuals diagnosed with acromegaly due to the increased mortality and morbidity seen with the disease.

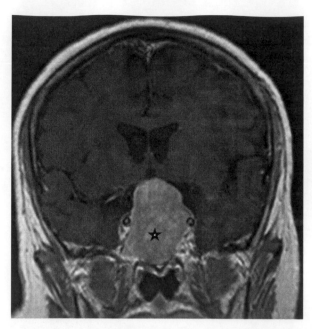

Figure 3.31: Contrast enhanced MRI of brain showing a large pituitary tumour (star) arising from the sella.

➤ The disease is best managed in specialist centres with close collaboration between an endocrinologist, a pituitary surgeon and possibly a radiotherapist.

➤ The aim of treatment is to reduce the growth hormone level to below 5 mU/L which has been proven to cause a reduction in mortality rate.

➤ Response to therapy is measured by assessing the growth hormone levels as well as serial IGF-1 measurements.

➤ Any features of hypopituitarism and diabetes or hypertension must be treated accordingly.

➤ Surgical management:

  o First line treatment is trans-sphenoidal surgery.

  o Results in clinical remission in around 90% of patients with micro-adenoma however only around 50% with a macro-adenoma.

  o Pituitary tissue is preserved as much as is possible.

  o Complications include infection (meningitis <5%) and hypopituitarism (10%).

  o Transfrontal surgery is now rarely indicated.

  o In the event of a massive macro-adenoma which is unlikely to be completely surgically resected, there may be a role for surgical debulking.

➤ Octreotide

  o A synthetic analogue of somatostatin

  o First–line medical therapy, used if surgery unsuccessful or not possible

  o Significantly reduces the level of growth hormone and IGF-1, with a response in around 60% of patients.

  o Usually given by subcutaneous depot injection monthly.

  o Very expensive although has few side effects apart from its association with gallstones as somatostatin inhibits gall bladder contraction.

➤ Dopamine agonists

  o Again, used if surgery unsuccessful or not possible.

  o Also have a use in tumour reduction prior to therapy such as surgery.

  o Achieves biochemical cure in relatively few patients (around 30%).

  o Cabergoline or bromocriptine are the most commonly used.

➤ Radiotherapy

  o Usually used following unsuccessful pituitary surgery in cases when medical therapy also unsuccessful.

  o Can also be used in conjunction with octreotide or a dopamine agonist as the biochemical response to radiotherapy is very slow and may take up to 10 years or even more.

  o The 'Gamma knife' is a highly focused stereotactic radiotherapy technique which is given as a single dose. This is becoming favoured over standard external beam radiotherapy given in multiple fractions.

  o Drawbacks are the length of time to achieve biochemical remission (years) and the side-effect of hypopituitarism (25% even with the gamma knife)

Prognosis:

➤ If left untreated, acromegaly leads to much reduced life expectancy with the majority of deaths occurring from heart failure, coronary artery disease, and secondary to hypertension.

➤ Aggressive management of both the primary adenoma and its sequelae such as hypertension, sleep apnoea and diabetes is improving both morbidity and mortality.

➤ A number of deaths occur as a result of malignancy such as colonic tumours.

ELECTROLYTE DISTURBANCES

Hypernatraemia

Defined as serum sodium > 145 mmol/L.

Epidemiology

Precise incidence unknown.

Aetiology

Almost always due to water loss or impaired ability to drink. Common causes in the hospital include infection, persistent vomiting, reduced oral intake in the unwell elderly patient and HHS. Rarer causes are diabetes insipidus and Mineralocorticoid excess e.g. in Conn's syndrome.

Pathophysiology

The pathophysiology is dependent on the aetiology.

Key features in the history/examination

- Any symptoms of infection
- Vomiting/diarrhoea
- Past history of diabetes
- Mobility (in the elderly)
- Assessment of hydration status shows:
  - o Hypotension (or postural hypotension)
  - o Skin turgor
  - o Dry mucous membranes

Investigations

Blood tests:

- FBC
- U&Es
- Inflammatory markers: CRP
- Glucose

Management

➢ Rehydration: The oral route is preferable and the aim should be to reduce the concentration by a rate of no more than 0.5 mmol/L per hour.

Prognosis:

➢ A full recovery is usual with careful fluid balance monitoring.

Hyponatraemia

Serum sodium (Na) of < 135 mmol/L.

Epidemiology

Precise incidence unknown, but thought to occur in up to 15% of in-patients.

Aetiology

Hyponatraemia may be divided into three forms:

Type	Diseases
Hyper-osmolar	Hyperglycaemia
Iso-osmolar	Pseudohyponatraemia (serum lipaemia or excess immunoglobins). Beware the sample taken from a 'drip arm' may also be pseudohyponatraemic
Hypo-osmolar	*Hypervolaemic* • Renal failure • CCF • Cirrhosis • Nephrotic syndrome *Euvolaemic* • Syndrome of inappropriate ADH secretion (SIADH) • Hypothyroidism • Psychogenic polydipsia *Hypovolaemic* • Diarrhoea (also high output stoma) • Vomiting • Sweating • Burns • Trauma • Diuretics • Salt-losing nephropathy • Addison's Disease

Table 3.64: Three forms of hyponatraemia

Pathophysiology

The serum and total body sodium levels are inextricably linked to water balance and hyponatraemia can be caused by a relative lack of sodium or excess of water. The average 70 Kg man has 42 L water (60% of body weight), made up in the following compartments:

- 28 L intracellular fluid
- 14 L extracellular fluid (of which 10.5 L is interstitial fluid and 3.5 L is intravascular fluid)

The usual osmolality (calculated as $2 \times [Na^+ + K^+] + Urea + Glucose$) is 280 mOsm/kg. Water balance is controlled by ADH which increases water resorption by stimulating the insertion of aquaporins, i.e. water channels, in the distal nephron and collecting duct. This is regulated by hypothalamic osmoreceptors and atrial baroreceptors. Sodium balance is controlled by the actions of ANP (reduces Na reabsorption) and aldosterone (increases Na reabsorption) on the kidneys.

3. Medicine

SIADH is seen only in euvolaemic states when diuretic use, Addison's disease and hypothyroidism have been excluded. Tests will reveal Hyponatraemia with a plasma osmolality < 270 mOsm/kg but an inappropriately concentrated urine with urine sodium > 20 mMol/L and urine osmolality > 300 mOsm/kg. Causes of SIADH include:

- Chest infection
- Malignancy: pancreas, gastric, lung
- Intracranial pathology, classically subdural haematoma but also meningitis, abscess and MS as well as post neuro-surgical intervention
- Drugs e.g. SSRI antidepressants

Key features in the history/examination

- Ultimately, depends on underlying aetiology
- Acute hyponatraemia:
  - Acute history of headache
  - Vomiting
  - Confusion
  - Seizures
  - Coma
- Chronic Hyponatraemia:
  - Insidious history of anorexia
  - Headache
  - Muscle cramps
  - Deteriorating cognitive function
- Assessment of fluid volume status may show fluid overload or fluid deficiency:
  - Fluid overload: raised JVP, dependent oedema and signs of pulmonary oedema
  - Fluid deficiency, dry mucous membranes, delayed capillary refill and postural or absolute hypotension

Further examination will be directed to help establish the underlying cause (see Figure 3.32).

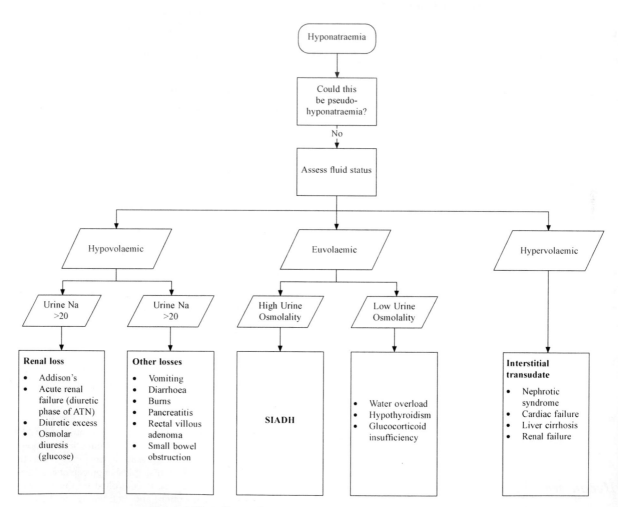

Figure 3.32: A diagnostic algorithm for the causes of hyponatraemia.

Investigations

Blood tests:

- FBC: get baseline values
- LFT: get baseline values
- Bone profile: get baseline values
- Glucose: get baseline values
- TFTs: get baseline values
- Plasma osmolality: get baseline values
- U&Es

Imaging:

- Chest X-ray
- CT brain: If subdural haemorrhage is suspected as a cause of SIADH

Others:

- Echocardiography
- Urinalysis: urine osmolality and sodium concentration
- ECG: if there is congestive cardiac failure.
- Other tests will be governed by the clinical scenario and the probable underlying cause.

Management

- ➢ Establish underlying cause and direct treatment accordingly.
- ➢ In the elderly there may a number of contributory causes.
- ➢ In chronic hyponatraemia beware of correcting serum sodium too quickly as there is a risk of central pontine myelinolysis: aim for an increase of no more than 0.5 mMol/L/hour.
- ➢ Frequent monitoring of sodium levels and an accurate fluid-balance record should be maintained.
- ➢ Any contributory drugs (especially diuretics or Citalopram): stopped or changed.

Acutely unwell and significantly symptomatic:

- ➢ IV NaCl. May require hypertonic saline with caution
- ➢ Add IV Furosemide, especially if at risk of fluid overload

Hypervolaemic hyponatraemia:

- ➢ Water restriction
- ➢ Diuretic use

Hypovolaemic hyponatraemia:

- ➢ IV normal saline

Euvolaemic hyponatraemia:

- ➢ Addison's: steroids
- ➢ Hypothyroidism: Levothyroxine

- ➢ Psychogenic polydipsia: fluid restriction

SIADH :

- ➢ Fluid restriction.
- ➢ If this does not work: Demeclocycline

Prognosis:

- ➢ A full recovery is usual if the underlying cause can be found and treated.

Hyperkalaemia

Defined as serum potassium > 5.5 mmol/L with severe serum potassium > 6.5 mmol/L.

Epidemiology

Precise incidence unknown.

Aetiology

The major causes of hyperkalaemia are:

- Renal failure
- Drugs: Angiotensin converting enzyme inhibitors, potassium sparing diuretics.
- Significant tissue breakdown e.g. rhabdomyolysis, tumour lysis
- Metabolic acidosis, causing a movement from the intracellular to the extracellular space
- Addison's disease
- Iatrogenic potassium overload
- Pseudohyperkalaemia: haemolysis of the blood sample

Pathophysiology

Potassium is one of the major cations in the body which is approximately 98% intracellular. The body's levels are predominantly regulated by the balance between GI absorption and renal excretion. Hyperkalaemia is classic cause of cardiac arrhythmias.

Key features in the history/examination

- Often asymptomatic, i.e. an incidental finding
- Symptoms often vague: fatigue, lethargy and generalised weakness
- Palpitations
- Trauma
- Drug history
- Risk factors for renal impairment e.g. history of hypertension and diabetes
- May be unremarkable
- Irregular pulse caused by ectopic beats

Investigations

Blood tests:

- U&Es: potassium level and evidence of renal impairment
- ABG: acid-base status
- Digoxin levels if taking Digoxin (hyperkalaemia increases Digoxin toxicity)

Others:

- ECG: shows changes that are progressive with increasing serum potassium, i.e. heart blocks, flattening of P waves, tenting of T waves, widening of QRS, ventricular tachycardia.

Management

Based on Resuscitation Council (UK) guidelines. It depends on degree of hyperkalaemia and hence the potassium levels should be carefully monitored. Patient with a mild to moderate hyperkalaemia should be on a cardiac monitor until the hyperkalaemia is resolved.

Mild (5.5–6.0 mmol/L):

- Stop drugs predisposing to hyperkalaemia
- Ensure adequate hydration
- Calcium resonium
- Consider furosemide

Moderate (6.0–6.5 mmol/L):

- Insulin/dextrose: typically 15 units actrapid in 50 mls 50% glucose over 15 minutes

Severe (> 6.5 mmol/L):

- Calcium chloride 10 mls 10% IV
- Salbutamol nebuliser
- Consider sodium bicarbonate
- Consider haemodialysis

In cardiac arrest:

- Calcium chloride 10 mls 10% IV
- Sodium bicarbonate 50 mls 8.4% IV
- Insulin/dextrose. Typically 15 units actrapid in 50 mls 50% glucose

Prognosis:

- The higher the potassium level, the greater the risk of VT and cardiac arrest, however with prompt and effective treatment a full recovery should be expected.

Hypokalaemia

Defined as serum potassium < 3.5 mmol/L. However moderate serum potassium levels are 2.5 to 3.0 mmol/L while severe serum potassium levels are less that 2.5 mmol/L.

Epidemiology

Precise incidence unknown.

Aetiology

Commonly due to urinary or GI loss of potassium. Clinical symptoms rarely occur unless serum potassium is less than 3.0 mmol/L. The main causes are:

- Decreased potassium intake
- Increased potassium entry into cells
- Increased potassium excretion
- Dialysis/plasmapheresis

Pathophysiology

Mechanism	Features
Decreased potassium intake	<ul><li>Rare</li><li>Associated with very restricted diets – low calorie protein diets</li><li>Anorexia nervosa</li><li>Increased potassium entry into cells</li><li>Potassium enters the cells in alkalosis</li><li>Catecholamines promote potassium in to the cell by increasing Na-K-ATPase activity</li><li>Salbutamol</li><li>Increased availability of insulin increased the activity of the Na-K-ATPase pump and promotes the entry of potassium into skeletal muscle and hepatic cells</li><li>Hypokalaemic periodic paralysis<ul><li>Rare</li><li>Characterised by potentially fatal paralysis and muscle weakness</li><li>Precipitated by stress, exercise and increased release of adrenaline, cortisol, aldosterone or insulin</li></ul></li><li>Increases in blood cell production<ul><li>May happen after administration of folic acid or B12 in megaloblastic anaemia</li><li>The administration of granulocyte-macrophage colony-stimulating factor in neutropenia</li></ul></li></ul>
Losses from GI tract from any cause	<ul><li>Vomiting</li><li>Diarrhoea</li><li>Ileus</li><li>Villous adenoma</li></ul>

Increased loss of potassium in urine	• Diuretics
	o Increase distal potassium delivery
	o Activate renin-angiotensin-aldosterone system
	o Increased potassium excretion
	o Problematic with loop and thiazide diuretics
	• Mineralocorticoid excess – primary aldosteronism
	• Salt-wasting nephropathies
	o Renal diseases with decreased proximal, loop or distal sodium reabsorption via similar mechanism to diuretics
	o Bartter's or Gitelman's syndromes
	o Tubulo-interstitial disease – Sjogren's syndrome or SLE
	o Metabolic acidosis
	o Hypomagnesaemia
	o Polyuria
Increased loss through sweating	• Exercise in hot climate
	• Cystic fibrosis
	• Burns and other dermatological conditions
Chronic alcoholism	

Table 3.65: Pathophysiology of hypokalaemia.

Key features in the history/examination

- Usually asymptomatic
- Presence of a likely cause – vomiting, diarrhoea, alcoholism
- Drug history, especially diuretic use
- Muscle weakness can sometimes be a feature of acute hypokalaemia
- With decreasing potassium, fatigue and cramps are a feature
- Most likely unremarkable

Investigations

Blood tests:

- U&Es
- TSH: hyperthyroidism is associated with hypokalaemic periodic paralysis
- ABG: in particular to measure the pH

Others:

- Urine potassium
- ECG: classical changes are ST depression, T wave flattening

and U waves. Alternatively AF or other arrhythmias may be seen.

Management

- ➢ Potassium replacement. Bearing in mind that since most of the body's potassium is intracellular, a reduction in serum potassium may reflect a significant total body deficit.
  - o Oral: for mild/moderate hypokalaemia. Each tablet contains around 12 mmol potassium and the taste is unpleasant and often induces nausea and vomiting in patients.
  - o IV: for moderate/severe hypokalaemia. The usual safe maximal replacement rate is 10 mmol/hour, or 20 mmol/hour via a central line with close cardiac monitoring.
- ➢ Cardiac arrest or peri-arrest: The Resuscitation Council's guidelines are 20 mmol/min over 10 minutes followed by a further 10 mmol over the next 10 minutes.
- ➢ During replacement regular monitoring of potassium levels are necessary
- ➢ Stop any causative drugs
- ➢ Replacement of magnesium if also low

Prognosis:

- ➢ Prompt and effective treatment is essential as hypokalaemia may progress to cause cardiac arrest.

Hypercalcaemia

Defined as calcium more than 2.6 mmol/L.

Epidemiology

It is a common, often incidental finding. 5% of hospitalised patients have hypercalcaemia.

Aetiology

Most cases are due to hyperparathyroidism (usually primary but can be due to secondary and tertiary) and malignancy. Most common malignancies are breast, lung, prostate, ovary, kidney and myeloma. Parathyroid hormone related peptide, osteolysis, vitamin D dependent (lymphoma) and ectopic PTH release are all involved in malignancies leading to hypercalcaemia. Other causes (10% of hypercalcaemia cases):

- Sarcoidosis
- Tuberculosis
- Drugs: thiazide diuretics, calcium/vitamin D, lithium
- Endocrine: thyrotoxicosis, acromegaly, hypoadrenalism
- Prolonged immobilisation
- Rhabdomyolysis (calcium low in the acute phase)
- Familial hypocalciuric hypercalcaemia

Pathophysiology

The pathophysiology is dependent on the aetiology.

Key features in the history/examination

- Asymptomatic (50%)
- Symptoms usually imply severe hypercalcaemia (>3.5 mmol/L)
- The classical symptoms:
  - o 'Bones': bone pain/fracture
  - o 'Groans' (GI): nausea, vomiting, constipation
  - o 'Stones' (Renal): polyuria/polydipsia; loin pain
  - o 'Psychic moans' (Psychiatric): depression/confusion
- Past or family history of cancer
- Cough, smoking history
- None (if mild)
- Dehydration
- Look for signs of underlying maligancy clubbing secondary to lung carcinoma, breast lump
- Erythema nodosum (sarcoid or TB)
- Reduced level of consciousness
- Seizures

Investigations

Blood tests:

- FBC
- U&Es: look for evidence of dehydration and renal impairment
- LFTs
- Glucose
- Mg^{2+}
- Inflammatory markers
- Bone profile
- PTH
- Consider myeloma screen (paired serum and urine protein electrophoresis for Bence-Jones protein) and PSA

Imaging:

- Chest X-ray
- AXR: may show renal stones
- Plain X-ray of any areas of bony pain
- Consider bone scan

Others:

- ECG: may show bradycardia and atrio-ventricular (AV) block.

Management

- ➢ IV fluid rehydration
- ➢ Furosemide will help calcium excretion but only once fully rehydrated
- ➢ Stop any calcium tablets and thiazide diuretics
- ➢ May need IV bisphosphonate (Pamidronate 60–90 mg) especially if refractory and painful
  - o After IV bisphosphonate it takes at least 72 hours before the calcium levels fall and the effects will last around three weeks. Beware re-treating too early as inevitably hypocalcaemia will be the consequence).
- ➢ Haemodialysis as a last resort treatment
- ➢ Monitor calcium levels and ensure decreasing
- ➢ Treat the underlying cause (e.g. parathyroidectomy, steroids for sarcoidosis, stop thiazide diuretics)

Prognosis:

- ➢ Very dependent on cause, but in the case of malignancy with bony metastases it will be poor
- ➢ Must be treated as it can result in cardiac arrest

Hypocalcaemia

Defined as calcium less than 2.1 mmol/L.

Epidemiology

Precise incidence unknown. It is present in 88% of critical ill patients admitted to Intensive Care Units.

Aetiology

Decreased levels of calcium in circulation can be due to:

- Vitamin D deficiency
- Chronic renal failure
- Hypoparathyroidism: Iatrogenic postsurgical hypoparathyroidism, HIV related, pseudohypoparathyroidism, idiopathic, autoimmune

Increased loss of circulating calcium can be due to:

- Rhabdomyolysis
- Acute pancreatitis

Drugs can also induce hypocalcaemia. Critical illnesses such as sepsis, burns and having multiple transfusions are known to cause hypocalcaemia as well as hypomagnesaemia.

Pathophysiology

Calcium levels are primarily controlled by parathyroid hormone (PTH) and Vitamin D. PTH is released from the parathyroid gland in response to low calcium and causes increases resorption from bone and increases 1-α hydroxylation of vitamin D. 1,25(OH)2-Vitamin D increases calcium resorption from the intestine and kidney.

Hypocalcaemia is mainly secondary to imbalance in calcium absorption, excretion and distribution.

Key features in the history/examination

- Lack of access to sunlight: elderly patients remaining indoors, religious dress reducing sun exposure
- Medical history: thyroid/parathyroid surgery,
- Paraesthesia: classically peri-oral but also fingertips and toes
- A range of behavioural changes and neuropsychiatric symptoms may be reported: cognitive impairment, depression, lethargy, irritability, anxiety and parkinsonism.
- Non-specific symptoms of fatigue and muscle weakness
- Abdominal pain: if pancreatitis suspected
- Chronic hypocalcaemia may well be asymptomatic
- Trousseau's sign: carpal spasm in response to ischaemia secondary to vascular occlusion with a blood pressure cuff for 3 minutes.
- Chvostek's sign: tapping over cranial nerve VII by the ear gives brief contraction/twitching of ipislateral perioral muscle resulting in contraction of a corner of the mouth.
- Carpo-pedal spasm

Features of chronic hypocalcaemia:

- Cataracts
- Extrapyramidal symptoms such as parkinsonism,
- Skin and hair changes
  - Dermatitis
  - Eczema
  - Hyperpigmentation
  - Psoriasis
  - Brittle hair with patchy alopecia
  - Brittle nails with transverse groove
- Dementia may be present in which case a Mini Mental Status Examination must be performed.

Investigations

Blood tests:

- U&Es
- Bone profile
- LFTs: albumin level
- Mg^{2+}
- More advanced tests such as PTH and Vitamin D levels if required

Others:

- ECG: may show prolonged QT interval, T wave inversion, heart block
- USS: of the kidneys is necessary if CRF is found.

Management

➢ Calcium gluconate (or chloride) 10 mls of 10% IV over 10 to 20 minutes. Repeated if necessary

➢ Treat any concurrent hypomagnesaemia
➢ Oral calcium and vitamin D supplements

Prognosis:

➢ Good prognosis if treated promptly
➢ Must be treated as it can result in cardiac arrest

Hypomagnesaemia

Defined as serum magnesium < 0.6 mmol/L.

Epidemiology

Incidence is unknown.

Aetiology

The control of magnesium homeostasis is the balance between gastrointestinal absorption and renal excretion. Unlike other ions there is no direct hormonal control over this, although PTH does increase GI absorption. Causes of hypomagnesaemia include:

- Malnutrition
- Alcohol dependence
- Refeeding syndrome
- Diarrhoea and vomiting (including high output stomas)
- Chronic diuretic use
- Bartter syndrome
- Total parental nutrition (TPN)
- Acute pancreatitis

Pathophysiology

The pathophysiology is dependent on the aetiology.

Key features in the history/examination

- Weakness
- Tremor
- Seizures
- Paraesthesia
- Nystagmus
- Tetany

Investigations

Blood tests:

- Mg^{2+}
- U&Es: hypomagnesaemia has many shared causes with hypokalaemia.
- Calcium: hypomagnesaemia impairs PTH secretion causing hypocalcaemia

Others:

- ECG: may show T wave changes, U waves and prolonged QT interval, ventricular ectopics, and Torsades de pointes.

Management

➢ Magnesium replacement – orally if asymptomatic or IV if severe/symptomatic

➢ Replacement of potassium and calcium if necessary

Prognosis:

➢ Good in detected and treated

Further reading and references

➢ www.addisons.org.uk

➢ Drivers Medical Group, DVLA (2009). *For Medical Practitioners. At a glance guide to the current medical standards of fitness to drive.*

➢ Resuscitation Council (UK) (2008). *Advanced Life Support* (5th Ed.)

PALPITATIONS

Differential diagnosis

Type	Disease
Arrhythmias	**Tachycardias**
	Long QT syndrome
	Bradycardias
	Atrial fibrillation (AF)
	Extrasystoles

Palpitations are an abnormal awareness of the heart beat. They are very common in General Practice, cardiology clinics and on the acute 'take'.

Tachycardia

Tachycardia is defined as a rate greater than 100 bpm. The management of palpitations caused by tachycardia depends on the underlying cardiac rhythm. There are two main categories of tachyarrhythmia; supraventricular/narrow complex (i.e. where the focus of rhythm is generated at or above the atrioventricular (AV) node) or ventricular/broad complex.

Narrow complex arrhythmias (QRS duration less than 120 ms/3 small squares):

- Sinus tachycardia
- AF with fast ventricular response
- Atrial flutter
- Atrial tachycardia

- AV nodal re-entrant tachycardia (AVNRT)
- AV re-entrant tachycardia (AVRT)

Ventricular tachycardias (QRS duration more than 120 ms/3 small squares):

- Monomorphic
- Polymorphic (e.g. Torsades de Pointes)

Epidemiology

Tachycardias are very common, especially sinus tachycardia and AF.

Aetiology and pathophysiology

There are many causes of tachycardia dependent on the specific type of tachycardia.

Sinus tachycardia:

A physiological response to a stressor e.g. sepsis, hypovolaemia, anxiety, pain and exercise. This is not managed by algorithm, but the underlying cause must be identified and treated. Common causes include:

- Hypovolaemia
- Drugs e.g. caffeine, alcohol, amphetamines
- Endocrine abnormalities e.g. hypoglycaemia, hyperthyroidism, phaeochromocytoma
- Anxiety and panic disorders
- Anaemia
- Sepsis
- Pregnancy
- After exercise

Atrial tachycardia:

- Originates in the atria but not the sino-atrial (SA) node
- Can be sustained
- Usually seen in structural heart disease
- Can be focal or a re-entrant circuit
- Sometimes multifocal, giving P waves of differing morphology

Atrial flutter:

- A macro re-entrant circuit in the atria, usually around the tricuspid valve, generating a very fast atrial response (typically 300 bpm).
- The AV node filters this, classically giving a 2:1 block and a ventricular response of 150 bpm
- Electrocardiogram (ECG) shows a 'saw-tooth' baseline, best seen in leads II, III, aVF and V1.
- 60% are precipitated by an acute intercurrent illness e.g. sepsis.

AVRNT:

- The most common form of supraventricular tachycardia (SVT).

- The AV node has two conduction pathways; a fast and a slow conducting. The fast usually dominates and has a longer refractory period.

- If a premature beat hits the AV node when the slow pathway is active but the fast pathway is still refractory, the slow pathway conducts the impulse to the ventricles but in addition the impulse is turned around within the AV node and is conducted back to the atria by the fast pathway (which is no longer refractory), initiating the SVT. This results in a retrograde p-wave that may be visible on an ECG.

- See Figures 3.36 and 3.41–3.43.

AVRT:

- An accessory pathway outside of the AV node is capable of conduction between the atria and ventricles.

- Most common is orthodromic: the impulse travels via the AV node then back to the atria via the accessory pathway.

- Less commonly antidromic: the initial conduction from the atria to the ventricles is via the accessory pathway, resulting in a broad QRS complex.

Wolff-Parkinson-White (WPW):

- Conduction from the atria to the ventricles via an accessory pathway generates a degree of ventricular pre-excitation.

- This is seen on the ECG as a shortened PR interval and a delta wave.

- Increased risk in AF: The usual filter to the ventricular response, the AV node, is bypassed by the accessory pathway giving a very rapid (250–300 bpm) 'pre-excited' AF.

- This is at high risk of degenerating into ventricular fibrillation (VF).

- See Figures 3.38–3.39 and 3.44.

Ventricular tachycardia:

- Always a very worrying sign!

- Always get senior help

- There is a high risk of degenerating into pulseless VT.

- See Figure 3.34.

Polymorphic VT

- Torsades de Pointes is usually non-sustained but risks degenerating into VF

- There is a characteristic ECG where the QRS complexes appear to twist around the axis

- It is associated with a long QT interval

- Other associations are with hypomagnesaemia and hypokalaemia, hence seen in alcoholics.

- See Figure 3.37.

Key features in the history/examination

- Onset and progression:
  - o When and how often do the palpitations occur
  - o How long do they last?
  - o Do they occur just occasionally or as sustained episodes?

- Fast or slow?

- Regular or irregular? It is often helpful to ask the patient to tap out the rhythm of the palpitations.

- Any associated symptoms – chest pain, dizziness or shortness of breath, collapse or loss of consciousness?

- Past history of tachycardias and hyperthyroidism

- Family history of abnormal heart rhythms (do any family members have pacemakers?) or sudden cardiac death.

- Drug history: prescribed, non-prescribed, illicit drug use, alcohol and caffeine intake.

- Assess tachycardic patients using the standard A to E approach advocated by the Resuscitation Council.

- Full cardiovascular examination

- Look for signs of sepsis and dehydration

- Examine the thyroid gland

Investigations

The key investigation in the assessment of a patient with palpitations is the 12 lead ECG. It is important to note whether the patient is experiencing palpitations at the time the ECG is taken. If no abnormalities are found on the 12 lead ECG, the patient may have a paroxysmal arrhythmia which may be detected on 24 hour ambulatory ECG monitoring or, if the palpitations do not occur frequently, an event monitor or implantable loop recorder.

ECG:

- 12 lead ECG

- 24 hour ambulatory ECG monitoring

Blood tests:

- FBC

- Renal function

- TFT

- Magnesium

- Glucose

- Cardiac enzymes

Others:

- Echocardiogram

- (Event Monitor or Implantable loop recorder)

There are three questions you need to consider when attempting to interpret the ECG of someone who presents with tachycardia:

3. Medicine

1. Are the QRS complexes narrow or broad?
2. Are there P waves?
3. Is it regular or irregular?

Management

➤ The management of tachycardia is summarised in the tachycardia algorithm from the Resuscitation Council.

➤ Look for the adverse signs early and seek senior help immediately if they are present.

➤ All patients should be constantly monitored and reassessed so that any deterioration in cardiac output may be recognised early.

➤ If DC cardioversion is required an anaesthetist will be needed to sedate or intubate the patient whilst this is happening.

➤ The precise number of joules required varies depending on the defibrillator used, so local policies should be known. The shock should be synchronised to avoid precipitating VF, but this is not unknown even with a synchronised shock.

Regular broad complex tachycardia (without compromise):

➤ If a decision needs to be made as to whether it is VT or SVT with aberrant conduction (e.g. SVT with left bundle branch block (LBBB)). It may be possible to see a previous ECG to help, or certain features on the ECG may imply VT (concordance, fusion and capture beats.) If in doubt it should be treated as VT and the usual management would be with amiodarone.

Irregular broad complex tachycardia (without compromise):

➤ More complicated and it would be very important for a FY doctor to get help if this is seen. Again a recent ECG will be invaluable to guide treatment.

➤ AF with bundle branch block should be treated as AF.

➤ Pre-excited AF, caused by WPW syndrome, is important to diagnose as treating this with drugs that slow AV node conduction may precipitate VT/VF. The best treatments are with amiodarone, flecanide or DC cardioversion. Drugs to be avoided include Digoxin, Diltiazem, Verapamil and Adenosine.

➤ Torsades de Pointes should be treated by stopping any medications which prolong the QT interval and ensuring that any hypokalaemia and hypomagnesaemia is corrected.

Regular narrow complex tachycardia:

Treated with vagal manoeuvres (blowing into a syringe is perhaps the easiest)

If unsuccessful then adenosine (6 mg, 12 mg, 12 mg).

	Narrow or broad	P waves	Regular or irregular
Sinus tachycardia	Narrow	Yes	Regular
Atrial tachycardia	Narrow	Yes but may be abnormal morphology	Regular
Atrial fibrillation	Narrow	No	Irregularly irregular
Atrial flutter	Narrow	May see sawtooth flutter waves	Regular (75, 100 or 150 bpm depending on level of block). Can be irregular if variable block
AVNRT/ AVRT	Narrow	May be seen after QRS complex due to retrograde conduction	Regular
Monomorphic VT	Broad – same amplitude	Can occasionally be seen, though no fixed relation to QRS	Regular
Polymorphic VT	Broad – varying amplitude	Can occasionally be seen, though no fixed relation to QRS	Regular

Table 3.66: ECG features of tachycardias.

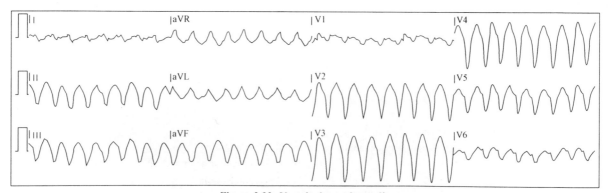

Figure 3.33: Ventricular tachycardia

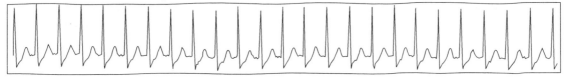

Figure 3.34: SVT in lead II.

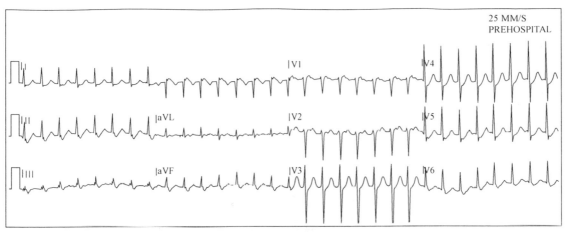

Figure 3.35: AVNRT.

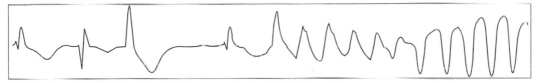

Figure 3.36: Torsades de Pointes.

> Push and flush the adenosine quickly as its half-life is only a few seconds.
> Warn the patient that it will make them feel truly awful – almost as if they are about to die – but that this will pass within a few seconds.
> Record a rhythm strip (using the printer on the defibrillator is usually the most convenient) whilst giving these treatments. (See Figure 3.42.)
> This has a good chance of cardioverting an SVT, and if the underlying rhythm is atrial flutter this will be unmasked and the diagnosis made.

Irregular narrow complex tachycardia:

> Is AF and the treatment is outlined in the AF section.

All rhythms:

> Following successful treatment for the tachycardia it is important to record the 12 lead ECG. This will show any underlying arrhythmia (e.g. Wolff Parkinson White syndrome, Brugada syndrome or long Q-T syndrome) which could predispose to future tachyarrhythmia.

> The patient will need referral to a cardiologist for ongoing medical management, consideration of electrophysiological studies and radiofrequency ablation to identify and break any aberrant conduction pathways and certainly any episodes of VT will need referral for consideration of an implantable defibrillator (ICD).

Long QT syndrome

Epidemiology

Estimated prevalence of 20/100,000.

Aetiology

• Congenital causes
  o Romano-Ward syndrome (autosomal dominant)

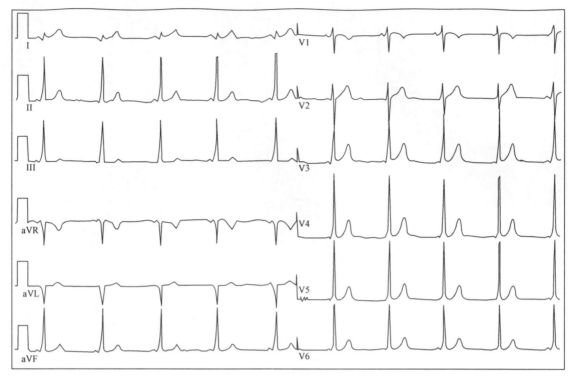

Figure 3.37: WPW.

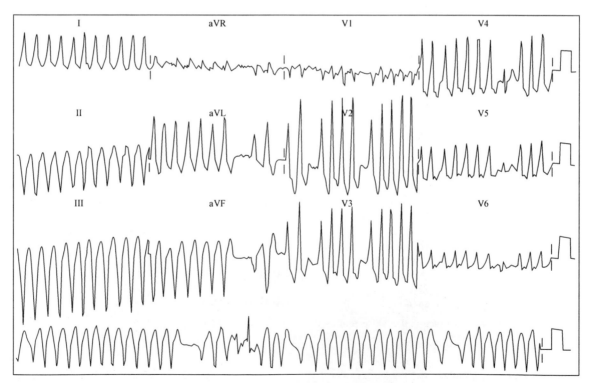

Figure 3.38: WPW with AF (pre-excited AF).

Adult Tachycardia Algorithm (with pulse)

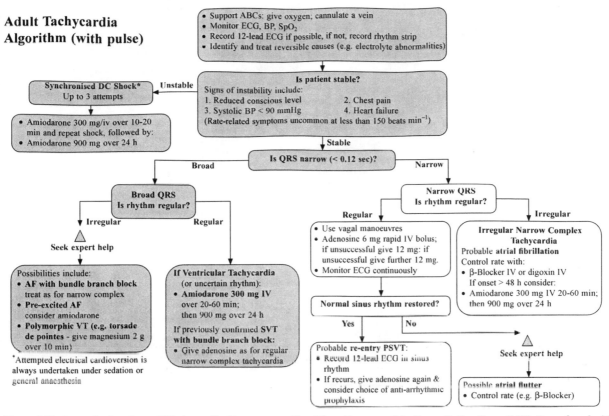

- Support ABCs: give oxygen; cannulate a vein
- Monitor ECG, BP, SpO$_2$
- Record 12-lead ECG if possible, if not, record rhythm strip
- Identify and treat reversible causes (e.g. electrolyte abnormalities)

Is patient stable?
Signs of instability include:
1. Reduced conscious level   2. Chest pain
3. Systolic BP < 90 mmHg   4. Heart failure
(Rate-related symptoms uncommon at less than 150 beats min^{-1})

Unstable →

Synchronised DC Shock*
Up to 3 attempts

- Amiodarone 300 mg/iv over 10-20 min and repeat shock, followed by:
- Amiodarone 900 mg over 24 h

Stable ↓

Is QRS narrow (< 0.12 sec)?

Broad ←   → Narrow

Broad QRS
Is rhythm regular?

Irregular   Regular

Seek expert help

Possibilities include:
- **AF with bundle branch block** treat as for narrow complex
- **Pre-excited AF** consider amiodarone
- **Polymorphic VT (e.g. torsade de pointes** - give magnesium 2 g over 10 min)

*Attempted electrical cardioversion is always undertaken under sedation or general anaesthesia

If Ventricular Tachycardia (or uncertain rhythm):
- **Amiodarone 300 mg IV** over 20-60 min; then 900 mg over 24 h

If previously confirmed **SVT with bundle branch block:**
- Give adenosine as for regular narrow complex tachycardia

Narrow QRS
Is rhythm regular?

Regular   Irregular

- Use vagal manoeuvres
- Adenosine 6 mg rapid IV bolus; if unsuccessful give 12 mg: if unsuccessful give further 12 mg.
- Monitor ECG continuously

Normal sinus rhythm restored?

Yes   No

Probable re-entry PSVT:
- Record 12-lead ECG in sinus rhythm
- If recurs, give adenosine again & consider choice of anti-arrhythmic prophylaxis

Irregular Narrow Complex Tachycardia
Probable atrial fibrillation
Control rate with:
- β-Blocker IV or digoxin IV
  If onset > 48 h consider:
- Amiodarone 300 mg IV 20-60 min; then 900 mg over 24 h

Seek expert help

Possible atrial flutter
- Control rate (e.g. β-Blocker)

Figure 3.39: Resuscitation Council Tachycardia Management Algorithm. *Courtesy of the Resuscitation Council UK. Reproduced with permission.*

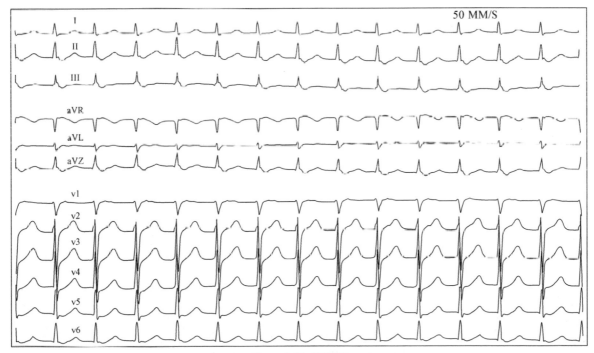

Figure 3.40: AVNRT.

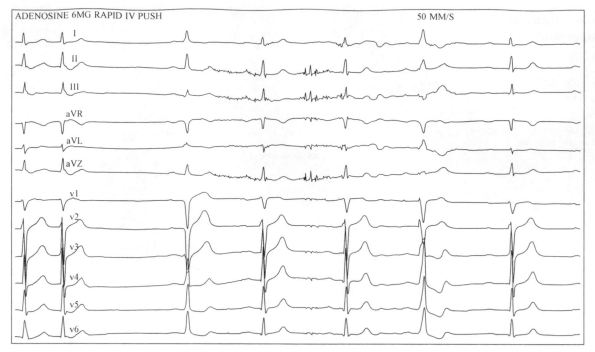

Figure 3.41: AVNRT terminating during adenosine iv push.

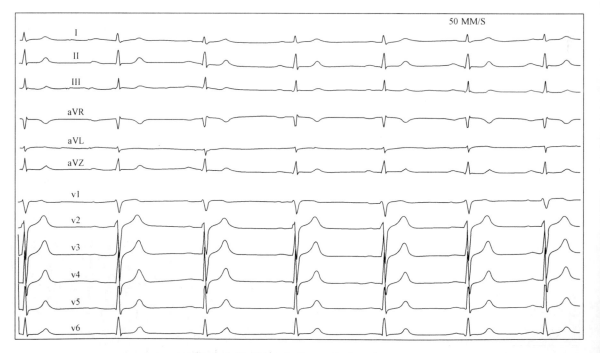

Figure 3.42: Sinus rhythm post-adenosine.

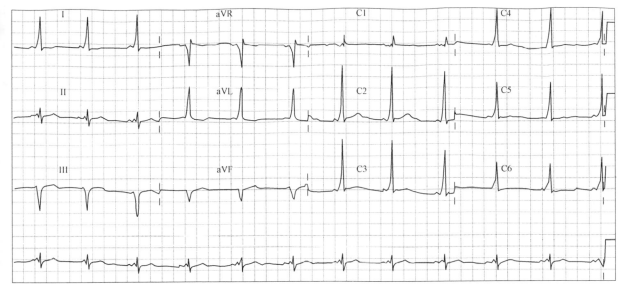

Figure 3.43: ECG of Wolff-Parkinson-White syndrome. Note the short PR interval and upsloping delta wave in the QRS complex.

- ○ Jervell, Lange-Nielsen syndrome (autosomal recessive, associated with deafness)

- ○ At least 12 genes associated with long QT syndrome (LQTS) have been discovered so far, and hundreds of mutations within these genes have been identified. Mutations in three of these genes account for about 75 percent of long QT syndrome:

  - ■ LQT1 – KCNQ1

  - ■ LQT2 – HERG

  - ■ LQT3 – SCN5A

- • Acquired causes include

- ○ Electrolyte imbalances (hypokalaemia, hypomagnesaemia and hypocalcaemia)

- ○ Drugs (eg Amiodarone, Sotalol, antihistamines and many more).

Pathophysiology

LQTS causes malfunction of cardiac ion channels. This tends to prolong the duration of the ventricular action potential (APD), which extends repolarisation, thus lengthening the QT interval. This abnormal repolarisation causes differences in myocyte refractory periods, meaning some parts of the myocardium might be refractory to subsequent depolarisation while others are ready.

Early after depolarisations (EADs - occur more commonly in LQTS) can be propagated to neighbouring myocytes due to differences in the refractory periods, leading to re-entrant polymorphic ventricular arrhythmias – Torsades de Pointes.

This may either revert spontaneously back to sinus rhythm causing syncope or degenerate to ventricular fibrillation causing sudden death.

EADs are caused by excessive prolongation of the action potential resulting in re-opening of certain L-type calcium channels during the plateau phase of the cardiac action potential.

In addition, sympathetic activity can increase the activity of the L-type calcium channels which increases the frequency of EADs. This provides a rationale for why the risk of sudden death in individuals with LQTS is higher during increased adrenergic states such as exercise or excitement.

Key features in the history/examination

- • Palpitations, syncope, seizures (sudden death) in the first 3 decades.

- • This is secondary to cardiac dysrhythmias, in particular VT and VF. These can be provoked by an external trigger e.g. a loud noise but commonly occur during sleep.

- • Onset and progression:

  - ○ when and how often do the palpitations occur?

  - ○ how long do they last?

  - ○ Do they occur just occasionally or as sustained episodes?

- • Regular or irregular? It is often helpful to ask the patient to tap out the rhythm of the palpitations.

- • Any associated symptoms: Chest pain, dizziness or shortness of breath, collapse or loss of consciousness?

- • Family history of abnormal heart rhythms (do any family members have pacemakers?) or sudden cardiac death.

- • Drug history: prescribed, non-prescribed, illicit drug use, alcohol and caffeine intake

- • Examination will be normal in most people

- • Check for hearing impairment

Investigations

ECG:

- 12 lead ECG: A resting ECG does not always demonstrate a prolonged QT interval, making diagnosis difficult.
- 24 hour holter monitor

On the ECG the QT interval will vary with heart rate, so the corrected QT interval must be calculated (QTc). Normally this will be automatically done by the ECG machine, but it can be calculated using the Bazett formula: QTc = QT/square root of RR interval. In adults a prolonged QTc is defined as >0.45 secs. See Figure 3.45.

Blood tests:

- Genetic testing is available via specialist clinics.

Cardiac stress test:

- May be necessary to unmask the LQTS.

Management

➢ Advice on lifestyle (avoid contact sports) and avoidance of drugs which prolong the QT interval.

➢ A beta-blocker can be used to shorten the QT interval.

➢ High risk cases can be fitted with an implantable defibrillator

Prognosis:

➢ Mortality can be as high as 70% over 10 years in untreated patients.

Bradycardia

Bradycardia is defined as a rate less than 60 bpm, with extreme bradycardia less than 40 bpm. Palpitations with bradycardia may be caused by a sinus bradycardia or a degree of 'block' in the normal conducting system of the heart; however the more usual presentation of bradycardias is with syncope or presyncope.

Aetiology

Causes of bradycardia and heart block include:

- Idiopathic: resulting from fibrosis of the conduction pathways
- Myocardial ischaemia (especially following inferior MI)
- Drugs which slow or block electrical conduction in the heart (e.g. beta-blockers, Digoxin and calcium channel blockers)
- Electrolyte disturbance (e.g. hyperkalaemia)
- Infective: Endocarditis with aortic root abscess, Lyme disease
- Infiltrative diseases: Sarcoidosis and amyloidosis
- Post cardiac surgery especially aortic valve replacement
- Physiological, especially in athletes

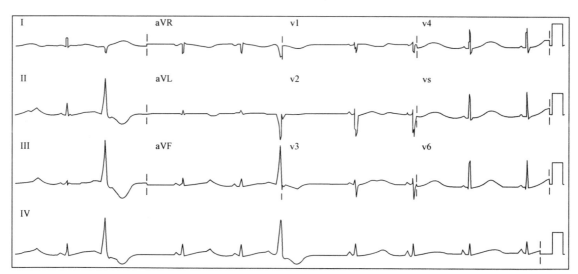

Figure 3.44: Long QT syndrome.

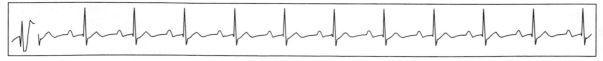

Figure 3.45: First degree heart block.

Pathophysiology

Heart block:

Heart block is a disturbance in the electrical conduction system below the level of the SA node that causes transient or permanent impairment of conduction of the normal electrical impulses. There are three degrees of heart block:

First degree: A prolonged PR interval (>200 msec or >5 small squares.) but all atrial impulses are conducted through to the ventricles. See Figure 3.46.

Second degree Mobitz type I (Wenckebach): The PR interval increases with each beat until the P wave fails to conduct to the ventricles leading to a dropped beat. The cycle then repeats itself.

Second degree Mobitz type II: the PR interval is constant but only a proportion of P waves are successfully conducted to the ventricles. See Figure 3.47.

Third degree or complete heart block: complete electrical dissociation between the atria and the ventricles. Although regular P waves and QRS complexes are seen, there is no association between them. The ventricular rate is typically 30–50 bpm. See Figure 3.48.

First degree and Wenckebach are relatively benign arrhythmias and may be found in fit young athletes. The level of the block is at the AV node, and consequently the QRS complexes are all narrow complex. No specific treatment is required unless it is drug-induced.

Mobitz type II and complete heart block are at risk of degenerating into a higher degree block or asystole. They are never physiological and should always be investigated and referred to a cardiologist. The level of block is below the AV node in the His-Purkinjie system. The precise level will determine the QRS morphology – if the block is in the bundle of His (25% cases) the QRS duration will be normal but the lower down the system the block, the wider the QRS and the greater the likelihood of degeneration. In third degree block there is no conduction and an alternative ventricular pacemaker generates the pulse, hence the QRS may well be wide.

Sick sinus syndrome (or SA node disease or tachy-brady syndrome) can cause both palpitations and syncope/presyncope. Usually idiopathic in origin, it can also be caused by ischaemic heart disease, cardiomyopathy and amyloidosis. It can be problematic to treat, as controlling the tachycardic element can worsen the bradycardic element. Sometimes a pacemaker is required to allow the tachycardia to be treated successfully with antiarrhythmic drugs.

Key features in the history/examination

- Onset and progression:
  - When and how often do the palpitations occur?
  - How long do they last?
  - Do they occur just occasionally or as sustained episodes?
- Regular or irregular? It is often helpful to ask the patient to tap out the rhythm of the palpitations.
- Any associated symptoms: Chest pain, dizziness or shortness of breath, collapse or loss of consciousness?
- Family history of abnormal heart rhythms (do any family members have pacemakers?) or sudden cardiac death.
- Drug history: prescribed, non-prescribed, illicit drug use, alcohol and caffeine intake.
- Findings are dependent on aetiology
- Pulse rate less than 60 bpm

Investigations

ECG:

- 12 lead ECG
- 24 hour ambulatory ECG monitoring

Blood tests:

- FBC
- U&Es: Checking for electrolyte abnormalities, in particular hypokalaemia
- Cardiac enzymes

Echocardiogram:

Others:

- Event monitor or Implantable loop recorder (Reveal device)

Management

➢ The management of bradycardia is outlined in the adjacent algorithm from the Resuscitation Council.

➢ Assess the patient using the standard A to E approach advocated by the Resuscitation Council.

➢ Look for the adverse signs and commence treatment with atropine

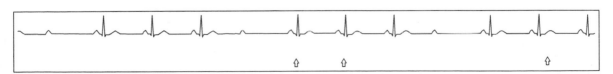

Figure 3.46: Mobitz type II heart block.

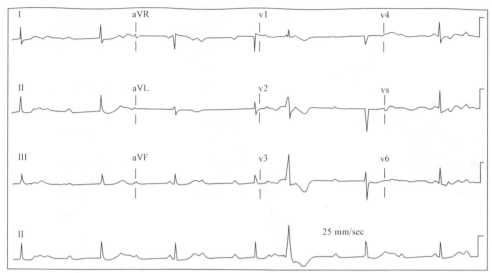

Figure 3.47: Complete heart block.

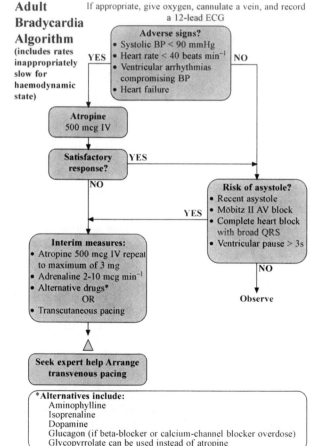

Adult Bradycardia Algorithm (includes rates inappropriately slow for haemodynamic state)

If appropriate, give oxygen, cannulate a vein, and record a 12-lead ECG

Adverse signs?
- Systolic BP < 90 mmHg
- Heart rate < 40 beats min⁻¹
- Ventricular arrhythmias compromising BP
- Heart failure

YES   NO

Atropine 500 mcg IV

Satisfactory response?   YES

NO

Risk of asystole?
- Recent asystole
- Möbitz II AV block
- Complete heart block with broad QRS
- Ventricular pause > 3s

YES

NO

Interim measures:
- Atropine 500 mcg IV repeat to maximum of 3 mg
- Adrenaline 2-10 mcg min⁻¹
- Alternative drugs*
  OR
- Transcutaneous pacing

Observe

Seek expert help Arrange transvenous pacing

*Alternatives include:
Aminophylline
Isoprenaline
Dopamine
Glucagon (if beta-blocker or calcium-channel blocker overdose)
Glycopyrrolate can be used instead of atropine

November 2005

Figure 3.48: Resuscitation Council Bradycardia Management Algorithm. *Courtesy of the Resuscitation Council UK. Reproduced with permission.*

> Senior help should be immediately sought.

> If the patient can be stabilised they should be reviewed by a Cardiologist to consider pacemaker insertion.

> If the patient cannot be stabilised then either a temporary pacing wire should be inserted or transcutaneous pacing commenced until a definitive pacemaker can be inserted.

> The decision to insert a permanent pacemaker is ultimately made by a Cardiologist in conjunction with the patient. Indications include a documented asystole of greater than three seconds or Mobitz type II/complete heart block.

Atrial fibrillation

Epidemiology

Atrial fibrillation affects about 1% of the population, but the prevalence dramatically rises with age, reaching 10% in those aged over 80.

Aetiology

- Hypertension
- Ischaemic heart disease
- Alcohol
- Hyperthyroidism
- Mitral valve disease (stenosis or regurgitation)
- Heart failure
- Sepsis
- Postoperative
- Electrolyte disturbance (hypokalaemia, hypocalcaemia and hypomagnesaemia)
- Cardiac tumours (e.g. atrial myxoma)
- 'Lone' AF (patients under 60 in whom no other cause is identified)

Pathophysiology

Atrial fibrillation is characterised by chaotic electrical activity within the atria which prevent their normal co-ordinated contraction which instead results in the uncoordinated fibrillation. Electrophysiological studies have shown that the commonest site for the initiation of AF is around the pulmonary veins. The electrical activity in the atria is conducted to the ventricles in an unpredictable way leading to irregularly irregular ventricular systole.

If atrial fibrillation persists electrophysiological remodelling occurs within the atria which favours continued fibrillation, making it harder for the heart to be cardioverted to sinus rhythm and so leading to permanent AF.

As the atria do not effectively contract in atrial fibrillation, ventricular filling depends almost entirely on passive filling during ventricular diastole which reduces cardiac output by 10–20%. In situations where passive filling of the left ventricles (LV) is impaired (e.g. in diastolic heart failure or restrictive cardiomyopathy), the onset of AF can prevent adequate cardiac output thus leading to decompensated heart failure.

In addition to the effects of atrial fibrillation on cardiac output, the lack of effective atrial contraction during the cardiac cycle results in stasis of blood in the atrial appendage and predisposes to thrombus formation in the left atrium. This may result in systemic thromboembolism including TIA or stroke, mesenteric ischaemia or acute limb ischaemia. In particular the risk of thromboembolism is greatest during the transition from AF to sinus rhythm and vice versa.

Classification:

Atrial fibrillation may be classified according to its duration and persistence. Management depends on whether the AF is of new onset (which may favour rhythm control) or prolonged and resistant to cardioversion (which may favour rate control and anticoagulation).

1. Paroxysmal: less than seven days in duration and terminates spontaneously

2. Persistent: more than seven days in duration and would potentially last indefinitely if not cardioverted

3. Permanent: more than seven days in duration but not possible to successfully revert to sinus rhythm

Key features in the history/examination

- Onset and progression:
  - o When and how often do the palpitations occur?
  - o How long do they last?
  - o Do they occur just occasionally or as sustained episodes?
- Fast or slow?
- Regular or irregular? It is often helpful to ask the patient to tap out the rhythm of the palpitations.
- Any associated symptoms: chest pain, dizziness or shortness of breath, collapse or loss of consciousness?

- Family history of abnormal heart rhythms (do any family members have pacemakers?) or sudden cardiac death.
- Drug history: prescribed, non-prescribed, illicit drug use, alcohol and caffeine intake
- An irregularly irregular pulse
- Absent 'a' waves in the JVP (owing to lack of atrial systole).
- Other features may be present depending on aetiology or complications (e.g. hypertension or signs of heart failure, valvular heart disease and hyperthyroidism).

Investigations

Blood tests:

These are not all U&E, so instead create bullet points as follows:

- U&Es: check for hypokalaemia.
- Mg: check for hypomagnesaemia.
- Bone profile: check for hypocalaemia.
- TFT

ECG:

- Irregularly irregular R-R interval and absence of P waves (an irregular baseline is seen in between the QRS complexes). If uncertain, compare the R-R interval between different QRS complexes with a piece of paper to see if they are the same or vary. See Figure 3.50.

Others:

Echocardiography: To establish systolic and diastolic heart function, look for any structural heart disease and measure left atrial size. An enlarged left atrium may make it more difficult to maintain sinus rhythm.

Management

There are two main aspects which need to be considered in managing patients with AF. The first is to optimise cardiac output. This may be achieved by either rhythm control to try to revert the heart back to sinus rhythm, or rate control to ensure that the ventricular rate is kept within normal limits in atrial fibrillation. The second is to consider anticoagulation to prevent the risk of subsequent thromboembolism.

Rhythm vs. rate control:

➤ The choice between rate and rhythm control of atrial fibrillation depends on whether it is paroxysmal, persistent or permanent, and on whether the atrial fibrillation is causing significant symptoms (e.g. palpitations or worsening heart failure). It should also be noted that some studies (e.g. AFFIRM) have demonstrated that in elderly asymptomatic patients there is no advantage of rhythm control over rate control in reducing mortality and may, in fact, increase morbidity owing to side effects from antiarrhythmic drugs.

➤ Broadly speaking, a rhythm control approach should be instituted for patients with paroxysmal AF and a rate control

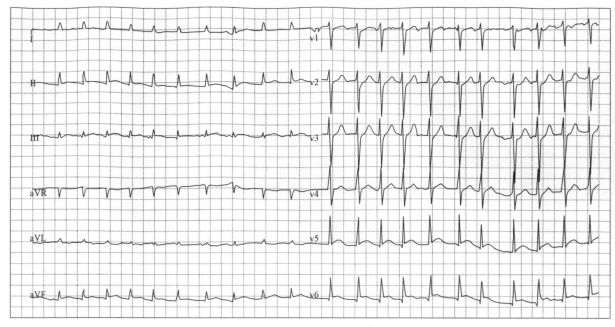

Figure 3.49: AF with fast ventricular response

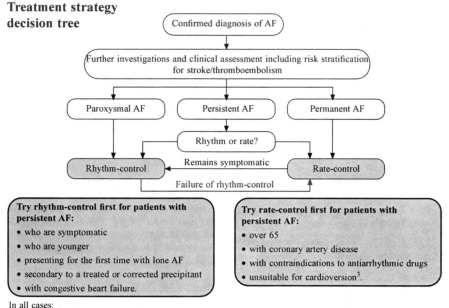

Treatment strategy decision tree

Confirmed diagnosis of AF

Further investigations and clinical assessment including risk stratification for stroke/thromboembolism

Paroxysmal AF   Persistent AF   Permanent AF

Rhythm or rate?

Rhythm-control   Remains symptomatic   Rate-control

Failure of rhythm-control

Try rhythm-control first for patients with persistent AF:

• who are symptomatic
• who are younger
• presenting for the first time with lone AF
• secondary to a treated or corrected precipitant
• with congestive heart failure.

Try rate-control first for patients with persistent AF:

• over 65
• with coronary artery disease
• with contraindications to antiarrhythmic drugs
• unsuitable for cardioversion[3].

In all cases:
– explain the advantages and disadvantages of each strategy to the patient before you decide which to use
– take into account comorbidities when deciding which to use
– use appropriate antithrombotic therapy.

[3]Patients unsuitable for cardioversion include those with: contraindications to anticoagulation; structural heart disease (e.g. large left atrium >5.5 cm, mitral stenosis) that precludes long-term maintenance of sinus rhythm; a long duration of AF (usually >12 months); a history of multiple failed attempts at cardioversion and/or relapses, even with concomitant use of antiarrhythmic drugs or non-pharmacological approaches; an ongoing but reversible cause of AF (e.g. thyrotoxicosis).

Figure 3.50: NICE management algorithm for the treatment strategy for AF patients. National Institute for Health and Clinical Excellence (2006) CG 36 *Atrial fibrillation: the management of atrial fibrillation*. London: NICE. Available from www.nice.org.uk/CG36. Reproduced with permission.

approach should be used for patients with permanent AF. The choice in persistent AF is less clear, but the NICE guidelines are very helpful in this circumstance.

➤ In all cases a clear underlying reversible cause (e.g. electrolyte disturbance or sepsis) should be sought and treated if possible.

Rhythm control in AF:

➤ Patients in new onset AF or persistent AF with significant symptoms often benefit from being reverted to sinus rhythm.

The method of achieving cardioversion and rhythm control depends on the onset of AF. If the patient is able to give a clear history of recent onset within 48 hours, a cardioversion attempt may be made immediately. However, if the history is not clear or onset is known to be beyond 48 hours previously, there is a risk of thrombus formation within the left atrium which may dislodge and embolise causing a stroke. In such cases, it is either necessary to therapeutically anticoagulate the patient with warfarin (with a target INR of 2.5) for one month before attempting cardioversion, or to perform transoesophageal echocardiography prior to

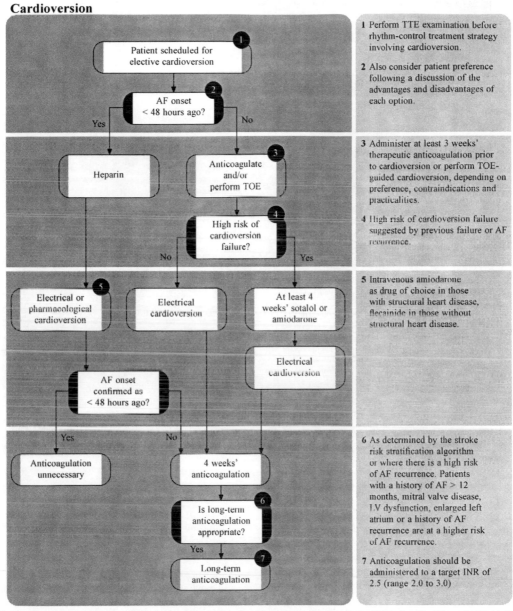

Cardioversion

1 Perform TTE examination before rhythm-control treatment strategy involving cardioversion.

2 Also consider patient preference following a discussion of the advantages and disadvantages of each option.

3 Administer at least 3 weeks' therapeutic anticoagulation prior to cardioversion or perform TOE-guided cardioversion, depending on preference, contraindications and practicalities.

4 High risk of cardioversion failure suggested by previous failure or AF recurrence.

5 Intravenous amiodarone as drug of choice in those with structural heart disease, flecainide in those without structural heart disease.

6 As determined by the stroke risk stratification algorithm or where there is a high risk of AF recurrence. Patients with a history of AF > 12 months, mitral valve disease, LV dysfunction, enlarged left atrium or a history of AF recurrence are at a higher risk of AF recurrence.

7 Anticoagulation should be administered to a target INR of 2.5 (range 2.0 to 3.0)

Figure 3.51: NICE management algorithm for cardioversion for AF patients. National Institute for Health and Clinical Excellence (2006) CG 36 *Atrial fibrillation: the management of atrial fibrillation*. London: NICE. Available from www.nice.org.uk/CG36. Reproduced with permission.

Rhythm-control treatment

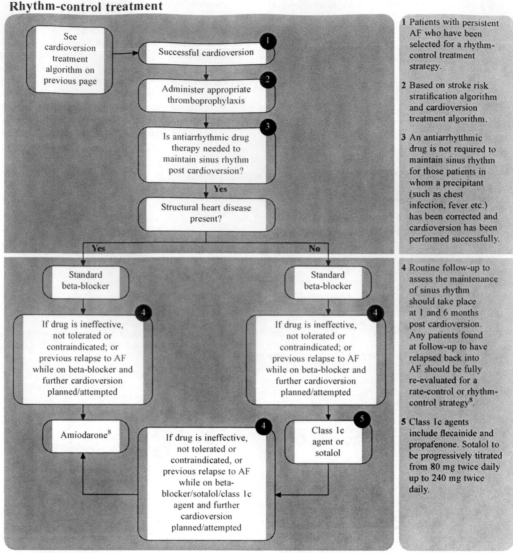

1 Patients with persistent AF who have been selected for a rhythm-control treatment strategy.

2 Based on stroke risk stratification algorithm and cardioversion treatment algorithm.

3 An antiarrhytthmic drug is not required to maintain sinus rhythm for those patients in whom a precipitant (such as chest infection, fever etc.) has been corrected and cardioversion has been performed successfully.

4 Routine follow-up to assess the maintenance of sinus rhythm should take place at 1 and 6 months post cardioversion. Any patients found at follow-up to have relapsed back into AF should be fully re-evaluated for a rate-control or rhythm-control strategy[8].

5 Class 1c agents include flecainide and propafenone. Sotalol to be progressively titrated from 80 mg twice daily up to 240 mg twice daily.

[8]If rhythm-control fails, consider the patient for rate-control strategy, or specialist referral for those with lone AF or ECG evidence of underlying electrophysiological disorder (e.g. Wolff-Parkinson-White [WPW] syndrome).

Figure 3.52: NICE management algorithm for rhythm-control for AF patients. National Institute for Health and Clinical Excellence (2006) CG 36 *Atrial fibrillation: the management of atrial fibrillation*. London: NICE. Available from www.nice.org.uk/CG36. Reproduced with permission.

cardioversion to rule out the presence of thrombus within the heart.

➤ Cardioversion may be performed pharmacologically or electrically. In patients with paroxysmal AF of less than 48 hours duration, either method may be employed although for patients with AF of longer than 48 hours duration elective electrical cardioversion (which may also be supplemented with rhythm controlling drugs beforehand) is the treatment of choice.

➤ Pharmacological cardioversion may be achieved with flecainide (in patients in whom structural heart disease has been ruled out) or amiodarone. Electrical cardioversion involves

synchronised DC shock (in a similar way to defibrillation in cardiac arrest) under a short general anaesthetic. The shock must be synchronised to the R wave as delivering the shock during the T wave could precipitate VF. The energy level used varies by defibrillator, so FY doctors should know the local policy.

➤ Following successful cardioversion, sinus rhythm may need to be maintained by continued use of antiarrhythmic drugs. Cardio-selective beta blockers (e.g. bisoprolol) are the first line choice for maintaining rhythm control. Where these fail to maintain sinus rhythm, other drugs such as flecanide, sotalol or amiodarone may be considered.

> Further electrophysiological intervention may be considered (e.g. electrophysiological studies and catheter ablation) to identify and treat the arrhythmogenic focus predisposing the patient to AF.

Rate control in AF:

> Where rhythm control has failed or is not feasible – patients in permanent AF and those in persistent AF where rate control is considered more appropriate – rate control is used. In most patients the first line choice for rate control is either a cardio-selective beta blocker such as bisoprolol or a calcium channel blocker such as diltiazem. The dose should be titrated up according to heart rate and blood pressure to provide adequate rate control. Digoxin should be used as add-on therapy if this fails to provide adequate control. Unless the patient has a sedentary lifestyle digoxin should be avoided as monotherapy as it only provides adequate rate control at rest and not during exercise.

Anticoagulation in AF:

> Long term anticoagulation should be considered in all patients with AF to reduce the risk of subsequent thromboembolic disease. Therapeutic anticoagulation in patients at risk of thromboembolism is usually achieved by starting aspirin (if at low risk of thromboembolism) or warfarin aiming to establish a therapeutic target INR of 2.5. The risk of thromboembolic stroke as a result of AF may be estimated using the CHADS-2 score (see Table 3.67), which should be used in conjunction

3. Medicine

Rate control for persistent and permanent AF

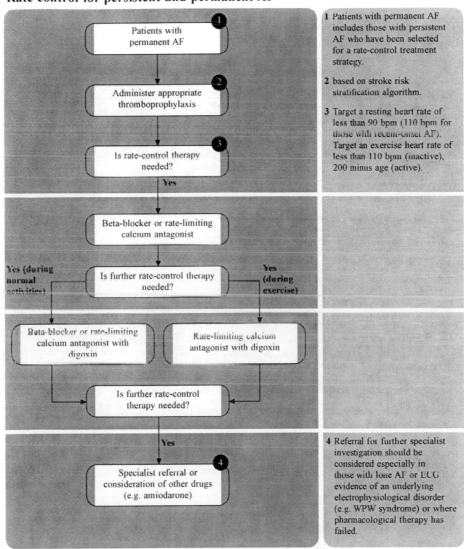

Figure 3.53: NICE management algorithm for rate control of AF patients. National Institute for Health and Clinical Excellence (2006) CG 36 *Atrial fibrillation: the management of atrial fibrillation*. London: NICE. Available from www.nice.org.uk/CG36. Reproduced with permission.

with the stroke risk stratification flow chart from NICE (see Figure 3.54).

Factor	Score
Congestive cardiac failure	1
Hypertension	1
Age >75 years	1
Diabetes	1
Previous stroke or TIA	2

Table 3.67: CHADS-2 score adapted from Gage, B. F, et al. JAMA (2001).

➤ Anticoagulation with aspirin should be considered in any patient with a score of 1 and warfarin should be considered in any patient with a score of 2 or more. The decision to start lifelong warfarin needs careful consideration and should be made with the patient only after discussing potential benefits and risks (e.g. bleeding) and taking into consideration any other co-morbidities (e.g. risk of falls). It should be noted that even if a patient has been successfully cardioverted to sinus rhythm, long term anticoagulation should still be considered in patients with paroxysmal or persistent AF in whom a reversible cause has not been identified owing to the risk of future relapse into AF and subsequent thromboembolic disease.

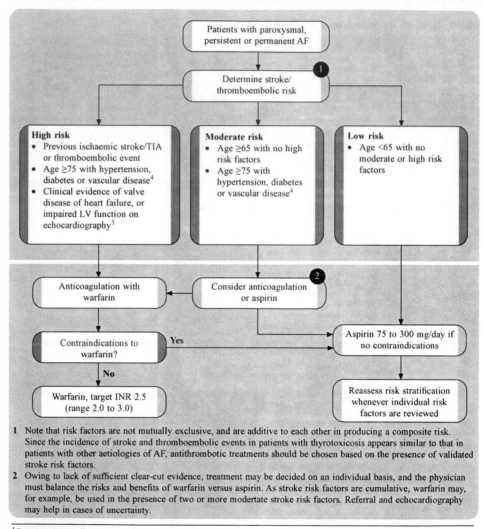

1   Note that risk factors are not mutually exclusive, and are additive to each other in producing a composite risk. Since the incidence of stroke and thromboembolic events in patients with thyrotoxicosis appears similar to that in patients with other aetiologies of AF, antithrombotic treatments should be chosen based on the presence of validated stroke risk factors.

2   Owing to lack of sufficient clear-cut evidence, treatment may be decided on an individual basis, and the physician must balance the risks and benefits of warfarin versus aspirin. As stroke risk factors are cumulative, warfarin may, for example, be used in the presence of two or more modertate stroke risk factors. Referral and echocardiography may help in cases of uncertainty.

[4]Coronary artery disease or peripheral artery disease.
[5]An echocardiogram is not needed for routine assessment, but refines clinical risk stratification in the case of moderate or severe LV dysfunction and valve disease.

Figure 3.54: NICE algorithm for stroke risk stratification in AF patients. National Institute for Health and Clinical Excellence (2006) CG 36 *Atrial fibrillation: the management of atrial fibrillation*. London: NICE. Available from www.nice.org.uk/CG36. Reproduced with permission.

CARDIOMYOPATHIES

Differential diagnosis

Type	Disease
Cardiomyopathy	**Hypertrophic cardiomyopathy (HCM)**
	Dilated cardiomyopathy (DCM)
	Restrictive cardiomyopathy (RCM)
	Arrthymogenic right ventricular cardiomyopathy (ARVC)
	Left ventricular non-compaction cardiomyopathy
	Takotsubo cardiomyopathy (TCM)

Cardiomyopathy is a term used to describe disorders of the heart with particular morphological and physiological characteristics.

This aim of this section is to give an overview of the pathophysiology and mechanisms responsible for the relevant clinical findings and to improve understanding of this often challenging group of diseases. It is important for an FY doctor to be able to ascertain the important features of the history and identify the characteristic examination findings. However, the management of cardiomyopathies is complex and requires early input from the Cardiology team and, if available, follow-up in a specialist heart muscle disease clinic.

Hypertrophic cardiomyopathy

Hypertrophic cardiomyopathy (HCM) is defined as the presence of increased ventricular wall thickness or mass in the absence of loading conditions (e.g. hypertension, aortic valve stenosis) sufficient to cause the observed abnormality.

Epidemiology

HCM is a clinically heterogeneous but relatively common autosomal dominant genetic heart disease. The prevalence is approximately 1:500 to 1:2,000 for the disease phenotype recognised by echocardiography and is therefore, probably the most frequently occurring cardiomyopathy.

HCM is the most common cause of sudden cardiac death in the young, including trained athletes and is an important substrate for heart failure disability at any age.

Morphologic evidence of disease is found by echocardiography in approximately 25% of first-degree relatives of patients with HCM.

Aetiology

Morphological subtypes:

According to the presence or absence of LV outflow tract obstruction, HCM can be defined as obstructive or non-obstructive.

- The obstructive variant of HCM is known as hypertrophic obstructive cardiomyopathy (HOCM). It was originally described as idiopathic hypertrophic subaortic stenosis (IHSS) or asymmetric septal hypertrophy (ASH).
- Apical hypertrophic cardiomyopathy is a non-obstructive variant of HCM, first described in the Japanese population and recently found to be more common in the UK Bangladeshi population.

Genetic:

Familial HCM occurs as an autosomal dominant Mendelian-inherited disease in approximately 50% of cases. Some, if not all, of the sporadic forms of the disease may be caused by spontaneous mutations. There are defects in several of the genes encoding for the sarcomeric proteins, such as myosin heavy chain, actin, tropomyosin, and titin.

Familial HCM is a genetically heterogeneous disease in that it can be caused by genetic defects at more than one locus. At least six different genes on at least four chromosomes are associated with HCM, with more than 50 different mutations discovered thus far.

In the young, HCM is often associated with congenital syndromes, inherited metabolic disorders and neuromuscular disease. Unlike the adult form of the disease, various patterns of inheritance are seen; Noonan and Leopard syndrome (autosomal dominant) and Friedreich's ataxia (autosomal recessive).

Wide variation exists in the phenotypic expression of a given mutation of a given gene, with variability in clinical symptoms and the degree of hypertrophy expressed. Phenotypic variability is related to the differences in genotype, with specific mutations associated with particular symptoms, the degree of hypertrophy, and the prognosis.

Abnormal calcium kinetics:

The actual causes of HCM include defects in the genes encoding for several of the sarcomeric proteins. Additional data link abnormal myocardial calcium kinetics and abnormal calcium fluxes from an increase in the number of calcium channels resulting in an increase in intracellular calcium concentration, which, in turn, may produce hypertrophy and cellular disarray.

Other causes:

- Abnormal sympathetic stimulation: Heightened responsiveness of the heart to the excessive production of catecholamines or the reduced neuronal uptake of noradrenaline might cause HCM.
- Abnormally thickened intramural coronary arteries: These do not dilate normally, which leads to myocardial ischaemia. This progresses to myocardial fibrosis and abnormal compensatory hypertrophy.
- Subendocardial ischaemia: this is related to abnormalities of the cardiac microcirculation that deplete the energy stores essential for the sequestration of calcium during diastole. Subendocardial ischaemia results in persistent interaction of the contractile elements during diastole and increased diastolic stiffness.

- Cardiac structural abnormalities: these include a catenoidal, or saddle-shaped, configuration of the septum, the mechanics of which result in fibre disarray and local myocardial cell hypertrophy.

Pathophysiology

Since the initial descriptions of hypertrophic cardiomyopathy, the feature that has attracted the greatest attention is the dynamic pressure gradient across the LV outflow tract. The pressure gradient appears to be related to further narrowing of an already small outflow tract (due to marked asymmetric septal hypertrophy and possibly an abnormal location of the mitral valve) by the systolic anterior motion of the mitral valve against the hypertrophied septum. The likely cause of this is a Venturi effect resulting from increased ejection velocity produced by the abnormal LV outflow tract orientation and geometry.

In addition, most patients have an abnormal diastolic function, whether or not a pressure gradient is present, which impairs ventricular filling and increases filling pressures; despite a normal or small ventricular cavity. These patients have abnormal calcium kinetics and subendocardial ischaemia, which are related to the profound hypertrophy and myopathic process.

Multiple mutations have been identified, with genotype-specific risks of mortality and degree of hypertrophy. Interestingly, the genetic basis of ventricular hypertrophy does not directly correlate with prognostic risk stratification. Patients with some mutations, such as specific tropomyosin substitutions, have only a mild degree of ventricular hypertrophy, with little or no LV outflow tract obstruction, but they still carry a disproportionately high risk of sudden death.

Key features in the history/examination

- **Dyspnoea:** The most common presenting symptom, occurring in as many as 90% of symptomatic patients. Dyspnoea largely is a consequence of elevated LV diastolic filling pressures (and transmission of those elevated pressures back into the pulmonary circulation). The elevated LV filling pressures principally are caused by impaired diastolic compliance as a result of marked hypertrophy of the ventricle.

- **Angina:** Typical symptoms of angina are quite common in patients with HCM and may occur in the absence of detectable coronary atherosclerosis. Impaired diastolic relaxation and markedly increased myocardial oxygen consumption are caused by ventricular hypertrophy that results in subendocardial ischaemia, particularly during exertion.

- **Palpitations:** Palpitations are common. These result from arrhythmias, such as premature atrial and ventricular beats, sinus pauses, atrial fibrillation, atrial flutter, supraventricular tachycardia, and ventricular tachycardia.

- **Orthopnoea and paroxysmal nocturnal dyspnoea (PND):** These are early signs of congestive heart failure and result from pulmonary venous congestion. While relatively uncommon they are observed in patients with severe HCM and result from impaired diastolic function and elevated LV filling pressure.

- **Peripheral oedema:** This is a late sign of congestive heart failure and results from elevated pulmonary venous pressures eventually causing elevated pulmonary arterial and right heart pressures.

- **Dizziness:** Dizziness is common in patients with HCM with elevated pressure gradients across the LV outflow tract. It is worsened by exertion and may be exacerbated by hypovolemia following high levels of exertion or increased insensible fluid loss (e.g. during extreme heat). Dizziness may occur as a result of manoeuvres, such as rapid standing or Valsalva during defecation, or certain medications, such as diuretics, nitroglycerin, and vasodilating antihypertensive agents, that decrease preload and afterload and increase the pressure gradient across the LV outflow tract. Dizziness may also be secondary to arrhythmia-related hypotension and decreased cerebral perfusion.

- **Pre-syncope and syncope:** Pre-syncope is a very common symptom and may occur with nonsustained atrial or ventricular tachyarrhythmias and is exacerbated by vagal stimulation. Syncope results from inadequate cardiac output upon exertion or from cardiac arrhythmia (either tachycardias or bradycardias). It occurs more commonly in children and young adults with small LV chamber size and evidence of ventricular tachycardia upon ambulatory monitoring. Syncope and presyncope identify patients at high risk of sudden death and warrant an urgent workup and aggressive treatment.

- **Sudden cardiac death:** This is the most devastating presenting manifestation of HCM. It has the highest incidence in preadolescent and adolescent children and is particularly related to extreme exertion. The risk of sudden death in children is as high as 6% per year, though is approximately 1.5% overall in large, unselected, non-referred case series. In more than 80% of cases, the arrhythmia that causes sudden death is ventricular fibrillation. Rapid atrial arrhythmias, such as fibrillation, supraventricular tachycardia, or Wolff-Parkinson-White syndrome may degenerate into ventricular fibrillation. Other cases result from ventricular tachycardia and low cardiac output collapse.

- **Precordial palpation:** Double apical impulse results from a forceful left atrial contraction against a highly noncompliant LV. This occurs quite commonly in adults. Triple apical impulse results from a late systolic bulge that occurs when the heart is almost empty and is performing near-isometric contraction. This is a highly characteristic finding of HCM; however, it occurs less frequently than the double apical impulse.

- **Heart sounds:**
  - Second heart sound usually is normally split, though in the setting of severe outflow gradients, can be paradoxically split (P2 before A2, due to delayed aortic valve closure)
  - S3 gallop is common in children, but it does not have the same ominous significance as in patients with aortic valve stenosis. When it occurs in adults, it indicates decompensated congestive heart failure.
  - Fourth heart sound (S4) is frequently heard and results from atrial systole against a highly noncompliant LV.
  - Ejection systolic crescendo-decrescendo murmur is usually present and is best heard between the apex and left sternal border and radiates to the suprasternal notch but not to

the carotid arteries or neck. The murmur and the gradient across the LV outflow tract diminish with any increase in preload (e.g. Mueller manoeuvre, squatting) or increase in afterload (e.g. handgrip). The murmur and the gradient increase with any decrease in preload (e.g. Valsalva manoeuvre, nitrate administration, diuretic administration, standing) or with any decrease in afterload (e.g. vasodilator administration).

o Pansystolic murmur of mitral regurgitation is heard at the apex and axilla in patients with systolic anterior motion of the mitral valve and significant LV outflow gradients.

o Early diastolic murmur of aortic regurgitation (AR) is heard in 10% of patients, although mild AR can be detected by Doppler echocardiography in 33% of patients.

- **Systemic examination:**
  o Brisk, jerky, or bisferiens pulse (a collapse of the pulse followed by a secondary rise). The carotid pulse rises quickly because of the increased velocity of blood through the LV outflow tract and into the aorta. The carotid pulse then declines in mid systole as the gradient develops. This is followed by a secondary rise in carotid pulsation during late systole.

  o Jugular venous pulse reveals a prominent a wave caused by diminished right ventricular compliance secondary to gross hypertrophy of the ventricular septum.

  o Pulmonary +/– peripheral oedema is relatively uncommon though may be observed in patients with severe HCM

  o It may occur as a result of a combination of impaired diastolic function and subendocardial ischaemia.

  o Systolic function in these patients may be well preserved.

Investigations

Blood tests:

- Genetic testing: This is becoming increasingly available in this disease setting. This can be used to identify asymptomatic family members with the same mutation as the proband.

ECG:

- Common findings include LV hypertrophy and ST-T wave abnormalities. Other findings observed on ECG include axis deviation (right or left), conduction abnormalities (P-R prolongation, bundle-branch block), sinus bradycardia with ectopic atrial rhythm and atrial enlargement. One mutation has been identified that is associated with both HCM and Wolff-Parkinson-White syndrome.

- Uncommon findings include an abnormal and prominent Q wave in the anterior precordial and lateral limb leads, short P-R interval with QRS suggestive of preexcitation, atrial fibrillation (poor prognostic sign), and a P-wave abnormality, including left atrial enlargement.

Imaging:

- **CXR**: Cardiac size may range from normal to significantly increased. Left atrial enlargement frequently is observed, especially in the context of significant mitral regurgitation. This is may give rise to a 'double-density' appearance.

- **Echocardiography**: This is very helpful in the diagnosis of HCM. Summary of echocardiography findings:
  o abnormal systolic anterior leaflet motion of the mitral valve
  o LV hypertrophy
  o small ventricular chamber size
  o septal hypertrophy with septal-to-free wall ratio greater than 1.4:1
  o left atrial enlargement
  o mitral valve prolapse and mitral regurgitation
  o decreased mid aortic flow
  o partial systolic closure of the aortic valve in mid systole.

- **Myocardial perfusion imaging**: Perfusion imaging with thallium or technetium (radionuclide), or gadolinium (cardiac MRI) may show reversible defects, mostly in the absence of coronary artery disease. These perfusion defects are more common in children and adolescents with a history of sudden death or syncope, which suggests that myocardial ischaemia may be a significant factor in the mechanism of the death of younger patients with HCM.

- **Cardiac MRI**: Will identify similar features as echocardiography but it also has the additional benefits of perfusion imaging and tissue characterisation with gadolinium.

Cardiac catheterisation:

- This procedure is useful to determine the degree of outflow obstruction, cardiac haemodynamics, diastolic characteristics of the LV, LV anatomy and, importantly, the coronary anatomy:
  o There will be a pressure difference between the LV and the aorta with left ventricular pressure higher than the aortic pressure. This gradient signifies the degree of obstruction
  o This pressure gradient may be quite labile and can vary between 0 and 175 mm Hg in the same patient under different loading conditions.

Electrophysiology studies:

- A diagnostic electrophysiology study may identify conduction abnormalities, sinus node dysfunction and the potential for inducible arrhythmias. The prognostic correlation of inducible arrhythmias with spontaneous clinical arrhythmias and/or sudden death, however, is not entirely clear.

Histology:

- Fibrosis is prominent and may be extensive enough to produce grossly visible scars.

- Myocardial hypertrophy and gross disorganisation of the muscle bundles result in a characteristic whorled pattern.

- Almost all patients with HCM will demonstrate cell-to-cell disarray and disorganisation of the myofibrillar architecture.

- Patients with HCM commonly have abnormal intramural coronary arteries, with a reduction in the size of the lumen and thickening of the vessel wall. This abnormality most frequently occurs in the ventricular septum and accompanies extensive fibrosis in the affected walls of the heart.

Management

➢ Patients should be advised to avoid strenuous activity such as intense sporting activities. This is particularly important for athletes.

Risk stratification:

➢ In all patients with hypertrophic cardiomyopathy it is essential to risk stratify in order to identify which patients are at risk for sudden cardiac death

➢ Tests: history, ECG, exercise test, Holter monitor, echocardiogram

➢ Major risk factors:
  - Prior cardiac arrest
  - Spontaneous sustained ventricular tachycardia (VT)
  - Family history of premature sudden cardiac death
  - Unexplained syncope
  - LV thickness > 30 mm
  - Abnormal blood pressure response to exercise (a failure to either augment and/or sustain a systolic blood pressure of > 25 mm Hg above the resting systolic blood pressure during exercise)
  - Non-sustained spontaneous VT on Holter or exercise

➢ If there is evidence of sustained or symptomatic VT or VF: ICD with or without Amiodarone is offered.

➢ If there is no evidence of sustained VT or VF, patients can be risk stratified as follows:
  - 0 risk factors: Reassure adults and reassess children
  - 1 risk factor: Individualise decision making based on presence of other factors
  - 2 risk factors: ICD with or without Amiodarone.
  - It is particularly important to note that the only proven therapy to decrease the risk of sudden cardiac death is an ICD implantation with or without Amiodarone.

Symptomatic management:

➢ The second aim of treatment (medical or surgical) is directed towards alleviating symptoms of dyspnoea, chest pain and syncope by decreasing the left ventricular outflow tract gradient by reducing ventricular contractility, increasing ventricular volume, increasing ventricular compliance and outflow tract dimensions

➢ Medical therapy is successful in the majority of patients.

➢ The following algorithm can be utilised according to symptom severity:
  - If no symptoms are present: No treatment required
  - If mild symptoms are present: Beta-blockers, calcium channel antagonists
  - If moderate to severe symptoms are present in non-obstructive HCM:
    - Beta-blocker or Verapamil
    - Diuretics should be use with caution as they reduce intravascular volume, decreasing amount of blood available to distend left ventricular outflow tract, leading to an increase in outflow tract obstruction.
    - Severe symptoms in non-obstructive HCM may actually be more difficult to treat because there is no obvious target (obstruction) to treat
  - If moderate to severe symptoms are present in obstructive HCM:
    - Beta-blocker or Verapamil
    - Add Disopyramide to Beta-blocker if symptoms and gradient persist
    - Invasive therapies – Surgical septal myectomy, alcohol septal ablation, pacemaker

➢ Surgical septal myectomy:
  - This is an open heart operation performed to relieve symptoms in patients who remain severely symptomatic despite medical therapy.
  - It has been performed successfully for more than 25 years.
  - Surgical myectomy decreases left ventricular outflow tract obstruction and improves symptoms.

➢ Mitral valve replacement: this is performed in patients with severe mitral regurgitation due to systolic anterior movement of the mitral valve, predominantly when it is associated with the development CCF or pulmonary hypertension.

➢ Alcohol septal ablation:
  - This a percutaneous technique that involves injection of alcohol into one or more septal branches of the left anterior descending artery, inducing a controlled myocardial infarction in the portion of the interventricular septum that involves the left ventricular outflow tract. This subsequently contracts into a scar and thins in size
  - This is a technique with results similar to the surgical septal myectomy procedure but is less invasive
  - In patients with high outflow tract gradients, alcohol septal ablation can reduce the symptoms of HCM
  - It is the procedure of choice for patients in whom surgical intervention would carry a high risk

➢ Ventricular pacing
  - Current guidelines for Device-Based Therapy of Cardiac Rhythm Abnormalities recommend permanent pacing for sinus nodal disease or atrioventricular block in patients with HCM.
  - Pacing can be used to cause asynchronous contraction of the LV, which moves the septum away from the outflow region thereby decreasing the gradient across the left ventricular outflow tract.

➢ Note: A reduction in LV outflow tract gradient does not

necessarily mean a reduction in vulnerability to ventricular arrhythmias and sudden death

➢ Cardiac transplantation: In cases that are refractory to all other forms of treatment, cardiac transplantation is an option.

Multidisciplinary care:

➢ Heart muscle disease clinics

➢ Pacemaker/ICD clinics

➢ Genetic screening and counselling

Dilated cardiomyopathy

Dilated cardiomyopathy (DCM) can be defined as the presence of left ventricular dilatation and left ventricular systolic dysfunction in the absence of abnormal loading conditions (hypertension, valve disease) or coronary artery disease sufficient to cause global systolic impairment. Right ventricular dilatation and dysfunction may be present but are not necessary for the diagnosis.

Epidemiology

The prevalence is approximately 1 in 5000 in the UK. It can affect both children and adults, but is most common in middle aged men. Familial disease is present in over 25% of patients in Western populations with predominantly an autosomal dominant inheritance

Aetiology

Inherited:

Familial dilated cardiomyopathy (DCM) has incomplete and age-dependent penetrance and is linked to a diverse group of more than 20 loci and genes. Like HCM, it is genetically heterogeneous.

The predominant mode of inheritance for dilated cardiomyopathy is autosomal dominant. This particular subset of DCM are caused by mutations in cytoskeletal, Z-band, nuclear membrane and intercalated disc protein genes, in addition to mutations in the contractile sarcomeric proteins, as seen in HCM. Research to determine further disease loci is ongoing.

Other inheritance patterns are less frequent:

• X-linked DCM

• X-linked diseases associated with DCM, e.g. Becker and Duchenne muscular dystrophies

• Autosomal recessive

• Inherited metabolic disorders associated with DCM, e.g. haemochromatosis

• Mitochondrial cytopathies

Non-inherited:

In this group there is a broad range of primary and secondary causes of DCM:

• Chronic excessive alcohol consumption

• Infections:

   o Viral endocarditis/myocarditis (coxsackie virus, adenovirus, parvovirus, human immunodeficiency virus [HIV])

   o Parasites

   o Protozoa

   o Chagas disease (most common cause in parts of South America)

• Drugs:

   o Anthracyclines (daunorubicin and doxorubicin)

   o Cocaine

   o Methamphetamine

   o Heavy metals

   o Cobalt

• High-output states:

   o Anaemia

   o Thyrotoxicosis

   o Tachycardias

• Collagen vascular disease

• Glycogen storage disease, type IV (Andersen disease)

• Thiamine deficiency and zinc deficiency

• Hypophosphataemia

• Amyloidosis

• Phaeochromocytoma

• Kawasaki disease

• Eosinophilic (Churg-Strauss syndrome)

• Pregnancy (see end of DCM section)

Pathophysiology

DCM may result from any conditions that promote cardiomyocyte injury or loss. It is characterized by ventricular chamber enlargement and systolic dysfunction with normal LV wall thickness. Ventricular enlargement and dysfunction generally leads to progressive heart failure with further decline in LV contractile function.

Sequelae include ventricular and supraventricular arrhythmias, conduction system abnormalities, thromboembolism, and sudden or heart failure-related death. Compensatory mechanisms associated with low cardiac output induce reflex upregulation of sympathetic tone and the renin-angiotensin axis, causing increased release of vasopressin, aldosterone, and atrial natriuretic peptide. Stimulation of these hormonal tracts results in volume expansion, which induces vasoconstriction. Vasoconstriction increases afterload that, in turn, decreases stroke volume. As cardiac output depends on stroke volume and heart rate, vasoconstriction ultimately can contribute to decreased cardiac output.

Key features in the history/examination

• It is important to determine the severity of disease, possible causes, and symptomatology. Symptoms are a good indicator of the severity of the disease.

• Past medical history:

   o Hypertension

   o Angina

   o Coronary artery disease

- o Anaemia
- o Thyroid dysfunction
- o Breast cancer
- o Prior history of heart failure or myocardial injury
- **Drugs:**
  - o Anthracyclines
  - o Cocaine
  - o Methamphetamine
  - o Heavy metals
  - o Cobalt
- **Social history:**
  - o Alcohol
  - o Tobacco
  - o Illicit drug use (cocaine)
- **Family history:** Cardiomyopathy or sudden cardiac death
- **Fatigue and dyspnoea:** The most common presenting symptoms. Dyspnoea initially will be on exertion
- **Palpitations:** Palpitations are common. These result from arrhythmias, such as premature atrial and ventricular beats, sinus pauses, atrial fibrillation, atrial flutter, supraventricular tachycardia, and ventricular tachycardia.
- **Orthopnoea and PND:** These are early signs of congestive heart failure and result from pulmonary venous congestion.
- **Peripheral oedema and increased abdominal girth:** This is a later sign of congestive heart failure and results from elevated pulmonary venous pressures eventually causing elevated pulmonary arterial and right heart pressures.
- **Dizziness:** This may be secondary to arrhythmia-related hypotension and decreased cerebral perfusion. Nonsustained arrhythmias often cause symptoms of dizziness, light headedness and presyncope, whereas sustained arrhythmias are more likely to lead to syncope, collapse, and/or sudden cardiac death.
- **Pre-syncope and syncope:** Pre-syncope is a very common symptom and may occur with nonsustained atrial or ventricular tachyarrhythmias and is exacerbated by vagal stimulation. Syncope and presyncope identify patients at high risk of sudden death and warrant an urgent workup and aggressive treatment.
- **Sudden cardiac death:** This may be a presenting manifestation of DCM, especially in the young. As with HCM, the most common arrhythmia that causes sudden death is ventricular fibrillation. Others cases result from ventricular tachycardia and low cardiac output collapse.
- **Precordial palpation:**
  - o Laterally and/or inferiorly displaced apical impulse due to ventricular dilatation
  - o Para-sternal (right ventricular) heave
- Heart sounds:
  - o Irregularly irregular rhythm due to atrial fibrillation
  - o S3 gallop is common, indicating decompensated congestive heart failure.

- o Pansystolic murmur of mitral regurgitation is heard at the apex and axilla in patients with significant left ventricular dilatation and secondary mitral annular dilatation
- Systemic examination:
  - o Elevated jugular venous pressure with a prominent a-wave and large cv waves, due to increased right heart pressures and significant tricuspid regurgitation respectively
  - o Goitre – thyrotoxicosis
  - o Pulmonary oedema or pleural effusion
  - o Hepatomegaly due to venous congestion or infiltrative disease
  - o Ascites due to portal hypertension
  - o Peripheral oedema
  - o Cyanosis
  - o Clubbing
  - o Muscle weakness with inherited dystrophies

Investigations

Blood tests:

- FBC: to investigate any cause of anaemia and treat iron deficiency anaemia. ACE inhibitors can cause leucopaenia in combination with allopurinol (gout prophylaxis).
- LFTs: results can be elevated, which may suggest alcoholic disease, haemochromatosis, hepatic congestion (nutmeg liver), and/or hepatic infarction due to hypoperfusion in inotrope-dependent patients.
- TFTs
- U&Es: an elevated creatinine level may represent a primary or drug-related aetiology (e.g. hypovolaemia, uraemia from ACE inhibitors). Hyponatraemia at the time of presentation has been found to be a marker of increased stimulation of the renin-angiotensin axis and of worsening of the disease course and prognosis.
- Cardiac biomarkers: the precise role of cardiac biomarkers is still being defined, however, there is evidence that patients who present with elevated markers experience more severe failure and higher mortality.
  - o Cardiac enzymes are useful for assessing acute or recent myocardial injury. Levels are markedly elevated in persons with muscular dystrophy.
  - o The measurement of plasma brain natriuretic peptide (BNP) is sensitive and specific in diagnosing heart failure. Changes in BNP level can reflect response to treatment.
  - o Magnesium levels should be closely followed because low levels may cause chronic hypokalaemia and predispose to arrhythmias such as atrial fibrillation.

ECG:

- This is helpful in identifying LV enlargement and estimating the other chamber sizes.
- Nonspecific ST-T wave changes and Q waves are characteristic.

- Atrial fibrillation or premature ventricular complexes are common
- An electrocardiogram showing AF increases the likelihood of heart failure. The absence of any electrocardiographic abnormality makes the diagnosis of heart failure unlikely
- LV hypertrophy or other chamber enlargement is often seen.
- Conduction delay, particularly LBBB, can be observed.

Imaging:

- **CXR**
  - Cardiomegaly may be observed. The absence of cardiomegaly on chest radiograph decreases the likelihood of heart failure
  - Depending on the severity of disease and the degree of medical control, signs of pulmonary oedema, upper lobe pulmonary venous congestion, Kerley B lines or frank interstitial infiltrates may be observed.
  - The presence of pulmonary vascular congestion and interstitial oedema on chest radiograph increases the likelihood of acute decompensated heart failure about 12-fold.

- **Echocardiography**
  - This may be indicated urgently when the cause of cardiac decompensation in the presence of findings suggestive of failure (e.g. raised JVP) is unclear. In this setting, the differential diagnosis may include pulmonary embolism or cardiac tamponade, and the echocardiogram can demonstrate right ventricular dilatation associated with pulmonary embolism or pericardial effusion with tamponade.

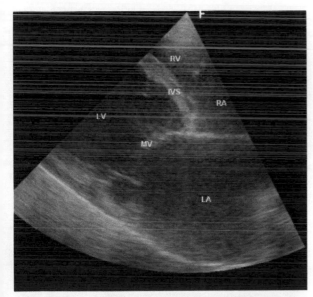

Figure 3.55: Echocardiogram of DCM (parasternal long-axis view) demonstrating a dilated left ventricle (LV) and left atrium (LA).

- Echocardiography is used to help differentiate dilated cardiomyopathy from restrictive and hypertrophic cardiomyopathy.
- Dilated chambers and thin walls are the most prominent features of dilated cardiomyopathy.
- Co-existent valvular dysfunction is easily identified
- **Cardiac MRI**
  - Compared to echocardiography, cardiac MRI is a more accurate test for identifying left ventricular thrombus, is the gold standard for assessing biventricular systolic function and allows tissue characterisation, including identification of scar/fibrosis
  - Approximately 30% of patients with DCM have midwall fibrosis as detected by late gadolinium-enhancement cardiovascular magnetic resonance (CMR).

Others:

- Urine pregnancy test
- Urine toxicology screen
- Histology: endomyocardial biopsy may be helpful in diagnosing myocarditis, connective tissue disorders, and amyloidosis.

Management

Risk stratification:

- Risk stratification of patients with dilated cardiomyopathy (DCM) in the era of device implantation is not well described. In DCM, mid-wall fibrosis determined by CMR is a predictor of the combined end point of all-cause mortality and cardiovascular hospitalisation. In addition, mid-wall fibrosis by CMR predicts sudden cardiac death/VT. CMR may therefore help in the risk stratification of patients with DCM, which may have value in determining the need for ICD therapy as primary prophylaxis for ventricular tachyarrhythmias (VT/VF).
- The presence of severe left ventricular systolic dysfunction (LVEF) < 30% may be sufficient to warrant ICD therapy as primary prophylaxis for ventricular tachyarrhythmias (VT/VF).

Medical management:

- Goals of treatment include symptom relief, improved cardiac output, shortened hospital stay, fewer hospital admissions, reversal of injury process, and decreased mortality
- ACE-inhibitors e.g. Ramipril
- Angiotensin II receptor antagonists, e.g. Candesartan
- Digoxin: A positive inotropic effect and ventricular rate control in AF.
- Loop diuretics: Furosemide or Bumetanide
- Thiazide diuretic: Bendroflumethiazide or Metolazone work in synergy with loop diuretics
- Cardioselective beta-blockers, e.g. Bisoprolol or Carvedilol

➢ Vasodilators: Hydralazine, IV GTN, ISDN and Hydralazine.

➢ Aldosterone antagonists: Spironolactone/Eplerenone

➢ Nesiritide: Recombinant DNA form of human BNP that dilates veins and arteries. Used temporarily in the management of decompensated heart failure.

➢ Anticoagulants (warfarin): Restrict to patients in atrial fibrillation, with artificial valves, and with known mural thrombus, as no benefit seen in other patient groups.

Cardiac resynchronisation therapy (biventricular pacing):

➢ Improves overall efficiency of cardiac function, if there is evidence of electrical dyssynchrony on ECG (broad LBBB with QRS duration >120 ms) and/or mechanical dyssynchrony on echocardiography (**inter-** and **intra-**ventricular dyssynchrony).

➢ Results in acute cardiac haemodynamic improvements, symptomatic benefits and more recent evidence demonstrates reduced mortality and hospitalisation rates compared to those achieved with optimal medical therapy.

➢ Lead positioning – right atrial lead, right ventricular lead, coronary sinus lead to pace the LV

➢ Resynchronization pacing generators have defibrillation capabilities (biventricular ICD)

➢ Current indications for cardiac resynchronization therapy are as follows:

o The presence of severe left ventricular systolic impairment.

o NYHA Class III or IV symptoms despite optimal medical therapy with ACE inhibitors, beta-blockers, and/or other appropriate pharmacologic measures.

o Evidence of significant inter or intra-ventricular conduction delay.

Surgical management:

➢ Various surgical options are available for patients with disease refractory to medical therapy. The following new surgical therapies are evolving for patients with end-stage heart disease.

➢ Left ventricular assist devices

o Portable electric left ventricular assist devices have been proven as the standard of care when a bridge to transplantation is needed.

o Left ventricular assist devices are being evaluated as permanent implantations in patients who are not candidates for heart transplantation (i.e. 'destination therapy'). Current limitations include high infection rates and mechanical malfunction.

➢ Partial left ventriculectomy (Batista procedure) for DCM: Reducing the LV diameter (Laplace law) in patients with dilated cardiomyopathy is thought to improve ventricular function.

➢ Heart transplantation: If all other management options fail to control symptoms

Prognosis:

o The severity of disease on initial diagnosis has been shown to be inversely proportional to the long-term survival.

o In general for DCM, the 60-day mortality rate following hospital admission due to an exacerbation of congestive heart failure (CHF) is 8–20% depending on the population studied.

Restrictive cardiomyopathy

Restrictive cardiomyopathy is defined as a myocardial disease characterised by restrictive filling and reduced diastolic volume of either or both ventricles with normal or near-normal systolic function and wall thickness. Increased interstitial fibrosis may be present.

Epidemiology

Least common type of cardiomyopathy accounting for approximately 5% of all cases of primary heart muscle disease.

Aetiology

• Idiopathic

• Familial:

o Often autosomal dominant inheritance. May be related to mutations in troponin I gene, desmin gene (associated with cardiac conduction defects and skeletal myopathy)

o Rarely autosomal recessive inheritance; haemochromatosis associated with HFE gene mutation or glycogen storage disease.

o X-linked inheritance; Anderson-Fabry disease.

• Infiltrative:

o Amyloidosis is the most common cause

o Glycogen storage disease

o Sarcoidosis

o Systemic sclerosis

• Endocardial pathology:

o Endomyocardial disease with hypereosinophilia (Loeffler endomyocarditis)

o Endomyocardial disease without hypereosinophilia (endomyocardial fibrosis (EMF)). This is most common in equatorial Africa. It may be related to drugs (e.g. Methysergide).

• Malignancy:

o Carcinoid heart disease

o Metastatic endocardial and myocardial infiltration

• Anthracycline toxicity

• Post-cardiac transplantation or mediastinal irradiation

Pathophysiology

RCM results in increased myocardium stiffness which causes ventricular pressure to rise precipitously with only small increases in volume. The increased LV diastolic stiffness (reduced compliance) leads to diastolic heart failure. The LV cannot fill adequately at normal diastolic pressures, leading to a reduction in cardiac output due to reduced left ventricular filling volume.

In the early stage of disease systolic function usually remains normal. Ventricular wall thickness is typically increased secondary to myocardial infiltration with amyloidosis, though not as pronounced as that observed in HCM. As the disease progresses, systolic function may begin to deteriorate. Reduced left ventricular filling volume leads to reduced stroke volume and low cardiac output symptoms (e.g. fatigue, lethargy), whereas increased filling pressures cause pulmonary and systemic congestion. Thus, restrictive cardiomyopathy (RCM) causes symptoms and signs of left- and/or right-sided failure as it affects both ventricles, but amyloidosis typically presents with predominant right-heart failure. Fibrosis encasing the sinoatrial or the atrioventricular nodes may result in complete heart block. Of note however, amyloid deposition in the bundle branches is rare.

RCM can be further sub-classified as obliterative (i.e. thrombus-filled ventricles) or non-obliterative/idiopathic.

Obliterative RCM is very rare. It may result from the end stage of the eosinophilic syndromes (Loeffler endomyocarditis), in which an intracavitary thrombus fills the left ventricular apex and hampers the filling of the ventricles. The fibrosis of the endocardium may extend to involve the atrioventricular valves and cause regurgitation. Chronic endomyocardial fibrosis (EMF) has a similar pathology though without eosinophila.

In idiopathic, or primary, RCM, progressive fibrosis of the myocardium but no thrombus formation occurs. This subtype lacks specific histopathological changes

Key features in the history/examination

- **Past medical history:**
  - o Radiation therapy
  - o Cardiac transplantation
  - o Chemotherapy
  - o Systemic disease
  - o See aetiology
- **Drugs:** Methysergide
- **Family history:** Cardiomyopathy or sudden cardiac death
- Fatigue and dyspnoea: The most common presenting symptoms, resulting from decreased stroke volume and cardiac output.
- **Palpitations:** These are common and are frequently due to atrial fibrillation, especially in idiopathic RCM due to gross atrial dilatation.
- **Angina:** Chest pain mimicking myocardial ischaemia can be observed, primarily in patients with amyloidosis, possibly due to myocardial compression of small vessels.
- **Orthopnoea and PND:** Results from pulmonary venous congestion causing pleural effusions (common in amyloidosis).

Orthopnoea may also result from ascites causing diaphragmatic splinting.

- **Peripheral oedema and increased abdominal girth:** Usually profound bilateral peripheral oedema due to right heart involvement.
- **Thromboembolism:** up to one third of patients may present with thromboembolic complications. Pulmonary emboli secondary to deep vein thrombosis and/or systemic emboli due to left atrial thrombus as a consequence of AF.
- **Pre-syncope and syncope:** Syncope can be due to a variety of causes.
  - o Conduction disturbances are particularly common in some forms of infiltrative RCM (not amyloidosis).
  - o Orthostatic hypotension secondary to a peripheral and/or autonomic neuropathy.
- **Sudden cardiac death:** Syncope and sudden death are common in amyloid light chain (AL) amyloidosis, but ventricular arrhythmias are uncommon. Electrical-mechanical dissociation is more common.
- **Precordial palpation:** Para-sternal (right ventricular) heave
- **Heart sounds:**
  - o Irregularly irregular rhythm due to atrial fibrillation
  - o S3 gallop is uncommon
  - o Pansystolic murmurs of mitral and tricuspid regurgitation, though usually not haemodynamically significant
- **Systemic examination:**
  - o Weight loss/cardiac cachexia
  - o Easy bruising, periorbital purpura, macroglossia (amyloidosis)
  - o Decreased pulse volume due to low cardiac output
  - o Elevated jugular venous pressure, with rapid x and y descents. Most prominent is the rapid y descent due to rapid atrial emptying
  - o Jugular venous pressure fails to fall on inspiration and may actually rise (Kussmaul sign)
  - o Pleural effusions: frequently bilateral and large in amyloidosis. Frank pulmonary oedema is rare
  - o Hepatomegaly (may be tender) due to venous congestion or amyloid infiltration
  - o Ascites due to portal hypertension
  - o Gross peripheral oedema

Investigations

Blood tests:

- FBC: With peripheral smear to identify eosinophilia.
- Renal function
- LFTs
- Haematinics: Serum iron concentrations, percent saturation of total iron-binding capacity, and serum ferritin levels to screen for haemochromatosis.

- Serum brain natriuretic peptide (BNP) level: recent data suggest that serum BNP levels are nearly normal in patients with constrictive physiology of heart failure and grossly elevated in patients with restrictive physiology, despite nearly identical clinical and haemodynamic presentations.

ECG:

- The findings on ECG depend on the stage of the disease and the specific diagnosis.
- May be normal or just show some non-specific ST-T wave changes
- Rhythm disorders (particularly AF) are common.
- Conduction abnormalities are uncommon in amyloidosis.
- Myocardial infiltration and/or small vessel induced ischaemia or infarction may give rise to a pseudo-infarct pattern
- Low QRS voltage is common in amyloidosis

Imaging:

- **CXR**: Cardiomegaly is often seen though is mainly due to gross atrial dilatation. Bilateral pleural effusions may also be identified.
- **Echocardiography**:
  - Ventricular size may be normal or reduced with normal wall thickness
  - However, diffuse ventricular hypertrophy is common with amyloidosis and other infiltrative diseases
  - Both atria will be markedly dilated.
  - Mural thrombus and cavity obliteration are seen in obliterative RCM
  - Abnormal myocardial texture seen as 'speckling' is characteristic of amyloidosis
  - Transmitral flow patterns and tissue Doppler imaging identify diastolic dysfunction
- **Cardiac MRI**: Detailed assessment of pericardial thickness and abnormal myocardial interstitium. There is a characteristic rapid emptying of the blood-pool gadolinium in RCM due to amyloidosis.
- **CT**: Similar to MRI in its ability to assess pericardial thickness. CT is better able to detect pericardial calcification as occurs in constrictive pericarditis

Cardiac catheterisation:

- Accentuated filling occurs in early diastole, which terminates abruptly at the end of the rapid filling phase. When pressure tracings are taken at this point, they show a characteristic diastolic dip and a plateau or a square-root sign.
- This dip and plateau or square-root sign of ventricular pressure is manifested in the atrial pressure tracing as a prominent descent followed by a rapid rise to a plateau.

Others:

- Cardiac biopsy:

  - Ventricular biopsy obtained from either the right or the LV has proved useful in certain cases in establishing whether endocardial or myocardial disease is present. This is especially useful when non-invasive studies have failed to establish a clear diagnosis.
  - Amyloidosis typically demonstrates apple-green birefringence when stained with Congo red and viewed under a polarizing microscope.
  - However, fine-needle aspiration of abdominal fat is easier and safer than myocardial biopsy to determine amyloidosis.
  - Liver biopsy is performed for the diagnosis of haemochromatosis.
  - Confirmation of the diagnosis of AL amyloidosis demands a search for a plasma cell dyscrasia (e.g. multiple myeloma)

Management

- ➤ Treatment goal is to reduce symptoms by lowering elevated filling pressures without significantly reducing cardiac output
- ➤ Unfortunately, current agents are not very effective in treating disorders of myocardial relaxation, therefore treatment is limited to:
  - Low dose thiazide or loop diuretics to reduce cardiac preload
  - Long-acting nitrates to reduce preload– e.g. isosorbide mononitrate or GTN patch
  - Digoxin – use with caution in amyloidosis as potentially arrhythmogenic
  - Anticoagulation for patients with a history of thromboembolism or atrial fibrillation.
  - Amiodarone – maintenance of sinus rhythm is important to preserve the atrial contribution to ventricular filling.

Targeted therapies:

- ➤ AL amyloidosis (primary systemic amyloidosis): Melphalan (anti-plasma cell therapy) may slow the progress of AL amyloidosis by stopping production of the paraprotein responsible for the amyloid formation.
- ➤ Loeffler endocarditis: in the early phase of the disease, corticosteroids, cytotoxic agents (e.g. hydroxyurea) and interferon to suppress the intense eosinophilic infiltration of the myocardium alongside conventional heart failure medication, improves symptoms and survival.
- ➤ Haemochromatosis: Chelation therapy or venesection is effective to decrease the iron overload.

Prognosis:

- ➤ The disease course varies depending on the pathology and treatment but is often unsatisfactory.
- ➤ The prognosis of patients with primary systemic amyloidosis remains poor, with a median survival of approximately 2 years

despite intervention with alkylating-based chemotherapy in selected cases.

➤ The importance of an accurate diagnosis of RCM is to distinguish it from constrictive pericarditis, which also presents with restrictive physiology but is frequently curable by surgical intervention (pericardiectomy).

Further reading and references

➤ Assomull RG, Prasad SK, Lyne J, et al. (2006). Cardiovascular Magnetic Resonance, Fibrosis, and Prognosis in Dilated Cardiomyopathy. *J Am Coll Cardiol.* 48: 1977–1985.

➤ Baker DW, Wright RF. (1994) Management of heart failure. IV. Anticoagulation for patients with heart failure due to left ventricular systolic dysfunction. *JAMA.* 23–30; 272(20): 1614–8.

➤ Epstein AE, Dimarco JP, Ellenbogen KA, et al. (2008) ACC/AHA/HRS 2008 guidelines for Device-Based Therapy of Cardiac Rhythm Abnormalities: executive summary. *Heart Rhythm*; 5(6): 934–55

➤ Elliott P, Andersson B, Arbustini E, et al. (2008) Classification of the cardiomyopathies: a position statement from the European society of cardiology working group on myocardial and pericardial diseases. *European Heart Journal.* 29(2): 270–276

➤ Gage, B. F., Waterman, A. D., Shannon, W., et al. (2001). Validation of clinical classification schemes for predicting stroke: Results from the national registry of atrial fibrillation. *JAMA,* 285(22), 2864–2870.

➤ National Institute for Health and Clinical Excellence (2006). *Atrial Fibrillation (CG036)*

➤ www.sads.org.uk/drugs_to_avoid.htm - Sudden arrhythmic syndrome website detailing drugs to avoid

➤ Maron BJ, Towbin JA, Thiene G, et al. (2006). American Heart Association; Council on Clinical Cardiology, Heart Failure and Transplantation Committee; Quality of Care and Outcomes Research and Functional Genomics and Translational Biology Interdisciplinary Working Groups; Council on Epidemiology and Prevention. Contemporary definitions and classification of the cardiomyopathies: an American Heart Association Scientific Statement from the Council on Clinical Cardiology, Heart Failure and Transplantation Committee; Quality of Care and Outcomes Research and Functional Genomics and Translational Biology Interdisciplinary Working Groups; and Council on Epidemiology and Prevention. *Circulation* 113: 1807–1816

➤ The Atrial Fibrillation Follow-up Investigation of Rhythm Management (AFFIRM) Investigators (2002). A Comparison of Rate Control and Rhythm Control in Patients with Atrial Fibrillation. *NEJM* 347: 1825–33.

➤ UK Resuscitation Council (2008). *Advanced Life Support (5th ed).*

➤ You JJ, Woo A, Ko DT, et al. (2007) Life expectancy gains and cost-effectiveness of implantable cardioverter/defibrillators for the primary prevention of sudden cardiac death in patients with hypertrophic cardiomyopathy. *Am Heart J.* 154(5): 899–907.

POISONING

Common poisons

Type of drug use	Poisons
Medicinal	**Paracetamol**
	Salicylates
	Opiates
	Benzodiazepines
	Tricyclic antidepressants (TCA)
Recreational	Cannabis
	Heroin
	Cocaine
	Ecstasy
	Gamma-hydroxybutyrate (GHB)
	Ampetamines
	Lysergic acid diethylamide (LSD)
	Ketamine

Poisoning in general

Epidemiology

Poisoning accounts for 10% of UK hospital admissions, about one third of which are due to Paracetamol. Although poisoning is a major cause of death in the under-50 year olds, less than 1% of those admitted to hospital die. Major causes of death are recreational drugs, antidepressants, Paracetamol and carbon monoxide.

Aetiology

Poisoning may be accidental, which is often the case in young children, or deliberate. Deliberate poisoning can either be as part of a completed suicide or an act of deliberate self-harm (DSH). On occasions poisoning can also be an act of terrorism or due to occupational, recreational, environmental and iatrogenic reasons.

Deliberate poisoning often involves more than one drug with alcohol being the commonest second agent. Poisoned patients will often admit to what they have taken, but the admitting doctor should keep an open mind, especially in patients with a reduced Glasgow coma score (GCS), and consider poisoning in the differential diagnosis.

Pathophysiology

The pathophysiology is dependent on the poison ingested.

Key features in the history/examination

• Causative agent: the signs and symptoms will depend on the nature of substance(s), amount and time taken. Look for

3. Medicine

any supporting evidence of the causative agent, e.g. packets of pills brought in by the patient, family and friends or the ambulance service.

- Past medical, drug and psychiatric history: in particular depression, previous episodes of DSH and medications which could produce toxicity.
- Indicators of suicidal intent
- Environment: the nature of the work/activity the patient was involved in, chemicals that were used in the processes, any Hazchem information.

Investigations

Blood tests:

- FBC
- U&Es
- LFTs
- Calcium
- Glucose
- Clotting
- Specific drug levels: Paracetamol and Salicylate should always be taken in the unconscious patient and in any patients in which there is any doubt about the medication that may have been taken. Digoxin and iron are also readily available if indicated. Other tests can be requested but take some time to obtain the results, e.g. Carbamazepine.
- Arterial blood gas (ABG): acidosis is very common in acute poisoning.

Imaging:

- CXR: especially if concurrent aspiration is suspected.

Others:

- Toxicology screen: may be required, but is not universally available.
- Dipstix tests: can be used to test for recreational drug use. These are expensive and not widely available in clinical areas.
- ECG: findings vary depending on the toxin

Management

This is dependent on the cause, however there is a general management to follow for all poisons.

Structured assessment:

- Use the A to E approach. (See Resuscitation chapter).
- Focus especially on the effects of the causative agent. For example looking for signs of hypotension, assessing the GCS and checking the ECG for QT prolongation in TCA overdose.

Supportive therapy:

- Correct hypotension with fluid replacement and vasopressors if required
- Control seizures and correct electrolyte imbalances
- Warm the patient if necessary
- Treat and manage hypoxia
- Protect the airway, potentially intubating the patient until the patient is capable of protecting their own airway.

Specific measures:

- Reducing absorption: activated charcoal can be used for a wide range of toxic agents, but is only beneficial if used within the first hour post ingestion. Gastric lavage, emesis and cathartics have no evidence to support an improvement in outcomes and may cause morbidity.
- Increasing elimination: urine alkalinisation can be beneficial in the treatment of salicylate poisoning.
- Antidotes: See Table 3.67 for more detail.

Poison	Antidote
Benzodiazepines	Flumanezil*
Beta-blockers	Glucagon
Calcium channel blockers	Calcium chloride
Cyanide	Hydroxocobalamin, dicolbalt edentate, sodium nitirite, sodium thiosulphate
Digoxin	Digibind
Heparin	Protamine sulphate
Iron	Desferrioxamine
Methanol, ethylene glycol	Ethanol
Nerve agents	Atropine, pralidoxime
Opioids	Naloxone
Paracetamol	N-acetylcysteine (NAC), methionine
Warfarin	Vitamin K

Table 3.67: Antidotes for common poisons. (*) antidote used only for the reversal of iatrogenic over-sedation.

Psychiatric assessment:

- Psychiatric assessment is necessary prior to discharge. Although not always intended as a suicide attempt, an act of DSH increases the likelihood not only of further episodes, but also of future completed suicide.
- Certain characteristics of the act may point to suicidal intent.
  - Evidence of premeditation
  - Suicide note
  - Precautions to avoid discovery

- o Act timed to avoid discovery
- o Not seeking help during or afterwards
- o Admission of suicidal intent
- o Older age
- o Male

➤ The patient should be sympathetically nursed in a bed which is easily observed and referred to psychiatric services as per local protocols.

The Foundation Year (FY) doctor will not be expected to know the specific effects, treatments and monitoring requirements of all possible poisonings. They will be expected to know the treatments of some common poisons and to know where to find the information required for all the others.

The British Association of Emergency Medicine produced a list of antidotes that should be stored in all Emergency Departments (ED) in 2006. In the EDs or Emergency Assessment Unit (EAU) you will have access to the following resources:

➤ Toxbase

➤ National Poisons Information Service

➤ British National Formulary (BNF)

Paracetamol

Epidemiology

Paracetamol poisoning is the commonest method of self-poisoning accounting for 50% of all cases.

Aetiology

Both deliberate self-harm (including attempted suicide) and accidental overdose are seen.

Pathophysiology

Paracetamol is conjugated in the liver to Paracetamol glucuronide and sulphate. 5–10% is oxidised by the cytochrome P450 enzymes into N-acetyl-p-benzoquinoncimine (NAPQI), which is highly toxic. This is normally detoxified by conjugation with glutathione. However, in overdose, the conjugation pathways are saturated resulting in large quantities of NAPQI and this depletes the glutathione stores leading to hepatocyte damage.

Key features in the history/examination

- The amount of Paracetamol ingested.
- The time since ingestion.
- Any other drugs taken with Paracetamol, especially alcohol.
- Risk factors for additional toxicity, e.g. liver disease, high alcohol consumption, eating disorders
- Patients with Paracetamol overdose are usually asymptomatic
- May report nausea, vomiting and anorexia

- In large overdoses there may be reduced level of consciousness and metabolic acidosis.
- In late presentation there may be signs of liver failure.

Investigations

Blood tests:

- Paracetamol and salicylate levels: taken at least four hours post ingestion
- LFTs
- Coagulation screen
- ABG: checking for metabolic acidosis

Management

Plasma Paracetamol levels should govern treatment. These should be taken at least four hours post ingestion and using the normogram available in the BNF administer the treatment. (See Figure 3.56).

➤ In the event of a large overdose, i.e. at least 12 g of Paracetamol in total or 150 mg/Kg, the treatment should begin immediately without waiting for blood levels.

➤ If there is doubt about the time that the overdose was taken then take bloods and commence NAC infusion.

➤ Dose of NAC administered should be:

- o 150 mg/kg over 15 minutes
- o 50 mg/kg over 4 hours
- o 100 mg/kg over 16 hours

➤ Treatment with NAC has been associated with mild elevation of the international normalised ratio (INR). Patients who have a marginally elevated INR, i.e. 1.3 or less, but normal transaminase levels (ALT or AST) after all three doses do not require further monitoring or treatment with NAC. If both the INR and transaminases are still elevated then repeat another bag of 100 mg/Kg over 16 hours.

➤ Approximately 5% of patients show symptoms of allergy to NAC with rash and wheeze. In this case the infusion should be stopped, chlorpheniramine given, and the infusion resumed at a slower rate.

➤ Kings College criteria for Paracetamol poisoning: these were developed to assist the early identification of poor prognosis associated with liver failure. If the patient fulfils these criteria, they should be referred to the local tertiary liver transplant unit as soon as possible. (See Table 3.68).

Arterial pH	< 7.3
Prothrombin time	> 100 seconds
Creatinine	> 300
Encephalopathy	Grade 3 or 4

Table 3.68: King's College criteria for Paracetamol poisoning.

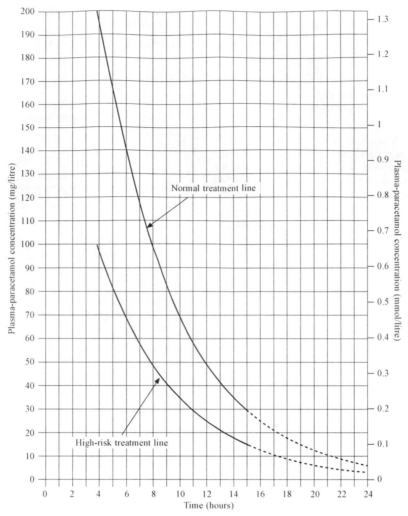

Patients whose plasma-paracetamol concentrations are above the **normal treatment line** should be treated with acetylcysteine by intravenous infusion (or, if acetylcysteine cannot be used, with methionine by mouth, provided the overdose has been taken **within 10–12 hours** and the patient is not vomiting).
Patients on enzyme-inducing drugs (e.g. carbamazepine, phenobarbital, phenytoin, primidone, rifampicin, alcohol, and St John's wort) or who are malnourished (e.g. in anorexia, in alcoholism, or those who are HIV-positive) should be treated if their plasma-paracetamol concentration is above the **high-risk treatment line**.
The prognostic accuracy after 15 hours is uncertain but a plasma-paracetamol concentration above the relevant treatment line should be regarded as carrying a serious risk of liver damage.
Graph reproduced courtesy of University of Wales College of Medicine Therapeutics and Toxicology Centre

Figure 3.56: BNF treatment normogram for Paracetamol overdose. *Courtesy of Professor P.A. Routledge, Cardiff University Therapeutics and Toxicology Centre*

Treatment by time:

0–4 hours:

➢ Consider activated charcoal if more than 12 g of Paracetamol has been ingested within the last hour.

➢ At four hours from ingestion, measure the plasma Paracetamol

concentration. It is not possible to interpret plasma concentrations measured at less than four hours

➢ NAC treatment may be considered immediately if more than 150 mg/Kg (or 12 g in an adult) – 75 mg/Kg if the patient has risk factors – of Paracetamol has been ingested whilst awaiting the four hour sample results.

4–8 hours:

➤ Measure plasma Paracetamol concentration.

➤ NAC treatment may be considered if more than 150 mg/Kg (or 12 g in an adult or 75 mg/Kg and the patient has risk factors) of Paracetamol has been ingested whilst awaiting the four-hour sample results.

➤ Assess treatment needs using the standard nomogram.

➤ Treatment must be started within eight hours for maximal benefit. If this is the case, the risk of liver or renal damage is insignificant.

➤ After NAC administration and the INR, creatinine, plasma bicarbonate and alanine aminotransferase (ALT) or aspartate aminotransferase (AST) levels are normal the patient can be discharged with advice to return to hospital if vomiting or abdominal pain occur.

8–15 hours:

➤ Give NAC especially if more than 150 mg/Kg (or 12 g in an adult or 75 mg/Kg to the patient has risk factors) of Paracetamol has been ingested.

➤ Measure plasma Paracetamol concentration, INR, creatinine and transaminase levels (ALT or AST).

➤ NAC may be discontinued if the patient is not at risk of liver damage, the INR, plasma creatinine and transaminases are normal, and the patient is asymptomatic. Do not discontinue if there is doubt about the overdose timing.

15–24 hours:

➤ Patients presenting at this time are much more likely to develop severe and potentially fatal liver damage. There is some evidence to suggest that the antidote may still offer some protection although not as much as when given early.

➤ Measure Paracetamol concentration, INR, creatinine, transaminase levels (ALT or AST) and ABG.

➤ The prognostic accuracy of the Paracetamol treatment graph after 15 hours is uncertain but a plasma-Paracetamol concentration above the relevant treatment line should be regarded as carrying a serious risk of liver damage and hence treatment administered.

Longer than 24 hours:

➤ Paracetamol levels are likely to be below the limit of detection even after substantial overdose. A measurable Paracetamol concentration indicates a significant overdose, a mistake in time of ingestion or a staggered overdose.

➤ Measure Paracetamol concentration, INR, creatinine, transaminase levels (ALT or AST) and ABG.

➤ Wait for the results before commencing treatment unless the patient is clearly jaundiced or has hepatic tenderness.

➤ Treat with NAC if INR is >1.3, the transaminases are elevated or there is an acidaemia.

➤ If significant liver dysfunction is found the local liver unit should be contacted for advice.

Prognosis:

➤ Liver transplant may be required for a few patients. Patients must be identified as early as possible, however, preferably on the second day.

➤ Current data indicates that an arterial pH <7.30, on the second or subsequent day after overdose is found in about 70% of cases with a poor prognosis.

➤ A combination of a prothrombin time of more than 100 seconds (INR 6.7), plasma creatinine concentration greater than 300 micromol/L and grade 3 or 4 hepatic encephalopathy is associated with a 17% survival rate.

➤ An increase in prothrombin time between the third and fourth days after overdose also indicates a poor prognosis.

➤ Liver transplantation is probably contra-indicated in patients with severe hypotension, severe cerebral oedema and serious infection.

Salicylates

Epidemiology

There were over 3,000 hospital admissions in England during 2007–2008 for salicylate poisoning.

Aetiology

Salicylate poisoning is usually due to aspirin overdose but it can be caused by the ingestion of oil of wintergreen.

Pathophysiology

A toxic dose of salicylate is >150 mg/Kg and severe toxicity is between 330–500 mg/Kg Doses of over 500 mg/kg are potentially lethal. The respiratory centre is stimulated to give tachypnoea with the resultant respiratory alkalosis. The acidic nature of salicylate gives a metabolic acidosis. There is also an uncoupling of the normal intracellular oxidative phosphorylation resulting in hyperpyrexia.

Key features in the history/examination

• How much aspirin was taken and when was it taken

• Any other toxins ingested

• Nausea and vomiting

• Abdominal pain

• Lethargy

• Tinnitus

• Dizziness

• Hyperthermia

• Tachypnoea

• Respiratory alkalosis

• Metabolic acidosis

- Hypoglycaemia
- Confusion
- Seizures
- Coma
- Examine for non-cardiogenic pulmonary oedema which has an increased risk in elderly and smokers with underlying chronic lung disease.

Investigations

Blood tests:

- Salicylate levels
- Baseline blood tests are required
- U&Es: may be raised if dehydrated from vomiting and hyperventilation
- Glucose
- ABG

Others:

- CXR

Management

➤ Activated charcoal is considered to be of use in the treatment of aspirin overdose.

➤ Repeated doses have been used, but this is not universally employed. After initial levels, repeat blood tests should be taken at three hour intervals until the serum salicylate level starts to decrease.

➤ Intravenous (IV) fluids to correct hypotension.

➤ Urine alkalisation may need to be instigated especially with severe acidosis. This can be achieved by using IV sodium bicarbonate (1.26%).

➤ Patients with severe toxicity are likely to require haemofiltration.

Opiates

Epidemiology

Opioid poisoning is an increasing problem. Morphine and diamorphine, as well as heroin are all drugs of abuse and accidental recreational overdoses are common. Deliberate poisoning is less common and iatrogenic overdose should always be considered in the deteriorating patient who has been prescribed opiates.

Aetiology

Opioids are common drugs of abuse in the forms of heroin, morphine and diamorphine. It is important to remember that opioids are commonly used analgesics in hospital patients and any patient that presents with the relevant clinical features on the wards should have their mediation charts checked.

Pathophysiology

Opioids act on the opioid receptors. Individuals have varying responses to opioids and hence doses that may be fine in one individual may cause an overdose in a sensitive individual. There are a number of common opioids, with significant variation in half-life. (See Table 3.69).

Opiate	Half-life (hours)
Morphine	3
Diamorphine	3
Codeine	3.5
Dihydrocodeine	4
Tramadol	6
Methadone	12–18

Table 3.69: Common opiates and their half-life.

Morphine is metabolised to morphine-6-glucuronide in the liver, which is excreted by the kidneys. Renal impairment can prolong the half-lives and increase the possibility of toxicity. The effects in overdose will also be potentiated by simultaneous ingestion of alcohol and other centrally acting drugs.

Key features in the history/examination

- Which opioid(s) were taken, when and by what route
- Any other toxins ingested
- Reduced respiratory rate
- Hypotension
- Bradycardia
- Pin-point pupils
- Reduced level of consciousness
- Vomiting and delayed gastric motility
- Needle and track mark in intravenous users
- Hallucinations
- Rhabdomyolysis in patients have been immobile for long periods

Investigations

Blood tests:

- FBC: check baselines
- U&Es: check baselines
- LFTs: check baselines

Others:

- ECG

Management

Conscious patient:

➤ A to E assessment

➤ Activated charcoal is a possibility if the overdose definitely occurred in the previous hour, ensuring airway protection.

➤ If the patient has clinical signs then observe them until fully awake.

➤ Consider giving Naloxone. The patient will then need observing for at least six hours.

➤ If the patient has no clinical signs then observe for at least four hours after ingestion of a standard release preparation or at least eight hours after a modified (slow) release preparation.

Unconscious patient:

➤ A to E assessment.

➤ Activated charcoal is a possibility if the overdose definitely occurred in the previous hour, ensuring airway protection.

➤ Administer 0.4–2 mg IV Naloxone and repeat the dose if there is no response within two minutes.

➤ Large doses (4 mg) may be required in a seriously poisoned patient. Intramuscular (IM) Naloxone is possible if necessary.

➤ Failure of a definite opioid overdose to respond to large doses of Naloxone suggests that another central nervous system (CNS) depressant drug or brain damage is present. Beware of an aggressive response from an opioid addict because their 'fix' is ruined when giving Naloxone.

➤ Naloxone has a short serum half life (30–80 minutes) in comparison to the opiates it reverses, so repeat doses or an IV infusion may be necessary.

➤ Observe the patient carefully for at least six hours after the last dose of Naloxone because further administration may be required.

Benzodiazepines

Epidemiology

Not as common as a drug of abuse, but very commonly used for sedative purposes in hospital. Often prescribed to patients with anxiety related disorders including depression.

Aetiology

The cause of benzodiazepine poisoning is usually iatrogenic.

Pathophysiology

There are a number of common benzodiazepines and they all have significant variation in half-life. (See Table 3.70). However their duration of action is less than the half-life. Benzodiazepines act on the gamma-aminobutyric acid (GABA) receptors. More specifically they are positive allosteric modulators of GABA-A

receptors and therefore potentiate the inhibitory effects within the CNS.

Benzodiazepines are very rarely fatal unless co-ingested with other CNS depressants.

Drug	Half-life (including active metabolites) (hours)
Flumazenil	1
Midazolam	1.8
Nitrazepam	10
Temazepam	20
Diazepam	36
Chlordiazepoxide	36

Table 3.70: Common benzodiazepines and their half-life.

Key features in the history/examination

• Which benzodiazepine(s) were taken, when and by what route

• Any other toxins ingested

• Drowsiness

• Respiratory depression

• Impaired balance

• Slurred speech

• Diplopia and nystagmus

• Bradycardia

• Hypotension

• Hypothermia

• Amnesia

• Ataxia

• Coma

Investigations

No specific investigations are required

Blood tests:

• Baseline blood tests are usually taken

• Paracetamol, salicylate and alcohol levels: may be taken

• ABG: if significant respiratory depression

Management

➤ Supportive management is the mainstay

➤ Flumazenil (200 micrograms) is the antidote for benzodiazepine but its use in overdose is controversial. It can be used with caution in the management of iatrogenic overdose but Flumazenil is not licensed for the management of deliberate overdose of benzodiazepines. This is due to the risk of inducing seizures that may not be controlled since this antidote acts as a competitive GABA-A antagonist.

Tricyclic antidepressants

Epidemiology

The incidence of TCA overdose is decreasing with the reduction in prescription numbers and a move towards the safer selective serotonin reuptake inhibitor (SSRI) class of antidepressants.

Aetiology

The most common cause of TCA overdose is due to suicide attempts.

Pathophysiology

TCAs have multiple effects which include blocking of monoamine oxidase (MAO) reuptake, anti-cholinergic action and blockade of ion channels in particular sodium ion channels. There are cardiovascular effects as a result of adrenoceptor blockade.

Key features in the history/examination

- Which TCA(s) were taken and when
- Any other toxins ingested
- Reduced level of consciousness
- Seizures
- Anticholinergic features such as dry mouth, blurred vision, urinary retention and constipation
- Dilated pupils
- Tachycardia
- Hypotension
- Cardiac conduction abnormalities: prolonged QT interval and atrio-ventricular (AV) nodal conduction delays
- Brisk reflexes
- Up-going plantars
- Hypoxia
- Bradypnoea and respiratory acidosis
- Metabolic acidosis
- Hypokalaemia

Investigations

Blood tests:

- Baseline blood tests
- ABG

Others:

- ECG

Management

- Activated charcoal if presenting within one hour
- IV fluid therapy to treat hypotension

- Inotropes may be necessary for hypotension treatment
- Monitor for respiratory depression. Intubation may be necessary.
- Cardiac monitoring
- Control seizures
- Sodium bicarbonate can be used in severe poisoning and may help control dysrhythmias
- If GCS <8 will require intensive care unit (ICU) referral and intubation to protect the airway.

Recreational drugs

It is likely that you will encounter patients admitted to hospital who are suffering from adverse reactions to the recreational use of drugs of abuse. It is useful to be familiar with some of the street terms that people may use to describe these drugs and the treatment required for them. (See Table 3.71).

Recreational drug	Street Name
Cannabis	Skunk, grass, dope, hash, gange
Heroin	H, horse, smack, junk, brown, gear, china white, skag
Cocaine	Coke, charlie, snow, white
3,4-methylenedioxymethamphetamine (MDMA)	Ecstasy, E, pills, doves, XTC, disco biscuits, Bruce Lees, echoes, hug drug, burgers, Smarties, magic beans, Mitsubishis, Rolexes, dolphins, snow ball, callies, eccies, little fellas, dids and yokes.
Gamma-hydroxybutyrate (GHB)	Liquid E, liquid X
Ampetamines	Speed, whizz, billy, uppers
Lysergic acid diethylamide (LSD)	Acid, sugar, trips, tabs, sid, Bart Simpsons, blotter, micro dots, liquid, Lucy, stars, lightening flash, paper mushrooms, rainbows, flash and hawk.
Ketamine	Special K, K, ket, super k, vitamin K, green, Mr Soft and techno smack.

Table 3.71: common recreational drugs and their street names.

Cocaine

Epidemiology

2.3% of population aged 16–59 regularly used cocaine in 2006–2007.

Aetiology

Cocaine is a very common recreational drug, taken orally, intravenously, by inhalation and intranasally. 'Body-packers' swallow packets of drugs, which can burst causing serious illness.

Pathophysiology

A CNS stimulant, inhibiting pre-synaptic re-uptake of MAO causes coronary artery vasospasm and can lead to myocardial ischaemia and infarction. It also causes cerebral artery vasospam and hence can lead to a stroke. Aortic dissection may result too.

Key features in the history/examination

- Palpitations
- Chest pain due to coronary artery spasm
- Hallucinations
- Agitation
- Pupil dilation
- Tachycardia
- Hypertension
- Hyperpyrexia
- Cardiac dysrhythmias
- Seizures

Investigations

Blood tests:

- Baseline blood tests
- Cardiac enzymes: especially if there is chest pain

Imaging:

- Abdominal X-ray (AXR): if body-packing is suspected
- Computer tomography (CT): thorax if dissection suspected

Others:

- ECG: looking for dysrhythmias and ischaemia

Management

➢ There is no specific antidote to cocaine and therefore treatment revolves around supportive measures.
➢ Benzodiazepines can control agitation and seizures.
➢ Hyperpyrexia should be treated by cooling
➢ Any patients complaining of chest pain must be treated as for acute coronary syndrome (ACS).

Ecstasy

Epidemiology

1.5% of population between ages of 16–59 used ecstasy in year 2006–2007.

Aetiology

Ecstasy is a common recreational drug.

Pathophysiology

MDMA cause the release of serotonin, dopamine and norephidrine from pre-synaptic terminals both in the central and peripheral nervous system. At the same time it binds and inhibits the reuptake of these neurotransmitters which increases the concentration at the synapse. Other effects include the increase in cortisol, prolactin, adrenocorticotrophic hormone (ACTH) and antidiuretic hormone (ADH). An increase in core body temperature regardless of ambient temperature is a serious complication. (See Table 3.72).

Complication	Features
Hyperthermia	Due to an intemperate environment and/or lack of hydration and/or lack of rest from physical activity.
Dehydration	Due to an intemperate environment and/or lack of hydration and/or lack of rest from physical activity.
Hyponatremia	Due to drug induced ADH release and/or excess compensatory intake of fluids. This is a rare complication.
Serotonin syndrome	Believed to be due to excess release of serotonin and sometimes triggered by co-administration of other serotonergic drugs.

Table 3.72: Serious complications of MDMA poisoning.

Key features in the history/examination

- Reports taking MDMA (may use slang).
- Time since ingestion
- Amount of fluid ingested
- Other activities engaged in since ingesting
- Urinary retention
- Abnormal pupil dilation
- Increased physical energy
- Tachycardia
- Hypertension
- Increased mean body temperature
- Trismus, i.e. inability to open the mouth.
- Bruxia, i.e. involuntary teeth grinding
- Gurning, i.e. projecting the lower jaw forward. This is usually caused by larger doses.
- Nystagmus

Investigations

Blood tests:

- U&Es: for checking sodium levels and for signs of dehydration

Others:

- ECG: to rule out dysrhythmias

Management

➢ The management of ecstasy overdose is supportive.

➢ Catheterisation for urinary retention

➢ Consider activated charcoal in large overdoses

➢ The serious complications require careful management in an ICU.

➢ Fluid administration needs to be very carefully monitored in these patients.

Further reading and references

➢ Bateman D.N., Vale A. (2007) *Poisoning*. Medicine Publishing, Oxford p 10–12.

➢ British National Formulary (57ed)

➢ www.collemergencymed.ac.uk

➢ Hoare J and Flatley J (2008) Drugs Misuse Declared: Findings from 2006/2007 British Crime Survey. *Home Office National Statistical Bulletin*

➢ www.npis.org

➢ O'Grady J.G., Alexander G.J., Hayllar K.M., et al. (1989). Early Indicators of prognosis in fulminant hepatic failure. *Gastroenterology* 97 (2): 439–45

➢ www.toxbase.org

RASH

Differential diagnosis

System/Organism	Disease
CNS	Meningococcal septicaemia/meningitis
Infection	Viral or fungal infection
Atopy/allergen-related	Dermatitis and eczema
Autoimmune	Psoriasis
Hormonal	Acne vulgaris
Fungal	Tinea (ringworm)
Others	Lichen planus
	Scabies
	Molluscum contagiosum
	Leprosy
	Erysipelas
	Bullous disease:
	Dermatitis herpetiformis
	Pemphigoid
	Pemphigus vulgaris
	Measles

Yeast	Pityriasis rosacea
	Pityriasis versicolor
Systemic	Skin manifestations of systemic disease
	Erythema nodosum
	Herpes simplex
	Drug-related rashes:
	Erythema Multiforme

The most important differential to consider in medicine is meningococcal septicaemia or meningitis.

Dermatitis and eczema

Epidemiology

Affects around 3% of the population, and 10% of children aged under 5 years suffer from this condition. It is a relapsing condition that often starts in infancy and continues into adulthood.

Aetiology

Results from a polygenetic pattern of inheritance and environmental influences. If one parent is atopic the risk for children developing the condition is 30% but this increases to 50% if both parents are affected. Strong detergents, chemicals and wearing woollen clothes can irritate the skin and exacerbate the condition in some individuals. The fur of cats and dogs as well as house dust mite may also worsen the condition. Dairy products can also precipitate the rash in particular in children.

Pathophysiology

There is inflammation of the skin in response to either an exogenous agent to which the individual reacts to or an endogenous process where the individual has an increased tendency to react to allergens in the environment. There is a strong hereditary component and patients have an inherited tendency to have altered immune responses to environmental allergens and families tend to have asthma, hay fever, conjunctivitis, or eczema.

There are three types of dermatitis:

- Contact dermatitis, which can be due to irritants or allergic reactions.
- Seborrhoeic dermatitis
- Atopic dermatitis

Key features in the history/examination

- A diffuse rash with patchy lesions which are irritating and occasionally painful. It is associated with erythema, oedema, dry and flaky skin.
- Associated initially with vesicle and bullae formation: these can burst and leave areas which are raw and weepy.
- Mostly affects the 'flexor areas', for example the front of the elbows and ankles, behind the knees and at the front of

the neck. This is reversed to involve the 'extensor areas' in individuals with pigmented skin.

- Pruritis tends to be the most common feature.
- Secondary bacterial infection may occur usually with Staphylococci. It causes crusting of the lesions and surrounding cellulitis.
- Where lesions are chronic there may be some scaling and resultant thickening of the skin known as lichenification.
- Lesions which are healed tend not to scar but may become pigmented.
- Histological findings may reveal an initial oedema of the epidermis which subsequently results in vesicle formation.
- When lesions involve the face or genital area there is significant oedema. However, vesicles tend to be more numerous on the palms and soles.
- Pitting and ridging of the nail-bed is a common associated feature.

Contact dermatitis (irritant):

- This results from a continuous exposure to either physical or chemical irritants such as industrial solvents.
- The history may be consistent with work exposure precipitating the rash.
- Occupations such as hairdressing and engineering pose a substantial risk for the development of this irritant form of contact dermatitis.

Contact dermatitis (allergic):

- Previous exposure and sensitisation to the allergen is required.
- A characteristic feature is that the rash will only be present in areas where there has been allergen exposure.
- A thorough history is key in delineating the responsible allergen followed by a patch test for all suspected cases to identify the causative agent.
- The most common allergens are:
  - Epoxy resins
  - Chromates
  - Nickel
  - Rubber
  - Dyes
  - Perfumes
  - Antibiotics (topical)
  - Plants
  - Antiseptics
  - Parabens (preservatives found in cosmetics and creams)

Seborrhoeic dermatitis:

- An erythematous, pruritic, and scaly rash which involves the greasy areas of the skin such as the scalp, eyebrows, nose and ear creases and around the head.

- Other regions classically involved are the axillae, inframammary areas and perineal regions.
- Nappy rash is a form of dermatitis secondary to prolonged ammonia exposure.

Atopic dermatitis:

- Atopic dermatitis is characterised by a predisposition to the development of a reaction to various allergens normally present within the environment. Features include asthma, rhinitis, conjunctivitis, and dermatitis.
- It affects up to 25% of individuals in the UK.
- Mainly presents in infancy and is accompanied by other atopic features.
- A positive family history is very common.
- The rash tends to affect the flexor areas and is pruritic and erythematous. Constant scratching especially in childhood can result in lichenification.

Investigations

Blood tests:

- Full blood count (FBC): White cell count may show eosinophilia.
- Serum IgE: levels are characteristically raised.

Others:

- Skin prick test: Performed using common environmental allergens and usually yields positive results.
- Skin swabs: may be necessary to confirm secondary infection of skin lesions.

Management

- The mainstay of management is to remove or reduce exposure to the responsible agent.
- Cotton clothing is best with avoidance of wool garments.
- Dietary changes such as a lactose-free diet have a small role in the routine treatment.
- Commercial soaps tend to contain irritants and hence bathing with only water or gentle soap substitutes is recommended.
- Potassium permanganate or oily baths, such as oilatum or balneum baths, can help with healing of lesions.
- Topical steroids will provide symptomatic relief.
- Dry and flaky skin will require aqueous or emollient cream application.
- Pruritus will be relieved with the use of sedating oral anti-histamine agents which are best taken at night to aid sleep.
- Topical Tacrolimus has recently been used for mild to moderate disease.
- For severe disease, systemic therapy with steroids or other immunosuppressants such as Ciclosporin or Azathioprine can be used.

3. Medicine

> Secondary infection of skin lesions is a frequent occurrence and oral antibiotics are required.
>> o Flucloxacillin is effective for *Staphylococci* infection and Penicillin V acts against *Streptococcus*.
>> o Erythromycin is used in Penicillin allergic patients.

Psoriasis

Epidemiology

Around 1–2% of individuals in the UK are affected. Usually affects two distinct age groups, either 16 to 22 years or 55 to 60 years. It can range from a mild form where it is not clinically obvious to a chronic and severe form where it may cause the patient to be incapacitated with severe aesthetic deformity. Occasionally it can present acutely and be life threatening.

Aetiology

Psoriasis is an autoimmune disease that is often associated with a positive family history. Its inheritance is polygenic as well as being influenced by environmental factors. Associated factors include:

- Infection, e.g. group A *Streptococcus*.
- Drugs, e.g. Lithium
- Ultraviolet light
- Alcohol abuse

Pathophysiology

A skin biopsy illustrates an increase in skin turnover. The granular layer is usually absent and the upper epidermis consists of polymorphonuclear abscesses. There will be capillary dilatation in the dermis too. There are several different types of psoriasis.

Chronic plaque psoriasis is the most common type. It characteristically involves pink/red scaly plaques on the extensor skin surfaces in particular the knees and elbows and may also involve the ears, scalp and lower back region. New psoriatic plaque lesions tend to form at sites of skin trauma which is known as Köbner's phenomenon. The lesions may be associated with pruritis or pain.

Flexural psoriasis usually presents at a later age. There are well-defined, erythematous, shiny plaque lesions mainly in the flexor areas such as the groin, underneath the breasts, and in the natal cleft. However, it is not associated with scaling.

Guttate psoriasis is mostly seen in children and young adults. Characteristically described as 'raindrop' type lesions, small circular or oval shaped plaque lesions appear around two weeks after a Streptococcal sore throat. It has a tendency to resolve spontaneously over a two month period even if no treatment is given.

Palmoplantar pustular psoriasis occurs with pustules confined to the hands and feet.

Erythrodermic and pustular psoriasis are the most severe forms, with diffuse and severe skin inflammation. Both forms may occur together in what is known as 'Von Zumbusch' psoriasis. These are potentially life threatening in nature. The associated features include malaise, pyrexia, and circulatory disturbance. The pustules contain a sterile collection of inflammatory cells.

Key features in the history/examination

Acute presentation:

- There may be multiple small skin lesions over the body, limbs, scalp, natal cleft and umbilicus.
- Lesions are round, silver and scaly in nature with an erythematous base.
- These lesions can be removed leaving small areas of bleeding (Auspitz sign).
- There is usually resolution over a two to four month period but a small number of patients will develop chronic lesions.
- Köbner's phenomenon may be seen.

Chronic presentation:

- Lesions (as described above) which mainly affect the extensor surfaces of the skin, in particular the back, elbows, knees and scalp.
- These lesions are characteristically symmetrical.
- Coarse pitting of the nail bed is often seen in such patients as well as onycholysis.
- If the flexor regions are involved the lesions have a different appearance as they are smooth and form confluent areas which are erythematous and associated with pruritus.
- Psoriatic arthropathy affects around 5–10% of individuals with psoriasis, and may predate the skin disease. Patterns of arthropathy vary and include:
  - o Asymmetrical involvement of the hands and feet
  - o Symmetrical arthropathy mimicking rheumatoid arthritis
  - o Sacroiliitis
  - o Arthritis mutilans

Investigations

This is a clinical diagnosis based on the appearance of the skin. There are no specific blood tests or diagnostic procedures for the disease.

Histology:

- Skin biopsy: May be performed in order to exclude other diagnoses. It will show clubbed Rete pegs if positive for the presence of psoriasis.

Management

Topical therapy:

> Salicylic acid: strength of 2–6% is available in a lotion or ointment. It helps to reduce the hyperkeratotic and scaly lesions and it can be used as an adjunct with coal tar or dithranol.

> Coal tar paste: is not commonly used in current practice because even though it is an effective therapy, it can be unpleasant to use as it can cause staining of the clothes and has an offensive odour. It is available in shampoo form and effective for scalp lesions. Baths in coal tar are very effective when there are extensive skin lesions.

> Dithranol: is a preparation which is applied to the skin lesions sparingly and then dressed ensuring adequate coverage. It is usually left on for up to two hours to ensure maximal benefit. However, it can cause irritation of the skin and hence a low strength preparation of 0.1% is used initially, gradually increasing to 5%. Unwanted effects such as staining of the skin, hair and clothes are expected.

> Calcipotriol: is a vitamin D analogue which is effective in mild to moderate psoriatic lesions.

Systemic therapy:

> Psoralens and ultraviolet A phototherapy (PUVA): is an effective treatment in clearing lesions and delaying the recurrence of the disease in chronic cases. However it has been associated with an increased risk of skin cancer.

> Retinoids: are vitamin A derivatives. Retinoid use is limited to severe cases which are resistant to other treatments. It can cause dry skin and lips associated with cracking and bleeding. Hair loss is also common. Other side effects include generalised myalgia, hepatic dysfunction, and hyperlipidaemia. Retinoids are also potentially teratogenic and therefore pregnancy must be avoided for two years after taking acitretin.

> Methotrexate and Ciclosporin: are reserved for use in very severe cases and require monitoring and supervision.

> Biological therapies: the use of drugs such as Infliximab and Adalimumab have been increased recently for psoriasis and psoriatic arthritis.

Prognosis:

> Most patients have an excellent prognosis and can live a relatively normal life with minimal disability. However, one in five patients have aggressive joint disease which may be very limiting upon their activities of daily living.

Acne vulgaris

Epidemiology

Acne vulgaris mostly affects individuals during puberty but the onset of the condition can occur up to the age of 40 years. It affects 85% people at some point during adolescence.

Aetiology

Acne vulgaris is typified by an increased size and activity of the sebaceous glands. The underlying aetiology of this is multifactorial. It is made more likely by environmental factors such as trauma, cosmetics and some medications (including topical corticosteroids). There is postulated a genetic influence which is polygenic in nature, with high concordance seen in twin studies.

Other influences are endocrine (hyperandrogenism), hence it is associated with polycystic ovaries in females (90%).

Pathophysiology

The rate of sebum production directly correlates with the severity of acne. Keratin can block the hair follicles and cause a build up of sebum which results in the characteristic blackheads known as 'comedones'. An inflammatory reaction is seen at the hair follicles, which is increased by colonisation with the bacterium *Propionibacterium acnes.*

Secondary bacterial infection of these blackheads can commonly occur.

Key features in the history/examination

- Acne vulgaris causes the following:
  - Seborrhoea
  - Comedones
  - Papules
  - Pustules
  - Nodules
  - Cysts
  - Scars
- The most common areas of distribution of skin lesions are the face, upper thorax, and shoulders.
- The skin tends to appear greasy and the lesion may result in scarring which persists into adulthood.

Investigations

This is mostly a clinical diagnosis based on the findings of history and examination. There are no formal investigations for the diagnosis of acne.

Management

> For adolescent-onset acne, the severity diminishes with time, so no treatment is required for the majority of sufferers. Keeping the face and other affected areas clean may help, but excessive washing is of no benefit.

> Control of hormone secretion with the combined oral contraceptive pill (OCP) is effective in females.

> Topical treatment with Benzoyl peroxide cream, antibiotics such as Erythromycin, topical retinoids or other topical keratolytics such as salicylic acid help with the skin lesions.

> Oral antibiotics such as Oxytetracycline or Erythromycin are given for at least six months and are effective in moderate disease.

> After failure of the above treatment, oral Isotretinoin, a vitamin A analogue, is useful for severe disease. However it is associated with side-effects such as dry skin, myalgia, hyperlipidaemia, and hepatic dysfunction. Due to its teratogenic potential, it cannot be used in pregnancy.

Tinea (ringworm)

Epidemiology

A common condition, in particular amongst children. It is heavily contagious and commonly transmitted via skin-to-skin contact or contaminated areas such as the shower or pool. Cats are known to be carriers of the common organisms.

Aetiology

Fungal organisms which are present within the skin's keratin layer are mostly responsible. These incluce *Trichophyton, Microsporum* and *Epidermophyton.* The fungus grows and multiplies over the skin, nails and scalp. Depending on the body site affected, tinae pedis, tinae cruris and tinae capitis can be diagnosed.

Pathophysiology

Fungal infection of the skin as described in the aetiology.

Key features in the history/examination

Tinea pedis:

- This is the most common form and involves the inter-digital skin, especially between the fourth and fifth metatarsals.
- The nails may also be involved
- The lesions are white, fissured and pruritic.
- Secondary infection with Streptococcus can develop and these are often recurrent.
- It may resemble atopic dermatitis especially when the lesions become diffuse and involve the soles and lateral feet borders.

Tinea cruris:

- This involves infection in the groin and the upper, inner thigh region
- Lesions appear raised, discrete and with an extending margin which is scaly.
- It may also be associated with pruritus.

Tinea capitis:

- This causes a localised area of hair loss with underlying scaling of the skin.
- Pre-pubertal children are mostly affected and hence it is spread easily by close contact.
- There may be circular patches of lesions which may be pustular.
- Secondary infection is common.

Investigations

Others:

- Wood's light examination: can be used to illustrate fluorescence of the lesions which is characteristic in tinea capitis.

Management

➢ For a localised problem, topical treatment with anti-fungals such as Imidazole, Clotrimazole, Miconazole, or Terbinafine is effective.

➢ For a widespread problem, systemic treatment may be necessary especially if there is hair or nail involvement. For example, oral Terbinafine or Itraconazole tends to be effective but they are only initiated following laboratory confirmation of the diagnosis.

Pityriasis rosea

Epidemiology

Young adults are mostly affected between the ages of 10 to 30 years. The incidence is estimated at between 0.1 to 3%. However, individuals of all ages as well as both males and females, are thought to be susceptible. It is an acute condition which tends to be self-limiting in nature.

Aetiology

Tends to occur in clusters amongst close contacts. Most cases are in the Spring and Autumn seasons with a relatively low rate of recurrence. It is thought that although no specific bacteria, fungus or virus has been implicated, human herpes virus 6 and 7 are thought to have a role.

Pathophysiology

The exact mechanisms which result in the initiation of the disease process are poorly understood.

Key features in the history/examination

- A 'herald patch' characteristically appears prior to the development of the rash. This is a distinct red brown oval shaped lesion which has a scaly appearance tends to appear over the abdomen or scapula.

- A pruritic macular rash follows the appearance of this lesion at around 1 to 2 weeks and tends to last up until 6 weeks.

  o It involves the trunk and the upper regions of the limbs (characteristically known as the 'christmas tree' distribution)

  o Lesions are oval shaped and have a scaly border.

  o Usually appears at the areas of the natural skin creases.

- Often occurs in clusters within families or in schools.

- Other accompanying features include headache, fever, nausea and fatigue.

Investigations

There are no specific investigations for diagnosis which is predominantly clinical in nature.

Management

➤ Usually self resolving within six weeks and therefore requires no specific treatment.

➤ Occasionally mild sedatives may be required to provide symptomatic relief as well as topical steroid preparations.

Lichen planus

Epidemiology

Lichen planus is not commonly encountered but it mostly affects middle-aged individuals. It tends to affect women more than men with a 3:2 ratio.

Aetiology

The cause is unknown but probable viral or autoimmune nature is suspected. Several drugs including anti-malarial drugs, gold, and anti-tuberculous drugs can produce similar lesions. Only half of the lesions resolve by around nine months.

Pathophysiology

The exact mechanisms which result in the initiation of the disease process are poorly understood.

Key features in the history/examination

• Presents with a pruritic and irritating rash involving the flexor surfaces of the forearm, wrist, trunk and ankles.

• Nail involvement is evident in up to 10% of patients.

• Distinct shiny papules are characteristic and usually purplish and polygonal in shape.

• Another feature is Wickham's striae, which are fine white lines with pass through the lesions.

• Lesions tend to form at areas of skin excoriation or injury (Köbner's phenomenon).

• There may be widespread lesions or a few and confined to one area.

• Other areas such as the oral mucosa or nails may be involved. Characteristically, a 'lace-like' appearance in the mouth is produced and this may be the only sign of the disease.

• Lesions usually resolve within six months, however recurrence is common.

Investigations

Histology:

• Skin biopsy: will show lymphoid infiltration of the epidermal basal cells which gives a classic saw-toothed appearance at the dermis-epidermis junction.

Management

➤ Topical treatment with steroids may provide symptomatic relief until the lesions subside.

➤ If lesions are extensive, they tend to be associated with severe pruritis which responds to systemic steroid therapy.

Rosacea

Epidemiology

Rosacea is three times more common in females and the peak incidence is between the age of 30 to 60 years.

Aetiology

It is precipitated by factors such as hot drinks, sunlight exposure, alcohol, and occasionally the use of topical steroids may cause an eruption.

Pathophysiology

Pathological mechanisms are unclear. A number of hypotheses exist, including vascular abnormalities, degeneration of the matrix of the dermis, certain environmental factors as well as microorganisms such as *Helicobacter pylori*. High levels of an abnormal form of the antimicrobial protein called cathelicidin have been reported in patients with rosacea. Studies are still ongoing in order to determine the role of this protein.

Key features in the history/examination

• The rash characteristically develops over the cheeks, nose, chin and forehead.

• The skin appears, red with papules and pustules as well as telangiectasia.

Investigations

The majority of patients with rosacea have very mild symptoms and therefore are not formally diagnosed or treated. It can mostly be diagnosed from clinical examination or with a trial of treatment in order to confirm the diagnosis when it is suspected. The diagnosis is often confused with acne vulgaris, however, it is important to bear in mind that rosacea primarily involves the face only.

Management

➤ Long-term use of oral antibiotics such as Oxytetracycline may be effective in suppressing the rash. It is usually given for two months followed by a rest period of two months prior to re-starting therapy.

Pityriasis versicolor

Epidemiology

A common skin infection affecting around 2 to 8% of the population at some stage. It mostly affects adolescents and young adults, especially where there is a warm and humid environment.

Aetiology

Pityriasis versicolor is a yeast infection usually due to *Pityrosporum orbiculare*. This is commonly found on the skin surface and growth is encouraged by a warm and humid environment.

Pathophysiology

The exact mechanisms which result in the initiation of the disease process are poorly understood.

Key features in the history/examination

- The trunk is involved with characteristic reddish-brown and scaly lesions which can vary in size and can form a confluent rash.
- It can result in depigmentation of the skin which can persist despite effective treatment.
- May give the appearance of vitiligo in patients with sun exposure as only the skin areas which are unaffected by the infection will be pigmented.

Investigations

Histology:

- Skin scrapings: Confirm the diagnosis.

Others:

- Wood's light examination: may also aid in diagnosis as it causes yellow fluorescence.

Management

- Selenium sulphide (2.5%), a topical anti-fungal medication, is the mainstay of treatment.
- Topical treatment with Imidazole may be required for long periods if the rash is severe.

Drug-related rashes

Epidemiology

Drug related rashes affect 1–2% of hospitalised patients.

Aetiology

Any drug can potentially cause a skin reaction, ranging from the trivial to life-threatening. The patient's medications must be considered as a cause in any patient presenting with a rash. The most common causes are:

- Oral and intravenous (IV) antibiotics, in particular the penicillins, are the commonest cause of a rash, which usually appears at around 10–12 days following treatment.
- Other common drugs that cause rashes include Penicillamine, Angiotensin converting enzyme (ACE) inhibitors, Allopurinol and Thiazides.

Pathophysiology

Different individuals may react in different ways to the same drug but the features of these rashes include:

- Maculopapular (morbilliform)
- Eczematous
- Urticarial
- Purpuric

Key features in the history/examination

Maculopapular rash:

- It is the most common presentation of a drug-related reaction and Penicillin is often the causative agent.
- There are features of flat coloured lesions of less than 1 cm in diameter combined with palpable lesions of less than 5 mm in diameter.

Urticarial rash:

- This rash is usually caused by penicillins and aspirins.
- Up to 2% of all patients receiving treatment with penicillin have a reaction.
- There is a cross-reaction in one in ten penicillin-allergic patients who are treated with a cephalosporin.
- It results from mast cell degranulation with histamine release as well as other vasoactive agents which cause erythema and oedema.
- Characteristically causes formation of pruritic erythematous wheals but widespread angio-oedema can also result.
- Skin reactions tend to be more common in adults as they will have had a previous exposure to the drug.
- Rarely, some patients have a serious anaphylactic reaction within minutes of drug exposure including hypotension, wheeze and arthralgia.
- Other drugs which may potentially cause an urticarial rash include:
  - ACE inhibitors
  - Barbiturates
  - Salicylates and non-steroidal anti-inflammatory drugs (NSAID)
  - Streptomycin
  - Sulphonamides
  - Tetracyclines
  - Phenothiazines
  - Chloramphenicol

Purpura:

- A rash resulting from capillary damage.
- Usually indicative of a severe drug reaction.
- Drugs which cause bone marrow suppression include gold and carbimazole resulting in thrombocytopenic purpura.

Investigations

- Investigations required are guided by the patients' clinical presentation.
- Essential to take a thorough history including a full drug history as well as any previous allergies.
- A careful clinical examination will indicate any investigations which may be required.

Management

- ➤ All likely drug precipitants should be stopped if at all possible.
- ➤ Symptoms of pruritus respond well to oral antihistamines and mild topical steroids.
- ➤ When patients have acute anaphylactic reactions (fortunately this is rare) they should be treated according to the Resuscitation Council (UK) guidelines. This involves IV fluid resuscitation, 0.5 mg Adrenaline IM injection (strength 1:1,000) as well as Chlorpheniramine and systemic steroids.

Erythema nodosum (systemic illness)

Epidemiology

Erythema nodosum is usually found in those aged 20 to 50 years and the male to female ratio is 1:5.

Aetiology

Erythema nodosum most commonly results from sarcoidosis (around a third of cases) but it may accompany Streptococcal infection such as in rheumatic fever. It is also a feature of tuberculosis, ulcerative colitis (UC) and Crohn's disease. It can result from drug use such as the sulphonamides, penicillins and salicylates. Often it is idiopathic. It is comonly recurrent in nature.

Pathophysiology

A panniculitis due to an immunological reaction to a variety of different causes.

Key features in the history/examination

- Characteristically there will be tender, erythematous, raised lesions on the shin which occasionally involves the thighs and upper limbs.
- The lesions change colour progressively similar to that of a bruise.
- Almost half of patients will also have arthropathy involving the lower limbs.

Investigations

Blood tests:

- If sarcoidosis is suspected, check calcium and serum ACE levels.

Imaging:

- Chest X-ray (CXR): look for bilateral hilar lymphadenopathy if sarcoidosis is suspected.

Management

- ➤ Treatment is directed towards the specific underlying cause of the disease.
- ➤ Mostly symptomatic management including bed rest, elevation of the legs and using compression bandages, wet dressings, as well as non-steroidal anti-inflammatory drugs.
- ➤ Where the cause is unknown, potassium iodide has been shown to be effective for persistent lesions.
- ➤ Corticosteroids are used in severe cases which are unresponsive to the standard treatment.

Herpes zoster/shingles (systemic disease)

Epidemiology

Worldwide, the incidence is between 1 to 3 cases per 1,000 per year, and 4 to 12 cases per 1,000 per year in those aged over 65 years.

Aetiology

Shingles is caused by the reactivation of the varicella zoster virus.

Pathophysiology

Shingles is often precipitated by immunosupression, which is increasingly likely in older age. Examples include acute intercurrent illness, diabetes, steroid (and other immunosuppressant) therapy and cancer.

Key features in the history/examination

- Characteristically there is a cluster of blistering lesions with an erythematous base. They can become filled with pus and subsequently crust over.
- They occur within the distribution of a nerve root and tend to cause pain and tingling prior to the appearance of the lesions.
- However it can involve more than one dermatome.
- The pain can be severe and intolerable.
- Prior infection with varicella zoster virus is necessary for the development of shingles as it remains latent within the dorsal root ganglia until reactivation occurs due to a reduced resistance in the host, for example, as a result of immunosuppression.
- The main complication is post-herpetic neuralgia where there is severe and persistent pain in the distribution of lesions. Eye symptoms may also arise if the ophthalmic nerve is involved.

Investigations

Diagnosis is primary made after visual inspection of the lesions.

Blood tests:

- Varicella zoster virus (VZV) specific IgM antibody: this is only present during chicken pox or herpes zoster and not when the virus is dormant.

Management

- ➢ Patients require isolation from susceptible individuals at least until the lesions are crusted over in order to minimise the risk of spread.
- ➢ Oral Acyclovir should be used to hasten healing of the lesions.
- ➢ Immunosuppressed individuals must be treated with IV Acyclovir.
- ➢ Analgesia is key in symptom relief.
- ➢ Antibiotics may be required if there is secondary bacterial infection.

Post-herpetic neuralgia:

- ➢ Symptoms of neuralgia are confined to the area of skin affected by the herpes zoster rash.
- ➢ The onset of pain tends to follow the healing and crusting over of lesions.
- ➢ Gabapentin, Amitriptiline and carbamezepine are commonly used and found to be most effective for neuralgic pain.

Dermatitis herpetiformis (bullous disease)

Epidemiology

Primarily a disease with onset in the second and third decades of life.

Aetiology

Dermatitis herpetiformis is seen in patients with gluten sensitivity. Up to 80% of individuals are positive for HLA B8.

Pathophysiology

IgA is deposited in the dermal papillae. Untreated, the severity varies according to the amount of gluten ingested.

Key features in the history/examination

- Intensely pruritic vesicular rash
- The buttocks are usually affected but the extensor aspects of the elbows and knees, the interscapular region and scalp can also be affected.

- Initially there are clusters of small urticarial blistering lesions which tend to be symmetrical in nature.

Investigations

Blood tests:

- IgA antibodies: Presence of IgA antibodies will be detected.

Histology:

- Skin biopsy: This will reveal the IgA deposits within the dermal papillae with the use of direct immunofluorescence.

These tests must be done prior to starting the patient on a gluten-free diet in order to avoid false-negative results.

Management

- ➢ A gluten-free diet is compulsory.
- ➢ Oral Dapsone is usually used.
- ➢ Sulphonamides can also be used for the skin lesions.
- ➢ Secondary infection with bacteria is common.

Pemphigoid (bullous disease)

Epidemiology

The incidence is approximately 5/100,000 per year and the elderly population is mostly effected. It is slightly more common in women than in men.

Aetiology

An autoimmune skin disease when bullae form as a result of an immune reaction where there is formation of autoantibodies targeting the type XVII collagen portion of hemidesmosomes. It will rarely involve the mucous membranes. There is infiltration of neutrophils, lymphocytes and eosinophils.

Pathophysiology

Lesions form at the basement membrane in-between the dermis and epidermis (deeper than in pemphigus vulgaris). There is deposition of IgG in the basement membrane.

Key features in the history/examination

- The limbs are mostly affected and often the trunk is affected too but rarely mucous membranes are involved.
- They may be a preceding pruritis over the skin prior to the onset of lesions.
- Tense bullae are seen (up to 3 cm) although these may be absent with signs of excoriation.
- Although lesions may form in areas of skin trauma, it does not break as easily as in pemphigus vulgaris.

- Nikolsky's sign will be negative.
- Patients tend not to become systemically unwell.

Investigations

Blood tests:

- Antibodies: Test for any atibodies against bullous pemphigoid antigens 1 (BPAG1) and bullous pemphigoid antigens 2 (BPAG2).

Management

➢ A referral to the dermatologist is required.

➢ Oral Prednisolone is usually sufficient for control of lesions and it may be used long-term in small doses.

Pemphigus vulgaris (bullous disease)

Epidemiology

A very rare condition nowadays with an incidence of less than 1/100,000 per year. It usually occurs in late-middle aged individuals.

Aetiology

An autoimmune disease where antibodies form against desmoglein which is responsible for the attachment of adjacent epidermal cells via attachment points known as desmosomes. Autoantibodies attack the desmogleins and cause separation of the cells, and hence the epidermis becomes unglued causing acantholysis. Blisters form which slough off and result in sores forming.

Pathophysiology

The epidermis is split above the basal layer and the epidermal cells degenerate. The tissue will be positive for IgG.

Key features in the history/examination

- Lesions are very superficial, large and lax.
- Most patients tend to present with extensive erosions of the skin with only a few progressing to form bullae.
- These lesions occur over the limbs and trunk regions.
- Oral lesions are common and may be the sole presenting feature initially.
- A differentiating feature is Nikolsky's sign where the superficial skin layer can be moved over the deeper skin layers causing the layers to breakdown and hence increasing susceptibility to infection.
- The break in the epithelium predisposes to infection.
- Lesions tend to occur where there has been a breach in the skin surface.
- Pain is often very severe.
- The patient may also present with systemic features of fever and feeling generally unwell.

Investigations

Histology:

- Skin biopsy: Characteristic features in the epidermis will be shown.

Management

➢ Referral to a dermatologist is required.

➢ Widespread disease may cause significant protein loss and so may need a dental review.

➢ High doses of steroids are required to control the lesions.

➢ Occasionally, Azathioprine and IV immunoglobulin therapy is indicated.

Erythema multiforme

Epidemiology

A common condition, with a peak incidence between 20 and 30 years.

Aetiology

The rash may be associated with drug therapy such as with Penicillin, Sulphonamides, Salicylates and Barbiturates. Infection with the herpes simplex virus for example can also result in characteristic lesions.

Pathophysiology

An immune-mediated condition, where IgM immune complexes are deposited in the superficial microvasculature of the epidermis and mucous membranes.

Key features in the history/examination

- A generalised disorder which manifests either as a skin disorder alone or with systemic features such as fever, sore throat, headache, arthralgia, diarrhoea and vomiting.
- The skin rash usually follows the symptoms, if present.
- Characteristics of the rash include an erythematous eruption which is of varying morphology. It may become bullous in nature.
- Usually the limbs are involved first and the rash then spreads to the trunk and eventually may involve the entire body.
- Patients' mouths should be examined as the buccal mucosa may be affected.
- Characteristic 'target' lesions usually occur late. These are concentric rings which are erythematous.
- Stevens-Johnson syndrome is a severe form of the disease where there are systemic features of the condition with multiple lesions in the oral cavity, conjunctiva, anal and genital regions.

Investigations

Diagnosis is clinical and based on the appearance of the skin lesions associated with the specific risk factors or associated pre-disposing conditions.

Histology:

- Skin biopsy: Microscopic examination of the tissue can also aid diagnosis when it is uncertain.

Management

- ➤ Usually resolves spontaneously within five to six weeks but recurrence is common.
- ➤ All drug treatment should be withdrawn as far as is possible.
- ➤ Mild topical steroids are effective in reducing symptoms of pruritus.
- ➤ Those with suspected Stevens-Johnsons syndrome will require systemic steroids to suppress and control the lesions.

Further reading and references

- ➤ National Institute for Health and Clinical Excellence (2004). *Frequency of application of topical corticosteroids for atopic eczema (TA81).*
- ➤ National Institute for Health and Clinical Excellence (2004). *Tacrolimus and pimecrolimus (TA82).*
- ➤ National Institute for Health and Clinical Excellence (2007). *Atopic eczema in children (CG057).*
- ➤ National Institute for Health and Clinical Excellence (2007). *Adalimumab for the treatment of psoriatic arthritis (TA125).*
- ➤ National Institute for Health and Clinical Excellence (2008). *Infliximab for the treatment of adults with psoriasis (TA134).*
- ➤ Resuscitation Council (UK) (2008). *Advanced Life Support (5th edition).*

SEIZURES

Differential diagnosis

System/Organ	Disease
Neurological	Epilepsy
	Structural brain lesion e.g. post-stroke, space occupying lesion (SOL) and tumour
Cardiovascular	Seizure-type activity during syncope
	Subarachnoid haemorrhage
	Intracerebral haemorrhage
Infective	Meningitis
	Encephalitis
	Abscess
Drugs/Toxins	Alcohol
Metabolic	Disorders of glucose, calcium, sodium
	Hypoxia

Seizures consist of abnormal sudden synchronous discharge of neurons in the cerebral cortex.

Epilepsy

A chronic condition characterised by recurrent, i.e. two or more, unprovoked seizures. There is more than one type of epilepsy and they all have differences in clinical features and the way they are managed. Diagnosis is usually made by a neurologist and the history plays a major part in this.

Epidemiology

Prevalence varies around the world but it is thought to be about 10/1000 in the UK with about 600,000 people in the UK having epilepsy. The overall incidence is 50/100,000 per year with bionodal peaks in younger and older age groups. However alcohol can precipitate epilepsy at any age.

Aetiology

Primary idiopathic epilepsy is likely to have polygenic underlying cause, but this is not well understood. Chromosomal causes exist as trisomy 21 sufferers have an increased tendency to epilepsy. Single gene inheritance is also seen with tuberous sclerosis (on chromosomes 9 and 16) and neurofibromatosis (on chromosomes 17 and 22) also having an increased tendency to epilepsy.

Cerebrovascular disease is the commonest cause of adult-onset epilepsy. The risk of seizures is greater with intracerebral haemorrhage than with ischaemia but the risk is greatest with subarachnoid haemorrhage. Perinatal insults such as hypoxia can also result in epilepsy. Cerebral infections can cause immediate or delayed epilepsy. Perinatal infections include cytomegalovirus (CMV) and *Toxoplasmosis gondii* while postnatal infections include bacterial meningitis, human immunodeficiency virus (HIV), malaria and cysticercosis.

Other causes of epilepsy include:

- Trauma
- Benign or malignant intracerebral tumours
- Neurodegenerative diseases
- Metabolic/toxic, the commonest of which is alcohol, can lead to epilepsy. Although alcohol can provoke fits in Wernicke-Korsakoff syndrome, hypoglycaemia, head injury, subdural haemorrhages (SDH) and withdrawal states, chronic alcohol ingestion can also cause unprovoked seizures.

Pathophysiology

The first fit:

A single fit does not make a diagnosis of epilepsy, but does warrant careful investigation. Making the diagnosis can be difficult, and a careful history and examination needs to be conducted. Unless the fit has happened in front of you and therefore you have observed the prodrome, the seizure and the aftermath, then the key will be a witness account. You must try hard to find and contact any witnesses, and if referring on to a neurology or 'first fit' clinic, please ensure you stress the importance of taking the witness along.

If the examination, blood tests and electrocardiogram (ECG) are normal it is safe to discharge the patient and perform the rest of the investigations and consider management as an outpatient in the first fit clinic. However some red flags necessitate admission:

- More than one seizure in 24 hours
- Failure to make a full recovery
- Focal neurological signs
- Pregnancy/post-partum seizures carry a risk of being the presentation of eclampsia or cerebral venous thrombosis.
- Evidence suggestive of intracerebral sepsis.

Classification:

Epilepsy can be classified into partial and generalised. Generalised seizures involve synchronised electrical discharge in both hemispheres and these seizures always involve impairment of consciousness. Partial seizures refer to focal electrical abnormalities within a part of the brain. However partial seizures can progress to become secondarily generalised. It is important to make a specific diagnosis as treatments and prognosis differ between different subtypes (see Table 3.73).

Type of epilepsy	Subtypes
Partial Seizures	**Simple Partial:** No loss of consciousness. Flushing and sweating. Feelings of fear, panic, sadness, happiness, or feeling detached from what's going on around you. Experiencing smells and tastes. Flashbacks. 'Deja vu' and 'jamais vu'.
	Complex Partial: Impairment of consciousness. Automatisms such as chewing, swallowing and lip-smacking. Staggering around and wandering off.
	Generalised: Temporal lobe epilepsy. – may be simple, partial, complex partial (if bilateral) or become secondarily generalised.
Generalised Epilepsy	**Absence Seizures:** Sudden loss of awareness, lasting only a few seconds, sometimes many times daily. Staring, eyelid flickering is seen. Formally called 'petit mal seizures'.
	Tonic: Rhythmical shaking of limbs and head. This may be a focal or generalised epilepsy
	Clonic: Stiffness and extension of limbs and neck. This may be a focal epilepsy with focal signs or generalised
	Tonic-clonic: The 'classical' seizure whereby there is an initial clonic phase followed by a tonic phase.
	Atonic: synonymous with 'drop attacks'.

Table 3.73: The different subtypes of partial and generalised seizures.

Key features in the history/examination

Prodrome:

- What was the patient doing at the time
- Standing/sitting/lying
- Unusual behaviour
- Unusual sensations/smells/tastes/colours
- Unusual movements
- Other symptoms e.g. pallor/palpitations

Fit:

- Injuries: lateral tongue bite more specific for seizure
- Urinary incontinence
- Loss of consciousness
- Witness description of seizure

Afterwards:

- What do you remember next?
- Duration of confusion
- Any focal neurology

Important to check:

- Past history (problems with birth, cerebral infections, stroke)
- Family history
- Drug history

The examination will most likely be normal between seizures, but a full neurological examination is mandatory.

Investigations

Blood tests:

- FBC
- U&Es
- LFTs
- Glucose, magnesium and calcium levels: are important to exclude a cause for the seizure.
- Creatinine kinase (CK) levels: are usually raised post-ictally.
- Prolactin: is not a reliable indicator.

Imaging:

- CT brain: to exclude underlying structural abnormality.
- MRI brain: more sensitive to exclude an underlying structural abnormality. The National Institute for Health and Clinical Excellence (NICE) considers this to be the neuroimaging modality of choice.

Others:

- ECG: to look for underlying cardiac arrhythmia.

- Electroencephalography (EEG): The inter-ictal EEG may be normal but it may show characteristic abnormalities such as the 3 per second spike and wave pattern seen in primary generalised epilepsy. It should be used as a tool to support the diagnosis where there is clinical suspicion and to help define the subtype of epilepsy.

Management

➢ Multidisciplinary management involving a Nurse Specialist, Consultant neurologist and General Practitioner (GP)

➢ Information and education to patients and their relatives in verbal and written form

➢ Patients should be empowered and involved in treatment decisions, and a management plan agreed.

➢ Information should be given about the possible side-effects of medications and the importance to withdraw them only under medical supervision.

➢ There are many on-line resources e.g. Epilepsy Action that patients may find useful.

➢ Advice needs to be given about driving. The patient needs to be informed that it is their responsibility to inform the Driver and Vehicle Licensing Agency (DVLA) and refrain from driving. This is best done in front of a witness and must be clearly documented in the medical notes.

➢ For an 'incidental' seizure on the ward in a known epileptic, it may be normal for them but it is important to ensure safety and privacy during the fit. Only intervene if the seizure is prolonged or unusual for them. This emphasises the importance of taking a good history, even if seizures are not the presenting complaint.

Pharmacological treatments:

Drug treatments should almost always be initiated and monitored by a specialist. Different medications are preferred in different subtypes of epilepsy and once interactions and side-effect profiles are taken into consideration, the precise management will be tailored to the individual. This has been shown in recent trials such as the 'Study of Standard and New Anti-Epileptic Drugs (SANAD), 2007'. Some examples of the current practice are:

➢ Partial seizures: Carbamazepine, Lamotrigine, Valproate

➢ Absence seizures: Lamotrigine, Valproate

➢ Tonic-clonic: Valproate, Lamotrigine, Carbamazepine, Levetiracetam, Phenytoin

Side-effects of pharmacological treatments:

All anti-epileptic drugs (AEDs) cause side-effects that range from trivial to serious. Patients should be made aware of these during discussions about management options.

➢ Common, non-specific: nausea and vomiting, diarrhoea and rash as well as ataxia and nystagmus in toxicity.

➢ Induction of the cytochrome P450 enzymes with Phenytoin, Carbamazepine and Phenobarbital. This is especially important

in patients taking Warfarin, Theophylline and the oral contraceptive pill (OCP).

➢ Carbamazapine: diplopia in toxicity

➢ Lamotrigine: Stevens-Johnson syndrome

➢ Phenytoin: gum hypertrophy

➢ Vigabatrin: visual field defects

Withdrawal of pharmacological treatments:

➢ This should always be done under the supervision of a specialist team.

➢ Should be done slowly and one drug at a time

➢ Risk of recurrence of seizures is greatest in the first six months and in the presence of a structural brain lesion.

➢ Again patients must be warned about stopping driving and referred to the DVLA guidelines.

Status epilepticus:

Classically defined as a seizure lasting longer than 30 minutes, or a series of seizures without regaining consciousness in between. However, since most seizures last less than two minutes there has recently been a move to define a seizure lasting longer than five minutes as impending status and treat. Status epilepticus is a medical emergency which, without prompt, effective treatment, carries a significant mortality. The longer the seizure is allowed to continue, the more refractory to treatment they become and the higher the risk of morbidity. The management would usually involve:

➢ Rapid A to E assessment, ensuring patent airway and intravenous (IV) access

➢ Local policies may differ, but a typical sequence of medications might be:

1. Lorazepam (or Diazepam) stat IV
2. Valproate, Phenytoin or Phenobarbitone IV infusion
3. Paraldehyde intramuscular (IM).
4. General anaesthetic

➢ IV glucose if hypoglycaemic

➢ Thiamine IV if alcohol is thought to be contributory

➢ Blood tests as stated in the investigations and also AED levels and arterial blood gas (ABG).

➢ Urine toxicology if appropriate

Pregnancy and epilepsy:

➢ Women of childbearing age should be given information in advance of commencing AED treatment.

➢ Many AEDs are enzyme-inducers and reduce the efficacy of oral contraceptive agents, in particular the progesterone only pill, so contraception failure is more likely.

➢ The risk of seizure-associated mortality is increased during pregnancy and the there is a 50% infant and 30% maternal mortality with status epilepticus. AEDs should therefore be continued during pregnancy.

> Pregnancy is related to an increase in seizure frequency. This is in part due to the fall in the levels of some AED during the second and third trimesters. This is particularly important with Lamotrigine.

> AEDs are linked to congenital malformations e.g. neural tube defects with Valproate use and a reduced IQ in childhood again, especially with Valproate

> Give folic acid supplementation

> Give vitamin K during the last four weeks of pregnancy

> Encourage registration with the UK Epilepsy and Pregnancy Register which aims to collate information about the frequency of major malformations in children whose mothers take AEDs.

> If status epilepticus occurs during labour an emergency caesarean section should be performed.

> Remember to reduce the dose of AEDs in post-partum if the dose had been increased during pregnancy.

> AEDs are found in breast milk but this should not be seen as a contraindication during breast-feeding.

Prognosis:

Epilepsy is a chronic condition which requires sensitive multidisciplinary management in view of the social implications, multiple side-effects of medications and issues around pregnancy.

It is associated with a raised standard mortality ratio (SMR), especially in the under 40s and those with severe epilepsy. This is thought to be due to:

> Sudden Unexplained Death in Epilepsy (SUDEP). The mechanism of this is not understood. Male sex and poor medication concordance increase the risk but it is not seen in idiopathic epilepsy in childhood.

> Accidental death e.g. trauma and drowning.

> Suicide, especially in severe and temporal lobe epilepsy.

Further reading and references

> Drivers Medical Group DVLA (2009). *At a glance guide to the current medical standards of fitness to drive.* Swansea.

> www.epilepsyandpregnancy.co.uk

> www.epilepsy.org.uk

> National Institute for Health and Clinical Excellence (2004). *The epilepsies: diagnosis and management of the epilepsies in adults in primary and secondary care (CG020).*

> Marson et al. (2007). The SANAD study. *Lancet* 369: 1000–1015.

WEAKNESS AND PARALYSIS

Differential Diagnosis

System/Organ	Disease
Common	**Stroke/Transient Ischaemic Attack**
	Multiple Sclerosis
	Guillain-Barré syndrome
	Motor Neurone Disease
	Myasthenia gravis
	Spinal cord compression/Trauma
Other	Vitamin deficiency
	Hyponatraemia
	Hypocalcaemia

Stroke/transient ischaemic attack

Stroke is now universally preferred to the terms 'cerebrovascular accident' or 'CVA', which now should not be used.

World Health Organization define Stroke as 'a clinical syndrome consisting of rapidly developing clinical signs of focal (or global in case of coma) disturbance of cerebral function lasting more than 24 hours or leading to death with no apparent cause other than a vascular origin.'

Transient ischaemic attack (TIA) has been traditionally defined as a focal neurological impairment lasting less than 24 hours, however it has been increasingly recognised that a cut-off of 1 hour is more appropriate.

Epidemiology

150,000 people per year have a stroke in the UK (approximately one every five minutes). It is the third biggest cause of death in the UK. With 900,000 people living in the UK with a disability related to stroke it is the most common cause of disability.

It is estimated that in England the annual incidence of TIA is 150–200 per 100,000 per year, however this is likely to be an underestimate as a number will go either unnoticed or unreported.

Stroke and TIA predominantly affects those over 65 but 1,000 people under the age of 30 suffer a stroke per year. One in four women and one in five men will have a stroke if they live to be 85.

Aetiology

There are two types of strokes; as shown in Table 3.74 below.

3. Medicine

	Ischaemic (85–90%)	Haemorrhagic (10–15%)
Modifiable risk factors	Smoking Hypertension Diabetes mellitus Hyperlipidaemia Atrial fibrillation Valvular heart disease Coagulopathy (e.g. antiphospholipid syndrome, Systemic Lupus Erythematosus (SLE)	Smoking Hypertension Diabetes mellitus Alcohol excess Drug treatments – i.e. anticoagulants
Unmodifiable risk factors	Increasing age Race – African, Asian, Afro-Caribbean Previous history of stroke/TIAIncreasing age	Amyloid angiopathy Race – African, Asian, Afro-Caribbean Berry aneurysms Arterio-venous malformation

Table 3.74: Risk factors for ischaemic and haemorrhagic stroke.

Pathophysiology

Acute ischaemic stroke is caused by a thrombosis, either from rupture of atherosclerotic plaque or from an embolus (e.g. caused by atrial fibrillation or carotid artery plaque). Both of these lead to an occlusion in an intracranial artery (most commonly the middle cerebral artery) causing ischaemia. An ischaemic stroke may also occur at a 'watershed' area between the distribution of 2 cerebral arteries (typically the middle and posterior) following a period of hypotension causing hypoperfusion of these areas. Haemorrhagic stroke is caused by vascular rupture leading to bleeding into either the subarachnoid space or an intra-paranchymal haemorrhage. An infarct may show 'haemorrhagic transformation' whereby the initial infarct triggers a secondary haemorrhage.

TIA shares a common aetiology and pathophysiology with ischaemic stroke.

Key features in the history/examination

- Time and date of onset of symptoms
- Duration of symptoms
- Risk factors for cerebrovascular disease
- Contraindications to thrombolysis
- Premorbid level of social functioning, e.g. walking, washing and dressing, existing care package
- Left or right handedness
- General examination
  - Pulse rate and rhythm
  - Cardiac murmurs
  - Neck Bruits
    - Peripheral pulses
    - Fundoscopy
- Gait
- Mini mental state examination if indicated
- Examine stroke using National Institute Health Stroke Scale (see Table 3.75)
- Examine TIA using the ABCD2 score (Table 3.76)
- Full detailed neurological examination required as a wide range of neurological findings may be present dependent on location of stroke (refer to Mini-CEX chapter)
- Examination will need to be repeated to document any recovery
- Strokes are commonly classified clinically using the Bamford/Oxford Community Stroke Project Classification (Table 3.77)

Item	Score range
Level of consciousness (LOC)	0–3
1a.LOC questions	0–2
1b.LOC commands	0–2
Best Gaze	0–2
Visual fields	0–3
Facial weakness	0–3
Motor arm	0–4 (right and left)
Motor leg	0–4 (right and left)
Limb ataxia	0–2
Sensory loss	0–2
Body Language	0–3
Dysarthria	0–2
Extinction and inattention	0–2

Table 3.75: National Institutes of Health Stroke scale items.

A	Age	> 59	1 point
B	BP on presentation	Systolic >139 mmHg or Diastolic >89 mmHg	1 point
C	Clinical Features	Unilateral weakness	2 points
		Speech disturbance without weakness	1 point
		Other	0 point
D	Duration	>59 minutes	2 points
		10–59 minutes	1 point
		<10 minutes	0 point
D	Diabetes	Presence	1 point

Table 3.76: ABCD2 Score.

OCSP	Clinical features	Vascular basis
Total Anterior Circulation Syndrome **20% of strokes**	Higher cortical dysfunction (visual neglect or dysphasia) and Hemiparesis in at least 2 of face/arm/leg and Homonymous hemianopia	Usually proximal middle cerebral artery or internal carotid artery
Partial Anterior Circulation Syndrome **35% of strokes**	Isolated higher cortical dysfunction or 2 out of: higher cortical dysfunction, hemiparesis, homonymous hemianopia	Usually branch middle cerebral artery occlusion
Posterior Circulation Syndrome **25% of strokes**	Isolated homonymous hemianopia or Brain stem (cranial nerve palsies). May have contralateral motor/sensory deficit Bilateral motor/sensory deficit or Cerebellar signs	Occlusion of vertebral, basilar, cerebellar or posterior cerebral artery
Lacunar Syndrome **20% of strokes**	Pure motor stroke or Pure sensory stroke or Sensorimotor stroke or Ataxic hemiparesis May be 'silent' and asymptomatic	Usually thrombosis occluding a smaller, deeper artery

Table 3.77: Bamford/Oxford Community Stroke Project Classification.

Sensori motor signs:

- Unilateral upper and lower limb weakness and facial drooping are indicative of stroke (One, two or all three of these may be present)
- Test for pronator drift
- Unilateral sensory impairment in upper and lower limb or face

Speech signs:

- Aphasia
- Dysphasia (expressive or receptive)
- Dysarythria

Opthalmic signs:

- Eye movements

- Visual neglect
- Partial visual field loss

Cerebellar signs:

- Ataxia
- Nystagmus
- Past-pointing
- Dysdiadochokinesis

The National Institutes of Health Stroke Scale has been developed to model the severity of the stroke. It is used in some clinical practice (e.g. The National Hospital for Neurology and Neurosurgery) as well as in research.

Investigations

Blood tests:

- FBC
- ESR
- U&Es
- LFTs
- Bone profile
- Thyroid function test (TFT)
- Glucose: to exclude hypoglycaemia as cause of symptoms
- Lipid profile
- If no clear cause for the stroke, especially in the younger age group, check thrombophilia screen, vasculitis and antiphospholipid screen and haemoglobin electrophoresis for sickle cell anaemia. Consider HIV testing with appropriate coinsetting

Imaging:

- Chest X-Ray

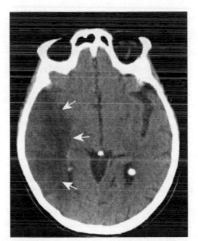

Figure 3.57: Non-contrast CT head showing a large area of hypo density in the Right temporo-parietal lobe (arrows) in keeping with an acute ischaemic infarct in the middle cerebral artery territory.

3. Medicine

- CT brain: to identify aetiology of stroke (see Table 3.74). An acute infarct may not be clearly visible.
- MRI brain may be required in cases of diagnostic doubt and especially in cases of brainstem stroke
- Carotid dopplers

Others:

- ECG – to check for dysrhythmia such as atrial fibrillation
- Echocardiography – this may be a 'bubble ECHO' to exclude a patent Foramen Ovale, especially if no risk factors found for stroke
- 24-hour tape if paroxysmal arrhythmia suspected

Management

Acute management of Ischaemic Stroke:

- A to E assessment
- Avoid use of oxygen therapy unless oxygen saturations are less than 94%
- Thrombolysis using alteplase following local policy – if onset of symptoms within three hours and no contraindications for thrombolysis. This may involve transport to a tertiary thrombolysis centre.

Acute management of haemorrhagic stroke:

- A to E assessment
- Avoid use of oxygen therapy unless oxygen saturations are less than 94%
- Discuss CT scan with Neuro-surgery – occasionally may be indication for surgical intervention. More often neurosurgeons will treat underlying cause such as arteriovenous malformations.

Acute Management of TIA:

- There will be a local protocol for the precise pathway to follow in the Emergency Department. Broadly:
- If ABCD2 score 3 or less, refer as outpatient to TIA clinic for investigation
- If ABCD2 score 4 or more, admit for urgent investigations
  - o This will include carotid Doppler (if appropriate) as the evidence suggests the earlier a carotid endarterectomy is performed, the greater the benefit

All patients with stroke are best managed on a multidisciplinary Stroke unit, which has proven to result in reduced death and disability. Interventions should include:

- Swallow assessment– if suspicious of a swallowing deficit, this should be initially assessed during the initial clerking procedure, and onward referral made to Speech and Language therapy (SLT) if required.
- Early mobilisation
- Early involvement of physiotherapy

- Early nutritional assessment and consideration of naso-gastric feeding if required
- Early detection and correction of physiological derangements – i.e. pyrexia
- Early discharge planning in a multidisciplinary setting.

A stroke can be a traumatic an upsetting experience for the patient and family. They will need sensitive support to understand the diagnosis and its implications, especially if the patient remains severely disabled by the stroke.

- Verbal and written information should be given about the diagnosis
- The patient and family should be involved as much as possible in treatment, goal-setting and discharge planning.
- Details of the stroke association and other national and local support groups should be given.

Secondary prevention – Stroke and TIA:

- Lifestyle changes including smoking cessation, exercise and weight loss
- Antiplatelet treatment: aspirin (clopidrogel in aspirin sensitivity) +/– dipyridamole.
- Lower blood pressure: follow British Hypertensive Society guidelines
- Lower cholesterol
- Consider anticoagulation with warfarin if atrial fibrillation cause of ischaemic stroke
- Carotid Doppler followed by carotid endarterectomy if indicated

Prognosis:

- TIA – overall risk of progression to full stroke within 3 months is 11% but is dependant on the ABCD2 score

ABCD2 Score	7 day mortality	3 month mortality
0–3	1%	3%
4–5	6%	10%
6–7	12%	18%

Table 3.78: 7 day and 3 month mortality according to ABCD2 score.

- Stroke – varies according to the clinical stroke syndrome as well as co-morbidities

	TACS		PACS		LACS		POCS	
	30 day	1 year	30 day	1 year	30 day	1 year	30 day	1 year
Death	40	60	5	15	5	10	5	20
Dependent	55	35	40	30	40	30	30	20
Independent	5	5	55	55	65	60	65	60

Table 3.79: Percentage mortality and morbidity post stroke, from the Bamford classification.

> ➢ Haemorrhagic – significantly higher mortality and morbidity than ischaemic stroke

Multiple Sclerosis

Epidemiology

Multiple sclerosis (MS) is predominantly a disease of young adults with a mean age of onset 29–33 years old. It affects more women than men with a male:female ratio of 3:2. There is a prevalence of 110 per 100,000 in UK and it is more common in Caucasians. 67% of patients present with relapsing remitting illness, 5–10% have benign disease course with infrequent relapses and 11% of patients have a gradual disease progression from outset.

Aetiology

MS is an auto-immune disease effecting the white matter in central nervous system (CNS) thought to be triggered by genetic and environmental factors. It is 20–40% more common in first degree relatives. Genes in Human Leucocyte Antigen and Interleukin region are thought to be involved.

Environmental factors implicated:

* Toxins
* Viral exposure – although none have been found to be causative
* Sunlight exposure

A diagnosis of MS is not made on the first presentation of focal demyelination. The first episode is considered a clinically isolated syndrome, a diagnosis of MS requires subsequent relapses involving different parts of the CNS. The exception is where radiology imaging demonstrates temporal and anatomical dispersal of demyelination. Refer to modified McDonald Criteria Table 3.80.

Relapses may be triggered by infections, post-partum changes, surgical procedures, trauma and stress.

Three clinical patterns of MS are recognised:

* Relapsing and remitting (80%)
* Secondary progressive
* Primary progressive

Pathophysiology

Relapsing remitting MS is believed to be an autoimmune disease mediated by T-cells against the myelin sheath although it appears that B-cells also play a part.

CD4 T cells become activated in the peripheral blood system and migrate across the blood-brain barrier where they react with the myelin sheath. This reaction causes the release of cytokines which activates macrophages and B-cells that cause inflammation and leads to the destruction of oligodendrocytes with demyelination of the axons.

Destruction of the myelin sheath leads to slowing in nerve conduction which leads to symptoms of relapse. Inflammation eventually subsides and sheaths remyelinate. However the axons do not completely recover and over time the axons may die, leaving progressive neurological deficits (secondary progressive disease).

Key features in the history/examination

There are a wide range of signs and symptoms dependent on the site of inflammation in the brain or spinal cord and residual physical dysfunction following previous relapses.

* Fatigue
* Weakness
* Clumsiness
* Visual disturbances
* Dizziness
* Poorly defined paraesthesiae
* 50% of patients present with weakness or numbness in one or more limb
* 25% with optic neuritis
* L'hermitte phenomenon – electric shock sensations in spine, arms or legs following flexion of neck
* Internuclear ophthalmoplegia may be present
* Optic atropy – optic disc pallor, decreased visual acuity, decreased colour vision, relative afferent papillary defect and central scotoma
* Diplopia
* Spasticity

Investigations

Blood tests:

* Baseline FBC, U&Es, LFTs
* ESR and CRP
* ANA, ANCA, Rheumatoid Factor, ENA and Anti-dsDNA
* TFTs
* B12
* Antiphospholipid and anti-cardiolipin antibodies

Imaging:

* MRI brain and spinal cord: are most important diagnostic test. Multiple hyperdense regions are seen, usually in the periventricular white matter, especially on the FLAIR sequences (see Figure 3.58).

Others:

* Lumbar Puncture: determine CSF cell count, protein and oligoclonal IgG (present in 98% of patients with MS)
* EEG: delayed visual evoked potentials demonstrated in 80–90% of patients

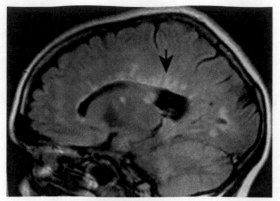

Figure 3.58: MRI of the brain showing increased finger like inflammatory changes in the periventricular white matter in keeping with multiple sclerosis.

Clinical presentation	Additional data needed
2+ relapses and evidence of 2+ objective lesions on MRI	None
1 relapse and evidence of 1 objective lesion on MRI	Positive CSF and 2+ lesions demonstrated on MRI or a further relapse
Insidious neurological progression suggestive of MS	Positive CSF and MRI evidence of: 9+ lesions in brain or 2+ lesions in spinal cord or 4–8 lesions in brain and 1 lesion in spinal cord

Table 3.80: Modified McDonald Criteria

Management

➢ Patient education, empowerment and participation in the decision-making process

➢ Support for patient, family and carers

➢ Provide information about support groups for instance the Multiple Sclerosis Society.

➢ Multidisciplinary involvement:

Neurologist	Physiotherapy
Occupational Therapist	Nurse specialist
Pain team	Psychologist

Acute exacerbations: corticosteroids (typically 0.5–1.0 g Methylprednisolone) either orally or IV.

Symptom treatment:

➢ Depression: selective serotonin reuptake inhibitor (Citalopram), selective serotonin norepinephrine reuptake inhibitor (Venlafaxine), tricyclic antidepressant (Amitriptyline)

➢ Pain: Gabapentin, Pregabalin, Amitriptyline

➢ Spasticity: Baclofen, Dantrolene, Diazepam, Tizanidine, Botulinum toxin, physiotherapy

➢ Bladder disturbance: Oxybutanin, Tolterodine, catherisation

➢ Tremor: Clonazepam, Primidone

➢ Erectile dysfunction: Sildenafil

Disease modification treatment:

➢ NICE guidelines recommend Nataluzimab for rapidly evolving and severe relapsing remitting MS- reduces relapses by 68%.

➢ NICE guidelines do not recommend the uses of interferon-beta and glatiramer acetate.

➢ In aggressive diseases that do not respond to Nataluzimab other immunosupressents may be used such as Cyclophosphamide.

Prognosis

The prognosis is improving with aggressive treatment of relapses, but it is still the case that ten years after diagnosis, 10% of patients are wheelchair-bound and around half are inable to maintain employment.

Guillain-Barré (Acute Inflammatory Demyelinating Polyradiculopathy)

Epidemiology

This is the most common neuromuscular cause of paralysis. There is a prevalence 1-2/100,000 per year with males being affected more than females. There are bimodal age peaks at 15–35 and 50–75.

Aetiology

Two thirds of patients have a history of recent gastro-intestinal or respiratory infection in proceeding 1–3 weeks. Infections include:

• *Camplyobacter jejuni*

• Heptatis B

• Cytalomegavirus

• *Mycoplasm pneumoniae*

• Epstein-barr virus

• Varicella-zoster

• HIV

Other risk factors include post-partum, malignancies such as lymphoma and vaccinations.

Pathophysiology

Cellular and humoral immune mechanisms are implicated in the development of the syndrome. It is proposed that the preceding infection leads to a production of antibodies to specific gangliosides and glycolipids. Antibodies react with myelin to cause demyelination.

Key features in the history/examination

- A rapidly progressive ascending weakness
- Weakness reported in 60% of cases in 1–3 weeks following infection reaching its peak at around 4 weeks after onset
- May report back pain or leg pain
- Reports of sensory loss starting in lower limbs
- Reports of paralysis starting in lower limbs
- Dyspnoea
- Shortness of breath
- The motor signs predominate the examination
- Ascending and symmetrical weakness varying in severity from minimal, to tetraplegia with respiratory paralysis.
- Hypotonia
- Absent or reduced reflexes
- Numbness or altered sensation, objective examination tends to find minimal changes
- Facial weakness

Autonomic changes can include the following:

- Tachycardia
- Bradycardia
- Facial flushing
- Paroxysmal hypertension
- Orthostatic hypotension
- Anhidrosis and/or diaphoresis

Respiratory muscle involvement, 40% of patients present with respiratory or oropharyngeal weakness:

- Dyspnoea
- Shortness of breath
- Slurred speech
- Dysphagia

Investigations

Blood tests:

- FBC
- U&Es
- Inflammatory markers – CRP and ESR
- Anti-GQ1b if Miller-Fisher variant suspected

Microbiology:

- If any evidence of ongoing infection, send relevant samples

Imaging:

- MRI (usually if diagnostic doubt)

Other:

- ECG: variety of arrhythmias
- Lumbar puncture: CSF will show elevated protein (may be absent in first week of disease)
- Nerve conduction studies
- Spirometry: vital capacity measurements govern the need for ventilation

Management

- ➤ Intubation and assisted ventilation in patients with respiratory weakness and paralysis necessary in around 30% of patients
- ➤ Plasma exchange – two to five session in a non-ambulant patient
- ➤ Immunoglobulin infusion – treatment of choice
- ➤ Intravenous Methylprednisolone in conjunction with immunoglobulin infusion may be used although studies have shown to be of no benefit

Recognition, treatment and prevention of complications are as important as any treatment:

- ➤ Monitor forced vital capacity 4 hourly (<15 ml/Kg indication for ventilation)
- ➤ DVT prophylaxis – anti-embolism stockings and low molecular weight heparin
- ➤ Physiotherapy
- ➤ Occupational Therapist
- ➤ Speech and language therapy for swallow assessment
- ➤ Pain – non-steriodal anti-inflammatory drugs, amitriptyline, carbamazepine, gabapentin, opiates

Prognosis:

- ➤ Mortality of 5%

Motor Neurone Disease

Epidemiology

This is a relatively rare disease with approximately 5,000 cases in the UK at any one time. There is increased risk with age and the incidence is highest between the ages 55 to 75. Motor neurone disease (MND) is 50% more common in males than females.

Aetiology

The cause and pathology behind MND is not very well understood. It is thought to be due to interplay between genetics and exogenous factors. Familial MND tends to have an earlier onset and about 20% of cases have mutations in the copper/zinc superoxide dismutase gene. Other genetic variants have been found but only in very small numbers.

Potential environmental factors

- Physical activity

- Smoking
- Mechanical and electrical injury
- Exposure to neurotoxins
- Occupations – farmer, military service, professional football

The symptoms of MND are caused by degeneration of Betz cells, pyramidal tracts, cranial nerve nuclei and anterior horn cells.

Type	Features
Amyotrophic lateral sclerosis (ALS)	75% of cases
	50% progress to bulbar
	Mixed upper and lower motor neurone clinical features starting in limbs
Progressive bulbar palsy (PBP)	20% of cases
	Most common in older women
	Poor prognosis
Progressive muscular atrophy (PMA)	5% of cases
	Lower motor neurone signs at onset
	More significantly common in men than women
	Over 50 years at onset
	Possible slower disease progress
Primary lateral sclerosis (PLS)	0.5% of cases
	Upper motor neurone signs at onset, often starting in lower limbs
	50% convert to ALS
	Survival over 10 years is common
Flail arm syndrome	Rare
	Proximal lower motor neurone weakness of arms
Flail leg syndrome	Rare
	Lower motor neurone weakness of legs

Table 3.81: The different types of MND.

Pathophysiology

Pathophysiology is dependent on the aetiology.

Key features in history/examination

Lower limb onset:

- Difficulty in walking
- Unsteadiness
- Foot drop
- Tendency to stumble
- Heaviness
- Stiffness in one or more limb

Upper limb onset:

- Loss of functional hand dexterity
- Poor grip
- Proximal arm weakness
- Muscle wasting particularly in the hands
- Fascilations especially of the large proximal limbs

Bulbar onset:

- Dysarthria
- Dysphonia with nasal, hoarse or tight voice
- Dysphagia

Respiratory onset:

- Breathlessness
- Orthopnea
- Hypercapnic features from overnight hypoventilation fatigue, reduced exercise tolerance, hypersomnolence and morning headaches

On examination concurrent upper motor neurone and lower motor neurone signs in the absence of sensory impairment or pain are suggestive of MND. However any combination of motor neurone signs may be elicited.

Upper motor neurone signs:

- Hypotonia
- Brisk reflexes
- Extensor plantar responses

Lower Motor Neurone signs:

- Muscle wasting
- Fasciculations
- Reduced/absent reflexes

Typically examination findings include:

- Wasting of tibialis anterior
- Wasting of small muscles of hands particularly first dorsal interosseous and thenar eminence
- Claw-like hand due to weakness of finer and wrist extensors
- Foot drop due to weak ankle dorsiflexion

No sensory signs are found

Investigations

Blood tests:

- CK: often up to four times normal level
- TFTs: to rule out hyperthyroidism and hyperparathyroidism which can mimic MND

- Serology: to rule out HIV and Lyme disease as both can mimic MND

Imaging:

- MRI: for upper motor neurone signs

Other:

- Lumbar puncture: in atypical presentation to exclude inflammatory or infiltrative disease
- Electromyography (EMG): can demonstrate the extent of the disease

Management

➤ Patient education, empowerment and participation in the decision-making process

➤ Information about support groups e.g. the Motor Neurone Disease Association.

➤ Requires multi-disciplinary approach likely to need input from:

Nurse specialists	Physiotherapy
Occupational Therapist	Speech and Language therapy
Dieticians	Respiratory physicians
Gastroenterologists	Palliative care team

Respiratory support:

➤ Non-Invasive Ventilation to support and prevent hypoventilation, less effective if poor bulbar function

➤ Early intervention found to be most effective

➤ Signs required are nocturnal desaturation, hypercapnia and forced vital capacity less than 50%

Nutritional Support:

Signs suggestive of need for intervention

➤ Aspiration

➤ Continued weight loss

➤ Choking episodes

➤ Tiring whilst eating

➤ Gastrostomy

➤ Discussed early if have bulbar symptoms

➤ Ideally performed when forced vital capacity is greater than 50%

➤ Pharmacology: Riluzole

  o NICE recommend for ALS form, often given for all forms

  o Prolongs survival by at least 3 months

  o Requires regular monitoring of liver function

Symptom relief:

➤ *Paroxysmal choking/laryngospasm:* sublingual lorazepam and positioning

➤ *Dyspnoea:* oral or nebulised morphine, sublingual lorazepam in conjunction with NIV

➤ *Difficulty coughing and clearing secretions:* nebulised saline, carbocysteine. Ensure adequate fluid intake. Suction and cough assist devices.

➤ *Spasticity:* baclofen, dantrolene, tizanidine

➤ *Cramps and fasciculations:* quinine, carbemazepine, diazepam and physiotherapy

➤ *Drooling:* hyoscine patch, amitriptyline, atropine, botulinum toxin to salivary glands

➤ *Constipation:* lactulose, docusate, movicol. Ensure adequate fibre and fluid

➤ *Emotional lability:* amitriptyline, SSRI

Prognosis:

➤ Variable from a number of months to 10 years

➤ Majority of patients survive 2–3 years from diagnosis

➤ Poor prognosis is linked to age at onset and respiratory or bulbar presentation

Myasthenia gravis

Epidemiology

The Incidence of Myasthenia gravis is about 10/100,000 per year. There is a bimodal distribution for age with a peak in the twenties (early onset) and a peak in the sixties (late onset). The early onset is more common in females whereas the late onset is more common in men.

Aetiology

Myasthenia gravis possibly has a genetic link. 75% of patients have some form of thymus abnormality and 50% of thymoma patients have Myasthenia gravis. Interestingly, Penicillin may induce or aggravate the disease.

There is a link to diabetes mellitus, thyrotoxicosis, rheumatoid arthritis and SLE. However most cases are idiopathic.

Pathophysiology

Majority of patients have auto-antibodies against the acetylcholine nicotinic post synaptic receptor (AChR). These actions reduce the number of receptors and block the sodium ion channel which leads to a reduction in neurotransmission and therefore fatiguable muscle weakness. Patients become symptomatic once acetylcholine receptors are reduced to 30%. It is thought that the thymus is the site of generation of auto-antibodies but it is not known what stimulates the production of these auto-antibodies.

Key features in the history/examination

- Generalised weakness
- Reduced exercise tolerance that improves with rest
- Initially symptoms may be intermittent occurring after repeated use of the muscle
- Full and accurate medication history – many medications may provoke exacerbations

Antibiotics	Macrolides
	Fluroquinolones
	Aminoglycaside
	Tetracycline
	Chloroquine
Anti-arrhythmic	Beta-blockers
	Calcium channel blockers
	Quinidine
	Lignocaine
	Procainamide
	Trimethaphan
Other	Lithium
	Chlorpromazine
	Muscle relaxants
	Levothyroxine
	Adrenocorticotropic hormone (ACTH)
	Corticosteroids

Table 3.82: Medications reported to exacerbate Myasthenia gravis.

- On examination 85% of patients have ptosis and diplopia (caused by a complex opthalmoplegia)
- The key element is the fatigueability: ask the patient to look upwards at your outstretched finger. The patient's eyelids will slowly droop over a few minutes as the muscles fatigue
- May have facial muscle involvement
  - Mild cases – weakness of eye or lip closure
  - Severe cases – may have expressionless face with slack muscles
- Neck muscle weakness may be present
- Limbs may have proximal rather than distal weakness
- Severe presentations may have bulbar and respiratory involvement
- Severe exacerbations:
  - Lack of tone in whole body
  - Unable to lift head from chest

  - Nasal quality to voice
  - Slack, expressionless face
  - Absence of gag reflex
  - Lack of cough and presence of pneumonia

Investigations

Blood tests:

- Serology: antibodies to AChR present in 50% of ocular patients, 85% of general patients

Imaging:

- CT: to check for thymus abnormality

Others:

- Electrophysiology: testing the reduction in evoked action potential following repetitive nerve stimulation to assist in the diagnosis. Increased 'jitter' seen in single fibre studies
- Tensilon test is rarely performed

Management

➤ Pyridostigmine: an acetylcholinesterase inhibitor

➤ Prednisolone: commencing may exacerbate symptoms so treatment should be started as an inpatient if bulbar or respiratory symptoms present

➤ May require other immunosuppression/steroid sparing agents e.g. azathioprine

➤ Thymectomy

Spinal Cord Compression

Epidemiology

Worldwide, trauma is the most common cause of spinal chord compression. There are 4,000 cases of metastatic spinal cord compression per year in the UK. 85% of spinal cord tumours are metastatic. Spinal epidural abscess is found in 2.8 cases per 10,000 admissions which is increasing due to increased intravenous drug use. Osteoporosis is the commonest cause of vertebral fractures leading to spinal cord compression.

Aetiology

Can occur as a result of:

- Spinal cord trauma
- Disc herniation
- Vertebral compression fracture
- Spinal tumour – either primary or metastatic
- Infection

Commonest causes of Vertebral compression fractures	Common tumours metastasising to bone	Infections
Osteoporosis	Breast	Discitis
Osteomyelitis	Bronchus	Pott's disease (Tuberculosis of spine)
Pathological fractures	Prostate	
Corticosteroid therapy (secondary osteoporosis)	Renal	Epidural abscess
Spinal subluxation		
Osteomalacia		

Table 3.83: Common causes of spinal compression.

Pathophysiology

Compression of the spinal cord is caused by either stretching (i.e. spinal cord subluxation) or pressure (i.e. tumour, disc herniation). Both lead to damage to the myelinated tracts and cell bodies in the spinal cord. The subsequent damage leads to reduction or cessation of sensation and motor functions.

Key features in history/examination

- Acute onset suggestive of trauma or disc herniation
- Chronic onset suggestive of malignancy or osteoporosis
- History of:
  - o primary tumour that metastasises to bone
  - o bone metastases
  - o intravenous drug use
- Numbness
- Parathesias – may be mild in early chronic forms
- Bladder and bowel dysfunction
- Signs of neurogenic shock may be present on examination in acute presentations
  - o Hypotension
  - o Bradycardia
  - o Warm, dry extremities
  - o Peripheral vasodilation
  - o Poikilothermia
  - o Decreased cardiac output
- Loss of motor function and sensation distal to the spinal level
- May have local deformity of spine
- Spinal tenderness may be present
- Hyper-reflexia

Investigations

Blood tests:

- FBC: to check for signs of infection

- ESR and CRP
- Bone profile

Microbiology:

- Blood cultures if infection is suspected
- Lumbar puncture if infection is suspected

Imaging:

- Chest X-ray: to rule out lung primary
- Spinal X-ray: to check for vertebral fracture
- CT spine
- MRI spine

Management

- ➢ Stabilisation and supportive treatment

Acute traumatic spinal cord injury:

- ➢ Immobilisation
- ➢ Decompression and stabilisation
- ➢ Corticosteroids – usually dexamethasone
- ➢ Prevention of further complications (DVT prophylaxis, gastric ulcer prophylaxis, physiotherapy)

Malignancy related options:

- ➢ Surgery to decompress
- ➢ Radiotherapy to shrink tumour
- ➢ Corticosteroids – usually dexamethasone
- ➢ Prevention of further complications (DVT prophylaxis, gastric ulcer prophylaxis, physiotherapy)
- ➢ Treatments may be combined or used on their own

Infection related:

- ➢ Antibiotics based on sensitivity of organism. Most effective if continued to 12 weeks
- ➢ Surgery
- ➢ Prevention of further complications (DVT prophylaxis, gastric ulcer prophylaxis, physiotherapy)

Prognosis:

- ➢ Malignancy related recurrence rate of 7–9% with multiple metastases increasing the risk
- ➢ Infection related: there is no reported risk of recurrence

Further reading and references

- ➢ Bamford J. Sandercock P, Dennis M et al. (1991) Classification and natural history of clinically identifiable subtypes of cerebral infarction. *Lancet* 337: 1521–6
- ➢ British Thoracic Society and Society of Cardiothoracic Surgeons

of Great Britain and Ireland Working Party; (2001) Guidelines on the selection of patients with lung cancer for surgery. *Thorax* 56: 89–108

➤ Johnson SC, Rothwell, PM, Nguyen-Huynh MN et al; (2007) Validation and refinement of scores to predict very early stroke risk after transient ischaemic attack. *Lancet* 369: 283–92

➤ www.mndassociation.org

➤ www.mssociety.org.uk

➤ National Institute for Health and Clinical Excellence (2002). *Multiple sclerosis – beta interferon and glatiramer acetate: guidance (TA32).*

➤ National Institute for Health and Clinical Excellence (2003). *Multiple Sclerosis (CG08).*

➤ National Institute for Health and Clinical Excellence (2007). *Alteplase for the treatment of acute ischaemic stroke (TA122)*

➤ National Institute for Health and Clinical Excellence (2007). *Multiple sclerosis – natalizumab (TA127).*

➤ National Institute for Health and Clinical Excellence. *Guidance of the use of Riluzole (Rilutek) for the treatment of Motor Neurone Disease. (TA20).*

➤ The Royal College of Physicians (2008). *National clinical guideline for stroke – (3rd Ed)*

➤ www.stroke.org.uk

➤ World Health Organisation (1978). Cerebrovascular Disorders (Offset Publications). Geneva

ACUTE ABDOMINAL PAIN

Differential diagnosis

System	Disease
Gastrointestinal	**Peptic ulcer disease**
	Acute intestinal obstruction
	Diverticulitis
	Colon cancer
	Acute appendicitis
	Meckel's diverticulum
	Mesenteric infarction
Hepato-biliary	**Biliary colic**
	Acute cholecystitis
	Ascending cholangitis
Pancreas	**Acute pancreatitis**
Spleen	**Splenic rupture**

System	Disease
Gynaecological	**Ectopic pregnancy**
	Ovarian torsion
Urinary tract	**Renal and ureteric calculi**
	Urinary tract infection (UTI)
	Urinary retention
Vascular	**Ruptured abdominal aortic aneurysm (AAA)**
	Aortic dissection
	Mesenteric infarction
Others	Haemorrhagic cyst
	Rectus sheath haematoma
	Retroperitoneal haemorrhage

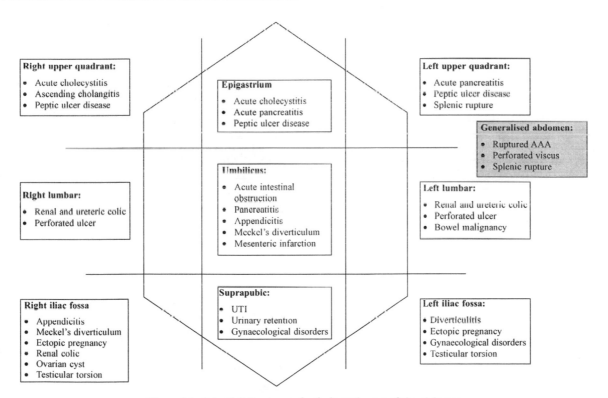

Figure 4.1: Potential diagnoses of pain in each area of the abdomen.

GASTROINTESTINAL STRUCTURES

Peptic ulcer disease

Epidemiology

Common sites of peptic ulcers include the duodenum and the stomach. Duodenal ulcers (70–80%) are more common than gastric ulcers, and usually occur in men between the ages of 35–55. Gastric ulcers occur later in life typically between 55–65 years.

Aetiology

Infection with *Helicobacter pylori* is the main cause of duodenal ulcers. It is present in approximately 80% of cases. *H. pylori* is a spiral shaped gram negative bacillus, with potent urease activity. It also releases cytotoxins which damage mucosal membranes. This degrades the stomach's defensive barrier and allows further damage of the mucosa by gastric acid.

Non-steroidal anti-inflammatory drugs (NSAIDs) are a known risk factor for the development of peptic ulceration. The effect is propagated through reducing the mucosal defences against gastric substances; by inhibiting the production of prostaglandins G_2 (PGG_2) and prostaglandin E_2 (PGE_2). Both PGG_2 and PGE_2 are involved in stimulating mucus secretion and encouraging blood flow to the gastric mucosa. Other risk factors include steroids, smoking and states of extreme physiological stress e.g. burns or major trauma.

Pathophysiology

Duodenal ulcers generally occur in the first part of the duodenum. They are commonly described as being either anterior or posterior. Anterior duodenal ulcers are prone to perforate while posterior duodenal ulcers tend to bleed. Malignancy in the duodenal region is rare.

Gastric ulcers tend to be larger than duodenal ulcers. Chronic gastric ulcers are commonly found on the lesser curve of the stomach. Large chronic ulcers can erode posteriorly into retroperitoneal structures such as the pancreas and the vasculature surrounding it.

Key features in the history/examination

- It is important to stress that gastric and duodenal ulcers cannot be differentiated on symptoms alone.
- Attack of epigastric abdominal pain, lasting for days to weeks with intermittent periods of complete relief is common. The pain can also radiate to the back.
- Onset of pain can occur immediately after a meal but typically occurs two hours after eating food. It is aggravated by spicy foods and relieved by milk.
- Associated symptoms include nausea and vomiting and heartburn.
- If there is chronic bleeding symptoms of anaemia can arise. However, in acute presentations haematemesis and malaena may also be seen.

- The abdomen is tender in the epigastric region. Whilst, a perforation would present with signs of localised or generalised peritonitis.

Investigations

Blood tests:

- Full blood count (FBC): may show anaemia secondary to bleeding.
- Serological testing: will identify the presence of antibodies to *H. pylori*. However, it can remain positive for 6–12 months after eradication. In such cases the urea breath test can be used.

Imaging:

- Double contrast barium meal: is performed, be it rarely, if endoscopy is not possible. This is useful to identify most ulcers and a hiatus hernia.

Endoscopy:

- Oesophagogastroduodenoscopy (OGD): is a very sensitive investigation which allows the oesophagus, stomach and the duodenum to be directly visualised and examined. If a gastric lesion is identified a biopsy is taken for analysis to differentiate between a benign and malignant lesion.
- Biopsy: performed during the endoscopy will identify the presence of the H. p*ylori*.

Others:

- Urease Campylobacter-like organism (CLO) test: involves the biopsy sample and a solution of urea being placed together with a pH indicator. Normally H. *pylori* splits the urea releasing ammonia and increases the pH of the solution. This can be seen as a colour change from yellow to red, indicating a positive result.
- Urea breath test: involves the patient ingesting a solution containing non-radioactive labelled urea. This breaks down to CO_2 in the patient's blood and hence by measuring the levels of CO_2 in the patient's breath before and after ingestion of the solution confirms the diagnosis.

Management

➢ First line management is medical
➢ Surgical management is reserved for complications, the most common being bleeding or perforation.
➢ General advice for patients is to avoid alcohol, smoking, stress, and the ingestion of NSAIDS (e.g. aspirin).

Medical management:

➢ **H. *pylori* eradication:**

○ The main principle of medical treatment is to eradicate the H. *pylori*.

o This is achieved with a one week course antibiotics and anti-acid drugs such as proton pump inhibitors (PPI).

o A typical regime of triple therapy consists of Amoxicillin, Clarithromycin, and Omeprazole.

o This eradicates H. *pylori* in approximately 90% of patients.

➢ Acid reduction:

o Reducing acid alone results in ulcer healing within 1–2 months of treatment. However if H. *pylori* is not eradicated ulcers will recur.

o Antacids can help to relieve symptoms, but the effect on ulcer healing is yet to be determined.

o H_2 receptor antagonists, such as ranitidine block H_2 histamine receptors therefore reducing gastric acid secretions. Most ulcers can be healed within a few weeks of taking these drugs. If these drugs are discontinued relapse is inevitable.

o PPIs such as Omeprazole inhibit hydrogen ion release from gastric Parietal cells. All peptic ulcers will heal usually within two weeks of taking these drugs and patients generally experience symptom relief within a few days. However, as with H_2 receptor antagonists, if treatment is stopped recurrence can occur.

➢ Barrier drugs (Sucralfate, Bismuth compounds): enhance mucosal defence mechanism by providing a protective layer on the epithelial surface.

Surgical management for duodenal ulcers:

➢ The incidence of elective operations for peptic ulcer disease has significantly reduced due to the emergence of PPIs. Surgery if still indicated aims to reduce the production of acid.

➢ Truncal vagotomy and pyloroplasty:

o This involves a section of the vagus nerve (which is involved in the secretion of gastric acid) to be transected at the level of the abdominal oesophagus.

o The lower 7 cm of the oesophagus should be cleared of nerve fibres to achieve a successful vagotomy

o Gastric dennervation may result in gastric stasis and require drainage via pyloroplasty.

➢ Selective and highly selective vagotomy:

o This is a similar procedure that aims to preserve innervation to the pylorus. However, this has a higher recurrence rate and is rarely performed.

Surgical management for gastric ulcers:

➢ The principle of surgical treatments are to remove the ulcer and the gastrin secreting zone. This involves the following procedures.

➢ Billroth I gastrectomy:

o The distal part of the stomach is removed and a gastroduodenal anastomosis is performed.

o Approximately 90% of gastric ulcers that are treated surgically are successfully managed with this procedure.

➢ Billroth II gastrectomy or Polya gastrectomy:

o This is performed if the Billroth I gastrectomy above is technically difficult.

o The antrum and the distal body of the stomach are removed, followed by closure of the duodenal stump. The remaining stomach is anastomosed to a small bowel loop (jejunum).

➢ Vagotomy and ulcer excision

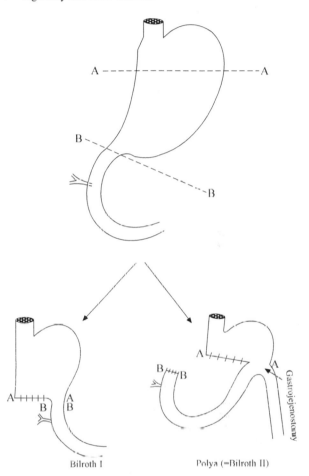

Figure 4.2: Billroth I and Billroth II gastrectomies. *Reprinted with Permission from Andrew Goldberg and Gerard Stansby, Surgical Talk, 2nd Ed, 2005, Imperial Colleague Press.*

Surgical management for perforated ulcers:

There are three surgical options for a perforated ulcer. These include:

➢ Abdominal washout and repair of the defect by approximation of ulcer edges or use of omental patch are the commonest practices for perforated duodenal ulcers.

➢ Excision of the ulcer

➢ Gastrectomy

Acute intestinal obstruction

Epidemiology

Intestinal obstruction can be divided into small and large bowel obstruction. Small bowel obstruction accounts for 5% of all acute surgical hospital admissions. The commonest small bowel presentations are adhesions (60%), malignancy (5%), and strangulated hernia (20%). Large bowel obstruction commonly arises due to colorectal malignancy and accounts for 15% of all cases.

Aetiology

The cause of obstruction can be classified according to the location, i.e. obstruction in the lumen, obstruction in the wall, or obstruction outside the wall. Some forms of obstruction are seen specifically in neonates and infants such as Hirschsprung's disease. (See Table 4.1).

Location of obstruction	Causes
Obstruction in the lumen	Faecal impaction, food bolus, tumour, gallstone ileus, foreign body.
Obstruction in the wall	Tumours, diverticulae, Crohn's disease, congenital atresia.
Obstruction outside the wall	Volvulus, strangulated hernia, adhesions, intussusceptions.
Obstruction in neonates and infants	Stenosis, imperforate anus, meconium ileus, Hirschsprung's disease, strangulated hernia.

Table 4.1: The classification of intestinal obstruction according to location and the causes of each type.

Pathophysiology

When a bowel lumen becomes obstructed, the bowel distal to the obstruction empties and the bowel proximal to the obstruction dilates usually with gas and fluid from the intestinal walls. Intestinal peristalsis increases in an attempt to overcome the obstruction. This inevitably results in intestinal colic.

Simple intestinal obstruction occurs when bowel is obstructed without the blood supply to the bowel being compromised. Strangulated obstruction, occurs when the blood supply to the affected segment of the bowel is acutely impaired.

In simple intestinal obstruction the increasing bowel distension can result in perforation directly due to increased pressure.

With bowel strangulation the blood supply is acutely impaired and ischaemia rapidly develops and weakens the mucosal layer of the bowel. This allows bacteria and associated toxins to leak into the peritoneal cavity, often leading to peritonitis. If the strangulation is not resolved gangrene can develop.

Key features in the history/examination

- There are four classic features of acute intestinal obstruction, i.e. **pain**, **vomiting**, **distension** and **constipation**.

- There is sudden onset of severe colicky abdominal pain.
- Central abdominal pain indicates small bowel obstruction.
- Lower abdominal pain suggests large bowel obstruction.
- The colicky pain may settle and become a constant dull pain.
- Vomiting is usually an early feature of small bowel obstruction.
- Nausea and vomiting are late features of large bowel obstruction.
- Vomiting may become faeculant in late obstruction as a result of bacterial decomposition of the contents of the obstructed bowel.
- Distension is dependent on the site of the obstruction. Often, there is typically more distension the more distal the obstruction.
- Absolute constipation is defined as passing no faeces or flatus. This is a sign of complete intestinal obstruction and it is an early feature of large bowel obstruction.
- Relative constipation is defined as the passing of flatus but not faeces.
- Signs may include pyrexia, dehydration, localised tenderness on palpation and visible peristalsis.
- Abdominal scars from a previous operation should lead to suspicion of adhesional intestinal obstruction.
- Bowel sounds are increased and 'tinkling' in nature.
- Rectal examination may identify an obstructing mass or faecal impaction.
- A collapsed rectum on the rectal exam suggests a mechanical obstruction, whilst a gas-filled rectum suggests pseudo-obstruction.
- There are specific features associated with strangulating obstruction:
  - Pyrexia and tachycardia
  - Colicky abdominal pain becoming constant
  - Increased abdominal tenderness and rigidity
  - Reduced or absent bowel sounds
  - Raised white cell count with bowel infarction

Investigations

Blood Test:

- FBC: may reveal a raised white cell count.
- Urea and electrolytes (U&Es): deranged as a result of dehydration
- Arterial blood gas (ABG): high lactate and metabolic acidosis are signs of bowel strangulation.

Imaging:

- Abdominal X-ray (AXR): loops of distended bowel are seen and a fluid level may be visible on an erect film. The dilated loops of small bowel obstruction are usually centrally placed with striation passing across the total bowel width known as valvulae conniventes. (See Figure 4.3).

An intramural diameter on abdominal X-ray of more than 3.5 cm diameter for small bowel, and 5 cm for large bowel, indicates obstruction.

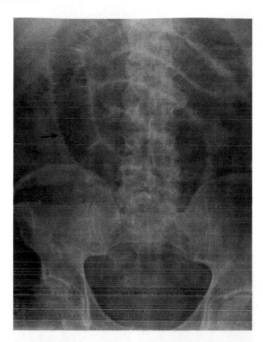

Figure 4.3: Plain film showing central dilated loops of small bowel (arrow) with relative paucity of gas in the large bowel in keeping with small bowel obstruction.

- The dilated loops of large bowel obstruction usually lie peripherally with haustra indentations not extending across the total width of large bowel. (See Figure 4.4).

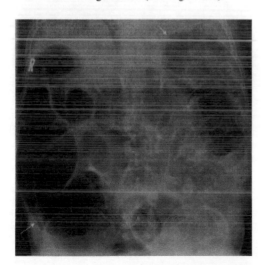

Figure 4.4: AXR of an 80-year-old woman who presented with abdominal distension and constipation. Note dilated peripheral loops of bowel (arrows) with a lack of complete haustral markings in keeping with large bowel obstruction.

- Barium follow through/ Barium enema: Barium sulphate is used with a series of X-rays to identify the level of intestinal obstruction. This is not indicated if perforation is clinically suspected.

- Computer tomography (CT): This will identify the specific site and cause of the bowel obstruction, and may provide evidence of bowel perforation.

Management

Immediate management:

➤ Acute intestinal obstruction is an emergency and usually requires urgent surgical intervention.

➤ Intravenous (IV) access and resuscitation:
  - ○ Large amounts of fluid sequestered in the gut, with losses from vomiting, means that a significant amount of fluid is required.

➤ Insertion of a nasogastric tube (NG):
  - ○ This allows decompression of the bowel
  - ○ Gastric contents are also emptied reducing the risk of aspiration.

➤ Insert a urinary catheter to accurately monitor fluid balance.

➤ Broad spectrum IV antibiotics in all cases of strangulation.

Surgical management:

➤ The surgical procedure of choice is an open midline laparotomy.

➤ The affected bowel is inspected carefully, to identify any non-viable areas.

➤ With non-viable bowel there is loss of peristalsis, loss of the normal sheen and green or black discolouration. There is also loss of pulsation of the blood vessels within the mesentery supplying the bowel. In the event of non-viable bowel being identified a resection is required.

➤ Small bowel obstruction:
  - ○ The small bowel is completely resected and a primary anastomosis is performed. This is usually a very successful procedure due to the good blood supply.

➤ Large bowel obstruction:
  - ○ If the obstruction is proximal to the splenic flexure, it is resected with a primary ileo-colic anastomosis.
  - ○ Left sided lesions are first resected, and the remaining bowel is brought out to the abdominal surface as a colostomy. The rectal stump can be oversewn as in a Hartmann's procedure or brought to the surface as a mucous fistula. A reversal procedure with anastomosis can be performed at a later date.
  - ○ In the event of bowel perforation and intra-abdominal contamination the risk of anastomotic breakdown is significantly higher. A stoma may be performed as a diversion, either instead of a bowel anastomosis or to protect one that was created.

4. Surgery

Diverticulitis

Epidemiology

Diverticulitis is often seen after the age of 50, with colonic diverticula being more common in western countries. They are usually found on the left colon (90% involving the sigmoid colon) but can affect the entire colon. Approximately 15% of patients with diverticulosis (having the presence of diverticula in the colon) develop acute diverticulitis.

Aetiology

Diverticula are protrusions of the mucosa and sub-mucosa through the muscle layers of the bowel wall. They may occur as a result of weakness of the bowel wall or increased intraluminal pressure. A lack of fibre in the diet has been associated with constipation causing a rise in intraluminal pressure, colonic wall muscle hypertrophy and increased segmentation.

Diverticulitis is caused by inflammation of one or more of these diverticula due to infection. Bleeding may occur as a result of inflammation of the bowel mucosa.

Pathophysiology

High intraluminal pressure is a result of hypertrophy of the muscle of the sigmoid colon. The points at which herniation occurs is where the mesenteric blood vessels penetrate the bowel wall. Diets low in fibre do not allow distension of the colon and therefore give rise to high intraluminal pressures.

Recurrent episodes of inflammation can lead to perforation resulting in abscess formation or generalised peritoneal contamination. Fibrotic healing of recurrent diverticulitis after inflammation can lead to colonic stenosis presenting as large bowel obstruction. Haemorrhage of diverticula occurs in approximately 15% of cases and fistula formation can arise.

45% of the diverticula are located in the sigmoid colon alone and 80% of are within the sigmoid and descending colon. The rest are found in the other parts of large bowel.

Key features in the history/examination

- Acute onset of lower abdominal pain, commonly on the left side.
- The pain becomes generalised and increases in severity with diverticula perforation.
- Associated symptoms include malaise, vomiting, and diarrhoea or constipation.
- Bleeding or mucus per rectum and symptoms of anaemia may be present too.
- Pyrexia in diverticulitis can occur.
- Lower abdomen and left iliac fossa tenderness with guarding.
- A mass may be palpated representing the sigmoid colon, which is tender and thickened.
- A tender mass may be palpated on digital rectal examination if the sigmoid has looped down into the pelvis.

- A perforated diverticulum produces signs of localised or generalised peritonitis.

Investigations

Blood tests:

- FBC: may reveal a raised white cell count.
- Inflammatory markers: check for elevated CRP.

Imaging:

- CT: is the investigation of choice in the acute phase. The Hinchey classification describes the severity of diverticulitis, whilst excluding other causes of abdominal pain.
- Double-contrast barium enema: can be used to view the whole of the large bowel and demonstrate stenosis, fistulas, and peri-colic abscesses. It is less invasive than endoscopy but small polyps or carcinoma may be missed. It is used as an outpatient investigation. (See Figure 4.5).

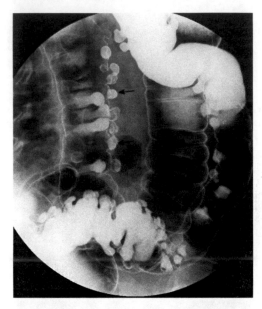

Figure 4.5: Single image from a barium enema examination showing multiple diverticular out- pouching from the large bowel (arrow) in keeping with colonic diverticulosis.

Endoscopy:

- Flexible Sigmoidoscopy: allows visualisation of the sigmoid colon. In acute attacks the procedure may be painful and the mucosa will be inflamed increasing the risk of iatrogenic perforation. It is commonly used once the acute attack has passed.
- Colonoscopy: the affected area of the colon may again be visualised and malignancy ruled out. The sigmoid colon may be rigid and narrow, making it difficult to pass the colonoscope through. Again it is an investigation used after recovery from the acute phase.

Management

Conservative management:

➢ IV access and resuscitation of the patient if necessary

➢ IV fluids

➢ Broad spectrum IV antibiotics (Penicillin and Metronidazole)

➢ Appropriate analgesia e.g. IV opioid and an anti-emetic

➢ Most acute attacks settle with conservative treatment

➢ Out-patient large bowel investigation once acute phase settled

Surgical management:

➢ A perforated diverticulum resulting in generalised peritonitis requires the patient to undergo an emergency laparotomy.

➢ A small localised perforation can be managed conservatively with IV antibiotics with or without CT guided drainage of a local collection.

➢ A further 10% of patients with recurrent attacks will also need surgical management.

➢ In an elective procedure the affected segment of bowel is removed and an end-to-end anastomosis is performed to allow continuity of the bowel.

➢ Obstruction requires a Hartmann's procedure and resection of the affected area. The rectum is closed and the left colon is brought out of the abdomen, and a colostomy is formed.

➢ Perforation: can be managed with a number of different procedures:

  o Laparotomy with an abdominal wash out and omental patch repair.

  o Primary resection and Hartmann's procedure

  o Primary resection and anastomosis. This is normally only practiced by colorectal surgeons.

Acute appendicitis

Epidemiology

This is one of the most common surgical emergencies requiring an operation. It has a lifetime prevalence of approximately 6–8%.

Aetiology

There is no single hypothesis for the cause of acute appendicitis. However there is a well known theory suggesting the lumen of the appendix becomes obstructed and then progresses to the development of a bacterial infection.

In the majority of cases the obstruction is a result of a faecolith, stricture or hypertrophy of lymphoid tissue within the appendiceal wall. A rare cause of acute appendicitis in the elderly includes, carcinoma of the caecum leading to obstruction of the appendix. Intestinal parasites (helminths and protozoas) have also been found to cause lumen obstruction in cases of acute appendicitis.

Pathophysiology

Acute appendicitis in some cases initially starts with mucosal inflammation and hyperplasia of lymphoid tissue, with a patent appendiceal lumen. If an infective organism is involved, an inflammatory response occurs, leading to an obstructed lumen. Intraluminal pressure increases as a result of continuous mucus and inflammatory exudate secretion. This leads to the obstruction of lymphatic drainage, resulting in mucosal oedema and ulceration. At this stage spontaneous resolution may occur particularly following a response to IV antibiotics. However, with progression, the appendix becomes distended, with the possibility of ischaemia developing within the appendix wall. The presence of ischaemia leads to bacterial spread through the submucosa resulting in acute appendicitis. If left untreated, this can lead to perforation and subsequent peritonitis.

Key features in the history/examination

• The classic presentation is of a central abdominal colicky pain (visceral), which later moves to the right iliac fossa. This is a result of inflammation of the peritoneum (somatic).

• The pain is usually aggravated by movement and relieved by lying still.

• With perforation of the appendix symptoms may resolve temporarily, due to relief of tension in the distended organ. The pain will then become greater in severity, resulting in the development of generalised peritonitis.

• Associated symptoms include anorexia and vomiting.

• Bowel habit may be altered with constipation being the usual symptom.

• Signs include pyrexia, tachycardia, foetor oris, right iliac fossa guarding, percussion tenderness and rebound tenderness (which is difficult to illicit if guarding is present).

• A painful digital rectal examination is a result of the appendix lying in the pelvic position, or the presence of pus in the pouch of Douglas.

• In late cases, presenting with generalised peritonitis, the abdomen is rigid, bowel sounds are absent, and the patient has a number of signs of sepsis.

Symptom	Early feature	Late feature
Pain	Peri-umbilical Pain	Moves to the right iliac fossa
Temperature	Apyrexial	Slight or high pyrexia
Pulse rate	Normal pulse rate	Raised as a response to temperature
Vomiting	Usually follows onset of pain	–
Anorexia	Constant	Constant

Table 4.2: The early and late features of acute appendicitis.

Specific signs associated with acute appendicitis:

➢ McBurney's point tenderness: tenderness at two thirds from the umbilicus to the anterior superior iliac spine.

4. Surgery

➢ Pointing sign: the patient points to where the pain initiated and to where it has now moved. This sign is not a commonly used sign and not very specific.

➢ Rovsing's sign: right iliac fossa pain on left iliac fossa palpation.

➢ Psoas sign: if the appendix is positioned on the psoas muscle, the patient will lie with the right hip flexed with aggravation of pain on hip extension.

➢ Obturator sign: when the hip is flexed and rotated, this results in spasm of the obturator muscle. If the appendix is inflamed and in contact with the obturator the patient will experience pain in the hypogastrium.

Investigations

The diagnosis of acute appendicitis is usually clinical, however routine investigations are performed.

Blood test:

• FBC: may reveal a raised white cell count

• U&Es: important particularly in the elderly patient with other co-morbidities.

Urinalysis:

• Urine dipstick: may show blood and leucocytes as a result of ureteric irritation and inflammation.

• Beta-human chorionic gonadotropin (HCG): to rule out pregnancy in all women of reproductive age.

Imaging:

• Erect CXR and AXR: used to exclude perforation or ureteric colic with a similar clinical presentation. Both of these are not indicated in young patients with good clinical signs of appendicitis.

• Abdomino-pelvic USS: if the diagnosis is unclear in a young woman then ovarian pathology i.e. ruptured cyst or ovarian torsion should be ruled out. Note that the USS cannot accurately identify the appendix unless it is markedly enlarged but it can highlight the presence of free fluid within the abdomen, which collaborates with a diagnosis of appendicitis.

• CT: this is 98% sensitive at diagnosing appendicitis, but is reserved for older patients where malignancy is suspected. Patients are exposed to a dose of high radiation, and so this is not a routinely used investigation.

Management

➢ Immediate management:

➢ IV access and resuscitation of the patient if necessary.

➢ Monitoring of blood pressure, heart rate, oxygen saturations, and urine output (via urinary catheter in seriously ill patients)

➢ IV fluids

➢ IV Paracetamol

➢ Appropriate analgesia, e.g. IV opioid and an anti-emetic

➢ The patient is to be kept nil by mouth (NBM)

➢ Pre-operative IV antibiotics are prescribed to reduce infective complications. They are given only after the diagnosis of appendicitis has been made and an operation is to follow

➢ Informed consent to operate is obtained

Surgical management:

➢ Definitive treatment is to perform an open or laparoscopic appendicectomy. The conventionally open appendicectomy is further described below.

➢ A transverse (Lanz) or grid iron incision is made in the right iliac fossa, centred at McBurney's point, (two thirds from the umbilicus to the anterior superior iliac spine). (See Figure 4.6)

➢ The incision is extended though the skin and the subcutaneous fat, until the external oblique is reached.

➢ The external oblique aponeurosis is incised. Next the internal oblique and transversus abdominis are split, after which the peritoneum is opened and the abdominal cavity is entered.

➢ The appendix and caecum are identified. In approximately 25% of cases the appendix is located in the retro-caecal position. The appendix has been occasionally found in other intra-peritoneal and extra-peritoneal positions.

➢ Once the appendix has been found, the mesoappendix (which includes the appendicular artery) is ligated and divided. The appendix is then excised at its base.

➢ The stump was traditionally buried with a purse-string suture, however there is little evidence it transfers any benefit. This type of suture is not performed with a laparoscopic appendicectomy.

➢ If there is severe contamination with pus and fluid, as in cases of a perforated appendix, an extensive washout should be performed and a drain sited.

➢ The abdominal layers are then individually closed.

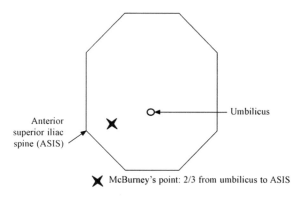

Figure 4.6: McBurney's point.

Meckel's diverticulum

Epidemiology

Meckel's diverticulum affects 2% of the population, of which inflammation is seen in 2% of these patients.

Aetiology

A Meckel's diverticulum is the remnant of the Vitello intestinal duct, which usually disappears by the end of embryological development. The apex is adherent to the umbilicus or attached via a fibrous cord.

Pathophysiology

It is located on the antimesenteric border, approximately 2 feet (60 cm) from the ileo-caecal valve of the small intestine. It has an average length of 2 inches. Therefore the rule of 2 (2%, 2 feet, 2 inches), helps with memory of this condition.

A Meckel's diverticulum is a true diverticulum encompassing all three layers of the intestinal wall, and possesses its own blood supply. It may contain ectopic mucosa, most commonly gastric or pancreatic. Such diverticulum, are at risk of perforation, haemorrhage, and intussusception.

Key features in the history/examination

- They can be asymptomatic
- Acute inflammation gives signs and symptoms similar to those of appendicitis.
- Perforation will present with shock and an acute abdomen.
- They can present with bleeding as a result of ulceration.
- Bleeding per rectum may be noted
- They can present as a volvulus or intussusception

Investigations

Meckel's diverticulum are usually an incidental operative finding, however certain investigations can aid the diagnosis.

Imaging:

- Technetium-99 scan: radioactive technetium is injected and then absorbed by the gastric mucosa. The stomach will be outlined and in 90% of cases the site of the Meckel's diverticulum will be identified.
- Barium follow through: will sometimes identify the diverticulum arising from the antimesenteric border.

Management

➢ If the patient presents to hospital in shock, with an acute abdomen, the patient must be immediately resuscitated.

➢ A Meckel's diverticulectomy is the only choice for definitive management.

HEPATO-BILIARY STRUCTURES

Biliary colic

Epidemiology

In western society 50% of women and 15% of men are diagnosed

with gallstones. After approximately five years, 10% of these cases become symptomatic.

Aetiology

Gallstones can give rise to biliary colic. There are three types of gallstones if classified by composition.

Bile pigment stones (5%): are seen in patients with excessive haemolysis e.g. due to sickle cell anaemia or thalassaemia. They are small, black, gritty, fragile, and are composed mostly of calcium bilirubinate. These stones are often found throughout the biliary tree, and in the ducts of patients with benign and malignant bile duct strictures.

Cholesterol stones (20%): are more common in those who are older, female, and with increased weight. They are typically solitary and oval in shape.

Mixed stones (75%): are composed mainly of cholesterol with varying amounts of calcium phosphate, calcium carbonate, calcium palmitate and proteins.

A typical sufferer of gallstones is said to be a 'fat, fertile, female of forty'. However, gallstones can occur in men, usually in the older age group. Cases have also been noted in childhood.

Pathophysiology

Biliary colic is the pain caused by muscle spasms of the gallbladder against a gallstone. This stone is usually lodged in the neck of the gallbladder (Hartmann's pouch) or the cystic duct.

Key features in the history/examination

- Severe continuous pain in the epigastrium or right upper quadrant, which may radiate to both costal areas and into the back or shoulders
- Associated symptoms include nausea and vomiting
- The patient is unable to lie still
- Pallor
- Tachycardia
- Epigastric and right upper quadrant tenderness on palpation
- Examination may be unremarkable as most attacks only last for approximately six hours, leaving the patient symptom free afterwards.

Investigations

Blood tests:

- FBC: may reveal a raised white cell count.
- Liver function tests (LFTs): are abnormal in cases of duct obstruction. In particular, high bilirubin and alkaline phosphatase (ALP) are seen.
- Amylase
- Renal function
- Glucose
- Clotting

4. Surgery

Imaging:

- Erect CXR: is done primarily to exclude a perforation.
- USS: gallstones may be seen.

Management

➢ IV access should be gained

➢ Monitoring of blood pressure, heart rate and oxygen saturations

➢ IV fluids

➢ Analgesia, e.g. IV opioid and an anti-emetic.

➢ A cholecystectomy can be arranged in a general surgical out-patient clinic once gallstones have been confirmed.

Acute cholecystitis

Epidemiology

Acute cholecystitis develops in 1–3% of patients with symptomatic gall stones. Approximately 10% of cases are identified in adults over the age of 60; 5% of which will result in gallbladder perforation.

Aetiology

Acute cholecystitis is inflammation of the gallbladder, commonly secondary to obstruction of the cystic duct by stones.

Pathophysiology

The inflammatory process of acute cholecystitis begins with either obstruction of the cystic duct or gallbladder neck by a calculus. This process may be initiated by a number of factors; the release of inflammatory mediators (e.g. prostaglandins), chemical irritation by bile acids, and a rise in intraluminal pressure.

A secondary bacterial infection may occur. The most common organism found is *Esherichia coli*; others include gram negative aerobic rods, anaerobes, and Enterocci.

Commonly, cystic duct patency is re-established within 4–7 days. Recurrent attacks of acute cholecystitis lead to fibrotic thickening of the gallbladder wall. This is a characteristic feature or chronic cholecystitis. If the cystic duct remains obstructed there is increased inflammatory cell infiltration within the wall of the gallbladder. This can lead to haemorrhagic necrosis, gangrene, and perforation.

Key features in the history/examination

- Right upper quadrant abdominal pain, which may radiate to the right side of the back and to the shoulder.
- The pain is severe and can last minutes to hours.
- The pain often starts at night, waking the patient.
- The pain may resolve; only to shortly follow with another attack of pain. This may be ongoing for a few weeks.

- If the pain does not resolve the infection progresses, leading to the patient becoming systemically unwell.
- Associated symptoms include vomiting and symptoms of dyspepsia.
- Early features are:
  o Pyrexia and tachycardia
  o Right upper quadrant tenderness and abdominal guarding on palpation.
- Murphy's sign: during palpation of the right upper quadrant the patient is asked to take a deep breath in. The inspiration causes the gallbladder to descend onto the palpating fingers and if this elicits significant pain the sign is positive. If this is repeated on the left side, no pain should be elicited.
- Late features are:
  o A palpable mass which is most likely the omental wall of the inflamed gallbladder or an empyema.
  o Rigid abdomen
  o Localised peritonitis or abscess formation, as a result of gallbladder perforation.

Investigations

Blood tests:

- FBC: may reveal a raised white cell count.
- Liver function tests (LFTs): are abnormal in cases of duct obstruction. In particular, high bilirubin and alkaline phosphatase (ALP) are seen.
- Amylase
- Renal function
- Glucose
- Clotting

Imaging:

- Erect CXR: is done primarily to exclude perforation.
- AXR: is not routinely performed
- USS: gallstones and a thickened gall bladder wall are seen. If the diameter of the common bile duct is greater than 7 mm, it suggests the presence of stones within the duct.
- Magnetic resonance cholangio-pancreatography (MRCP): the biliary tree is visualised and calculi may be detected. (See Figure 4.7)
- Endoscopic retrograde cholangio-pancreatography (ERCP): this is more invasive than an MRCP with the added risk of precipitating pancreatitis. It involves endoscopic access of the bile duct, enabling visualisation of any calculi within the duct. If calculi are seen they can be removed at the same time, via a sphincterotomy. (See Figure 4.8).

Others:

- Electrocardiography (ECG): to rule out atypical presentation of ischaemic heart disease.

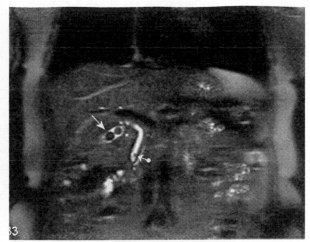

Figure 4.7: Magnetic resonance cholangio-pancreatography (MRCP) reveals gallstones in the gallbladder (straight arrow) and common hepatic ducts (round ended arrow).

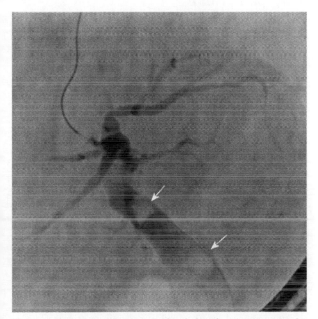

Figure 4.8: Endoscopic retrograde cholangio-pancreatography (ERCP) showing a dilated common bile duct with multiple filling defects (arrows) in keeping with gallstones.

Management

Immediate management:

➤ IV access and resuscitation of the patient.

➤ Monitoring of blood pressure, heart rate, oxygen saturations, and urine output (urinary catheter).

➤ IV fluids

➤ Analgesia, e.g. IV opioid and an anti-emetic.

➤ The patient is to be kept NBM.

➤ Broad spectrum IV antibiotics

➤ Once there are signs of reducing inflammation, (The patient is apyrexial, and has a normal heart rate), oral fluids and fat free diet is recommended.

➤ 80–90% of cases will settle with conservative treatment over 24–48 hours. These patients are readmitted 6–8 weeks later for an elective laparoscopic cholecystectomy.

➤ The remaining 10% of cases will require urgent surgery.

➤ There is an increasing trend towards performing a cholecystectomy during the acute phase, as adhesions are yet to occur, making dissection easier.

➤ When there is biochemical or imaging evidence of stones in the common bile duct an on-table cholangiogram could be performed to locate the stones. They can then be retrieved laparoscopically or with an ERCP.

Surgical management:

➤ Laparoscopic cholecystectomy is usually offered.

➤ To gain access to the peritoneal cavity, the peritoneum is exposed at the umbilicus and a blunt trochar is inserted. Carbon dioxide is used for abdominal insufflation.

➤ The camera (laparoscope) is inserted through the umbilical port and three further ports are sited under direct vision. The three sites include the epigastrium, the right costal margin, and the right flank. These ports allow access for additional instruments and graspers.

➤ The first step is to retract the gallbladder upwards; lifting the liver and allowing full visualisation of the gallbladder.

➤ The neck of the gallbladder is dissected off the liver.

➤ Callot's triangle (cystic duct, the common hepatic duct, and the inferior border of the liver edge) is identified, as the cystic artery is often located within this area.

➤ The cystic duct and artery are clipped and divided above a further two clips.

➤ The gallbladder is dissected off the liver and removed through the umbilical port.

➤ The gallbladder bed is irrigated with normal saline.

➤ Haemostasis is ensured.

➤ Carbon dioxide is removed from the abdomen and the ports are removed.

➤ The fascia and skin at the umbilicus are sutured

➤ A drain may be sited if there are concerns regarding bleeding from the hepatic bed.

Ascending cholangitis

This is a condition in which there is an ascending bacterial infection of the common bile duct stone within the biliary tree. If confirmed this is a medical emergency.

Epidemiology

In the Western world around 15% have gallstones in their gallbladder but many remain asymptomatic. In 2–3% of cases these will present with severe complications of pancreatitis or ascending cholangitis.

Aetiology

The predisposing factors to cholangitis are common bile duct stones, benign or malignant biliary strictures, and pancreatic or duodenal tumours. It has been identified that cholangitis can occur following biliary reconstructive surgery and with bile duct instrumentation (e.g. ERCP).

Pathophysiology

Ascending cholangitis arises following bile duct obstruction causing biliary stasis and resultant bacterial infection. During periods of biliary obstruction the pressure within the biliary system rises. This increases the potential for stagnant contaminated bile to infect the bile duct and enter the blood stream causing septicaemia. This is a medical emergency, which can rapidly progress to systemic inflammatory response syndrome (SIRS) leading to multi-organ failure.

Key features in the history/examination

- Patients present with jaundice, rigors, and abdominal pain; known as Charcot's triad.

- Pyrexia and signs of sepsis may be present, e.g. tachycardia, sweating and low blood pressure.

- Clinical signs of jaundice, (Skin pigmentation and yellowing of the sclera).

- Tenderness in right upper quadrant with or without the presence of a positive Murphy's sign.

Investigations

Blood tests:

- LFTs: may be deranged with an obstructive picture (elevated bilirubin and ALP levels).

Microbiology:

- Blood cultures: should be sent when patients have a significant pyrexia or evidence of sepsis. The commonest bacteria associated with ascending cholangitis are the gram negative bacilli (E. *coli*, Klebsiella and Enterobacter) and the gram positive *Enterococcus*.

Imaging:

- USS: of the abdomen confirms dilated bile ducts and in some cases a MRCP is used to more accurately delineate the site of biliary obstruction.

Management

➢ Rehydration

➢ IV antibiotics

➢ Urgent biliary drainage (endoscopically or percutaneous transhepatic drainage). The timing of intervention depends on the clinical condition of the patient and ideally 24–48 hours after the initiation of IV antibiotics. However in cases of worsening sepsis relief of the biliary obstruction may be required urgently to prevent further deterioration.

➢ ERCP is the favoured procedure which enables retrieval of bile duct stones, biopsy of sites of potential malignancy, and the deployment of plastic or metal stents in areas of narrowing.

➢ In cases where ERCP is not suitable (high proximal biliary obstruction or tight stricture) a percutaneous transhepatic cholangiography is performed. This entails passing a tube for drainage from skin to bile duct under ultrasound guidance.

PANCREAS

Acute pancreatitis

Epidemiology

Acute pancreatitis is relatively common, and accounts for approximately 3% of all cases of abdominal pain admitted to hospital in the UK. This disease has a mortality of 5–10% of all cases, of which one third of patients will die in the early acute phase from multi system organ failure.

Aetiology

The two common causes of acute pancreatitis include gallstones and alcohol, accounting for 60% and 20% of patients. A useful pneumonic, 'GET SMASHED' is used to identify the causes of acute pancreatitis:

- Gallstones: present in half the cases seen in the UK

- Ethanol: is the commonest cause of recurrent pancreatitis

- Trauma: blunt or crush injury disrupting the parenchyma or ducts

- Steroids

- Mumps: other infections including coxsackie B

- Autoimmune diseases: vasculitis, systemic lupus erythematosus (SLE)

- Scorpion venom: rare and not seen in the UK

- Hyperlipidaemia/hypothermia/hypercalcaemia

- ERCP

- Drugs: e.g. azathioprine and thiazides

Pathophysiology

In acute pancreatitis, pancreatic enzymes (trypsin, lipase, amylase), are released and activated resulting in auto-digestion of the pancreas. The process of pancreatitis occurs in a four stage process.

4. Surgery

1. The patient presents with hypovolaemic shock as a result of oedema and fluid shifts within the abdomen. The pancreas releases fluid and enzymes into the peritoneal cavity. This leads to the auto-digestion of fats and the subsequent development of necrosis.

2. The blood vessels are affected by the autodigestion, leading to haemorrhage into the retroperitoneal space. This tracking of blood-stained fluid may result in bruising at the abdominal flanks (Grey Turner's sign) or bruising at the umbilicus (Cullen's sign).

3. Ongoing inflammation progresses to necrosis of all or part of the pancreas and enzymes leak into the blood stream causing systemic effects.

4. The necrotic areas become infected resulting in a high rate of mortality.

Key features of the history/examination

- Rapid onset of pain occurring over minutes and lasting for hours or even days

- Pain is constant and severe

- Typically the pain is in the epigastrium with radiation to the centre of the back

- Frequent vomiting is an associated symptom.

- On observation the patient may look well or extremely ill

- Tachypnoea, tachycardia, and hypotension may be present

- Mild jaundice as a result of common bile duct obstruction by the oedematous pancreatic head or gallstones.

- Tenderness on abdominal palpation, especially over the epigastric region, with or without guarding.

- Bluish discolouration at the flanks and umbilicus is uncommon but it can develop over a few days.

- In 10–20% of cases a pleural effusion is present.

- Positive shifting dullness for the presence of ascites is a rare occurrence.

Investigations

Blood tests:

- FBC: may show a raised white cell count

- Amylase: will be grossly elevated in the acute phase

- Pancreatic lipase: is a more accurate marker than amylase as it has a longer half-life.

- LFTs

- U&Es: renal function should be determined

- Calcium: hypocalcaemia which can lead to tetany

- Inflammatory markers: CRP is a good marker of progress of acute pancreatitis

- Glucose: will be raised

- ABG: Hypoxia can develop in severe cases.

Imaging:

- CXR: a pleural effusion may be seen.

- AXR: a colon 'cut off' sign and a renal 'halo' sign may be seen.

- USS: of the abdomen is required to diagnose gallstones and whether there is dilatation of the common bile duct.

- CT: to assess disease severity, and identify any pseudocysts/fluid collection, which may require drainage. The visualisation of free fluid and air within pancreatic tissue indicates pancreatic necrosis. The Royal Society of Radiologists (RCR) guidelines suggest CT is not indicated for the first 72 hours as these features present later (See Figure 4.9).

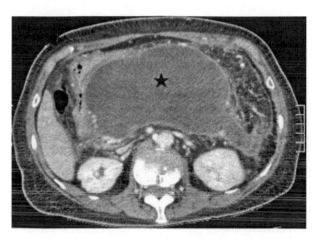

Figure 4.9: CT showing a large cystic collection in the anterior abdomen (star) with thick walls. This patient was recently discharged from the hospital after treatment for acute pancreatitis. Features are in those of a large pancreatic pseudocyst.

Others:

- ECG: arrhythmia and absent T waves.

Management

➢ There are two common multifactorial scoring systems used to assess the severity of the condition over the first 48 hours; Glasgow Imrie criteria and Ranson score. (See Table 4.3).

Management for a mild attack:

➢ Conservative management is appropriate

➢ The patient is kept NBM

➢ IV access and IV fluids

➢ Frequent observation

➢ The patient can be managed on the general surgical ward

Management for a severe attack:

➢ Score ≥ 3

Glasgow Imrie Criteria	Ranson Score
• Age greater than 55 years old	***On admission:***
• Blood glucose > 11 mmol/L	• Age greater than 55 years old
• Serum lactate dehydrogenase (LDH) > 500 IU/L	• Blood glucose > 11 mmol/L
	• Serum LDH > 500 IU/L
• aspartate aminotransferase (AST) > 200 IU/l	• AST > 200 IU/L
	• White blood count > 16 × 10^9/L
• White blood count > 16 × 10^9/L	***Within 48 hours:***
• Blood urea > 16 mmol/L	• Blood urea > 16 mmol/L
• Serum calcium < 2 mmol/L	• Serum calcium < 2 mmol/L
	• Arterial pO_2 < 8 kPa
• Arterial pO_2 < 8 kPa	• Base deficit < –4 mmol/L
• Albumin < 32 g/L	• Haematocrit fall > 10%

Table 4.3: The Glasgow Imrie criteria and Ranson score for assessing acute pancreatitis. One point is given for each criterion and if there is a score of three or more it indicates severe pancreatitis.

➢ Regular observations and aggressive management is required

➢ The patient is kept NBM

➢ High flow oxygen

➢ IV access and IV fluids as above

➢ NG tube

➢ IV analgesia: morphine titrated according to response.

➢ Give an anti-emetic: Cyclizine or Metoclopramide

➢ Monitor urine output with a urinary catheter

➢ An identified biliary cause needs an urgent ERCP and sphincterotomy.

➢ Expert help and transfer patient to high dependency unit (HDU)/intensive care unit (ICU) if necessary. May require inotropic support in severe sepsis.

➢ Nutritional support in the form of enteral or parenteral nutrition, early in the disease is important. Enteral feeding by naso-jejunal route has been shown to have lower complications but may require endoscopic placement.

➢ Drainage of pseudocysts may be required

➢ Surgery is avoided in the initial acute attack. However it may be necessary for the patient to undergo debridement of the necrotic pancreas (necrosectomy), later in the disease particularly with infected necrosis.

➢ If gallstones are identified on USS a laparoscopic cholecystectomy should be considered once the attack has settled.

➢ Most patients are treated with conservative management, however there are a few individuals who develop multi-organ failure and die as a result.

SPLEEN

Splenic rupture

Epidemiology

This is the commonest internal abdominal injury caused as a result of non-penetrating trauma.

Aetiology

Splenic rupture should be suspected after any trauma, especially injury to the left upper abdominal quadrant. If the overlying ribs are fractured this should increase clinical suspicion of a splenic rupture.

Key features in the history/examination

Splenic rupture can have different presentations:

Haemorrhagic shock:

• This is a result of complete splenic rupture

• The spleen may have avulsed from its pedicle

• Death may occur rapidly

• Pallor

• Prolonged capillary refill time

• Drowsy and lethargic

• Tachycardic and hypotensive

Acute abdomen:

• Over a period of hours, the patient may complain of abdominal pain.

• The pain can be generalised or increased in the left flank.

• There is often referred left shoulder tip pain (Kehr's sign).

• Generalised or left sided abdominal tenderness on palpation

• Guarding and rigidity may be present

• Abdominal distension

• Bruising of the abdominal wall may be seen

Delayed rupture:

• This can occur hours to days after the injury

• This is a result of an enlarging splenic haematoma which suddenly ruptures.

• Such cases are rare as a result of USS on initial admission to hospital, where a haematoma if present will be identified.

Investigations

A diagnosis of a ruptured spleen is made clinically after a brief history and examination. If there is massive haemorrhage the surgeon may decide to proceed for an urgent laparotomy. If the patient is stable there may be time to perform a few specific investigations.

Imaging:

- CXR: rib fractures and a raised left hemi-diaphragm may be seen. Injury to the left lung (haemothroax or pneumothorax) may be apparent.

- AXR: the gastric bubble may be displaced to the right while the splenic outline and psoas shadow may not be seen. If there is a haematoma present in the spleen, the splenic flexure of the colon may be displaced downwards.

- CT: of the abdomen will detect any injury to the spleen (e.g. laceration). Intra-abdominal fluid can be seen and damage to surrounding organs and structures can be identified.

Others:

- Urinalysis: the presence of haematuria may be suggestive of renal damage.

Management

Immediate management:

➤ IV access and resuscitation of the patient with haemorrhagic shock.

➤ IV fluids

➤ Blood products when available

➤ Appropriate analgesia, (IV opioid and an anti-emetic)

➤ The patient is to be kept NBM

➤ In a haemodynamically stable patient with a low grade splenic injury confirmed on CT, conservative management with close observation may be appropriate.

Surgical management:

➤ If a patient is requiring resuscitation with blood products, an emergency splenectomy will be the next step.

➤ If a small laceration has been identified it may be possible to salvage the spleen. In most circumstances a splenectomy is performed.

Post splenectomy:

➤ After a splenectomy has been performed patients are in an immunocompromised state.

➤ These patients should be given *Pneumoccal, Haemophilus* type B, and meningitis A and C vaccines.

➤ They should also receive annual flu vaccines

➤ They must take the antibiotic Penicillin V for two years post splenectomy

➤ If at any point the patient suspects they may have an infection, antibiotics (e.g. amoxicillin) should be started.

GYNAECOLOGICAL STRUCTURES

Ectopic pregnancy

Epidemiology

Ectopic pregnancies are defined as a fertilised ovum that has implanted outside the uterine cavity. It is becoming increasingly common, and in the UK alone it affects 1 in 60–100 pregnancies. Of these women approximately 10% will go on to have another ectopic pregnancy.

Aetiology

No specific cause has been identified to account for ectopic pregnancies. Any factor which has been found to damage the fallopian tubes can account for a tubal ectopic pregnancy. Other risk factors include assisted conception, pelvic and tubal surgery.

Pathophysiology

Ectopic pregnancies can occur at different sites. It affects less than 1% of pregnancies however there is an increase in risk with previous salpingitis and the use of intrauterine coil devices (IUCD).

The most common site is in the fallopian tube (95%). Other sites include the cervix, cornu, ovary, and abdominal cavity. (See Figure 4.10). With a tubal ectopic pregnancy the fallopian tube is unable to withstand the invasion of trophoblastic tissue. This results in bleeding into the lumen, which can result in rupture of the trophoblast. This leads to intra-peritoneal blood loss, which can be fatal. However, ectopic pregnancies can abort naturally without causing any symptoms.

Key features in the history/examination

- Sudden onset of pain

- Initial colicky abdominal pain which later becomes constant

- If a tubal ectopic pregnancy is present, the pain may be isolated to the right or left iliac fossa.

- Abnormal dark vaginal bleeding

- Collapse

- Shoulder tip pain (suggesting intra-peritoneal blood loss)

- Tachycardia and hypotension (as a result of blood loss)

- Abdominal palpation may demonstrate guarding and rebound tenderness

- Vaginal examination may reveal:
  o Cervical excitation
  o Tender adnexae
  o Uterus is small for the expected gestational age
  o Closed cervical os

4. Surgery

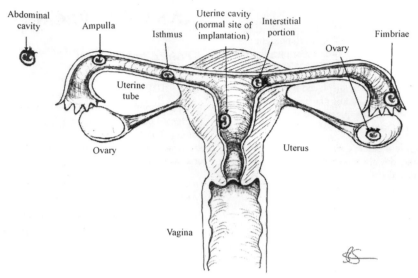

Figure 4.10: Sites of ectopic pregnancy.

Investigations

Blood test:

- FBC
- Group and save and cross-match
- Serum beta-HCG: more than 1000 IU/L should show an intrauterine pregnancy on USS. In a viable pregnancy the serum beta-HCG rises by more than 66% in 48 hours (Usually the beta-HCG level doubles). If the levels are rising slowly or falling, an ectopic or non-viable pregnancy may be present.

Urinalysis:

- Beta-HCG: should be performed in all women of reproductive age.

Imaging:

- USS: may not visualise the ectopic pregnancy. It should identify an intrauterine pregnancy but if the uterus is empty the potential diagnosis is early gestation, a complete miscarriage or an ectopic pregnancy.

Management

Management of acute presentation:

- ➢ IV access and IV fluids
- ➢ Monitoring of blood pressure, heart rate, and urine output via a urinary catheter
- ➢ Analgesia e.g. IV opioid and an anti-emetic
- ➢ The patient is to be kept NBM.
- ➢ Transfusion of packed red cells may also be required
- ➢ A laparotomy is the treatment in the haemodynamically unstable patient with a salpingectomy (removal of the tube) performed.

Management of sub-acute presentation:

- ➢ A laparoscopic procedure is performed
    - ○ Salpingostomy is the removal of the ectopic pregnancy from the tube
    - ○ Salpingectomy is the removal of the fallopian tube
- ➢ This reduces hospital stay and aids faster patient recovery
- ➢ If the ectopic pregnancy has not ruptured, is < 35 mm in diameter, and serum beta-HCG is less than 5,000 IU/mL, a single dose of methotrexate can be given. Further doses may be required if unsuccessful. To ensure complete resolution, serial beta-HCG levels are performed every 48 hours until levels are low or undetectable.
- ➢ With small and unruptured ectopic pregnancies, and reducing beta-HCG levels, no active treatment is required and the patient is managed conservatively.

Ovarian torsion

Epidemiology

Ovarian torsion can occur at any age. However approximately 70% of cases are seen in women less than 30 years of age. 17% of cases have been identified in those who are pre-menarchal or postmenopausal. It is a disease which is often difficult to diagnose. The most common pathologies involved are haemorrhagic cysts, serous cystadenoma, and a benign teratoma.

Aetiology

A number of factors have been identified as a cause of ovarian torsion. Torsion usually occurs as a result of an anatomical change or abnormality.

If it occurs in a young child the ovary is commonly normal, and the abnormality is usually a long fallopian tube or an absent mesosalpinx. During pregnancy an enlarged corpus luteum cyst predisposes to ovarian torsion. Women undergoing fertility treatment have an increased risk of ovarian torsion due to the increased number of luteal cysts, which increase the volume of the ovaries. Approximately 50–60% of cases involve an ovarian tumour.

Pathophysiology

Ovarian torsion typically occurs in an enlarged ovary and is usually unilateral. If there are ovarian masses involved in the case of torsion, they are commonly greater than 4–6 cm in size. Torsion can occur with masses of a smaller size.

Key features in the history/examination

- Sudden onset, severe, unilateral abdominal pain.
- The severity of the pain increases over time.
- The pain can radiate to the back, pelvis or thigh.
- The pain is described as a sharp and stabbing pain
- The pain is exacerbated by exercise or movement
- Associated symptoms include nausea, vomiting and fever.
- Pyrexia and tachycardia are noted
- Abdominal palpation may identify a tender, unilateral, adnexal mass
- Signs of peritonitis are seen in late cases, as a result of necrosis of the ovary

Investigations

Imaging:

- USS: of the pelvis may show an ovarian enlargement that may be an ovarian mass or cyst.
- CT: is a sensitive investigation and enlarged ovaries and pelvic masses can be identified. It can also rule out any other cause of lower abdominal pain.

Management

A senior gynaecologist must be consulted early if ovarian torsion is a differential diagnosis, despite normal investigations.

➤ IV access and IV fluids

➤ Analgesia e.g. NSAIDs or opioids

➤ Laparoscopy is the surgical procedure of choice. This procedure confirms the diagnosis and also treats it.

➤ The procedure involves uncoiling the ovary and possible fixation of the ovary to the pelvic wall (oophoropexy).

➤ If on visualisation there is peritonitis or tissue necrosis the ovary and fallopian tube may be removed (salpingo-oophorectomy).

➤ With early diagnosis and treatment there is excellent prognosis

URINARY TRACT STRUCTURES

Renal and ureteric calculi

Epidemiology

Renal tract calculi are common, with 50% of cases presenting between 30 and 50 years of age. It has a prevalence of 0.2% of the entire population.

Aetiology

Urinary tract calculi can occur without any explanation but there are three main predisposing factors.

1. Inadequate drainage (or stasis) of urine seen in cases of hydronephrosis or bladder diverticulum.

2. Increased amount of the normal constituents of urine, leading to supersaturated urine, which predisposes to calculi formation. This is seen in populations who have moved to intemperate climates, where dehydration is a problem. Increased excretion of calcium may be noted in the urine which may be secondary to hypercalcaemia, as seen in hyperparathyroidism. In conditions such as gout, or post chemotherapy in patients with leukaemia, there is increased uric acid production. This commonly results in uric acid stone formation. The levels of oxalate are also increased in patients whose diets consist of strawberries, leafy vegetables, and tea.

3. The presence of abnormal constituents in urine. For example foreign bodies (stents, non-absorbable sutures, fragments of a urinary catheter) present in the urinary tract are associated with renal calculi. UTIs with obstruction may result in the production of epithelial slough. UTIs also tend to alter the urinary pH and precipitate stone formation (e.g. calcium phosphate stones). Cystine stone formation may occur as a result of an inborn error of amino acid metabolism.

Pathophysiology

There are three main constituents of urinary tract calculi; oxalate stones (60%), phosphate stones (30%), and uric acid and urate stones (5%).

Oxalate stones are most common. They have a hard, sharp surface that can damage the urinary epithelium. This results in bleeding from the tract causing the stones to appear black.

Phosphate stones are usually composed of calcium, ammonium, and magnesium phosphate. They are described as hard, chalky and white. These stones are associated with a staghorn calculus and commonly found in patients with UTIs.

Uric acid stones and urate stones are hard and brown with a smooth surface. Pure uric acid calculi are radiolucent.

Key features in the history/examination

- Pain is commonly the first symptom to be noted
- Severe ureteric colic can occur if the stone impacts at the pelvic-ureteric junction, or moves down the ureter

- The pain is described as a dull loin pain
- The pain radiates from the loin to the groin
- The pain is constant with episodes of increased waves of pain.
- Renal pain is noticed posteriorly in the renal angle.
- This pain is exacerbated by movement
- If the pain radiates to the tip of the penis this can indicate a bladder stone
- Some calculi may be asymptomatic
- Associated symptoms include nausea, vomiting, sweating and fever.
- The patient appears restless and cannot lie still.
- The lateral abdominal muscles are rigid
- On palpation there is tenderness over the renal angle
- Percussion over the kidneys may illicit pain

Investigations

Blood test:

- FBC
- U&Es
- Calcium: raised serum calcium
- Phosphate levels
- Uric acid levels

Urinalysis:

- Blood may be present
- Nitrates and leucocytes suggest a possible UTI

Imaging:

- Kidney-ureter-bladder (KUB): AXR of the kidneys, ureters, and bladder may show calculi in 90% of cases. (See Figure 4.11).
- Intravenous urogram (IVU): where IV contrast allows the anatomy of the renal tract to be visualised as well as identifying hydronephrosis and calculi. An IVU film must be compared to the plain KUB but contraindications include contrast allergy, pregnancy, asthma, renal failure and patients taking metformin. (See Figure 4.12).
- CT: A spiral, non-contrast CT scan is fast and more sensitive in identifying renal calculi when compared to an IVU. It can also diagnose and rule out other differential diagnoses, including ovarian cysts, and an aortic aneurysm. (See Figure 4.13).
- Dimercaptosuccinic acid (DMSA) scan: uses Technesium 99 and Dimercaptosuccinic acid to identify renal scarring. Tumours and trauma can also be detected.

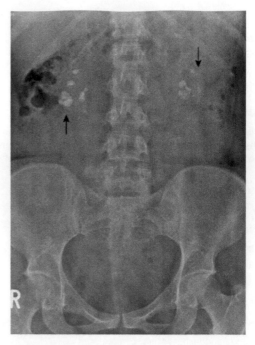

Figure 4.11: Plain X-Ray of the abdomen showing bilateral multiple dense renal calculi (arrow).

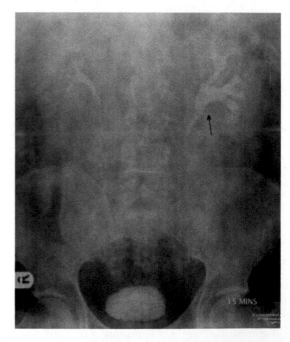

Figure 4.12: A 15 minute film from an IVU study showing delayed excretion of contrast from left kidney (arrow) with dilated pelvicalyceal system compared to the right side in keeping with mild hydronephrosis on the left.

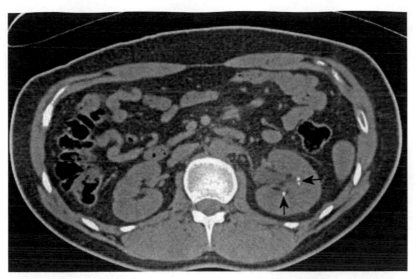

Figure 4.13: CT KUB examination showing three calculi in the left kidney (arrows). The right kidney is normal.

Management

Conservative management:

➤ IV access

➤ Analgesia e.g. Morphine, Pethidine, rectal Diclofenac

➤ Encourage oral intake

➤ Ureteric stones less than 5 mm in size usually pass spontaneously

Long-term management:

➤ Ureteric stones:

  o If the stone remains in the ureter and will not pass spontaneously intervention may be necessary.

  o Extracorporeal shock wave lithotripsy (ESWL) is used to shatter the stone. The resultant smaller fragments can then be allowed to pass spontaneously.

  o Ureteroscopy is the endoscopic removal of the stone. A dormia basket is used under direct visualisation to remove the stone. If the stone is too large for the basket the stones are fragmented using a laser.

  o Open surgery, called ureterlithotomy is used to gain access to the ureter, percutaneously to remove the ureteric stone.

➤ Renal stones:

  o These can also be managed with ESWL. If this is unsuccessful stones can be removed via a percutaneous nephrolithotomy (PCNL)

  o PCNL is a procedure in which a hollow needle is introduced to the renal parenchyma. A wire is then passed through the needle and acts as a guide for the dilator to expand the passage to the kidney. A nephroscope is introduced through this track to identify any stones and remove them under direct vision.

  o Open surgery may be required to remove the stone, but this is very rare.

➤ In septic patients with an obstruction

  o An emergency percutaneous nephrostomy tube is inserted

  o IV antibiotics are given

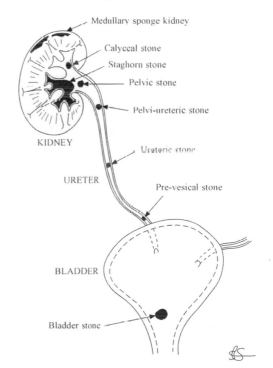

Figure 4.14: Common sites of renal and ureteric stones.

➤ All patients should be encouraged to increase their oral intake to produce dilute urine.

➤ Indications for the removal of renal and ureteric calculi are as follows:

　o Recurrent attacks of renal and ureteric colic

　o Large stone

　o An enlarging stone

　o Bilateral obstruction of the kidney

　o Obstruction of a solitary kidney

VASCULAR STRUCTURES

Ruptured abdominal aortic aneurysm

Epidemiology

An abdominal aortic aneurysm (AAA) is found in 2% of the population at autopsy. In 90% of cases they are found below the renal arteries (Infra renal). It has an incidence of 5% in patients with known coronary artery disease. AAAs can rupture anteriorly (20%) into the peritoneal cavity, and the remaining rupture posteriorly (80%) into the retroperitoneal space.

Aetiology

An AAA is defined as a greater than 50% increase in the normal aortic diameter (>3 cm in diameter). It is the commonest type of aortic aneurysm. Risk factors include: increasing age, smoking, atherosclerosis, hypertension, connective tissue disorders such as Marfan's syndrome and syphilis infection.

Pathophysiology

Elastin is a component of the connective tissue of the aorta which provides its tensile strength. In the normal human aorta there is gradual reduction in the amount of elastin in the distal portion of the aorta compared with the proximal segment. The walls in a AAA have histologically shown elastin fragmentation and degeneration.

Risk factors for heart disease such as atherosclerotic plaques weaken artery walls, and disrupt the integrity of the tunica media. Smoking also hardens the arterial walls and predisposes vessels to damage.

Connective tissue disorders such as Marfan's syndrome and Ehlers-Danlos syndrome predispose patients to AAAs. Syphilis infection results in mycotic aneurysms but this is rarely seen today.

Key features of the history/examination

• Severe and sudden onset generalised abdominal pain

• Severe back pain with radiation to the groin should prompt AAA to be ruled out, especially with suspected cases of renal colic.

• Associated symptoms include nausea, vomiting, cold legs and sweating

• Signs of shock (cold, clammy, tachycardia and hypotension) will be present

• Periods of loss of consciousness

• Absent femoral pulses in one or both groins

• A pulsatile mass on abdominal palpation

• A radial-radial delay is a well known but rare sign of dissection involving the thoracic aorta.

Investigations

Investigations should only be performed if the patient is haemodynamically stable, or if there is reasonable doubt about the diagnosis. Any delay in treatment may be fatal.

Blood tests:

➤ Crossmatch 6–8 units of blood

➤ FBC

➤ U&Es

➤ Glucose

➤ LFTs

➤ Clotting

Imaging:

• AXR: an aneurysm may be difficult to palpate either due to the patient being hypotensive, or the presence of a large retroperitoneal aneurysm. A plain film will show calcification in the wall of the aneurysm and loss of the 'psoas shadow'.

• CT: of the abdomen is needed if the patient is known to have an aneurysm and presents with abdominal pain and is normotensive. A CT scan would be the most useful investigation to identify a leak. A CT scan can identify relevant anatomy such as the relationship of the aneurysm to the renal arteries and involvement of the common iliac vessels. It can provide information regarding the aortic angulation and dimensions, which are paramount if endovascular aneurysm repair (EVAR) is to be considered. This investigation will not differentiate between an uncomplicated aneurysm and one that is about to rupture.

• CXR

Others:

➤ ECG

Management

Immediate management:

➤ 50% of patients with a ruptured AAA die prior to reaching hospital.

➤ Two large bore venous cannulas in both antecubital fossa

➤ Blood is sent for investigations.

➤ Infusion of normal saline or volume expanders is administered to raise the systolic blood pressure, however not allowing it to go higher than 90–100 mmHg. Too much fluid replacement may lead to further bleeding by dilution of blood products.

➤ IV analgesia (Morphine titrated to patients response)

➤ IV antiemetic (e.g. Cyclizine 50 mg)

➤ A urinary catheter is inserted to monitor input/output of fluid

➤ Informed consent is obtained for surgery

➤ The patient should be transferred to theatre immediately.

Surgical management:

➤ Definitive treatment for a ruptured aneurysm is an operation

➤ Open surgical procedure is the traditional approach

➤ The neck of the aneurysm is clamped below the renal arteries

➤ An artificial graft is sutured inside the aneurysm sac

➤ The graft is either a straight graft, sewn down to above the bifurcation of the aorta, or a bifurcated graft sewn onto each iliac artery.

➤ EVAR repair for ruptured AAA is done in some research centres but is not recommended routine practice under the current National Institute for Health and Clinical Excellence (NICE) guidelines.

➤ With this procedure there is significant mortality and morbidity, including acute renal failure, myocardial infarction (MI), and distal embolisation.

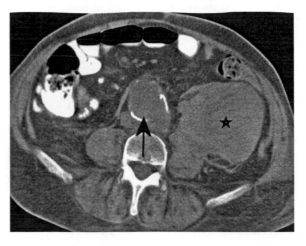

Figure 4.16: Non – contrast CT of the abdomen showing a large left retroperitoneal haematoma (star) secondary to the rupture of an AAA (arrow). *Courtesy of Mr. Ravivarma Balasubramaniam*

Aortic dissection

Epidemiology

Aortic dissection is a problem affecting adults mainly between the ages of 50 and 70 years. It is the most common emergency affecting the aorta.

Aetiology

The aortic wall is weakened by cystic medial degeneration and thus causing splitting of the wall to occur. Patients with atherosclerosis, hypertension and Marfan's syndrome are predisposed to aortic dissection.

Pathophysiology

Aortic dissection comprises of a tear in the aortic wall allowing blood to dissect between the middle and outer layers of the tunica media and adventitia, creating a false passage. This false passage may rupture internally into the true lumen of the aorta creating a double lumen. If the aneurysm ruptures externally, it can result in cardiac tamponade and fatal haemorrhage. When the aortic layers separate, the lumen can become obstructed which leads to end-organ ischaemia.

Aortic dissections can be classified into Stanford type A and type B dissections. Type A occurs in two thirds of all cases and affects the ascending aorta as well as the arch of the aorta. Type B occurs in one third of all cases and affects the descending aorta only. (See Figure 4.17).

Key features in the history/examination

• Sudden onset chest pain

• The pain can radiate to the arms, neck or abdomen

• Typically there may be a tearing interscapular pain

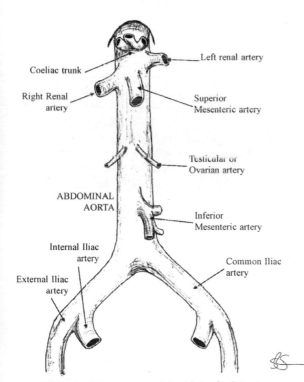

Coeliac trunk

Right Renal artery

Left renal artery

Superior Mesenteric artery

Testicular or Ovarian artery

ABDOMINAL AORTA

Inferior Mesenteric artery

Internal Iliac artery

Common Iliac artery

External Iliac artery

Figure 4.15: Anatomy of the Abdominal Aorta.

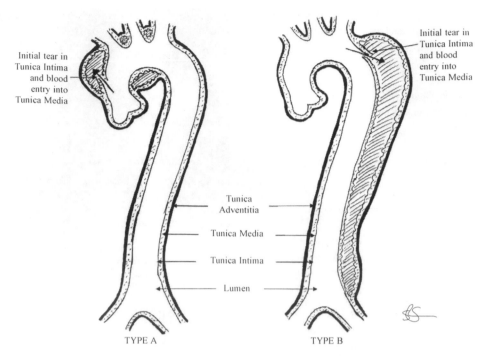

Initial tear in Tunica Intima and blood entry into Tunica Media

Initial tear in Tunica Intima and blood entry into Tunica Media

Tunica Adventitia

Tunica Media

Tunica Intima

Lumen

TYPE A

TYPE B

Figure 4.17: Type A and type B Aortic dissection.

- A new diastolic murmur (representing aortic regurgitation) is auscultated
- Pulseless cold legs from femoral artery occlusion.
- Oliguria from renal artery occlusion.
- Paraplegia or hemiplegia as a result of vertebral artery or carotid artery occlusion.

Investigations

Imaging:

- CXR: widening of the mediastinum is seen with the loss of aortic knob silhouette. A pleural effusion (haemothorax) may also be present.
- CT: identifies the origin of the dissection, and the extent of the dissection. (See Figure 4.18).

Others:

- Echocardiogram: may demonstrate an intimal flap. The presence of a pericardial effusion and aortic regurgitation can also be detected.
- ECG: inferior ECG changes from dissection of coronary orifices.

Management

Management of type A dissection:

➢ Surgery is the recommended treatment of this type of dissection

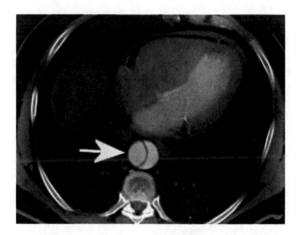

Figure 4.18: CT axial image of the chest showing a clear dissection flap in the descending thoracic aorta (arrow).

➢ A median sternotomy is performed to open the chest cavity
➢ The femoral artery is cannulated
➢ Venous drainage occurs either from the femoral vein or right atrium
➢ Cardiopulmonary bypass is initiated
➢ The aorta is cross-clamped and cut open
➢ If an intimal tear has been identified, this section of the ascending aorta is resected and a synthetic graft (Dacron) sited.

➤ The aortic valve may need replacing and is often done using a composite graft consisting of a valve and tube.

➤ This procedure should prevent further dissection

Management of type B dissection:

➤ Medical treatment is first line in type B dissection

➤ Hypotensive drugs are used to reduce the systolic blood pressure to prevent further dissection (usually to 100–120 mmHg)

➤ Thrombosis of the dissected segment may then occur.

➤ Surgery may be an option if the patient experiences increased pain indicating possible rupture, if neurological symptoms develop and if the aneurysm is increasing in size on serial CXRs.

Prognosis:

➤ Surgical complications include haemorrhage (20%), renal failure (20%), paraplegia (11%), MI (30%) and death (15%).

➤ Two thirds of surviving patients will die within seven years as a result of cardiac and cerebrovascular disease.

Mesenteric Infarction

Epidemiology

Mesenteric ischaemia accounts for 1–2% of all gastrointestinal diseases. It is typically a disease of adults over the age of 50 and is a cause of 0.1% of all hospital admissions.

Aetiology

Acute intestinal ischaemia can occur as a result of arterial, venous, central, or peripheral vascular disease. The superior mesenteric vessels are the vessels most likely to be affected by emboli or thrombus.

Typically, emboli lodge at the branch of the middle colic artery (first large branch of the superior mesenteric artery). Mesenteric emboli can arise from the left atrium in atrial fibrillation (AF), a mural thrombus after an MI, atheromatous plaque from an aortic aneurysm, and mitral valve vegetation. Mesenteric arterial thrombosis is usually secondary to atheroma but arterial occlusion can also be a result of post aortic dissection. Mesenteric venous thrombosis may occur as a result of pre-existing diseases including, portal hypertension, sickle cell disease, women on the contraceptive pill, and thrombophillia.

Pathophysiology

The blood supply to the gut can be divided into three main parts. The foregut (stomach and duodenum) receives blood via the coeliac artery, the mid-gut (jejunum to distal transverse colon) receives blood via the superior mesenteric artery (SMA), and the hind-gut (remaining gut) receives blood via the inferior mesenteric artery.

Haemorrhagic infarction occurs with both arterial and venous occlusion but ischaemic infarction can occur with or without occlusion of the vessels. Thrombosis is commonly the cause of occlusion at the origin of the SMA.

The originating site of the middle colic artery is the usual site where emboli are found.

The mucosal layer of the intestinal wall has little resistance to ischaemic injury, and therefore results in an oedematous intestine and mesentery. Bloodstained fluid then tracks into the bowel lumen and peritoneal cavity. Eventually gangrene and perforation of the ischaemic bowel occurs.

With small occlusions the patient may remain asymptomatic as result of collateral circulation.

Key features in the history/examination

• Sudden onset of colicky abdominal pain

• Central abdominal pain

• The severity of pain increases with time

• Associated symptoms include rectal bleeding, persistent vomiting and frequent defaecation

• Evidence of recent MI, cardiac arrhythmia, and peripheral vascular disease should increase suspicion of mesenteric ischaemia

• Signs of hypovolaemic shock may be present

• On abdominal palpation there may be mild tenderness in the early stages, with guarding and a rigid abdomen in the later stage

• A tender mass may be palpated, which represents the infarcted bowel (rare)

• Classically, the pain is disproportionate to the examination findings

Investigations

There are no specific laboratory investigations that are diagnostic of mesenteric ischaemia.

Blood tests:

• FBC: will show a significantly raised white cell count

• Group and save, and cross-match

• ABG: Metabolic acidosis and raised lactate may be present

Imaging:

• Erect CXR: to exclude perforation

• AXR: thick intestinal walls may be seen

• CT: scan is not diagnostic but able to identify the site of bowel inflammation. It helps to exclude other differential diagnosis.

• Mesenteric angiogram: can differentiate between embolic, thrombotic or non-occlusive ischaemia and also diagnose mesenteric vein thrombosis.

Others:

- ECG: Acute MI or cardiac arrhythmias may be revealed.

Management

- ➤ Resuscitation is essential in all shocked patients.
- ➤ In early cases an SMA arteriotomy and embolectomy may be performed.
- ➤ If the entire supply to the mesentery has been affected (the small intestine and right side of colon) the situation is usually fatal.
- ➤ Infarction of the large bowel alone is rare, but is managed with a transverse colectomy (if the ischaemia is confined to the transverse colon).
- ➤ Surgical management involves resecting the affected bowel. The viable bowel is then inspected the next day with a second look laparotomy.
- ➤ Postoperative anticoagulation is required to prevent further emboli.
- ➤ If successful it is important to address patient nutrition. Often patients will require permanent parenteral nutrition.

Further reading and references

- ➤ Addiss DG, Shaffer N, Fowler BS, et al. (1990). The epidemiology of appendicitis and appendectomy in the United States. Am J Epidemiol 132: 910–925.
- ➤ Bulstrode CJK, Russell RCG, Williams NS (2000) *Bailey & Love's Short Practice of Surgery* (23 Ed.). Arnold.
- ➤ Calne R, Ellis H, Whatson C (2002). *Lecture Notes on General Surgery.* (10 Ed.) Blackwell Publishing.
- ➤ Goldberg A, Stansby G (2006). *Surgical Talk: Revision in Surgery* (2 Ed.). Imperial college press.
- ➤ Gurusamy KS, Samraj K (2009). Early versus delayed laparoscopic cholecystectomy for acute cholecystitis (Review). The Cochrane Collaboration. John Wiley & Sons LT.
- ➤ Hospital appendicitis episode statistics: financial year 2004. Department of Health. UK. www.hesonline.nhs.uk
- ➤ Humes DJ, Simpson J (2006). Clinical review: Acute appendicitis. *BMJ* 2006; 333.
- ➤ Impey L (2004). *Obstetrics and Gynaecology.* (2 Ed.) Blackwell Publishing.
- ➤ Indar AA, Beckingham IJ (2002). Clinical review: Acute cholecystitis. *BMJ* 325: 639–643.
- ➤ Mergener K, Baillie J (1998). Forthnightly review: Acute pancreatitis. *BMJ* 316: 44–48.
- ➤ Miller NL, Lingeman JE (2007). Clinical review: Management of kidney stones. *BMJ* 334: 468–472.
- ➤ Munoz A, Katerndahl D (2000). Diagnosis and management of acute pancreatitis. *American Family Physician* 63.
- ➤ Urbach DR, Stukel TA (2005). Rate of elective cholecystectomy and the incidence of severe gallstone disease. *CMAJ* 172(8): 1015–9.
- ➤ Weintraub NL (2009). Understanding Abdominal Aortic Aneurysm. *NEJM* 361: 1114–1116.
- ➤ www.surgical-tutor.org.uk
- ➤ Yasuhara H. (2005). Acute Mesenteric Ischemia: The challenge of Gastroenterology. *Surgery Today.* Vol 35 (3).

RECTAL BLEEDING

Differential diagnosis

System	Disease
Upper gastrointestinal tract	Bleeding duodenal ulcer
Lower gastrointestinal tract	**Haemorrhoids**
	Anal fissure
	colorectal tumours
	Diverticular disease
	Ulcerative colitis (UC)
Others	Trauma
	Angiodysplasia

Haemorrhoids

Epidemiology

This condition is extremely common and occurs in up to 50% of the adult population.

Aetiology

Haemorrhoids can be idiopathic but hereditary forms are seen too. Hereditary haemorrhoids are often seen in members of the same family. A theory of possible congenital weakness of the vein walls has been suggested. Leg varicose veins and haemorrhoids have been found to occur simultaneously.

The superior rectal veins lie within the connective tissue of the ano-rectum and drains into the inferior mesenteric vein. These veins engorge during increased abdominal pressure (commonly defaecation).

Haemorrhoids are defined by their origin in relation to the dentate line which delineates the transition point from columnar epithelium above, to squamous below.

Predisposing factors can result in congestion of the superior rectal veins. These risk factors include:

- Straining due to constipation
- Pelvic tumour
- Pregnancy
- Use of purgatives
- Rectal carcinoma
- Enteritis and colitis can exacerbate haemorrhoids

Pathophysiology

Haemorrhoids were once described as dilated veins in relation to the anus. This definition has expanded to haemorrhoids being vascular cushions containing a branch of the superior rectal artery and vein.

Haemorrhoids can be described as external or internal in relation to the anus. External haemorrhoids are covered by skin and found below the dentate line, whereas internal haemorrhoids are covered by mucous membrane and found above the dentate line. Interio-external haemorrhoids, is a term given to those internal haemorrhoids that prolapse.

Once the patient is placed into the lithotomy position major piles are located at the 3, 7, and 11 o'clock position. Each individual haemorrhoid can be divided into three parts:

- The pedicle: this is found at the ano-rectal ring, and is covered by a pale pink mucosa.
- The internal haemorrhoid: is bright red or purple and originates from just above the dentate line.
- External associated haemorrhoid: this is covered by a layer of skin. If fibrosis has not occurred, blue veins are visible through this layer.

There are four grades of haemorrhoids as described in Table 4.4.

The complications of haemorrhoids include:

- Strangulation
- Thrombosis
- Ulceration and gangrene
- Fibrosis

Grade	Features
First degree	They do not prolapse from the anus but can bleed
Second degree	These do prolapse on straining or defecation, but reduce spontaneously
Third degree	These haemorrhoids prolapse and can only be manually replaced by the patient
Fourth degree	These haemorrhoids prolapse and are irreducible

Table 4.4: The different grades of haemorrhoids.

Key features in the history/examination

- Bleeding is the most common symptom and it arises early in the disease. The blood is bright red and is seen around the motion not mixed in, i.e. on the toilet paper or splashed onto the toilet pan
- Mucous discharge is commonly associated with prolapsed haemorrhoids
- Pruritus is almost always present following discharge
- Haemorrhoids are often painless, but thrombosed strangulated external haemorrhoids, become increasingly swollen and very painful. These are defined as a perianal haematoma formed from the rupture of a subcutaneous vein
- If pain is present without an identifiable external haemorrhoidal component, then other conditions should be considered

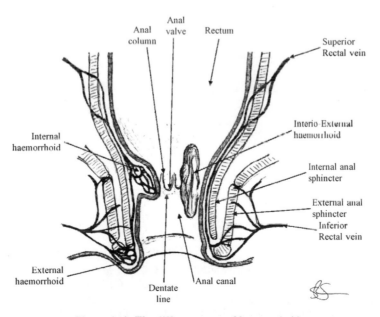

Figure 4.19: The different types of haemorrhoids.

- Prolapse occurs late in the disease and is seen in second to fourth degree haemorrhoids
- Symptoms of anaemia can occur as a result of profuse bleeding, but this is rare and other bowel pathology must be ruled out first
- Ensure there are no palpable masses associated with the colon and exclude exacerbating factors such as a pregnant uterus, pelvic mass and enlarged liver
- Prolapsed piles are easily identified on rectal examination but internal haemorrhoids cannot be palpated

Investigations

Endoscopy:

- Proctoscopy: a proctoscope passed through the anus shows large prolapsed haemorrhoids encompassing tissue from above and below the dentate line.
- Sigmoidoscopy: this is performed to exclude any lesion further up the rectum e.g. polyp or tumour.
- Colonoscopy: This is performed if a further lesion has been identified. A biopsy can be taken from the lesion.

Management

Conservative treatment:

- The patient should be advised to avoid straining when passing stool.
- Encourage increased oral intake
- A bulk laxative can be offered
- Thrombosed, strangulated haemorrhoids can be treated with topical Lidocaine gel, ice packing, and analgesia.

Sclerotherapy:

- This method of treatment is suitable for first and second degree haemorrhoids.
- 2–3 mls of 0.5% phenol in almond oil (sclerosing agent) is injected above each haemorrhoid.
- The injection is painless and further injections may be required at monthly intervals.

Haemorrhoid banding:

- Large first and second degree haemorrhoids are not suitable for injection therapy and are treated with banding.
- Tight elastic bands are placed at the base of the haemorrhoid pedicle. These are done above the dentate line otherwise they can be very painful.
- The bands result in necrosis of the haemorrhoids, which spontaneously detach, after a few days.
- Only two haemorrhoids at one time should be banded.
- This can be performed as a day case/out-patient procedure.

Haemorrhoidectomy (operative management):

- This procedure is performed for third or fourth degree haemorrhoids
- It is carried out under general anaesthesia.
- The traditional scalpel method or stapled method can be used.
- An alternative procedure is the minimally invasive Doppler-guided haemorrhoidal artery ligation of the terminal branches of the superior haemorrhoidal artery.
- Early complications of a haemorrhoidectomy include pain, acute urinary retention and reactionary haemorrhage.
- Late complications of a haemorrhoidectomy include secondary haemorrhage, anal stricture and an anal fissure.
- Post-operative advice for the patient should be:
  - Regular analgesia
  - Bulk laxatives
  - Warm baths
  - Dry and sterile dressings should be applied as necessary
  - Out-patient follow up in 4–6 weeks

Anal fissures

Epidemiology

Anal fissure occurs predominantly in young to middle-aged adults and show no gender predominance.

Aetiology

An anal fissure is described as a longitudinal tear of the squamous epithelium lining the lower half of the anal canal from the anal verge to the dentate line. 90% of all fissures are found at the posterior site in the midline. It is not fully understood as to why this is the common site of occurrence, however it is thought that as a patient defecates, majority of the pressure is applied to the posterior anal tissues.

Anterior anal fissures are more common in women, especially in those who are multi-parous. This is thought to be a result of damage to the pelvic floor following perineal tears during labour.

Anal fissures can be a complication of inflammatory bowel disease, usually Crohn's disease. The development of an anal fissure is a recognised complication following haemorrhoid surgery.

After the initial formation of an anal fissure the pain experienced on defecation results in anal sphincter spasm, which extends the fissure line. This leads to the development of a spasm-fissure cycle.

Pathophysiology

Anal fissures can be acute or chronic. Acute anal fissures have a significant tear through the skin of the anal margin. The tear extends through the anal canal and there will be slight skin induration and oedema. There may also be spasms of the anal sphincter muscle.

In chronic anal fissures there is inflammation and induration of the fissure margins. The base of the fissure or lower border of the internal sphincter muscle may consist of scar tissue and in long term cases; fibrosis develops as well as continuous contraction of the sphincter muscles. In addition there is an increased risk of infection, abscess, and fistula formation.

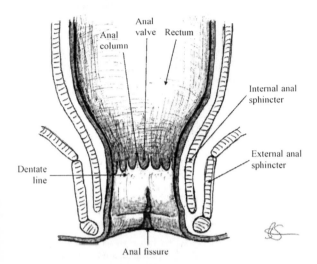

Figure 4.20: Anal fissure

Key features in the history/examination

- Pain occurs on defecation and it is sharp and stinging in character. It lasts 1–2 hours after the stool has been passed and as a result of anticipated pain the patient usually avoids passing stool.
- Pruritus occurs in around half of all patients.
- Bleeding is usually minimal and only noticed when wiping with tissue paper.
- A small amount of discharge may be noticed
- The anus should be examined but digital rectal examination may not be possible as a result of extreme pain.
- The buttocks may be separated and the fissure identified by gently parting the anal margin.
- The rectum may be examined and the fissure palpated with application of local anaesthetic.
- A sentinel pile may be identified in association with the fissure. This occurs due to the base of the fissure becoming oedematous and hypertrophied.

Investigations

The diagnosis of an anal fissure is confirmed with clinical examination. No additional investigations are required.

Management

Conservative management:

- Patients are advised to avoid straining on defecation

- Bulk laxatives can be prescribed
- Topical anaesthetic such as Xylocaine gels can be prescribed.
- Topical nitrates (e.g. 0.2% glyceryl trinitrate paste) may be useful. Nitric oxide has been found to act as a muscle relaxant, causing relaxation of the internal sphincter.
- If all methods have failed, operative management will be the next step.
- Botulinum A toxin can be injected into the external anal sphincter to break the spasm-fissure cycle. This is less invasive and has a lower rate of faecal incontinence compared to sphincterotomy.

Dilatation of the sphincter:

- This is the simplest procedure performed under general anaesthesia.
- The index and middle finger are placed into the anus where the edges are parted, and the anus is dilated.
- It is important to not overstretch the anal sphincter as this can lead to incontinence.
- This is not a favourable procedure due to the high incidence of subsequent incontinence.

Anal sphincterectomy:

- The internal sphincter is divided and separated from the fissure
- This can be achieved in the right or left lateral positions
- This is a procedure more suited for acute anal fissures.
- There is again a small risk of incontinence for which patients are counselled.

Further reading and references

- Acheson AG, Scholefield JH (2008). Clinical review: Management of haemorrhoids. *BMJ* 336: 380–383.
- Goldberg A, Stansby G (2006). *Surgical Talk: Revision in Surgery* (2 Ed.). Imperial college press.
- Hass P, Fox T, Hass G (1984). The Pathogenesis of haemorrhoids. Disease of the colon and rectum 27(7).
- Nelson R (2007). A Review of Operative Procedures for Anal Fissure. *Journal of gastrointestinal Surgery* 6: 284–289.

HAEMATURIA

Differential diagnosis

Classification	Disease
Infections	Urinary tract infection (UTI)
	Tuberculosis
Cancers	**Renal tumours**
	Bladder cancer

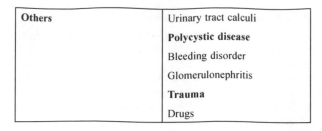

Others	Urinary tract calculi
	Polycystic disease
	Bleeding disorder
	Glomerulonephritis
	Trauma
	Drugs

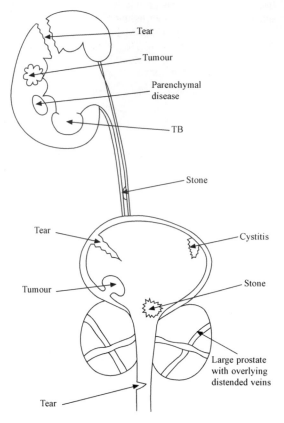

Figure 4.21: The different causes of haematuria.

Renal tumours

Epidemiology

Renal tumours are very uncommon and tend to present in adults over the age of 40. Male to female ratio is 2:1. Renal cell carcinoma or hypernephroma accounts for 2% of all adult malignancies. Wilms' tumour in children accounts for 8% of childhood cancers.

Aetiology

The aetiology is unknown but there are factors associated with the development of renal tumours. Carcinogens have been identified as a risk factor for transitional cell carcinoma. Those with chronic renal stones are at risk of developing squamous cell carcinoma (SSC). Renal cell carcinoma is associated with Von Hippel-Lindau disease and smoking is also a known risk factor.

Pathophysiology

Renal tumours can be benign (e.g. cysts) or malignant. Malignant tumours can be primary or secondary. While secondary tumours are rare, primary tumours can be classified as those arising from the pelvis and those from the kidney.

Tumours arising from the pelvis can either be transitional cell carcinomas, SSCs or papillomas. Transitional cell carcinomas are extremely malignant and occur where there is transitional cell epithelium present. SSCs commonly progress from squamous metaplasia.

There are two principal malignant tumours of the kidney, i.e. hypernephroma (Grawitz tumour) and nephroblastoma (Wilms' tumour). (See Table 4.5).

Tumour	Features
Hypernephroma (Grawitz tumour)	• This accounts for 80% of all renal tumours • It has associations with familial conditions such as Von Hippel-Lindau disease, and tuberous sclerosis. • The tumour originates from the renal tubules and macroscopically looks like a large vascular mass, in either or both poles of the kidney.
Nephroblastoma (Wilms' tumour)	• It is a childhood tumour usually affecting children below five years of age. • Bilateral tumours are seen in 5–10% of tumours. • These tumours are thought to originate from embryonic mesodermal tissue. • There are known association with congenital anomalies such as macroglossia, and aniridia. • These tumours are large, pale when cut into sections, and contain haemorrhagic areas.

Table 4.5: Features of hypernephroma and nephroblastoma.

Key features in the history/examination

- The different tumours can present with varying signs and symptoms
- Shortness of breath and pathological fractures suggest metastasis
- Renal colic

- Anorexia and weight loss

- Pallor (anaemia)

- Hypertension

- A mass palpated in the loin (see Table 4.6)

- Varicocele is present in 1% of cases where the tumour has spread along the renal vein obstructing the testicular vein

- Transitional cell carcinoma can be asymptomatic or present with painless haematuria

- Hypernephromas only occur in 11% of cases and generally patients only present in advanced disease. It may present with a classic triad of loin pain, loin mass and haematuria

Features of the kidney	Features of the spleen
• The kidney is ballotable	• The spleen is notched
• The kidney moves down vertically on inspiration	• The spleen moves towards the right iliac fossa on inspiration
• The kidney is resonant to percussion as a result of the overlying bowel.	• The spleen is dull to percussion as there is no bowel overlying it.

Table 4.6: How to differentiate a kidney from the spleen.

Investigations

Blood tests:

- FBC

- U&Es

- LFTs

- Calcium

- Clotting

- Group and save

Urinalysis:

- Urine dipstick: to demonstrate haematuria

- Cytology: for transitional cell carcinomas only

Imaging:

- CXR: to identify metastases (cannonball metastases)

- IVU: will identify filling defects, hydronephrosis and any renal mass.

- USS: may identify a mass and it can distinguish between solid and cystic tumours. The involvement of the inferior vena cava can be determined.

- CT: Is a useful investigation for staging the tumour and allows assessment of the other kidney.

- Magnetic resonance imaging (MRI): can show renal vein or vena caval tumour thrombosis.

Management

➤ Nephroureterectomy is the procedure of choice with transitional cell carcinomas. This involves removal of the entire renal tract on the affected side.

➤ Laparosopic or open radical nephrectomy is performed for large nephromas with a normal functioning kidney on the other side. It may be necessary to approach this procedure through the chest which increases the risk of pneumothoraces.

➤ A partial nephrectomy can be considered in small tumours of less than 4 cm and in those patients with a single functioning kidney. The local recurrence rate is < 10%.

➤ With the presence of metastatic disease chemotherapy and radiotherapy is offered as palliative care.

Prognosis:

➤ Nephroblastomas have an 80% survival rate for the first five years in children less than one. Recurrence commonly occurs within the first year but it is unlikely after 18 months.

➤ In operable hypernephromas there is a 70% survival after three years and 60% after five years. The five-year survival with metastatic disease is 20%.

Bladder cancer

Epidemiology

Bladder cancer usually occurs in adults over the age of 65 years. It has an incidence of 1 in 5,000 in the UK, affecting four times as many men than women.

Aetiology

The aetiology remains unknown but there are a number of predisposing factors associated with bladder cancer:

- Smoking

- Pelvic irradiation

- Industrial toxins from the dye industry such as beta-naphthylamine

- Chronic bladder irritation due to schistosomiasis, calculi or chronic infection

- Urachal remnants, e.g. embryological remnants between the umbilicus and the bladder

Schistosomiasis is associated with SSC with a peak age of incidence between the sixth and eight decades. The male to female ratio is 3:1.

Pathophysiology

90% of bladder cancers are transitional cell carcinomas. They can be solid, papillary, or both. SSC accounts for 7% and adenocarcinoma (AC) accounts for 2% of bladder cancers. The tumour can spread directly to the rectum, vagina, prostate, and uterus. Renal failure can result due to obstruction of the ureters, leading to hydronephrosis. However the liver and lung are the common sites for metastatic disease

4. Surgery

Stage	Level of spread
Ta	Confined to the mucosa
T1	Lamina propria is invaded
T2	The muscle is involved
T3	The perivesical fat is involved
T4	The tumour has invaded beyond the bladder to adjacent organs or to the pelvic wall

Table 4.7: Tumour, node and metastasis (TNM) staging.

Grade	Differentiation
G1	Well differentiated
G2	Intermediate differentiation
G3	Poorly differentiated

Table 4.8: Grading of tumours.

Key features in the history/examination

- Commonly patients are asymptomatic
- Painless haematuria
- Urinary symptoms include dysuria, urgency and frequency
- Acute urinary retention can result due to bladder neck obstruction
- Abdominal pain in the suprapubic or pelvic regions
- Shortness of breath suggests metastatic lung disease
- Signs of anaemia (pallor)
- Palpable mass
- Palpable lymph nodes
- Hepatomegaly
- Examination can often be normal with no identifiable signs

Investigations

Blood tests:

- FBC
- U&Es
- LFTs
- Calcium
- Clotting
- Group and save

Urinalysis:

- Urine dipstick: to demonstrate haematuria
- Cytology: for transitional cell carcinomas only

Imaging:

- CXR: to identify metastases

- IVU: will identify filling defects, hydronephrosis and any other renal masses.
- USS: may identify a mass and it can distinguish between solid and cystic tumours. The involvement of the inferior vena cava can be determined.
- CT: is the investigation of choice for staging the tumour
- MRI: again this can show renal vein or vena caval tumour thrombosis.

Management

- ➤ All tumours must be resected via transurethral resection of the bladder tumour (TURBT) under general anaesthesia. The tumour can then be staged and graded.
- ➤ Stage Ta, T1, T2 and Grade G1, G2:
  - o Intra-vesical chemotherapy is administered via a urinary catheter that has been inserted into the bladder and held there for approximately one hour. Patients have a repeat cystoscopy 8–10 weeks after chemotherapy.
  - o Intra-vesical immunotherapy using Bacillus Calmette-Guérin (BCG) has been shown to be more effective than chemotherapy in treating recurrent disease. However, with this treatment there are increased local and systemic side effects.
  - o All patients are followed up with regular cytoscopies at six months to one year intervals.
- ➤ Stage T3, T4 and Grade G3:
  - o Radical radiotherapy
  - o Cystectomy with the formation of an ileal conduit.

Operative management:

- ➤ Prior to the operation patients must be counselled with regards to the possible outcome of impotence and absent ejaculation after the procedure.
- ➤ Patients should be seen by a stoma nurse specialist, who should provide education about the stoma bags.
- ➤ Pre-operatively the bowel preparation is given to empty the bowel. Prophylactic antibiotics and low dose heparin is also prescribed.
- ➤ A low midline incision is made down to the symphysis pubis.
- ➤ The liver and retroperitoneum are inspected for metastatic disease.
- ➤ A bilateral pelvic lymphadenectomy is performed.
- ➤ The blood vessels passing to the bladder from the side wall are ligated, and the posterior ligaments of the bladder are ligated.
- ➤ The ureters and urethra are mobilised and then divided.
- ➤ The ligaments lateral to the prostate, are divided and the bladder is removed.
- ➤ The ureters are implanted into the small bowel and an ileo conduit is formed. This passage allows urine to pass from the ureters into a urostomy bag.

Prognosis:

➢ The five year survival rate is described in Table 4.9.

Stage	5 year survival rate
Ta/T1	70–80%
T2	40–50%
T3	25%
T4	Patients are dead with one year

Table 4.9: Five-year survival rates for bladder cancer.

Polycystic disease

Epidemiology

Adult polycystic kidney disease usually presents in those aged between 30 to 60 years. It accounts for 8–10% of all end-stage renal disease (ESRD).

Aetiology

This is a congenital condition which is inherited as an autosomal dominant trait. Polycystic kidney disease in children involves autosomal recessive inheritance and usually presents with renal failure. The aetiology of all renal cysts remains unknown.

Pathophysiology

Multiple cysts are present throughout the renal parenchyma. The cysts are different in size and can contain clear fluid, or coagulated blood.

Other cysts, associated with polycystic kidney disease include liver cysts (30%) and cysts in the lungs, spleen and pancreas (10%). There is also a well known association with intracranial berry aneurysms.

Key features in the history/examination

- Abdominal mass: commonly bilateral
- Loin pain: is characteristically a dull, constant ache. Severe pain may result if there is haemorrhage into the cysts.
- Urinary symptoms include urinary retention and dysuria
- Symptoms of uraemia: headache, anorexia and fatigue. There may also be drowsiness and vomiting.
- Drowsy and lethargic
- Loin tenderness on palpation
- Irregular and knobbly kidney enlargement
- Hypertension (75%)
- Pyrexia and tachycardia with an infection

Investigations

Blood tests:

- U&Es: urea and creatinine are elevated in renal failure

Urinalysis:

- Urine dipstick: may reveal a UTI or haematuria.

Imaging:

- USS: can identify multiple renal cysts in adults. It is less useful in children as a result of the smaller sized renal cysts.
- IVU: the contrast will outline elongated and narrow calyces.

Management

➢ Medical treatment is required for the management of renal failure and the associated hypertension.

➢ This may involve treatment with dialysis.

➢ Other complications such as anaemia and infection are usually best treated under the care of a nephrologist.

➢ A nephrectomy is performed if there is chronic loin pain, recurrent infections, haematuria and large kidneys.

➢ A bilateral nephrectomy may be necessary to control severe hypertension.

Trauma

Epidemiology

In the UK 90% of renal trauma is due to blunt trauma. Approximately 40% of these patients have associated intra-abdominal injuries.

Aetiology

Injury to the kidney can result from a direct blow to the loin or it can be a penetrating wound. Crushing injury to the abdomen in road traffic accidents can also affect the kidneys.

Pathophysiology

The degree of damage can vary from mild bruising or a capsular haematoma to complete rupture of the kidney. The kidney may also be avulsed partially or completely from its vascular pedicle.

Key features in the history/examination

- Loin pain
- Haematuria
- Abdominal distension is secondary to an ileus, as a result of a retroperitoneal haematoma
- Examination may only reveal tenderness over the loin/renal angle on palpation. There are no other specific signs on examination.
- With blunt trauma, other organs are often involved, for example the liver and spleen. Signs and symptoms may arise as a result of damage to these organs.

Investigations

Urinalysis:

- Urine dipstick: macroscopic haematuria may develop a few hours post injury.

Imaging:

- IVU: the contrast medium used may be found outside the renal border or the medium may illustrate rupture/damage to the renal calyces. A normal kidney will also be identified on the opposite side.
- USS: may identify a renal tear. Other injuries such as liver and spleen damage may also be detected.
- CT: is used in all trauma patients with penetrating trauma, blunt trauma or macroscopic haematuria, and with patients in hypovolaemic shock.

Management

Immediate management:

- ➢ IV access and resuscitation if the patient is shocked
- ➢ If there is macroscopic haematuria the patient should be advised to bed rest and avoid physical activity until the urine becomes clear.
- ➢ Analgesia
- ➢ Hourly observations must be recorded
- ➢ Antibiotics can be prescribed to prevent an infection from developing.
- ➢ All urine samples must be checked
- ➢ An urgent IVU is organised

Surgical management:

- ➢ Surgery may be required if there is progressive blood loss and an enlarging mass is identified in the loin.
- ➢ 95% of cases are managed conservatively
- ➢ An operation is performed to control and stop the bleeding, and conserve renal tissue.
- ➢ A nephrectomy is only performed if:
  - ○ There is life-threatening haemorrhage
  - ○ Severe hypertension continuously after the renal trauma
  - ○ The patient is symptomatic a few months after the trauma and there is little or no function in the damaged kidney. This is usually due to renal calculi or recurrent UTIs.
- ➢ Complications include bladder outlet obstruction as a result of clots, renal hypertension, and renal artery aneurysm.
- ➢ Renal embolisation can be performed to treat the haemorrhage. This is only performed following specialist advice.

Further reading and references

- ➢ Kaufman DS, Shipley WU, Feldman AS (2009). Bladder Cancer. *Lancet* 374.
- ➢ Parchment-Smith C, (2006). Essential Revision Notes for Intercollegiate MRCS: Bk. 1. PasTest.
- ➢ Parchment-Smith C, (2006). Essential Revision Notes for Intercollegiate MRCS: Bk. 2. PasTest.
- ➢ Kanani M, Elliott M, (2003). Applied Surgical physiology vivas. Cambridge University Press.

URINARY RETENTION

Differential diagnosis

Sex	Disease
Both	**Acute urinary retention**
	Urethral stricture
	Post-operative urinary retention
	Renal tract cancer
	Urinary tract infection (UTI)
	Multiple sclerosis
	Drugs
	Constipation
	Prolapsed intervertebral disc
Male	**Benign prostatic hyperplasia (BPH)**
	Prostate cancer
	Phimosis
	Paraphimosis
Female	Retroverted gravid uterus

Acute urinary retention

Epidemiology

Acute urinary retention is very common. It is often seen post operatively.

Aetiology

Urinary retention can be acute, chronic, or acute on chronic. The general causes of acute urinary retention are described in Table 4.10.

No obstruction	Local causes
• Postoperative	• Obstruction in the urethral lumen due to calculi or a blood clot
• Pain	
• Central nervous system (CNS) conditions such as multiple sclerosis or a spinal tumour.	• Abnormal wall pathologies e.g. stricture
	• Compression from outside the wall e.g. prostatic enlargement, faecal impaction, pelvic tumour, or a pregnant uterus.
• Drugs such as Tricyclic antidepressants (TCA), and anticholinergics	

Table 4.10: The causes of acute urinary retention.

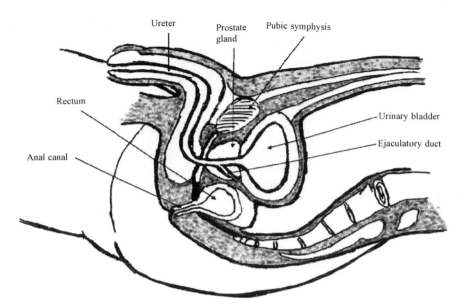

Figure 4.22: Anatomy of the male prostate.

Key features of the history/examination

- Patients usually present with reduced or no passage of urine for several hours.
- Lower abdominal pain, which can be severe in acute retention
- Signs of dehydration
- The patient may be pyrexial
- Suprapubic tenderness on palpation
- A palpable bladder which is dull to percussion
- Rectal examination may reveal an enlarged or hard prostate. If there is reduced anal tone and reduced sacral sensation, this may be a sign of cauda equina syndrome which is a surgical emergency!
- CNS/peripheral nervous system (PNS) examination should be carried out to assess for neurological causes of urinary retention.

Investigations

Blood tests:

- FBC: may show a raised white cell count
- U&Es: may be deranged
- Prostate specific antigen (PSA) level: determined before a rectal examination, if assessing for prostate cancer. This will be falsely elevated in UTIs, acute prostatitis and following urethral instrumentation.

Urinalysis:

- After urethral catheterisation may show a UTI.

Imaging:

- CXR: to identify metastatic disease
- KUB: to check for urinary tract calculi
- USS: to assess the residual volume in the bladder and to look for any bladder abnormalities. Back pressure leading to hydronephrosis may be present with resultant dilated renal calyces and ureter.

Management

- ➢ Try to mobilise the patient whilst running water from the tap. If this fails a urinary catheter should be inserted.
- ➢ Once the catheter has been sited document the residual volume, and monitor hourly urine output.
- ➢ After two unsuccessful attempts, consult a senior colleague who may attempt insertion of a urethral catheter or choose to site a suprapubic catheter.
- ➢ Antibiotics may be given to the patient to treat a UTI or to cover the infection risk of inserting a catheter.
- ➢ IV fluids may be required if the serum electrolytes are deranged.
- ➢ A trial without catheter (TWOC) should not be attempted within the first 24 hours after its insertion, due to the risk of going back into retention.
- ➢ Some centres will organise urodynamics prior to TWOC if they have a residual greater than two litres.
- ➢ The underlying cause must be identified and treated.

Urethral stricture

Epidemiology

The true incidence of urethral strictures is unknown. However there is an increase in the rate of stricture disease after the age of 55.

Aetiology

Urethral strictures may be congenital or acquired.

Type	Disease
Congenital	Meatal stenosis in hypospadias
Acquired	Trauma: mainly blunt trauma or instrumentation. This is common.
	Previous urethral or prostatic surgery
	Infection secondary to *Chlamydia/Gonococcal* urethritis
	Perineal injury
	Pelvic fractures
	Balanitis xerotica obliterans (BXO)

Table 4.11: The causes of urethral strictures.

Pathophysiology

The pathophysiology is dependent on the aetiology.

Key features in the history/examination

- Hesitancy
- Poor stream or spraying of urine
- Post micturition dribbling
- Painful ejaculation
- On examination the urethra should be palpated through the penis and do not forget to examine the urethral meatus.

Investigations

Imaging:

- Urethrogram: will identify the site of the stricture.
- USS: of the urethra will assess the stricture and identify the presence of fibrosis. This can aid in determining the risk of recurrence.

Endoscopy:

- Cysto-urethroscopy: this procedure can assist with treatment of the stricture, by performing dilatation of the stricture under direct vision. Dilatation can be carried out with metal dilators, gum-elastic bougies, or with self-dilators (e.g. catheters).

Others:

- Urodynamic investigations: the peak flow rate is reduced (Peak flow less than 10 ml/sec) and there is a prolonged micturition time.

Management

➢ Intermittent dilatation:
  o This is mainly symptomatic management and not a long term cure, as there is a poor success rate with a high recurrence rate.
  o This method of treatment is performed aseptically using a number of dilators to stretch the urethra.
  o Complications include a false passage, infection and septicaemia.

➢ Optical urethrotomy:
  o The stricture is cut under direct vision, using a knife passed through the sheath of the urethroscope.
  o This is suitable for short strictures
  o The stricture is cut at the 12 o'clock position, taking care not to cut the vascular areas of the corpus spongiosum, surrounding the urethra.
  o There is a 50% recurrence rate with this procedure but the recurrence rate can be reduced further with post operative intermittent dilatation.

➢ Urethroplasty:
  o This is the procedure used for recurrent strictures
  o The stricture is resected with an end-end anastomosis and ideally the patient should not have any instrumentation via the urethra in the three months following the procedure.

Post-operative urinary retention

Urinary retention can occur after any surgical operation

Epidemiology

The incidence of post-operative urinary retention can range from approximately 10–55% depending on the type of procedure they have undergone.

Aetiology

It is common to see urinary retention after an operation involving the anal canal and perineal region. As a result, a urinary catheter is placed prior to the end of the procedure. Other common problems include:

- Patients find it difficult to pass urine lying down or sitting in bed
- Urinary retention may be missed in sedated patients
- Elderly male patients have a history of prostatic obstruction therefore making urinary retention a common occurrence

Key features in the history/examination

- The patient has undergone surgery under general anaesthesia in the previous 24–48 hours
- The patient may complain of lower abdominal pain and the inability to pass urine
- There is suprapubic tenderness and a palpable bladder on abdominal palpation
- There is a dull note with percussion over the bladder

Investigations

The diagnosis is usually made from your clinical findings.

Imaging:

- Bladder scan: this can be found on the general surgical and urology wards. It is performed on the ward and scans the bladder, quantifying the residual volume of urine within the bladder.

Management

- ➤ The patient should be reassured
- ➤ Running tap water can often help
- ➤ If allowed, a warm bath is also helpful
- ➤ If after many attempts the patient has not passed urine a temporary urinary catheter may have to be inserted.

Benign prostatic hyperplasia

Epidemiology

This is a condition affecting men over the age of 50 years. Approximately 50% of these men will have histological changes of BPH and 15% will complain of urinary symptoms.

Aetiology

The prostate consist of three lobes. It is the inner zone of the prostate that enlarges resulting in compression of the urethra. There are two known theories for BPH. The hormone theory suggests that the prostate gland enlarges as a result of reduced amounts of testosterone and increased amounts of oestrogen. The increased amount of oestrogen causes hyperplasia. The neoplastic theory suggests that the enlargement of the prostate occurs due to a benign neoplasm.

Pathophysiology

The prostate consists of glandular and stromal tissue. Through its lifetime it is influenced by hormonal change, which can result in enlargement of the gland. In addition the prostate may be enlarged due to proliferation of epithelial and stromal tissue which then obstructs the urethra within the gland.

Enlargement of all of the three lobes of the prostate can lead to obstruction of the urethral lumen leading to urinary outflow obstruction.

Urinary outflow obstruction can result in

- Bladder stones as a result of urinary stasis
- Bladder diverticula
- Bladder trabeculation as a result of bladder hypertrophy
- UTI
- Back pressure on the ureters can lead to hydronephrosis and eventual renal failure

Key features in the history/examination

- Obstructive urinary (voiding) symptoms include poor stream, straining, hesitancy, terminal dribbling and sudden onset of abdominal pain if there is acute urinary retention.
- Detrusor instability (storage) symptoms include frequency, urgency and nocturia.
- Symptoms of renal failure are headache, confusion and lethargy.
- Signs of uraemia are dry furry tongue, confusion and pallor.
- Abdominal palpation may reveal a large bladder that is dull to percussion and tenderness if there is acute urinary retention.
- Rectal examination may reveal an enlarged smooth prostate. The lateral lobes are enlarged with a sulcus between the lobes. The examination should be performed after the bladder has been emptied because the gland is pushed down with a full bladder and therefore appears larger than it actually is.

Investigations

Blood tests:

- FBC: may show anaemia as a result of uraemia
- U&Es: will be deranged in renal failure
- PSA: is an indicator for prostate carcinoma. Levels less than 4.0 ng/mL are normal but if levels are more than 4.0 ng/mL then a transrectal ultrasound scan (TRUS) can be performed. Multiple biopsies can be taken under TRUS guidance.

Urinalysis:

- Urine dipstick: to look for infection
- Mid-stream urine (MSU): to look for infection

Imaging:

- KUB or USS: the upper urinary tract can be visualised to identify any complications such as hydronephrosis. An enlarged bladder may be identified. Residual volume of the bladder can be measured after urination.

Others:

- Urodynamics: A urine flow test is performed in which the patient passes urine into a flow meter; at least 200 mls of urine is required. A graph of urinary volume against time is formulated. A peak flow rate of less than 10 ml/sec suggests detrusor instability or obstructed urinary flow.

Management

Conservative management:

➤ It is feasible to offer conservative treatment in those patients with minimal symptoms

➤ General advice with regards to fluid intake such as limiting fluid intake in the evening.

➤ Simple bladder training involving asking the patient to hold his urine for a further ten minutes from the point in which he would normally want to void.

➤ These patients would be reviewed in outpatient clinic in six months time.

➤ Approximately 65% of patients will not improve and will return with worsening symptoms.

Pharmacological management:

➤ This is the treatment of choice in those with moderate to severe symptoms. Patients with storage symptoms benefit most. Combined medical therapy is acceptable practice.

➤ α-adrenergic antagonists (e.g. Tamsulosin, Alfuzosin):
   - They act by causing relaxation of smooth muscle of the bladder neck and prostate, improving symptoms of obstruction.
   - They are faster acting when compared with 5α-reductase inhibitors.
   - Postural hypotension is a significant side effect.

➤ 5α-reductase inhibitors (Finasteride):
   - A competitive selective inhibitor of 5α-reductase
   - These drugs prevent the conversion of testosterone to its active form, dihydrotestosterone (DHT), therefore reducing the volume of the prostate.
   - They have fewer side effects than α-adrenergic antagonists.

Surgical management:

➤ A significant number of men will decide to undergo surgical treatment due to the substantial improvement noted in operative management in comparison to medical management. Medical management is however, the treatment of choice for those who have failed conservative treatment and who do not want to undergo surgery.

➤ Pre-operative counselling may be necessary to inform patients of the complications:

➤ Retrograde ejaculation occurs in 65% of men following the procedure.
   - 5% of men will suffer with erectile impotence.
   - 15% of patients will require a further procedure in 8–10 years.
   - Mortality rate is less than 0.5%.

   - Complications include urethral stricture, sepsis, haematuria, urinary incontinence, UTI and transurethral resection (TUR) syndrome which is hyponatraemia and confusion as a result of absorption of large volumes of irrigating fluid.

➤ Transurethral resection of the prostate (TURP):
   - The patient is placed in the lithotomy position so that a cystoscope can be passed through the urethra to visualise the prostate.
   - A diathermy cutting loop is used to resect the lateral and middle lobes from the bladder neck.
   - Coagulation of bleeding points is simultaneously achieved with diathermy.
   - Hyponatraemia is avoided by using 1.5% isotonic glycine for irrigation.
   - A three way catheter is sited at the end of the procedure to continue irrigation of the bladder until the outflow is pink.
   - The prostate chippings are weighed and sent for histology.

➤ Open prostatectomy:
   - A retropubic approach is used to resect very large prostates (80–100 g)

➤ Newer treatments include:
   - Laser prostatectomy
   - Transurethral microwave thermotherapy using radiating heat therapy to cause sterile necrosis of the prostate tissue.
   - The effectiveness of these newer treatments in comparison to the traditional TURP remains unknown.

Phimosis

Epidemiology

Phimosis is very common in young boys, however it can present later in adult life. The true incidence of pathological phimosis in uncircumcised adult males is 1%.

Aetiology

The causes of phimosis include trauma, forceful retraction of the prepuce or recurrent balanitis. It can occur as a congenital lesion but this is rare.

Pathophysiology

Phimosis is the gross narrowing of the preputial orifice. In adult life it may present as a result of balanitis xerotica obliterans, in which the foreskin becomes thickened and will not retract. Patients may complain of painful intercourse, cracking or bleeding of the foreskin and infection.

Key features in the history/examination

- Ballooning of the prepuce on micturition
- Urinary flow is represented as a dribble
- Pain during sexual intercourse

Investigations

The diagnosis is made clinically and therefore no investigations are performed.

Management

➢ Antibiotics should be given if there is an infection present.

➢ A circumcision is performed if indicated.

➢ Indications in adults are balanitis, splitting of a tight frenulum, and prior to treatment in penile carcinoma.

➢ Indications in infants and young boys include phimosis and parental request due to religious or social beliefs.

➢ Procedure in an infant:

    o A surgical circumcision can be performed or alternatively a plastibell device is used.

    o The foreskin is mobilised and retracted

    o A device known as the plastibell (ring) is slipped over the glans penis.

    o The foreskin is then ligated and any redundant foreskin is cut away and discarded.

    o The plastibel separates 5–8 days postoperatively.

    o A dorsal slit can be performed in acute cases for immediate relief.

Paraphimosis

This is a condition where the foreskin has retracted beyond the glans, and cannot be replaced.

Epidemiology

Paraphimosis is common during infancy and adolescence. It has an incidence of approximately 1% in males over the age of 16 years.

Aetiology

Common causes include failure to replace the foreskin following urinary catheterisation insertion, masturbation, sexual intercourse, and occasionally during urination.

Pathophysiology

Venous and lymphatic drainage from the glans is obstructed, resulting in oedema and swelling. This may be followed by ischaemia of the glans.

Investigations

The diagnosis is made clinically and therefore no investigations are performed.

Management

➢ Manual reduction is first line treatment

➢ Before attempting this procedure the swelling must be reduced by using ice bags and gentle pressure or aspiration of the glans with a needle. A dorsal slit of the prepuce under local anaesthetic will relieve the pressure

➢ If manipulation fails a circumcision may be required

Further reading and references

➢ Barry MJ, Roehrborn CG (2001). Clinical Review: Extracts from 'Clinical Evidence' Benign Prostatic Hyperplasia. *BMJ* 323: 1042–1046.

➢ Kanani M (2002). Surgical Critical Care vivas. Cambridge University Press.

➢ Bulstrode CJK, Russell RCG, Williams NS (2000). *Bailey & Love's Short Practice of Surgery* (23 Ed.). Arnold.

➢ Calne R, Ellis H, Whatson C (2002). *Lecture Notes on General Surgery*. (10 Ed.) Blackwell Publishing.

➢ Goldberg A, Stansby G (2006). *Surgical Talk: Revision in Surgery* (2 Ed.). Imperial college press.

➢ Mundy AR (2006). Review: Management of urethral strictures. *Postgraduate Medical Journal* 82: 489–493.

LIMB PAIN

Differential diagnosis

Pathology	Disease
Venous	**Varicose veins**
	Venous leg ulcers
	Venous thrombosis
Arterial	**Arterial leg ulcers**
	Acute limb ischaemia
	Arterial stenosis
	Chronic limb ischaemia
Others	**Compartment syndrome**
	Small vessel disease

Varicose veins

Epidemiology

Varicose veins are dilated superficial veins that affect 20% of the western population. 2% of these go on to develop associated skin changes, which can lead to ulcer formation.

Anatomy

There are two venous systems in the lower limbs. Both ensure blood from the skin and muscles of the legs is returned to the trunk.

Superficial venous system:

- The long (great) Saphenous vein extends from just anterior to the medial malleolus along the medial aspect of the thigh.

- This drainage system involves the dorsum of the foot up until the Sapheno-femoral junction in the groin.

- The short (small) Saphenous vein is placed laterally and drains into the popliteal vein behind the knee.

- This venous system does not involve the deep fascia, and only takes an active role in venous drainage of the skin and superficial tissue.

Deep venous system:

- This consists of a group of veins within the deep fascia, which surround the leg muscles.

- Smaller venous tributaries drain behind the knee into the popliteal vein.

- Once the popliteal vein ascends, it becomes the femoral vein.

- As the femoral vein reaches the inguinal ligament it becomes the external iliac vein.

- After this point venous return occurs through the common iliac vein, the inferior vena cava, and finally entering the right atrium.

Perforators:

- These are veins which allow communication between the deep and superficial veins.

- These perforating veins contain valves to prevent back flow from the deep to the superficial veins.

Calf pump:

- When the calf muscle contracts blood from the deep veins is pushed up towards the heart.

- Valves present in these veins prevent blood from falling back down the deep veins.

- When the calf muscles relax, blood flows from the superficial veins into the deep veins, awaiting calf muscle contraction.

- The calf muscles therefore work as a pump.

Aetiology

Varicose veins occur as a result of dysfunction of the valves in the veins of the legs. The exact mechanism is unknown but two theories have been proposed. Primary valve incompetence or structural weakness of the venous walls resulting in dilatation and valve disruption, are thought to be the cause.

If both parents have been affected by varicose veins, off-springs have an 80% chance of developing them as well. Environmental factors include standing on the heels all day, usually for occupational reasons. Pregnancy can cause varicose veins as a result of the oestrogen and progesterone causing smooth muscle relaxation of the leg veins. Other environmental factors include previous deep vein thrombosis (DVT), abdominal or pelvic mass, ascites, obesity and constipation.

Pathophysiology

Varicose veins are thought to be a result of increased pressure within the superficial venous system. A patient at rest will have equal pressures in the superficial and deep venous systems. A patient carrying out any activity has increased pressure in the deep venous system. If the venous valves of the superficial system are incompetent, these veins will not be protected from the high pressures and varicosities will result.

It is thought that first a small gap is found between the vein wall and the valve leaflets (valve cusps). This gap increases in size allowing increased reflux of blood flow. Over time there is degeneration of the valve cusps, after which they will completely disappear. This vein below the valve will dilate and can increase by five times its normal size.

Key features in the history/examination

- Can be asymptomatic
- Leg discomfort or cramp-like pain
- Skin changes or ulcerations
- Ankle swelling
- Pruritis
- Patients may complain for cosmetic reasons

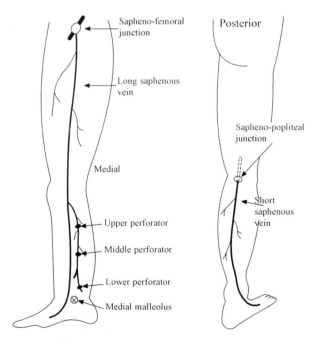

Figure 4.23: Deep and Superficial venous drainage of the lower limb. *Reprinted with Permission from Andrew Goldberg and Gerard Stansby, Surgical Talk, 2nd Ed, 2005, Imperial Colleague Press.*

- Classically described as 'long, tortuous and dilated' veins in the leg
- Initially noted on the calves
- Small veins can have a diameter of 0.5 mm and appear purple/red in colour.
- Larger veins are noted with a diameter of 1–3 mm. If the Saphenous veins are affected the diameter can range from 5–15 mm.
- Skin changes include pigmentation, eczema, ulceration, lipodermatosclerosis (wax like skin), and heamosiderin deposit (blue/purple discolouration caused by loss of red cells into the tissue due to increased venous pressure).

Trendelenburg's test:

1. This test is used to identify reflux of blood from the deep to the superficial veins.

2. With the patient lying flat the superficial veins are emptied by elevating the leg.

3. A tourniquet is applied to the upper thigh (occlusion of superficial venous system at level of tourniquet).

4. The patient is then asked to stand up.

5. If the veins remain empty it can be safely assumed that the Sapheno-femoral junction is incompetent and is the cause of the superficial venous reflux.

6. If the tourniquet does not control the varicose veins and allows the vein to fill with blood, the test can be repeated with the tourniquet placed lower down the leg until the point of control is reached.

Table 4.12: The procedures involved in the Trendelenburg's test.

Tap test:

1. Fingers from one hand are placed over the Sapheno-femoral junction

2. A distal varicose vein is then tapped

3. A transmitted thrill may be felt over the Sapheno-femoral junction if incompetent.

4. This occurs as there will be a column of blood in the vein due to the absence of vein valves.

Table 4.13: The procedure involved in the tap test.

Site of Incompetence	Distribution
Sapheno-femoral junction	Long Saphenous distribution
Mid-thigh perforators	Short Saphenous distribution
Sapheno-popliteal junction	Short Saphenous and medial calf perforator distribution
Medial calf perforators	Mixed picture

Table 4.14: Distribution of varicose veins as a result of the site of incompetence.

Investigations

Blood tests:

- FBC: baseline levels
- U&Es: baseline levels
- Clotting: baseline levels
- Group and save

Imaging:

- Doppler USS: This is used to exclude arterial disease and detect venous reflux. The Doppler probe is placed over the Sapheno-femoral junction and the venous flow in the common femoral vein is identified. The calf on the same side is gently squeezed to accelerate blood flow from the Saphenous vein up the Sapheno-femoral junction into the common femoral vein. A sound such as 'whoosh' is heard. When the calf is released a sound to illustrate reverse flow may be heard. An abnormal prolonged second 'whoosh' indicates valve incompetence as blood flows back unrestricted.

- Colour duplex scanning: This test outlines the veins of the legs. It can identify valve and perforator incompetence and it will confirm if the deep venous system is patent. This is essential before the patient is considered for any superficial venous avulsion.

- Venography: A tourniquet is placed around the ankle and the superficial veins are occluded. Then a contrast medium is injected into the dorsum of the foot, where it will be passed through the deep venous system. Multiple X-rays are taken and any reflux through the deep and perforating veins can be seen. This used to be the gold standard test, but is used less frequently due to the development of non-invasive methods and the increased risk of reaction to the contrast medium.

- Plethysmography: this investigation uses light transmission to assess filling of the veins. A probe is placed on the skin and light transmission through this assesses venous filling on the skin surface. The filling of the vein through light transmission represents the pressure of the superficial leg veins. This test can be repeated with application of a tourniquet to identify which set of veins have been affected.

Others:

- ECG should be done prior to any operative procedure

Management

Conservative management:

➢ The underlying cause must be treated, e.g. lose weight or treat the constipation.

➢ Compressive support stockings: provides symptomatic relief and the progression of varicose veins is reduced.

➢ Injection sclerotherapy: A sclerosing agent (sodium tetradecyl sulphate) is injected into the veins. Then foam pads are applied firmly after the procedure to provide compression for two weeks. Eventually the vein is replaced with a fibrous cord.

4. Surgery

➤ Laser coagulation: can be used to treat small varicose veins.

Operative management:

➤ Operative treatment is usually offered to those with Saphenofemoral incompetence and/ or major perforator incompetence. These operations can be performed as day cases.

➤ Trendelenburg procedure (high tie): the long Saphenous vein is ligated at its entry point into the femoral vein and all its tributaries are ligated. This procedure has a high recurrence rate.

➤ Short Saphenous vein ligation: the short Saphenous vein is ligated deep in the popliteal fossa.

➤ Multiple avulsions: multiple stab incisions are performed to strip individual varicose veins.

➤ Ligation of perforators: this procedure is performed for calf and ankle perforators.

➤ Endovenous laser ablation (EVLA): this works by means of thermal destruction of venous tissues. USS is used to map out the venous system and guide cannulation of the affected vein. The treatment is less invasive than the traditional high tie and has equal if not lower recurrence rates.

➤ Post-operative management involves compression bandages being applied to reduce bruising. After 1–2 days the bandages are removed and replaced with compression stockings. These stockings can be removed to allow the patient to shower.

➤ Post operative complications include:
  o Bruising and pain
  o Haematoma
  o Wound infection
  o Nerve damage e.g. In particular the Saphenous, Sural and Common Peroneal nerves can be damaged
  o DVT
  o Recurrence of varicose veins
  o Lymphoedema

Venous leg ulcers

Epidemiology

Venous leg ulcers are the most common type of leg ulcers, accounting for 80% of cases in the western community. Around 10% of leg ulcers are due to arterial disease, with 5–10% a result of mixed venous and arterial pathology.

Aetiology

Venous ulcers are thought to arise as a result of the constant high blood pressure within the veins of the lower legs due to venous insufficiency. Risk factors include increasing age, obesity, immobility, varicose veins, and a previous history of a DVT.

Pathophysiology

Venous ulcers can arise as a result of superficial or deep venous incompetence. This commonly is a result of valvular incompetence resulting in abnormal blood flow and venous congestion. These ulcers are seen proximal to the medial or lateral malleolus, typically along the medial gaiter region. There are often associated signs of long-standing venous disease, such as oedema, haemosiderin deposition, lipodermatosclerosis and varicose veins.

Other types of leg ulcers include arterial ulcers, neuropathic ulcers, traumatic ulcers, ulcers due to systemic disease, and neoplastic ulcers. Leg ulcers can frequently be of mixed pathology, i.e. venous/diabetic/arterial.

Key features in the history/examination

• Patients may complain of pain, swelling and altered sensation.

• Varicose veins may be present

• Peripheral pulses should be palpated and a complete peripheral vascular examination should be performed.

• Neoplastic changes along the edge of a long standing venous ulcer can occur (e.g. Marjolin ulcer)

• On examination the sensation may be altered in the limbs and ulcerated areas. Peripheral neuropathy is commonly seen with diabetic foot ulcers.

• Doppler ankle-brachial blood pressure should be measured

VARICOSE VEINS

NORMAL VEINS

Incompetent valves causes reflux of blood

Long, tortuous, dilated veins

Normal valves allow blood flow in one direction

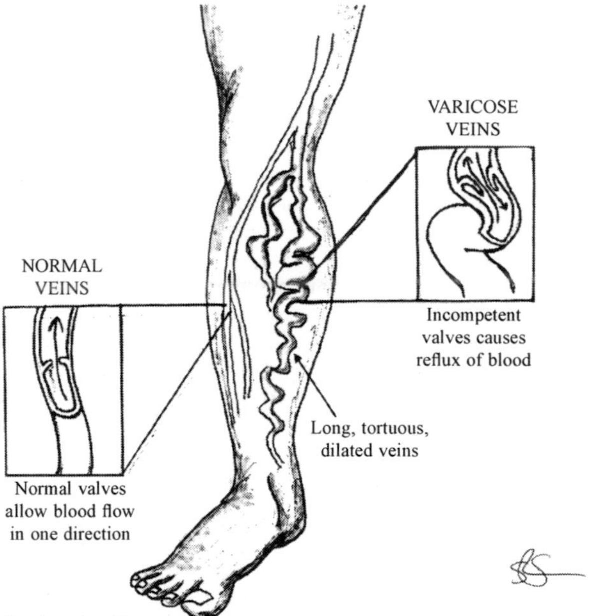

Treatment options:

Conservative:
Compressive support
Stockings
Injection Sclerotherapy
Laser coagulation

Operative:
Trendelenburg procedure (High tie)
Short Saphenous vein ligation
Multiple avulsions
Ligation of perforators
Endovenous laser ablation (EVLA)

Figure 4.24: Varicose veins and their management.

Investigations

These are important to assess the type of ulcer, especially when attempting to distinguish between venous and arterial ulcers.

Blood tests:

- FBC: baseline levels
- U&Es: baseline levels
- Clotting: baseline levels
- Group and save

Imaging:

- Duplex USS: this is required to assess the severity of arterial disease and the extent of collateral circulation.
- Angiography: this is also required to assess the severity of arterial disease and the extent of collateral circulation.

Others:

- Ulcer biopsy: this can identify venous or arterial disease. Malignancy can also be detected.

Management

- ➢ In venous ulcers occurring as a result of superficial venous incompetence, surgical removal of the associated varicose veins has been proven to promote ulcer healing.
- ➢ Patients with deep venous incompetence and those who are unfit for surgery should be managed conservatively.
- ➢ Venous ulcers can heal sufficiently if kept clean.
- ➢ Patients who are bed-bound are advised to keep their feet elevated to reduce the high venous pressures.
- ➢ Antibiotics are only prescribed if an ulcer has become infected or if there is surrounding cellulitis.
- ➢ Most of the patients affected are elderly and are unable to manage these ulcers on their own. This can lead to prolonged ulceration and further complications.
- ➢ In these cases it is appropriate to use four layer pressure bandages, which act to empty the superficial veins, encouraging the calf pump to work.
- ➢ With large ulcers, skin grafting may be an option to encourage ulcer healing.
- ➢ District nurses are usually responsible for changing the bandages once or twice a week.
- ➢ After an ulcer has healed the incompetent veins do not spontaneously resolve and therefore recurrence is common.
- ➢ Patients should therefore continue to wear elastic compression stockings, and elevate their limbs.

Arterial leg ulcers

Epidemiology

Approximately 10% of leg ulcers are due to arterial disease with 5–10% a result of mixed venous and arterial pathology.

Aetiology

Arterial ulcers result from an inadequate blood supply due to peripheral vascular disease, diabetes mellitus or trauma. Atherosclerosis is the major contributing factor to arterial ulcer formation. Other arterial vascular diseases that can cause ulcers include Raynaud's disease, Buerger's disease, scleroderma and rheumatoid vasculitis. Radiation and electrical burns can also result in arterial leg ulcers.

Pathophysiology

The initial ischaemia causes tissue necrosis which leads to the formation of arterial ulcers but then these ulcers fail to heal due to an inadequate blood supply. Arterial ulcers are often found at the most distal site of the circulation such as the tips of toes.

Key features in the history/examination

- Clinical history of intermittent claudication or rest pain of the lower limbs indicates the presence of peripheral vascular disease. Patients normally describe a cramp like pain in the lower limbs on walking a particular distance which is relieved with rest.
- Arterial ulcers are usually very painful and pain may be leg position-dependent, i.e. aggravated by leg elevation.
- Surrounding skin is hairless and shiny
- Nails are thickened due to fungal infection
- Foot may appear pale, mottled or purple depending on the extent of ischaemia.
- Cool limb on palpation with delayed capillary refill
- Distal foot pulses may be absent or weaker
- Features of arterial ulcer see Table 4.15

Arterial ulcer	Venous ulcer
Distribution on pressure areas of the foot. Common sites include heel, head of 5th metatarsal, tips of toes, ball of foot.	Distribution along the gaiter region (medial aspect of foot).
Painful	Can be painless
Punched out appearance with steep edges	Superficial with gently sloping ragged edge
Pale bloodless sloughy dry base.	Red velvety granulation tissue at the base and the ulcer margin has a slight blue rim.
Surrounding skin may be pale, shiny and hairless	Surrounding skin shows evidence of venous insufficiency such as varicose veins, lipodermatosclerosis and haemosiderin deposition.

Table 4.15: Showing classical features of arterial and venous ulcers.

4. Surgery

Investigations

These are important to assess the type of ulcer, especially when attempting to distinguish between venous and arterial ulcers.

Blood tests:

- FBC: baseline levels
- U&Es: baseline levels
- Clotting: baseline levels
- Group and save

Imaging:

- Angiography: is required to assess the severity of arterial disease and it also provides a treatment option.
- Doppler USS and Duplex USS: indicate the degree of arterial flow. Ankle brachial pressure index (ABPI) will demonstrate if there is a peripheral vascular disease component. The pressure at the ankle should be the same as the brachial artery pressure with the patient in the supine position. (See Table 4.16).

ABPI	Severity
1	Normal
0.8–0.9	Some arterial insufficiency but not enough to cause symptoms.
0.41–0.8	Correlates with claudication symptoms
< 0.4	rest pain

Table 4.16: The integrity of arterial blood flow as indicated by ABPI. Note diabetics can have heavily calcified vessels providing a falsely elevated ABPI reading

Others:

- Ulcer biopsy: This can identify venous or arterial disease. Malignancy can also be detected.

Management

Treatment for arterial ulcers is to improve the arterial circulation to the ulcer site thereby encouraging tissue healing.

Medical management:

- Medical management will reduce the chance of disease progression but alone is unlikely to achieve complete ulcer healing.
- Smoking cessation
- Anti-platelet drugs (Aspirin, Clopidogrel)
- Cholesterol reducing drugs (Statins)

Surgical management:

- Before progressing on to surgical treatment the sites of arterial stenosis must first be identified by an arteriogram.

- Percutaneous angioplasty and stent placement are performed to open up the site of stenosis. The durability of these procedures is poor and most patients eventually require surgical management.
- Bypass grafting using synthetic material or autogenous vein is the standard surgical treatment. Aorto-iliac bypass, femoral-popliteal bypass, and distal bypasses are the main types of operations for arterial insufficiency.

Acute limb ischaemia

Acute limb ischaemia is a surgical emergency which can result in the patient losing a limb if they do not receive immediate treatment.

Epidemiology

There are approximately 5,000 cases per year in the UK.

Aetiology

The causes of an acutely ischaemic limb include thrombosis, embolism, trauma, aortic dissection, aneurysms and iatrogenic causes. However, thrombus and emboli are the two most common causes of sudden limb occlusion.

Pathophysiology

Thrombosis accounts for 60% of all cases. The main cause for this is plaque rupture within an already stenosed vessel. Predisposing factors for thrombosis include dehydration, malignancy, hyperviscosity and thrombophilia.

An embolism accounts for 30% of all cases of acute limb ischaemia. An embolism is an abnormal mass of un-dissolved tissue that passes in the blood stream from one part of the circulation to another. A fluid or solid particle lodges within the vascular system, where the embolus diameter is greater than the diameter of the blood vessel. Predisposing factors for emboli include thrombus, atheroma, tumour, foreign body, air, cholesterol and a hypercoaguable state (e.g. protein C or S deficiency, polycythaemia, malignancy). Emboli commonly arise from a mural thrombus, mitral stenosis, and as a result of cardiac arrhythmias (e.g. AF). Emboli can lodge in any organ and cause ischaemia (e.g. limbs, brain, spleen, kidneys, lungs, and mesenteric vessels).

Thrombus	Emboli
• History of intermittent claudication or rest pain • Onset occurs over hours • Signs of chronic vascular disease • The artery is hard to touch • No audible bruits	• History of recent MI and AF • No intermittent claudication • Onset occurs over seconds to minutes • No history of evidence of vascular disease • The artery is soft to touch • Audible bruit

Table 4.17: How to differentiate between a thrombus and emboli

Key features in the history/examination

- Severe pain
- Loss of sensation or having numbness
- Cold limbs
- Unable to move toes
- There are six well known signs of an acutely ischaemic leg. These are known as the 6Ps. (See Table 4.18).

Pain	The pain is severe
Pallor	A salvageable limb is white, then mottled and blanches. A non-salvageable limb is mottled, non-blanching, with a fixed dark colour.
Parasthesiae	This is associated with poor prognosis.
Pulselessness	A Doppler probe is used to verify this.
Paralysis	The patient is unable to move their toes
Perishing cold	Cold limb

Table 4.18: The 6Ps associated with acute limb ischaemia.

Investigations

The diagnosis is made clinically as without imminent treatment the patient may lose a limb.

Management

Immediate management:

- ➤ Senior involvement must be early
- ➤ Analgesia e.g. morphine
- ➤ IV access and fluids
- ➤ NBM
- ➤ IV heparin (5,000 units stat)
- ➤ Angiogram: only in those patients with incomplete ischaemia.
- ➤ If acute limb ischaemia is due to thrombosis:
  - ○ Thrombolysis e.g. tissue plasminogen activator (tPA) or streptokinase
  - ○ Angioplasty and stenting
  - ○ Emergency reconstruction with or without a fasciotomy
  - ○ Amputation
- ➤ If acute limb ischaemia is due to an embolus:
  - ○ Embolectomy with a Fogarty catheter
  - ○ On table thrombolysis with unsuccessful embolectomy
  - ○ Emergency reconstruction with or without fasciotomy
  - ○ Amputation

Thrombolysis:

- ➤ Arteriography of the affected limb is performed.
- ➤ At the end of the procedure a narrow catheter is passed into the blocked vessel.
- ➤ A thrombolytic agent (streptokinase, tPA, urokinase) is administered into the vessel through the catheter.
- ➤ This procedure should occur in HDU, ICU, or the theatre.
- ➤ Regular angiograms are performed to monitor clot lysis.
- ➤ Streptokinase can take up to 48 hours and tPA can take up to 24 hours for complete lysis to occur.
- ➤ Contraindications include a recent stroke and pregnancy.

Embolectomy:

- ➤ Local or general anaesthesia can be used
- ➤ The artery with the clot is exposed and then supported and held with rubber tube or sling.
- ➤ A longitudinal or transverse incision is made and the clot and embolus is removed.
- ➤ Fogarty catheterisation is a balloon catheter passed over a guide wire and advanced through the embolus. The balloon is inflated and the embolus and thrombus are removed through an arteriotomy.
- ➤ The affected artery is then flushed with heparin-saline solution and distal pulses are assessed to determine success of procedure.
- ➤ Post-operative management involves:
  - ○ 48 hours of heparin infusion
  - ○ Long term anticoagulation with warfarin is initiated
  - ○ Following the acute management of an ischaemic limb, investigations should be performed to identify the possible source of the emboli. These may include echocardiography, 24-hour tape and USS of the aorta (and distal vessels if necessary to rule out an aneurysm).
- ➤ Post-operative complications include:
  - ○ Reperfusion injury: when oxygen is reintroduced to the vessels, oxygen free radicals can damage vessel endothelium. This can result in compartment syndrome, acidosis, hyperkalaemia and shock
  - ○ Compartment syndrome needs to be treated with a fasciotomy
  - ○ Chronic pain

Compartment syndrome

Epidemiology

The incidence varies according to the aetiology. However, it is commonly associated with limb fractures.

Aetiology

Causes of compartment syndrome are as follows:

- Fracture with subsequent haemorrhage (e.g. tibial or forearm fractures)
- Ischaemic reperfusion following injury
- Vascular puncture

- IV drug injection
- Tight fitting casts
- Prolonged limb compression
- Crush injuries
- Burns
- Vigorous exercise

Pathophysiology

Compartment syndrome is caused by increased tissue pressure in a fascial compartment impairing blood circulation to the muscles and nerves.

The normal mean interstitial tissue pressure is near 0 mmHg in non-contracting muscle. A pressure elevation of 30 mmHg or more, results in compression of small vessels in the tissue, reducing nutrient blood flow and causing ischaemia and pain.

The commonest fascial compartments involved are the forearm and the leg. In the lower limbs, the anterior (extensors), posterior (flexors of the ankle), and peroneal (evertors) may be affected.

Key features in the history/examination

- Pain: is out of proportion to the injury sustained and is aggravated by stretching of the muscles in the involved compartment.
- Pale: the limb is pale tense swollen and shiny
- Poikilothermia (cold): cool on palpation and there is a general tenderness to the affected compartment.
- Parasthesia: occurs in the cutaneous nerve distribution of the affected limb.
- Paralysis: is normally a late finding when significant muscle ischaemia has occurred.
- Pulseless: initially in compartment syndrome the distal circulation and pulses are normal. Loss of the pulse in the affected limb is a late finding and often indicates the time for limb salvage is passing.

Investigations

The diagnosis is made on the clinical history and examination.

Others:

➢ Pressure gauge: the intra-compartmental pressure can be tested by using a pressure gauge cannulated into the affected tissue. Generally an intra-compartmental pressure of more than 30 mmHg indicates compartment syndrome and a fasciotomy will be required.

Management

➢ Removal of cast or bandages if present
➢ Surgical treatment with fasciotomy to decompress the affected limb. In the calf this involves two incisions; a lateral incision to free the peroneal and anterior compartments and a medial incision to free the superficial and deep posterior compartments.

Prognosis:

➢ If compartment syndrome is left untreated it will eventually cause tissue hypoxia and necrosis. This will result in loss of the affected limb as well as rhabdomyolysis, causing acute renal failure.

Further reading and references

➢ Hiatt WR (2001). Medical treatment of peripheral arterial disease and claudication. NEJM 344: 1608–1621.
➢ London N, Nash R (2000). Clinical review: ABC of arterial and venous disease – Varicose veins. BMJ 320: 1391–1394.
➢ Parchment-Smith C (2002). Surgical Short Cases for the MRCS Clinical Examination. PasTest.

LUMPS

Differential diagnosis

Structure	Disease
Skin	**Sebaceous cyst**
	Benign naevi
	Lipoma
	Neurofibroma
	Papilloma
	Kaposi's sarcoma
	Basal cell carcinoma (BCC)
	Bowen's disease
	Squamous cell carcinoma (SSC)
	Malignant melanoma
Neck	**Thyroglossal cyst**
	Goitre
	Thyroid cyst
	Primary thyroid tumour
	Solitary thyroid nodules
	Thyroid carcinoma
	Branchial cyst
	Branchial sinus
	Dermoid cyst
	Carotid body tumour
	Pharyngeal pouch
	Salivary gland neoplasm
	Acute parotitis
	Cystic hygroma

Breast	Breast cancer
	Fibroadenoma
	Breast lipoma
	Breast cyst
	Abscess
	Haematoma
Groin and scrotum	**Incompletely descended testis**
	Testicular torsion
	Hydrocele
	Varicocele
	Epididymal cyst
	Spermatocele
	Testicular carcinoma
	Epididymo-orchitis
	Saphena varix
	Femoral artery aneurysm
	Haematoma
	Lipoma of the cord
	Inguinal lymph nodes
Hernias	**Inguinal**
	Femoral
	Incisional
	Umbilical
	Para-umbilical
	Epigastric
	Spigelian
	Obturator
	Lumbar
	Sciatic

SKIN

Sebaceous cyst

Epidemiology

Sebaceous cysts are extremely common. They present between the age of 20–30 years, and have been found to be twice as common in men than women.

Aetiology

Sebaceous cysts can arise due to blocked sebaceous glands, trauma or surgical disruption, swollen hair follicles and increased production of testosterone. Infection with human papilloma virus (HPV) has also been associated with such cysts.

Hereditary conditions such as Gardner's syndrome and basal cell naevus syndrome can result in the formation sebaceous cysts.

Pathophysiology

Sebaceous cysts are sometimes referred to as epidermoid cysts. They occur following obstruction to the mouth of the sebaceous gland and can arise at any site where sebaceous glands are present. Therefore, they are typically found on the scalp, face, scrotum and vulva. They do not occur on the soles of the feet or the palms of hands.

Key features in the history/examination

- The cyst is a round swelling attached to the skin
- It moves freely with the skin over deeper lying structures.
- The cyst is fluctuant
- A central punctum is often diagnostic of a sebaceous cyst
- The cyst usually contains 'cheesy' material which has an offensive smell
- Superimposed infection is a common complication
- Ulceration of the cyst can look like a SSC, which is known as 'Cocks peculiar tumour'.
- A sebaceous horn may form as a result of leakage and drying of the cyst contents.

Investigations

Usually the diagnosis is based on the clinical signs and symptoms. However, in cases of suspected malignancy, the lump should be excised and sent to histopathology for analysis.

Management

- ➢ With uncomplicated sebaceous cysts surgical resection is the best option.
- ➢ Under local anaesthetic, a small ellipse incision is made around the cyst and punctum.
- ➢ The cyst capsule is identified and removed as an intact lesion.
- ➢ The entire wall must be removed to prevent recurrence.
- ➢ The cyst should always be sent for histology to confirm diagnosis
- ➢ If there is infection and inflammation of the cyst, an incision and drainage procedure is performed. The capsule wall remains and needs to be resected at a later date otherwise the cyst will recur.

Benign naevi

Epidemiology

These are more common in fair skinned individuals.

Aetiology

Benign naevi can be congenital (as a result of embryological anomalies), and therefore are present from birth. Acquired benign naevi develop later in life and often occur as a result of sun exposure.

Pathophysiology

Melanocytes are clear cells found in the basal layer of the epidermis. Melanocytes arise from the embryonic neural crest and it is these cells which produce the brown pigment melanin. If these cells increase in number within the layers of the skin, they develop into benign pigmented naevi (moles).

Type	Feature
Dermal naevi	• Also known as the common mole • Appearances can vary as the naevus can be light or dark in colour, flat or raised, and with hair present or absent. • These naevi can occur at most sites of the body, with the palms, soles, and scrotum being exceptions. • All of the melanocytes are found within the dermis. • These naevi do not progress to malignancy.
Junctional naevi	• The melanocytes are distributed within the basal layer of the epidermis, with projections into the dermis. • They can vary in colour, ranging from light brown to black. • These naevi are mostly smooth, flat, and do not have any hair present. • They can occur anywhere on the body, including the soles, palms and genitalia. • These naevi do carry potential for malignant change.
Compound naevi	• These consist of features of both dermal and junctional naevi. • Clinically they appear similar to dermal naevi and therefore, it can be difficult to differentiate between the two.
Malignant melanoma	• See Insidious onset section.

Table 4.19: The different types of naevi.

Investigations

Benign naevi are diagnosed with the information gained from the clinical history and examination. If malignant change is suspected a biopsy should be taken and sent for histological analysis.

Management

➤ Treatment in the form of surgical excision may be considered for cosmetic purpose.

➤ It may also be considered if the naevi is causing problems such as irritation when rubbed by clothing, or trauma from shaving.

➤ All lesions excised are sent for histological analysis.

Lipoma

Epidemiology

Lipomas are the most common benign subcutaneous tumours, affecting 1% of the population. It can arise at any age but is often seen in adults between 40 – 60 years old.

Aetiology

The aetiology is unknown.

Pathophysiology

These can be defined as benign tumours consisting of adipose tissue and can occur anywhere in the body where fat is present. They are the commonest type of benign tumour. Multiple lipomas are seen in a condition called Dercum's disease, which is a familial condition.

Large lipomas can develop into liposarcomas and calcification can also occur in the long term.

Type	Site
Subcutaneous	Often seen on the shoulders or back, but can occur anywhere.
Subfascial	They are seen under the palmar or plantar fascia. If left alone they can erode into the underlying bone.
Sub synovial	Commonly found in the knee and have often been mistaken for a baker's cyst.
Intra-articular	Rare benign lipoma originating from the joint synovium. Can restrict joint range of movement.
Intermuscular	Common in the thigh and shoulders
Parosteal	Can occur under the bone periosteum.
Subserous	These can be found under the pleura, and also in the retroperitoneal cavity.
Submucous	These are rare but can occur under the mucous membranes of the respiratory and gastrointestinal tracts. E.g. tongue, larynx, and intestine.
Central nervous system	These lipomas can occur at any point within the extradural space, the spinal cord, and the brain.
Intraglandular	There have been cases of breast, pancreatic, and renal lipomas.
Retroperitoneal	The retroperitoneal tissue is a site for large lipomas. They are very rare.

Table 4.20: The classification of lipomas and their features.

Key features in the history/examination

- They are soft fluctuant swellings
- Usually painless
- The swellings are mobile and not fixed to the overlying skin or deeper structures

Investigations

This is usually a clinical diagnosis. However, investigations can be performed if the diagnosis is uncertain and a malignancy is suspected.

Imaging:

- USS: to delineate the characteristic of the lump macroscopically.

Others:

- Fine needle aspiration (FNA): can provide definitive histological diagnosis if the lumps are considered to be suspicious.

Management

➢ Excision of a lipoma is only considered if the patient is symptomatic, with a painful lump or simply finds the lump unsightly.

➢ All projections from the lipoma must be removed.

➢ Haemostasis must be achieved to prevent a haematoma forming post-operatively.

NECK

Thyroglossal cyst

Epidemiology

Thyroglossal cysts are one of the common congenital cystic abnormalities of the neck. They account for approximately 70% of all congenital neck abnormalities. These cysts can affect patients at any age, however almost 50% of patients are diagnosed before the age of 20 years.

Aetiology

During embryological development the thyroid gland starts at the base of the tongue and progresses to its final position at the lower midline aspect of the neck. Remnants of the thyroid can be left behind at any point and it is this remnant that is known as the thyroglossal cyst.

Pathophysiology

The different sites of the tract at which a thyroglossal cyst can occur include:

- Under the foramen caecum

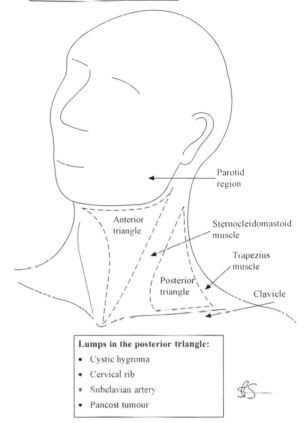

Lumps in the anterior triangle:
- Thyroglossal cyst
- Dermoid cyst
- Branchial cyst
- Carotid body tumour

Parotid region

Anterior triangle

Sternocleidomastoid muscle

Trapezius muscle

Posterior triangle

Clavicle

Lumps in the posterior triangle:
- Cystic hygroma
- Cervical rib
- Subclavian artery
- Pancost tumour

Figure 4.25: Lumps in anterior and posterior triangles of the neck.

- In the floor of the mouth
- Suprahyoid
- Subhyoid
- On the thyroid cartilage
- At the level of the cricoid cartilage

Key features in the history/examination

- The cyst is found in the midline of the neck and moves up when the tongue is protruded
- The cyst also moves on swallowing

Investigations

This is usually a clinical diagnosis. However, investigations can be performed if the diagnosis is uncertain and a malignancy is suspected.

4. Surgery

Imaging:

- USS

Others:

- FNA: can be used to differentiate benign and malignant tumours

Management

➢ The cyst should be surgically excised due to the increased risk of infection.

➢ In most cases the entire thyroglossal tract is removed.

➢ Complications arise when the infected cyst is mistaken for an abscess and incised. This can result in the formation of a thyroglossal fistula.

Goitre

Epidemiology

Thyroid nodules are seen in approximately 5% of middle-aged women. They are more common in women than in men and can give rise to a goitre. Solitary nodules appear to be more common than multinodular goitres. Globally iodine deficiency is one of the leading causes of a goitre.

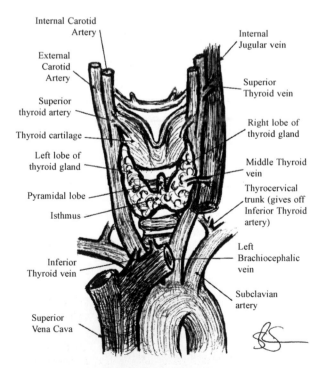

Figure 4.26: Thyroid gland anatomy and its blood supply.

Anatomy

- The thyroid gland develops from the thyroglossal duct in the pharynx.
- The gland weighs about 20–25g.
- The blood supply is extensive with many anastomoses between the thyroid arteries and branches of the tracheal and oesophageal arteries.

Aetiology

A normal thyroid gland should not be palpable. A goitre can be defined as a generalised enlargement of the thyroid gland. There are a number of different types of goitres (see Table 4.21).

Goitre	Features
Simple Goitre	• Diffuse hyperplastic e.g. physiological, pubertal, and pregnancy • Multinodular goitre
Toxic	• Diffuse e.g. Graves' disease • Multinodular • Toxic adenoma
Neoplastic	• Benign • Malignant
Inflammatory	• Autoimmune e.g. chronic lymphocytic thyroiditis, and Hashimoto's disease
Granulomatous	• De Quervain's thyroiditis
Fibrosing	• Riedel's thyroiditis
Infective	• Acute e.g. Bacterial and viral thyroiditis • Chronic e.g. Tuberculosis (TB)

Table 4.21: The features of the different types of goitres.

This section will concentrate on the clinical aspects of simple goitres. The common causes of a simple goitre include the lack of iodine in the diet and hormonal stimulation of the thyroid gland.

Dietary iodine deficiency is endemic in mountainous areas such as the Himalayas and the Alps. Derbyshire in the UK has also been found to have reduced amounts of iodide in the water supply and food. Other low land areas including the Congo and Nile valley have a lack of iodide in the soil.

The thyroid gland can be stimulated by thyroid stimulating hormone (TSH) as a result of low levels of thyroid hormones or even a pituitary adenoma.

Diffuse hyperplastic goitres are seen in childhood and are found in the endemic areas mentioned above. This type of goitre also occurs at times of increased metabolic need (e.g. pubertal goitre) and during stressful situations (e.g. pregnancy). Nodular goitres can consist of a single nodule, but more commonly contain multiple nodules. These nodules can be cystic, colloid, and haemorrhagic.

Pathophysiology

Diffuse hyperplasia of the goitre can occur as a result of continuous growth stimulation. The lobules of the thyroid contain follicles which are involved in the uptake of iodine. If the stimulation to the thyroid gland is stopped the goitre can regress. Occasionally, there is intermittent stimulation of the goitre which results in segments of active and inactive lobules of the thyroid gland.

Active lobules develop and become increasingly vascular which may progress to haemorrhage and central necrosis. These necrotic lobules combine together and form colloid filled nodules. This process is repeated and a nodular goitre is formed.

Key features in the history/examination

- Patients can present with symptoms of thyroid disease.

- Retrosternal goitres may be asymptomatic or produce symptoms such as dyspnoea with cough and stridor, dysphagia, hoarseness, and neck vein engorgement.

- The nodules in the neck are visible and on palpation are smooth and firm.

- The goitre is painless

- The goitre moves on swallowing

- If the nodules are hard, painful, and irregular a carcinoma may be present

Investigations

Blood tests:

- TFTs: serum thyroid hormones (T3 and T4) and Thyroid stimulating hormone (TSH) levels are detected.

- Autoantibody titres: this will help to identify autoimmune thyroiditis.

Imaging:

- CXR: may illustrate a calcified mass and tracheal deviation.

- Isotope scan: the nodules can be referred to as 'hot' (overactive), 'warm' (active) or 'cold' (underactive). If a hot nodule is present, it takes up the isotope, but the surrounding thyroid tissue does not. This occurs as the nodule is producing increased amounts of thyroid hormone and therefore suppressing TSH secretion, resulting in inactive thyroid tissue. If a warm nodule is present it takes up the isotope and the thyroid tissue also takes up the isotope. If a cold nodule is present it does not take up any of the isotope. This is not a first line investigation.

- USS: this can be performed to identify any masses and illustrate some of the clinical features of the nodule/mass.

Management

- In endemic areas improvements have been seen with the introduction of iodised salt to the diet.

- Diffuse hyperplastic goitres can be reversed by giving thyroxine for a few months.

- Nodular goitres cannot be reversed. Most patients with a nodular goitre are asymptomatic, and therefore an operation is not required.

- However, surgery may be performed for cosmetic reasons, if there is tracheal compression, toxic goitre, and if there is suspicion of malignancy.

- A total thyroidectomy and lifelong thyroxine replacement can be offered.

- A partial thyroid resection with conservation of functioning thyroid tissue is also possible.

Branchial cyst

Epidemiology

They are the commonest congenital cause of neck lump and are bilateral in 2–3% of all cases. The exact incidence of branchial cysts is unknown. The majority of patients present between the age of 15 and 25 years, but cases later in middle age have also been identified.

Aetiology

During foetal development at approximately five weeks, four branchial clefts (grooves), develop on each side of the neck. In between these clefts are branchial arches which contain a central cartilage. The first cleft progresses and becomes the auditory meatus. The second, third, and fourth clefts regress and normally disappear. Branchial cysts arise due to failure in the normal regression of these branchial clefts.

Pathophysiology

A branchial cyst, sinus or fistula, usually develop from remnants of the second branchial cleft.

Key features in the history/examination

- Site: branchial cysts are found on the upper neck. More specifically the upper and middle third of the anterior border of the sternocleidomastoid muscle

- The swelling is fluctuant but may be difficult to palpate in the early stage

- It may transilluminate

- If there is a superimposed infection the swelling will be tender and erythematous. The swelling is lined with squamous epithelium and contains cholesterol.

- Failure of the distal end of the branchial cleft to fuse can result in a branchial fistula or sinus. This appears as a small dimple on the skin, normally at the junction of the middle and lower third of sternocleidomastoid. Mucus may discharge intermittently from the sinus or fistula.

Investigations

A clinical diagnosis is made following a history and examination.

Others:

- FNA: can be performed on any swelling and if cholesterol crystals are seen under the microscope, the diagnosis is confirmed.

Management

➢ Surgical removal is the recognised treatment.

➢ During the procedure close attention must be paid to the surrounding structures, as the hypoglossal, accessory and mandibular branch of the facial nerves are in close proximity.

➢ If the cyst is not resected it is prone to developing recurrent infections.

Dermoid cyst

There are two different types of dermoid cysts known as inclusion and implantation cysts. (See Table 4.22)

Type	Features
Inclusion dermoids	<ul><li>These are congenital lesions and are found at sites of embryological fusion. E.g. midline of the neck, root of the nose.</li><li>The lesions are described as swellings that are not attached to the overlying skin.</li></ul>
Implantation dermoids	<ul><li>These lesions are associated with penetrating trauma.</li><li>They are usually seen in the hands as subcutaneous swellings.</li><li>These dermoids occur due to the introduction of epidermal tissue under the skin.</li></ul>

Table 4.22: The features of inclusion and implantation dermoid cysts.

Pharyngeal pouch

Epidemiology

This is a condition that affects approximately 1 in 200,000 people in the UK. It is often seen in adults over the age of 60 years, with a greater prevalence in men than in women.

Anatomy

- The upper part of the respiratory and oesophageal passage is where the pharynx is situated.

- The pharynx is a fibromuscular tube along the length of the base of the skull to the sixth cervical vertebrae.

- It is divided into three different parts; the nasopharynx, oropharynx, and hypopharynx.

- The nasopharynx lies anterior to the first cervical vertebrae and it opens anteriorly into the nose. During the action of swallowing the nasopharynx is closed off from the oropharynx.

- The oropharynx contains the tonsils and the posterior third of the tongue.

- The hypopharynx is found above the epiglottis, and the inferior border of the hypopharynx is the lower border of the cricoid cartilage.

- The hypopharynx leads into the oesophagus.

Aetiology

The true aetiology is unknown, but may involve increased lower oesophageal tone due to gastro-oesophageal reflux, or neuromuscular dysfunction.

Pathophysiology

A pharyngeal pouch occurs as a result of the protrusion of the mucosa and submucosa through a weak area of the posterior pharyngeal wall, known as Killian's dehiscence. Killian's dehiscence is located between the thyropharyngeus and circopharyngeus muscles.

The fibres involved in this area of the wall and the upper oesophagus form the oesophageal sphincter.

Key features in the history/examination

- Halitosis

- Patients may feel like they have an object or lump in their throat.

- Dysphagia.

- Regurgitation on swallowing may occur, after bending, or turning in bed.

- Occasionally liquid and food may aspirate resulting in aspiration pneumonia and lung abscess formation.

- At night patients may awake with a feeling of throat tightness or a coughing fit.

- With the pouch increasing in size patients will complain of:
  - Gurgling noises on swallowing
  - A swelling in the neck which gurgles on palpation (Boyce's sign)
  - On drinking the swelling becomes noticeable
  - Weight loss as a result of difficulties in swallowing.

Investigations

Imaging:

- Barium swallow: the barium will clearly outline the pouch and the upper oesophagus
- Video fluoroscopic study: will provide detail on the contraction waves of the pharynx, and the oesophageal sphincter
- CXR: to exclude aspiration pneumonia

Management

Surgery is only an option if the oesophageal sphincter has been affected and the patient has developed significant symptoms of dysphagia.

Pre-operative management:

- ➢ Assessment of the cardiovascular and respiratory systems
- ➢ Provision of appropriate nutritional supplements
- ➢ Chest physiotherapy
- ➢ Antibiotics

Operative management:

- ➢ A pharyngoscope is used to identify the pouch
- ➢ A NG tube is inserted in to the oesophagus, which is important for postoperative nutrition.
- ➢ The oesophagus may initially be difficult to identify with the endoscope as the opening is significantly smaller when compared to the opening of the pouch. The NG tube aids identification of the oesophagus.
- ➢ The pharyngeal pouch is packed with proflavin soaked ribbon gauze, in order to help identify the neck of the pouch.
- ➢ Two different types of neck incisions can be made; either a transverse crease incision or a lower neck incision at the anterior aspect of the sternocleidomastoid muscle.
- ➢ The muscle and carotid sheath are retracted laterally.
- ➢ The trachea and larynx are retracted medially.
- ➢ Next the middle thyroid vein is divided
- ➢ Above the inferior aspect of the thyroid cartilage is where the retropharyngeal space is accessed.
- ➢ The pouch is found behind the lower pharynx.
- ➢ Dissection of the pouch is carefully performed back to the Killian's dehiscence where it originated from.
- ➢ The pouch can then be resected and the pharynx sutured in two layers.
- ➢ A drain is usually sited.
- ➢ The patient is fed through the NG tube usually for 3–7 days.
- ➢ An alternative is endoscopic stapling/ diathermy of the pharyngeal pouch (Dolman's procedure). Some literature suggests this method has a higher recurrence rate (5–7%).
- ➢ Complications include infection, recurrent laryngeal nerve palsy (hoarse voice), pharyngeal fistula, oesophageal stenosis, and recurrence of the pharyngeal pouch.

Salivary gland neoplasm

Epidemiology

Salivary gland neoplasms account for approximately 1% of all head and neck tumours. The incidence is around 1.5 per 100,000 people and they normally present in the sixth decade of life.

Aetiology

There is currently no defined aetiology for salivary gland neoplasms. However a clear association has been made with radiation therapy.

Pathophysiology

The salivary gland contains the parotid, the submandibular, the sublingual and other smaller salivary glands. Approximately 75% of salivary tumours are found in the parotid gland and of these 80% are benign (pleomorphic adenoma). They can be classified as benign and malignant tumours:

Benign tumours:

- Pleomorphic Adenoma: 80% are found in the parotid region however, they can also be present in the submandibular, sublingual, and accessory salivary glands. The patient may complain of a slow growing lump in the parotid area, which is hard and well defined. Treatment consists of wide excision of the tumour or complete removal of the salivary gland in cases of a large tumour.
- Adenolymphoma (Warthin's tumour): this accounts for approximately 10% of parotid tumours. These tumours are soft and have a cyst like appearance. Local excision of the tumour provides excellent results.

Malignant tumours:

- Adenoid cystic carcinoma: is the most common malignant tumour to affect the salivary glands. It arises more frequently in the smaller salivary gland and is slow growing. It often spreads along the nerve sheaths and can present with facial pain or facial nerve palsy. This type of tumour does not metastasise early and lymph node spread is uncommon.
- Adenocarcinoma (AC): makes up 10% of submandibular and minor salivary gland tumours. In around 20% of cases, lymph nodes are involved at the initial presentation.
- Mucoepidermoid tumours: these are the commonest salivary neoplasm in children. They arise mainly in the parotid gland and metastasise to lymph nodes and later to the lungs and brain.

Key features in the history/examination

- Slow growing and enlarging painless lump
- Facial nerve paralysis may be present
- Cervical lymphadenopathy which indicates metastasis

4. Surgery

Investigations

Blood tests:

- FBC
- Inflammatory markers: check for erythrocyte sedimentation rate (ESR)
- Thyroid function tests (TFTs)
- Antibodies: antibodies such as anti-Ro and anti-La should be used to rule out autoimmune disease such as Sjögren syndrome.
- Rheumatoid and antinuclear factors: to rule out autoimmune causes

Imaging:

- CT or MRI: provides information on the extra-glandular extension of the tumour.

Others:

- FNA: provides tissue histology, but a negative result does not exclude malignancy.

Management

- ➢ The aim of surgery is to fully resect the tumour leaving a margin of macroscopically normal tissue, whilst preserving the facial nerve. Salivary gland tumours respond poorly to chemotherapy and it is only considered in palliative cases.
- ➢ Superficial parotidectomy: the superficial parotid lobe is resected only. This is not suitable if there is involvement of the deep lobe.
- ➢ Total conservative parotidectomy: complete removal of the parotid gland with preservation of the facial nerve.
- ➢ Total radical parotidectomy: complete removal of the parotid gland with the facial nerve.
- ➢ Submandibular gland surgery: this follows similar principles to parotid gland surgery. A small tumour can be removed by wedge resection. More extensive tumours require radical submandibular gland excision. If the tumour directly involves surrounding nerves they may need to be sacrificed. This is commonly the hypoglossal and lingual cranial nerves.
- ➢ Neck dissection: this is required if there is nodal disease or a high grade tumour present.
- ➢ Post-operative radiotherapy is indicated if there is:
  - ○ Residual disease
  - ○ Evidence of extra capsular lymph node spread
  - ○ Adenoid cystic tumour
  - ○ Surgery for recurrent tumour
  - ○ High grade tumours

Cystic hygroma

Epidemiology

Cystic hygroma is rare in the adult population, however is present in approximately 1 in 6,000 to 16,000 live births.

Aetiology

Cystic hygroma has an unknown aetiology. However, 90% of these are a result of a congenital abnormality presenting in children less than two years of age.

Pathophysiology

A cystic hygroma is a lump identified in neonates or early infancy. It is commonly present at birth and on rare occasions causes obstruction during labour. It is a type of lymphangioma that occurs as a result of sequestration of the lymph sacs from the lymphatic system. These cysts contain clear fluid.

Approximately 60% of cases involve the neck, but other sites affected include the axilla and chest wall.

Key features in the history/examination

- Site: found in the posterior triangle or axilla
- It is a soft swelling and cannot be compressed
- It is superficial to underlying muscle and arises from the subcutaneous tissue
- When a child coughs or cries the swelling increases in size
- The swelling is translucent when transilluminated

Investigations

Imaging:

- USS: pre-natal diagnosis can be made during routine antenatal care of the mother
- CT: this is contraindicated in pregnancy and is therefore rarely used

Management

- Cystic hygromas have been known to spontaneously regress
- If this does not occur the cystic hygroma should be surgically excised
- During the procedure care must be taken to avoid damage to surrounding structures, especially neurovascular structures
- Surgical resection is the definitive treatment of these swellings, however recurrence can occur

GROIN AND SCROTUM

Incompletely descended testis

Epidemiology

3% of all testicles at birth are undescended. The incidence falls to 1% after one year. Undescended testes are commonly seen in premature babies, who have an incidence of 30%.

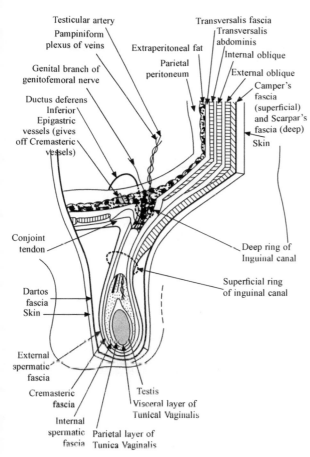

Testicular artery
Pampiniform plexus of veins
Extraperitoneal fat
Genital branch of genitofemoral nerve
Ductus deferens
Inferior Epigastric vessels (gives off Cremasteric vessels)
Conjoint tendon
Dartos fascia
Skin
External spermatic fascia
Cremasteric fascia
Internal spermatic fascia

Transversalis fascia
Transversalis abdominis
Internal oblique
Parietal peritoneum
External oblique
Camper's fascia (superficial) and Scarpar's fascia (deep)
Skin
Deep ring of Inguinal canal
Superficial ring of inguinal canal
Testis
Visceral layer of Tunical Vaginalis
Parietal layer of Tunica Vaginalis

Figure 4.27: The inguinal canal and scrotum.

Aetiology

Undescended testes commonly arise from a local defect during development.

Pathophysiology

An incompletely descended testis can be normal until the age of six years. After the onset of puberty the undescended testis develops poorly in comparison to intra-scrotal structures. Histological examination identifies immature tissue and destructive changes. This results in the absence of spermatogenesis and also increases the risk of developing testicular cancer.

Key features in the history/examination

- Pain in the presence of trauma
- Sterility is common in bilateral cases
- Inguinal hernia resulting in torsion or epididymo-orchitis
- If the testis is not palpable at any site on examination, further investigation is required

- The testis may be found in the extraperitoneal cavity of the abdomen, just above the internal inguinal ring
- The testis may also be situated in the inguinal canal, which can either be palpated or not
- Another site for an undescended testis is the superficial inguinal pouch
- The scrotum in nearly all cases is under-developed and appears flat

Investigations

The diagnosis is usually made on clinical examination.

Imaging:

- USS or MRI: are used to identify the testes

Management

➢ All undescended testes will require surgery
➢ An orchidoplexy is not usually performed until the age of two years when it is safe to anaesthetise the child

Operative management:

➢ A short incision over the deep inguinal ring is made
➢ The external oblique muscle is divided to expose the inguinal canal
➢ The testis and the spermatic cord are mobilised
➢ With a sufficient length of the cord the testis can be placed back into the scrotum without any tension of the cord
➢ A finger is used to stretch the empty scrotum allowing enough space for the testis
➢ The testis must be secured in the scrotum
➢ An absorbable suture can be used to anchor the testis to the fundus of the scrotum. However commonly a pouch (dartos pouch) is created between the dartos muscle and the skin, with the dartos muscle then preventing the testis from retracting out of the scrotum

Testicular torsion

Epidemiology

Torsion of the testis is relatively uncommon, as a normal fully descended testis should be secure and unable to rotate. It can occur at any age, but is commonly seen between the ages of 10 and 25 years. A higher incidence has been found in patients with an undescended testis.

Aetiology

Inversion of the testis is the most common cause of testicular torsion. The testis is found to be rotated and in a transverse position. If there is high attachment of the tunica vaginalis, the testis will hang within the tunica. The testis is often described as

4. Surgery

hanging like a 'bell-clapper' within the tunica vaginalis (intra-vaginal torsion). If the epididymis is separated from the body of the testis, torsion can occur. This type of testicular torsion does not involve the spermatic cord.

If any of the abnormalities above are present, activities such as straining, sexual intercourse, and lifting heavy weights may result in torsion.

Pathophysiology

Torsion of the testis prevents blood flow to the testis, resulting in infarction. Blood stained fluid exudes into the tunica vaginalis. There is irreversible infarction after a few hours without any treatment.

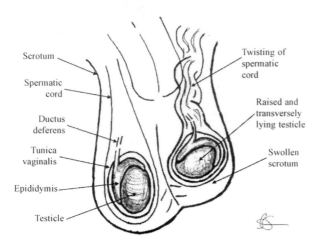

Figure 4.28: Testicular torsion.

Key features in the history/examination

- Sudden onset of severe pain in the groin and lower abdomen. The nerve supply for the testis is from the T10 sympathetic pathway, which is why the patient experiences abdominal pain

- Associated symptoms include vomiting

- On palpation of the scrotum the testis may be swollen and the testis may be lying high

- The testis will be tender

- Thickened spermatic cord on palpation

- The overlying scrotal skin becomes red and oedematous, which is a late sign.

Investigations

Testicular torsion is a urological emergency. Therefore diagnosis is made on clinical examination, without any formal investigations. The patient is prepared for emergency theatre.

Management

➢ Within the first hour the testis maybe manipulated gently. If this is successful, arrangements can be made for surgery to fix the testis in place, and prevent further episodes of torsion. However if this is not possible surgical exploration of the scrotum is essential.

➢ A scrotal incision is made to visualise the testis and cord

➢ The cord is untwisted and the testes are examined for viability

➢ If viable the testis is fixed with non-absorbable sutures to the tunica vaginalis (scrotal wall) otherwise called the 3-point fixation method. Alternatively the testis can be fixed with the creation of a dartos pouch and Jaboulay procedure which entails everting the tunica vaginalis.

➢ The opposite testis should also be fixed at the same time, due to the knowledge that most anatomical defects are likely to be bilateral.

➢ If the testis is non-viable and completely infarcted it should be removed. If the testis is removed the patient can be counselled about prosthetic replacement, at a later date.

Hydrocele

This is an abnormal or excessive collection of serous fluid within the tunica vaginalis.

Epidemiology

A hydrocele is estimated to affect 1% of the male population.

Aetiology

Primary hydroceles are idiopathic and arise in children and the elderly. Secondary hydroceles are associated with an abnormal testis. The testis is surrounded by a serosal sac, which becomes filled with inflammatory or malignant exudates. Causes include:

- Trauma (Haemorrhagic)

- Epididymo-orchitis/ Tuberculosis

- Testicular tumour

- Obstruction of the lymphatic drainage of the scrotum.

Pathophysiology

There are four main types of hydrocele, i.e. vaginal hydrocele, congenital hydrocele, infantile hydrocele, and hydrocele of the cord.

In a vaginal hydrocele, a patent processus vaginalis is present but there is no communication with the peritoneal cavity. The swelling is painless, and therefore patients present late. The testis may be palpated within the hydrocele, however if the sac is tense a USS may be required to identify the testis. The swelling can be transilluminated. 5% of indirect inguinal hernias have a vaginal hydrocele on the same side.

In a congenital hydrocele, there is a connection between the patent processus vaginalis and the peritoneal cavity and therefore fluid form the hydrocele can drain back into the peritoneal cavity. Most hydroceles are congenital and are noted in children aged 1–2 years.

Infantile hydroceles are found along the testis to the internal inguinal ring and do not enter the peritoneal cavity.

Hydrocele of the cord is rare. There is a smooth swelling close to the spermatic cord and this is often mistaken for an inguinal hernia. If the testis is gently pulled down, the swelling moves in a downward direction.

Investigations

Imaging:

- USS: can assess for a hydrocele and identify an abnormal testis, which may require surgery.

Management

- ➢ Most hydroceles resolve spontaneously and therefore can be conservatively managed in infants. Approximately **80%** of new born males have a patent processus vaginalis but most close within 12 months.

- ➢ An operation will be required if the hydrocele has not resolved after one year.

- ➢ A hydrocele with a normal testis can be treated with aspiration (straw-coloured fluid), however recurrence may occur.

- ➢ Lord's operation is where the tunica vaginalis is placated with interrupted absorbable sutures.

- ➢ Jaboulay's procedure is where the hydrocele sac is everted, with the opening secured with sutures.

Varicocele

Epidemiology

Varicocele is defined as dilatation of the veins of the testis and arises in approximately 20% of the male population.

Anatomy

- The group of veins that drain the testis and the epididymis make up the pampiniform plexus. (See Figure 4.27)

- There are fewer veins along the inguinal canal and at the inguinal ring

- These veins join together and form the testicular veins

- The left testicular vein drains into the left renal vein

- The right testicular vein drains into the inferior vena cava; just below the right renal vein

- A collateral venous drainage system of the testes, occur via the cremasteric veins into the inferior epigastric vessels

Aetiology

It has been found that 95% of cases are associated with the left side, as a result of the angle of left testicular vein emptying into left renal vein and lack of anti-reflux valves. The dilated veins in the varicocele are the cremasteric veins. If the patient is diagnosed with a left renal tumour this can cause obstruction of the left testicular vein resulting in a varicocele.

Key features in the history/examination

- Varicocele can be asymptomatic

- Patients may complain of an uncomfortable dragging sensation in the scrotum. The discomfort is worse when not wearing any underwear

- Varicoceles are associated with increased infertility and are commonly diagnosed following investigation for infertility

- On palpation with the patient standing, the scrotum feels like a 'bag of worms'

- The affected side of the scrotum may hang lower compared to the normal side

- On lying down the veins empty and the testis can be palpated

Investigations

The diagnosis is usually made on clinical examination.

Management

- ➢ Conservative treatment is the mainstay of treatment

- ➢ An operation is only indicated if the patient is symptomatic with pain or unexplained infertility

- ➢ A laparoscopic or open procedure is performed to ligate the testicular vein along the inguinal canal

- ➢ Recurrence is common as a result of the collateral venous supply

- ➢ Percutaneous embolisation of the internal spermatic vein via cannulation through the femoral vein is an alternative option. This method is normally reserved for recurrent disease

Epididymal cyst

Epidemiology

Epididymal cysts are common and are usually found in middle-aged individuals. These cysts are rare in children.

Aetiology

Epididymal cysts occur as a result of cystic degeneration of epididymal or para-epididymal structures.

Pathophysiology

The cysts are filled with clear fluid. They are typically found bilaterally, with multiple cysts present.

Key features in the history/examination

- The cysts feel like a bunch of grapes on palpation
- They are fluctuant and transilluminable
- In most cases they are separate from the testis

Investigations

Imaging:

- Scrotal USS: this will confirm the diagnosis of an epididymal cyst. Aspiration of fluid from the cyst is occasionally performed, however this is rarely useful.

Management

➢ The cysts are multi-locular and therefore aspiration is not an option.

➢ Surgical removal of the cysts is possible if it is causing the patient discomfort.

Epididymo-orchitis

Epidemiology

Males between the age of 14 and 35 years are commonly affected.

Aetiology

Epididymo-orchitis is inflammation of the epididymis and testis. The causes include the mumps virus, sexually transmitted infections, (*Chlamydia trachomatis* and *Neisseria gonorrhoea*), complicated UTI, and following an operation involving the prostate or urethra.

Pathophysiology

The primary infection of the urethra, prostate or seminal vesicles spreads to the globus minus of the epididymis.

Key features in the history/examination

- Fever
- Sweaty
- Urethral discharge
- Dysuria
- Swelling of the epididymis and the testis
- Tender on palpation
- The scrotum appears red and shiny
- This can progress to the formation of an abscess, with pus discharging through the scrotal skin

Investigations

Blood tests:

- FBC

- U&Es
- Inflammatory markers: CRP

Urinalysis:

- Urine dipstick
- MSU

Imaging:

- USS: to look for an abscess

Others:

- Urethral swab

Management

➢ In the acute phase bed rest is advised

➢ A positive *Chlamydia* infection requires a course of Doxycyline (100 mg once a day) or a one of dose of Azithromycin.

➢ If no organism has been identified a broad spectrum antibiotic (Levofloxacin or Ofloxacin) should be prescribed. A two-week course is usually sufficient, or until the inflammation has settled.

➢ Systemic illness warrants hospitalization and coverage with IV Ampicillin and Gentamicin.

➢ Analgesia is important

➢ A sling is made from adhesive tape to support the scrotum between the thighs.

➢ Incision and drainage may be required if an abscess is present.

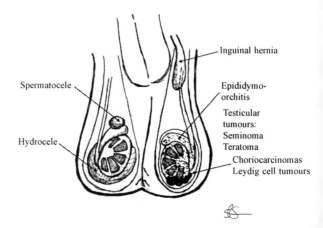

Figure 4.29: The common scrotal lumps.

HERNIAS

A hernia is defined as the protrusion of a viscus through an abnormal defect in the wall of its containing compartment. Some hernias are more common than others. The most common are inguinal hernias (75%), umbilical hernias (15%), and femoral hernias (8%).

There are three parts to a hernia, the sac, the coverings, and the sac contents. The hernial sac is an out-pouching of the peritoneum comprising of a mouth, neck, body, and fundus. When the neck is narrow strangulation of bowel can occur. However, the body of the sac varies in size and may or may not be occupied. The coverings are taken from the layers of the abdominal wall. It is through this that the sac passes. What occupies the sac is referred to as the contents. This may be omentum, intestine, a section of the bladder, ovary, diverticulum or peritoneal fluid.

Type of hernia	Features
Reducible	• The hernial sac can be returned to its original cavity
Irreducible	• The contents of the sac cannot be returned to its cavity • This is commonly a result of adhesions between the sac and its contents • Irreducibility predisposes to strangulation
Obstructed	• This hernia is irreducible and the lumen of the bowel is obstructed by the hernia neck • The blood supply to the bowel is not affected • On examination an obstructed hernia cannot be differentiated from a strangulated hernia
Strangulated	• The blood supply to the contents of the hernia has become compromised • Initially the venous system is occluded but with increasing pressure the arterial supply becomes compromised. In a very tight hernia neck the arterial supply can become directly occluded. The contents then become ischaemic and progress to gangrene formation • A femoral hernia is at a greater risk of strangulation due to its narrow neck
Sliding	• This is a type of hernia in which a segment of the sac is formed by the bowel
Richter's hernia	• This is identified as a hernial sac containing only a segment of the circumference of the intestine

Table 4.23: Classification of hernias.

Inguinal hernia

Epidemiology

The incidence of inguinal hernias in newborn babies is 4%. This increases to 30% in premature babies. Approximately 8–15% of patients with this hernia will present to the accident and emergency department with bowel obstruction and strangulation.

Anatomy

See Figure 4.27 for the anatomy of the inguinal canal.

The inguinal canal:

• The inguinal canal is approximately 3.75 cm long and it extends downwards and medially from the deep inguinal to the superficial inguinal ring.

• The inguinal canal has four bordering structures:

  o The anterior wall consists of the external oblique aponeurosis and the internal oblique.

  o The posterior wall consists of the transversalis fascia and the conjoined tendon.

  o The roof of the canal contains the internal oblique which arches from front to back.

  o The floor of the canal represents the inguinal ligament.

The superficial inguinal ring:

• This is found in the external oblique aponeurosis.

• It is approximately 1.25 cm above and lateral to the pubic tubercle.

The deep inguinal ring:

• This ring is found 1.25 cm above the inguinal ligament, and is midway between the anterior superior iliac spine and the pubic tubercle (mid-point of the inguinal ligament).

• At the posterior and medial aspect of the deep inguinal ring the inferior epigastric vessels will be found.

Aetiology

Inguinal hernias can either be congenital or acquired. Congenital abnormalities such as a patent processus vaginalis can predispose to hernias. The acquired causes all tend to produce a rise in intra-abdominal pressure. This will increase the chance of developing a hernia. An increase in intra-abdominal pressure can be due to:

• Chronic cough

• Straining on defecation

• Prostatism or difficulty micturating

• Pregnancy

• Obesity

• Ascites

• Excessive or repetitive muscular effort

Previous hernia and hernia repairs tend to weaken the abdominal wall and hence predispose to developing hernias in the future. Smoking is also associated with the development of a hernia.

4. Surgery

Pathophysiology

An inguinal hernia can be palpated above and medial to the pubic tubercle. They can be classified into a direct and indirect hernia. (See Table 4.24)

Direct hernia	Indirect hernia
• This hernia passes directly through the posterior wall of the inguinal canal • This is medial to the inferior epigastric vessels • This is a common hernia in the elderly population • These account for 35% of inguinal hernias • Direct hernias rarely extend to the scrotum	• This hernia passes through the internal ring, lateral to the inferior epigastric vessels • It can extend down the canal along the side of the spermatic cord into the scrotum • This is the most common type of hernia (65%) in the young adult • 55% are right sided hernias and 12% are bilateral

Table 4.24: Features of direct and indirect hernias.

Key features in the history/examination

- Groin pain can be present

- Radiation of the pain to the testicle

- When the patient coughs a bulge may appear

- If palpated a cough impulse can be felt

- It may often be best to examine the hernia with the patient standing as gravity enables the hernia to become visible

- A hernia which is identified as being above and medial to the pubic tubercle is an inguinal hernia.

- Bowel sounds may be heard over the hernia

- Always examine the scrotum to identify scrotal involvement

- To differentiate between a direct and indirect hernia, the hernia is reduced and pressure applied over the deep inguinal ring. The patient is then asked to cough or strain. If the hernia is controlled this is an indirect hernia, and if the hernia is revealed it is a direct hernia. This examination diagnoses the correct type of inguinal hernia in only a third of cases. The only definitive method is intra-operatively.

Investigations

The diagnosis is usually made following clinical examination.

Management

➢ If patients are fit to undergo surgery, an operation is the best available treatment. This can be performed as an open or laparoscopic procedure.

Inguinal herniotomy:

➢ This is recommended in children

➢ The hernial sac is opened and the contents are reduced.

➢ No mesh is used making it suitable for growing children.

Inguinal herniotomy and repair (herniorrhaphy):

➢ The hernial sac is excised

➢ The internal inguinal ring and transversalis fascia are repaired.

➢ The posterior wall of the inguinal canal is then reinforced:

  o This can be achieved by the Shouldice repair, which involves securing the transversalis muscle to the posterior wall with a nylon suture (no mesh repair).

  o The Lichenstein repair can also be used to reinforce the posterior wall with a nylon or polyprolene mesh.

  o This mesh technique is tension free and is the treatment of choice.

Post operative management:

➢ Most hernia operations can be performed as a day case procedure by either open or laparoscopic methods.

➢ The patient can be discharged with analgesia and laxatives if required.

➢ Scrotal support and wound care advice is given.

➢ Patients are advised to refrain from strenuous exercise or manual labour for 4–6 weeks.

Conservative management:

➢ In those patients who are unsuitable for surgical repair (e.g. elderly, other co-morbidities) may be prescribed a truss to support the hernia.

➢ However these hernias can progress to strangulation and require an emergency operation.

Femoral hernia

Epidemiology

These hernias usually occur in the middle aged and elderly population. They account for almost 7% of all groin herniae. Approximately 50% of femoral hernias are diagnosed when they present to the accident and emergency department.

Anatomy

- The femoral canal is 1.25 cm long, and extends from the femoral ring to the opening of the Saphenous vein.

- It contains fat and lymphatic vessels.

  o The femoral canal is surrounded by a number of structures:

  o The anterior wall is composed of the inguinal ligament

  o The posterior aspect is represented by Astley Cooper's (ileo-pectineal) ligament, the pubic bone, and the overlying pectineus muscle fascia.

o The medial aspect consists of the lacunar ligament.

o The lateral aspect is composed of a thin septum which separates the canal from the femoral vein.

Aetiology

The causes are all acquired and are again associated with an increase in intra-abdominal pressure. An increase in intra-abdominal pressure can be due to:

- Chronic cough
- Straining on defecation
- Difficulty in micturition
- Pregnancy
- Obesity
- Straining of muscles

Pathophysiology

The hernia passes down the femoral canal until the opening of the saphenous vein. Whilst inside the walls of the femoral canal, the hernia is narrow. However, once the hernia has passed through the saphenous opening it can dilate and distend. This increases the likelihood of an irreducible hernia which is at risk of strangulation.

Key features in the history/examination

- Painless lump in the groin
- The lump is below and lateral to the pubic tubercle
- Femoral hernias are often irreducible on examination
- If the patient presents with strangulation they will be in extreme pain
- On examination the lump will be hot, red, tender, and irreducible

Investigations

The diagnosis is usually made following clinical examination. USS, CT, or MRI may help with the diagnosis.

Management

➤ All femoral hernias are treated surgically due to the risk of strangulation.

➤ A low approach (Lockwood) is taken where an incision is performed over the hernia. The femoral sac is excised and the repair is then performed which involves suturing the inguinal ligament to the pectineal ligament.

➤ In an emergency the femoral hernia is repaired using the high approach (McEvedy) with the incision being made over the inguinal region. This allows closer examination of the bowel which can be difficult with a low approach. The repair is performed as above.

Others

Hernia	Key features in the history/examination	Management
Incisional	• Occurs through a previous acquired defect e.g. operative scar • Asymptomatic • Can be large and unsightly	➤ Conservative ➤ Surgical repair e.g. mesh repair
Umbilical	• These are seen in infants • Congenital and acquired • Asymptomatic but unsightly	➤ 95% resolve spontaneously ➤ Surgical repair after the age of three years.
Para-umbilical	• These are seen in adults • Defect in the linea alba, above and below the umbilicus • Risk or irreducibility and obstruction	➤ Surgical repair with or without a mesh
Epigastric	• Defect in the linea alba • The hernia contains omentum • Pea-sized swelling • Risk of strangulation	➤ Operative repair with or without a mesh
Spigelian	• Rare • The hernia occurs through the linea semilunaris • The hernia is found between the abdominal wall layers	➤ Surgical repair
Obturator	• A lump can be felt within the femoral triangle. • The hernial sac is found extending through the obturator canal. • Risk of obstruction and strangulation • Referred pain can be felt over the medial aspect of the knee Surgery can treat the obstruction	➤ The defect cannot be sutured
Lumbar	• Occur post loin incisions	➤ Conservative methods e.g. corset ➤ Surgical mesh repair
Sciatic	• The hernia is seen through the greater sciatic foramen • Presents as small bowel obstruction	➤ Surgical repair

Table 4.25: The other types of hernias.

4. Surgery

Further reading and references

➤ Aly A, Devitt PG, Jamieson GG (2004). Evolution of surgical treatment for pharyngeal pouch. Br J Surg 91: 657–664.

➤ Davenport M (1996). ABC of General Surgery in Children: Lumps and swellings of the head and neck. British Medical Journal 312: 368–371.

➤ Hatton R, Patel M, Devendra D (2009). Thyroid swellings. British Medical Journal 339: 563.

➤ Ivaz S, Lloyd-Hughes H, Oakeshott P, et al. (2009). Malignant melanoma. BMJ 339: 3078.

➤ Mannu GS, Odutoye T (2008). The pharyngeal pouch. Student BMJ 16: 616.

➤ Mehanna HM, Jain A, Morton RP, et al. (2009). Clinical Review: Investigating the thyroid nodule. BMJ 338: 733.

➤ Mehta MR (2000). Cystic Hygroma: Presentation of two cases with a review of the literature. Indian Journal of Otolaryngology and Head & Neck Surgery 52.

➤ Pavlidis TE (2009). Current opinion on laparoscopic repair of inguinal hernia. Surgical Endoscopy.

➤ Prasad KC, Dannana NK, Prasad SC (2006). Thyroglossal duct cyst: an unusual presentation. Ear, Nose & Throat Journal.

➤ Purushotham S, Gauray K, Bhattacharyya K (2006). Pharyngeal pouch: associations and complications. European Archive of Otorhinolaryngology 263: 463–468.

➤ Sandlow J (2004). Pathogenesis and treatment of varicoceles. BMJ 328: 967–968.

ORGANOMEGALY

Differential diagnosis

Organ	Disease
Hepatic	Hepatomegaly
Spleen	Splenomegaly

Hepatomegaly

Epidemiology

The epidemiology is dependent on the aetiology

Aetiology

The aetiology of hepatomegaly can be classified into five categories. (See Table 4.26)

Pathophysiology

The pathophysiology is dependent on the aetiology.

Key features in the history/examination

- The enlarged liver is palpated below the right costal margin

Type	Diseases
Congenital	• Polycystic disease • Riedals lobe
Cirrhosis	• Portal and biliary • Haemochromatosis
Inflammatory	• Alcoholic hepatitis • Viral hepatitis • Autoimmune hepatitis • Liver abscess (See Figure 4.32) • Leptospirosis (Weil's disease)
Haematological disease	• Hodgkin's and non-Hodgkin's lymphoma • Leukaemia • Polycythaemia
Metabolic conditions	• Amyloid • Gauchers disease

Table 4.26: Classification of hepatomegaly.

- Gross hepatomegaly is identified when the liver extends over to beneath the left costal margin
- The liver moves with respiration
- The liver is dull to percussion
- If a liver is palpable there may be associated splenomegaly and lymphadenopathy

Investigations

Investigations should be tailored to individual differential diagnoses.

Blood tests:
- FBC
- U&Es
- LFTs
- Clotting
- Amylase
- Glucose
- Hepatitis screen
- Serology

Imaging:
- USS: of the liver
- CT: of the abdomen

Others:
- Liver biopsy
- Urine dipstick: check for bilirubin

Management

➢ The indications for a liver transplant include:

    o Estimated survival of less than one year

    o Signs and symptoms such as ascites, lethargy, pruritus resulting in poor quality of life.

➢ Some of the conditions suitable for a liver transplant include the autoimmune diseases, and liver hepatitis.

➢ Contraindications to liver transplant:

    o Primary liver carcinoma and metastatic disease

    o Secondary metastatic liver disease

    o Current alcohol abuse

    o Sepsis

    o Cardiac, pulmonary and cerebral disease

Splenomegaly

Epidemiology

The epidemiology is dependent on the aetiology.

Actiology

The netiology of splenomegaly can be classified into five categories. (See Table 4.27)

Type	Disease
Infections	• Viruses: glandular fever • Bacterial: typhoid and septicaemia • Protozoal: malaria, kala-azar, schistosomiasis • Parasitic: hydatid
Haematological conditions	• Leukaemia: chronic myeloid leukaemia (CML), chronic lymphocytic leukaemia (CLL) • Lymphoma: non-Hodgkin's and Hodgkin's lymphoma • Myelofibrosis: idiopathic thrombocytopenic purpura (ITP), polycythaemia rubra vera • Haemolytic disease: spherocytosis
Metabolic conditions	• Storage disease: Gaucher's disease, Niemann-Pick disease
Splenic masses	• Tumours • Cysts • Abscesses
Portal hypertension	• Cirrhosis • Hepatitis (rare) • Infection e.g. schistosomiasis • Portal vein thrombosis

Table 4.27: Classification of splenomegaly.

Pathophysiology

The pathophysiology is dependent on the aetiology.

Key features in the history/examination

• Mass palpable below the left costal margin

• Descends on inspiration towards the right iliac fossa

• The mass is dull to percussion

Investigations

This is dependent on the aetiology but a basic screen would be appropriate for all causes.

Blood tests:

• FBC

• Clotting

• Serology

Imaging:

• USS

• CT: of the abdomen

Management

➢ Each different cause can have varying presentations and require individual diagnostic tests. Specific management is dependent on the actual cause.

➢ A splenectomy however may be the appropriate treatment if certain criteria are met:

    o Splenic rupture

    o Haematological disease e.g. haemolytic anaemia

    o Tumours

    o If required as part of another procedure e.g. radical gastrectomy for gastric carcinoma.

Further reading and references

➢ Ramachandran R, Poole A, (2003) *Clinical Cases and OSCEs in Surgery (MRCS Study Guides)*. Churchill and Livingstone.

INSIDIOUS ONSET

Differential diagnosis

System/Organ	Disease
Skin	**Basal cell carcinoma (BCC) (rodent ulcer)** **Bowen's disease** **Squamous cell carcinomas (SCC)** **Malignant melanoma**

4. Surgery

Neck	Thyroid cancer
Breast	Breast cancer
Alimentary canal	Oesophageal cancer
	Colon cancer
Hepato-biliary	Hepato-cellular cancer (HCC)
	Cholangiocarcinoma
	Gallbladder cancer
Pancreas	Pancreatic carcinoma
Urological and groin	Renal carcinoma
	Bladder cancer
	Prostate cancer
	Testicular cancer

Basal cell carcinoma (rodent ulcer)

Epidemiology

Basal cell carcinoma (BCC) is the commonest type of skin cancer, affecting adults between the ages of 40–79 years.

Aetiology

Sunlight exposure and irradiation are well known predisposing factors

Pathophysiology

90% of tumours are identified on the face, commonly around the eyes, nasolabial folds, and the scalp hairline. However the tumour can occur on any part of the body. Metastatic disease is very rare.

Key features in the history/examination

- The tumour itself is a raised lesion with rolled edges. It is classically described as a pearly nodule with overlying telangiectasia (fine blood vessels).
- The tumour is slow growing and results in long term ulceration.
- Microscopically the cells involved arise from the basal layer. The tumour advances with surrounding tissue destruction. In some cases underlying bone and facial structures may be damaged and distorted.
- 26 types of BCC have been identified but often, it is only five that are clinically diagnosed; nodular (50%); superficial (10%); cystic (8%); pigmented (6%); and morpheic (2%).

Investigations

- The diagnosis is usually made following clinical examination. However, a biopsy should be sent to confirm the diagnosis.

Management

- Treatment consists of complete surgical excision of the lesion with adequate resection of the margins.

- Surgery gives patients an 85–95% chance of a cure.
- In early cases or those unsuitable for surgery, superficial radiotherapy is offered with a success rate of approximately 90%.
- In advanced disease the only option is surgical removal.
- Follow-up is not usually necessary if tumour margins on histology are clear.
- However, patients with the familial condition known as Gorlin's syndrome are predisposed to developing further BCC's, and therefore warrant close follow-up.

Bowen's disease

Epidemiology

The elderly population is typically affected.

Aetiology

This is defined as an intra-epidermal SCC. A viral aetiology has been suggested, due to the presence of HPV DNA identified in some lesions.

Pathophysiology

The lesions appear as flat, red, scaly, or crusted plaques. It is often difficult to clinically distinguish Bowen's disease from solar keratosis. If the lesion is left untreated 3–5% of patients will progress to malignancy.

Management

- If the diagnosis is uncertain a biopsy can be performed for histological confirmation.
- Local treatment involves cryotherapy or curettage and cauterisation.
- Radiotherapy and chemotherapy can be used with positive results.
- If local management of the superficial lesion has failed to treat deeper structures, recurrence is often seen. Eventually this may progress to invasive SCC.
- The treatment of choice is surgical excision.

Squamous cell carcinoma

Epidemiology

- SCC is a malignancy affecting the elderly and Caucasian population.

Aetiology

Solar keratosis and Bowen's disease are predisposing conditions to SCC. Other risk factors include sunlight/ultraviolet irradiation, infection with HPV (types 6, 11, 16, 18), exposure to carcinogens such as tar and soot, and chronic ulceration.

Pathophysiology

SCC is a malignant tumour arising from pre-malignant lesions. They are less common than BCC's, but are more malignant. The tumour spreads locally and via the lymphatic system.

Key features in the history/examination

- Ulcerated lesion
- Raised and everted edges
- A central scab is present

Investigations

An incisional or punch biopsy is performed to confirm the diagnosis.

Management

➢ Wide local excision (WLE) of the tumour is the treatment of choice.

➢ Radiotherapy is offered with inoperable tumours or post-operatively to ensure complete eradication.

Malignant melanoma

Epidemiology

Malignant melanoma accounts for 10% of all skin cancers. It is a cancer affecting the Caucasian population and is responsible for most deaths from skin cancer.

Aetiology

Exposure to sunlight (ultraviolet radiation) is a well known risk factor. Skin conditions such as albinism and xeroderma pigmentosa are associated with malignant melanoma. Those patients with pre-existing junctional or compound naevi have also been shown to develop this cancer.

Pathophysiology

There are five different presentations of malignant melanoma; superficial spreading, nodular, lentigo maligna, acral lentiginous, and amelanotic. Malignant melanoma can spread to the lymph nodes, lungs, liver, and brain.

Key features in the history/examination

Superficial spreading:

- This is the most common presentation
- The lesion can occur anywhere on the body
- Usually a palpable lesion, with an irregular border and varied pigmentation.
- Common sites include the legs in females and the torso in males.

Nodular:

- This lesion is typically seen in the younger population, and can be found on any part of the body.
- It is considered the most malignant lesion.
- The naevi is a pigmented nodule, with a smooth surface, and irregular border.
- The nodule can bleed and ulcerate.

Lentigo maligna:

- This type of lesion is seen in the elderly population.
- It is commonly seen on the face of the patient, however can occur anywhere on the body.
- The lesion appears as a flat, brown and irregular pigmented patch

Acral lentiginous:

- These lesions are found on the extremities of the patient e.g. the palms of the hands and soles of the feet.
- This is the type of cancer seen in dark-skinned races.

Amelanotic:

- The lesion appears pink with pigmentation at the base.
- This type of cancer may present with lymph node metastasis.

Signs suggesting a malignant change of a melanoma include an increase in size, increase in irregularity or change in shape, and increased or irregular pigmentation. Bleeding, ulceration, pain, itching, and a diameter of greater than 5 cm are also associated with a malignant change.

Investigations

Clinical examination should arouse suspicion of a malignant lesion. Further investigations are required to confirm the diagnosis.

Others:

Complete excisional biopsy: ensuring a 2 mm margin is performed to make a diagnosis. The melanoma is then staged using the Clarks system (Table 4.28) or the Breslow thickness system. (Table 4.29)

Stage	Features
I	Involves the epidermis
II	The tumour goes through the epidermis and into the papillary dermis
III	The tumour invades the papillary dermis
IV	Reticular dermis is then invaded
V	The tumour finally invades the subcutaneous

Table 4.28: Clarks staging system to look at the depth of tumour invasion in relation to the layers of the skin. The five-year survival for stage II or less is approximately 90%.

4. Surgery

Management

➢ Surgical resection is the first line treatment.

➢ The lesion is completely excised with a minimum margin of 1.0 cm and a maximum margin of 2.0 cm.

➢ Excision beyond the deep fascia is not performed.

➢ In certain cases the margins may be adapted for cosmetic or structural reasons.

➢ It is thought that malignant melanomas have an immunological component. Therefore, some success has been observed with immunotherapy (gamma-interferon or interleukin-2).

➢ Radiotherapy does not have a role in the treatment of the tumour. However, chemotherapy has been used in some cases of melanoma.

➢ Regional lymphadenopathy needs careful assessment. If the lymph nodes are not palpable they are managed conservatively with close observation. If there is palpable lymphadenopathy a surgical clearance is performed.

➢ Patients are closely followed up in the outpatient clinic due to the risk of disease recurrence.

Depth (mm)	Five-year survival
< 0.75	> 95%
0.75–1.5	90%
1.5–4.0	70%
> 4.0	< 50%

Table 4.29: The five-year survival rate according to the Breslow's staging system, which incorporates the thickness and depth of the tumour.

Thyroid cancer

Epidemiology

Thyroid neoplasms have an incidence of 3.7 per 100,000 per year. The relative incidences of thyroid carcinoma differ with each type of neoplasm. (See Table 4.30)

Tumour	Incidence
Papillary carcinoma	70%
Follicular carcinoma	17%
Medullary carcinoma	5%
Malignant lymphoma	2–5%
Anaplastic carcinoma	1–2%

Table 4.30: The incidence of the different types of thyroid carcinomas.

Aetiology

Papillary carcinoma is linked with accidental thyroid irradiation in childhood. Follicular carcinoma has been found to be prevalent in areas where goitres are endemic, (e.g. populations with a low dietary iodine intake), or occur as a result of excess TSH activity. Medullary carcinoma has been associated with familial conditions and other malignancies including multiple endocrine neoplasia (MEN) 2, phaeochromocytoma, and neurofibromas. Malignant lymphomas are associated with autoimmune thyroiditis.

Pathophysiology

Papillary carcinoma is commonly seen in young adults and even children. These tumours consist of a mixture of papillary and colloid follicles and are slow growing and multifocal. Papillary carcinomas tend to invade locally and spread via the cervical lymphatics.

Follicular carcinomas are seen in middle-aged adults. These tumours tend to be solitary and encapsulated. They spread via blood to the lungs and bone. Lymph nodes are affected late in the disease.

Medullary carcinomas can occur in any age group. These tumours arise in para-follicular C-cells and can be multifocal. They secrete calcitonin which can be used as a tumour marker. Medullary carcinomas metastasise via the lymph nodes.

Anaplastic carcinoma is a carcinoma of the elderly population. It is rapidly growing and extremely aggressive. These tumours spread via local infiltration and the lymphatic system.

Key features in the history/examination

• Thyroid swelling

• Enlarged cervical lymph nodes

• Hoarseness as a result of a recurrent laryngeal palsy.

• Dysphagia may occur if the tumour causes extrinsic compression of the oesophagus.

Investigations

Most thyroid carcinomas are suspected on clinical examination. There is no investigation which is completely diagnostic of a carcinoma. This can only be achieved with surgical exploration and excision. However some useful investigations should be considered.

Blood tests:

• Thyroid antibody titres: are sometimes raised in thyroid carcinoma

• Serum calcitonin: > 0.08 ng/ml is suggestive of medullary carcinoma

Imaging:

• USS: commonly used imaging modality in thyroid disease but unable to differentiate benign and malignant nodules.

Others:

FNA: is the most important tool in diagnosing thyroid cancer. The procedure can be performed in the out-patient setting under local anaesthesia. A minimum of three biopsies are recommended to minimise false negative results. USS can be used to improve the accuracy of FNA.

Management

Papillary carcinoma:

> Total thyroid lobectomy is the removal of the affected lobe.
> If there is lymph node spread or the lesion is greater than 1cm a total thyroidectomy is performed with block dissection of the lymph nodes
> The thyroid must be suppressed (reduce TSH) post surgery by giving thyroxine (T4).
> These tumours are iodine sensitive therefore radioiodine can be given to treat recurrent and metastatic disease.
> Annual thyroglobulin measurements can be performed to identify recurrence.

Follicular carcinoma:

> Total thyroid lobectomy
> Total thyroidectomy is performed if there is vascular invasion
> Radioiodine and thyroid suppression is also indicated

Medullary carcinoma:

> Total thyroidectomy
> Lymph node clearance as involvement is usually present
> Calcitonin should be measured at follow up. Raised levels indicate metastatic disease.

Anaplastic carcinoma:

> A total thyroidectomy can be performed. However, most patients present late and have a mean survival of 6–8 months.
> Palliative radiotherapy is performed in selected cases to de-bulk the tumour.
> If there is airway obstruction a tracheostomy or tracheal stenting may be required.

Post-operative complications:

Haemorrhage:

> Acute haemorrhage post operatively can lead to airway obstruction, which is a life-threatening complication
> The patient will inevitably need intubation.
> The surgical clips are removed
> The deeper sutures may need to be cut to release the haematoma.
> The patient is taken back to theatre for exploration of the wound.

Recurrent laryngeal nerve injury:

> Along the posterior aspect of the thyroid gland is where the recurrent laryngeal nerve if situated.

> Unless the nerve is identified it is at risk of injury, especially when ligating the inferior thyroid artery.
> Unilateral nerve injury can result in hoarseness. However, if both recurrent laryngeal nerves are injured this may cause acute airway obstruction.

Damage to the parathyroid glands:

> This can occur following accidental injury or reduced blood supply.
> If there is significant damage, hypocalcaemia will result and present as tetany.
> Tetany can be demonstrated by Chvostek's sign (Twitching of the muscles of the face when the facial nerve is tapped), and Trousseau's sign (the upper arm is compressed with a blood pressure cuff causing carpal spasm).
> Treatment is with oral calcium supplements or a slow infusion of calcium gluconate.

Hypothyroidism:

> Surgery can result in reduction of thyroid tissue, leading to hypothyroidism.

Breast cancer

Epidemiology

In the UK breast cancer affects one in ten women, with approximately 20,000 new cases a year. The incidence of breast cancer continues to rise, however a reduction in the mortality has been noted.

Aetiology

Previous breast cancer and a family history of breast cancer are strong risk factors. A first degree relative with breast cancer doubles the risk. The inheritance is autosomal dominant in 5–10% of cases. Breast cancer 1 (BRCA1), breast cancer 2 (BRCA2) and p 53 genes have been identified in patients with breast cancer.

Oestrogen exposure due to a greater number of menstrual cycles is a risk factor for breast cancer. This is noted in early menarche, late menopause, or pregnancy after the age of 30 years.

There is a small increased risk of breast cancer with oestrogen-only hormone replacement therapy (HRT). The risk of breast cancer is doubled with oestrogen-progesterone HRT. Continuous use of the oral contraceptive pill (OCP) for greater than four years is also associated with an increased risk of breast cancer.

Other risk factors include exposure to radiation, alcohol use and a diet high in saturated fats.

Pathophysiology

Breast cancer can be referred to as *in situ* or invasive. If the cancer is *in situ* it carries a possibility of being curable as the ductal basement membrane has not been breached.

Non-invasive ductal carcinoma *in situ* (DCIS) is a pre-malignant lesion. Mammograms classically show microcalcification. Unifocal lesions may be treated with lumpectomy (localised excisions), but widespread lesion are commonly treated with a mastectomy. If left without any treatment the lesion can progress to invasive breast cancer. Non-invasive lobular carcinoma *in situ* (LCIS) is less common than DCIS and is usually multi-focal.

Invasive ductal carcinoma is the commonest type of breast cancer. It is usually noted as a hard lump. Other cancers include invasive lobular carcinoma, invasive medullary carcinoma (which accounts for approximately 5% of all breast cancers and is seen in younger patients), and invasive papillary carcinoma.

Paget's disease presents as an eczema-type skin condition on the nipple, where the skin involved may ulcerate and bleed. This usually represents an underlying malignancy and therefore should be investigated further.

Key features in the history/examination

- Lump that is firm and painless is usually noted by the patient.
- Nipple discharge
- Nipple retraction and breast tissue distortion
- Bone pain and abdominal pain may represent metastatic disease
- It is important to examine all lumps in the same manner. Some of the features of breast cancer include:
  - Firm, irregular lump
  - Asymmetry of the breasts
  - Nipple retraction/discharge
  - Skin tethering
  - The breast may have the appearance of the skin of an orange. This is known as Peau d'orange.
  - Fungating lesion
  - Axillary lymphadenopathy
  - Hepatomegaly suggests metastatic disease

Investigations

All women who are referred with a breast lump receive a triple assessment. This type of assessment aims to identify 95% of breast cancers. The triple assessment is composed of a detailed history and examination, radiology (mammography and USS), and FNA cytology (or core biopsy).

Mammography:

- The breasts are compressed between two plates
- Craniocaudal and oblique views of the breast are taken
- Breast cancer will be illustrated as a white spiculated lesion with microcalcification.
- Approximately 10% of cancers are missed with mammography.

Ultrasound scan:

- This is used together with mammography

- It does not identify microcalcification
- It is not a useful tool for screening for breast cancer
- It is useful in identifying cysts

Fine needle aspiration:

- If a lump has been identified FNA is performed.
- A 10 ml syringe and green needle is inserted into the lump and an aspirate is obtained.
- The sample is placed onto a slide and sent to pathology, where the slide is stained using haematoxylin and eosin.
- The results are divided into cytology codes. (See Table 4.31)
- Breast cysts usually disappear on aspirating with the needle.

Cytology code	Description
C1	Insufficient sample
C2	Benign cells
C3	Uncertain diagnosis
C4	Probable breast cancer
C5	Breast cancer

Table 4.31: The cytology codes.

Core biopsy:

- If breast cancer is suspected and the FNA results are inconclusive (C1-C3), the lump may be removed or a core biopsy is performed.
- Local anaesthetic is injected
- A scalpel blade is used to puncture the skin overlying the lump
- A core biopsy needle is pushed into the lump and a sample is removed
- Core biopsy can be performed with ultrasound guidance
- Patients return to clinic after a few days for the results

After a diagnosis of breast cancer has been made other investigations may be performed.

Blood tests:

- FBC
- LFTs
- U&Es
- Alkaline phosphatase (ALP)

Imaging:

- CXR: to look for metastatic disease.
- Liver USS: for staging of cancer
- Bone scan: for staging of cancer
- CT scan: for staging of cancer

Management

Breast cancer treatment depends on a number of factors including; clinical staging of the disease, morbidity of the patient undergoing the surgery, and the patient's choice to treatment options.

Staging of Breast cancer:

➢ Staging of the breast cancer is carried out using the clinical staging process (Table 4.32) or the tumour-node-metastasis (TNM) classification (Table 4.33)

Stage	Clinical features
Stage 1	• The growth is mobile • Confined to the breast • No lymph node involvement
Stage 2	• Clinical findings of stage 1 • Mobile axillary lymph nodes on the same side
Stage 3	• The tumour is fixed to the underlying muscle • The lymph nodes may have become fixed
Stage 4	• The tumour is now completely fixed to the chest wall • Metastatic disease is present • There may be opposite breast involvement

Table 4.32: Clinical staging of breast cancer.

TNM classification	Features
Tumour	T1: Tumour < 2 cm T2: Tumour 2–5 cm T3: Tumour 5–10 cm T4: Tumour > 10 cm, chest wall fixation and skin involvement
Node	N0: No nodes N1: Mobile lymph nodes on the same side of the breast lump N2: Fixed lymph nodes on the same side N3: Supraclavicular/Infraclavicular lymph node involvement
Metastases	M0: No metastases M1: Metastatic disease (liver, bones, and lungs)

Table 4.33: The TNM staging of breast cancer.

Operative management:

➢ Operative management is offered in early breast cancer.

➢ Clinical stages 1 and 2 can be treated surgically. Surgery should be avoided in stages 3 and 4.

➢ Wide local excision (WLE) followed by radiotherapy treatment five days a week for five weeks is usually the common choice of treatment. This provides patients with a better cosmetic outcome.

4. Surgery

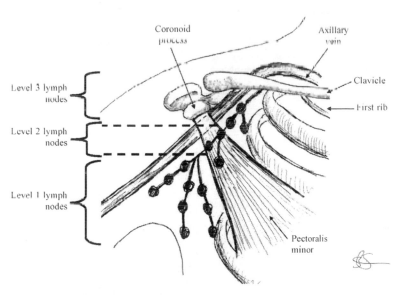

Figure 4.30: Axillary lymph nodes.

- ➤ Mastectomy is preferred for larger tumours or multifocal disease. The patient may choose to have a mastectomy over WLE however, radiotherapy is not possible here.

- ➤ Survival rates are the same for WLE and mastectomy.

- ➤ It is important to identify lymph node involvement in the disease to complete the staging of breast cancer. To achieve this, a number of different procedures can be performed at the time of surgery.

- ➤ Axillary sampling:
  - o The lower axillary nodes are removed
  - o If these nodes are involved in the disease process; axillary clearance or radiotherapy will be performed

- ➤ Axillary clearance involves the clearance of lymph nodes at different levels. (See Figure 4.30)
  - o Level 1: Lymph nodes are removed up to the axillary vein
  - o Level 2: Lymph nodes are removed up to the medial border of the pectoralis minor
  - o Level 3: Lymph nodes are removed up to the border of the first rib

- ➤ Sentinal node mapping:
  - o The sentinel node is the first node that the lymph fluid from the breast drains into.
  - o Blue dye or a radioisotope is injected and using a probe the sentinel node can be identified.
  - o The sentinel node is removed on frozen section, and if it is clear of disease no further nodal removal is required.
  - o Complications of surgery include wound infection, haematoma, seroma and Lymphoedema.

Medical management:

- ➤ Systemic treatment of early breast cancer can be adjuvant or neo-adjuvant (before surgery) therapy. This may consist of radiotherapy, chemotherapy, and endocrine treatment.
  - o Radiotherapy: can be directed at the breast, chest wall, and axilla. It is commonly used for palliative care of the patient.
  - o Chemotherapy: is useful for large tumours or recurrent diseases. Neo-adjuvent chemotherapy is given prior to surgery.
  - o Endocrine treatment: Tamoxifen (partial oestrogen receptor agonist) and Arimidex (aromatase enzyme inhibitor) both reduce the risk of new or contralateral disease.

- ➤ Both monotherapy and combination therapy can be used in the treatment of breast cancer.

- ➤ There are other newer drugs potentially available for the treatment of breast cancer. Herceptin (Taxane) is a humanised monoclonal antibody which binds to human epidermal growth factor receptor 2 (HER2), i.e. an oncoprotein. These newer drugs are still under development and are currently not available on the National Health Service (NHS).

Management of advanced breast cancer (Stage 3 and 4):

- ➤ Management is dependent on the individual status of the disease in each patient.

- ➤ Local recurrence should be managed with radiotherapy, further excision of the tumour, and regional chemotherapy.

- ➤ Metastasis to the bone should be managed with analgesia, radiotherapy, and bisphosphonates.

- ➤ Metastasis to the brain should be managed with radiotherapy, steroids and rarely surgery.

- ➤ All patients with advanced disease must be provided with a palliative care package and appropriate support.

Breast screening:

- ➤ Introduced to the UK in 1988 after publication of The Forrest Report.

- ➤ Women aged 50–65 are invited every three years to undergo a mammogram.

- ➤ Two-view mammogram is usually used

- ➤ Triple assessment is performed if required

Oesophageal cancer

The oesophagus is a muscular tube transporting food from the mouth to the stomach. It is approximately 25 cm in length and spans from the cricoid cartilage (C6) to the cardiac orifice of the stomach (T10). The epithelium of the oesophagus is stratified squamous up to the level of the gastro-oesophageal junction.

Epidemiology

Oesophageal cancer is the ninth commonest cancer in the UK with a lifetime risk of 1 in 64 for men and 1 in 116 for women. The disease tends to occur in people over the age of 40 years. Worldwide distribution shows a higher preponderance to Russia and Asia, in particular China.

Aetiology

There are two main histological types of oesophageal cancer: SCC and AC. The risk factors associated with SCC and AC are described in Table 4.34.

Adenocarcinoma	Squamous cell carcinoma
Barrett's oesophagus	Tobacco use
Gastro-oesophageal reflux (GOR)	High alcohol
Obesity	Vitamin C & A deficiency
Cigarette smoking	Coeliac disease
High alcohol intake	Oesophageal strictures
	Achalasia

Table 4.34: The associated risk factors of AC and SSC.

Pathophysiology

SCC tends to occur in the upper two thirds of the oesophagus whilst, AC is found in the lower third portion. The incidence of SCC has remained relatively stable in the western population over the last two decades however, that of AC has been on the increase. The cancer metastasises initially to the peri-oesophageal lymph nodes and adjacent structures such as the tracheo-bronchial tree, aorta, and recurrent laryngeal nerve. The liver and lungs are affected late in the disease.

Key features in the history/examination

- Dysphagia and/or odynophagia: patients normally give a history of progressive dysphagia initially with solid food and later progressing to liquids.
- Retrosternal discomfort
- Aspiration pneumonia and coughing during ingestion.
- Hoarse voice due to recurrent laryngeal nerve palsy.
- Anaemia
- Weight loss
- Massive haematemesis
- Cachexia
- Lymphadenopathy, in particular the supraclavicular nodes (Virchow's node)
- Hepatomegaly may be present with liver metastasis

Investigations

Imaging:

- Barium swallow: is sensitive at detecting oesophageal strictures and intra-luminal masses.
- Endoscopic USS: is most sensitive test in determining depth of tumour invasion and involvement of peri-oesophageal lymph nodes (T & N staging)
- CT chest and abdomen: provides important information on metastatic spread to lungs and liver and gives information on tumour involvement with adjacent structures.
- Positron emission tomography (PET) scan: is a relatively new imaging modality that assists in identifying bone and lymph node involvement.

Endoscopy:

- Oesophago-gastro-duodenoscopy: allows direct visualisation and biopsy of the tumour. All patients undergo this investigation to confirm the histology.

Management

- Surgical resection is offered to all patients who are medically fit for surgery with no significant metastatic disease. Only about 30% of oesophageal cancers are appropriate for resection and the overall five-year survival in the UK is approximately 25%.

- Patients with contraindications to surgery should be managed with palliative care. Such patient are those with:
  - Metastatic involvement to N2 nodes or solid organs e.g. liver or lung.
  - Invasion to adjacent organs such as the aorta, tracheo-bronchial tree or pericardium
  - Severe cardio-respiratory diseases (forced expiratory volume in 1 sec (FEV_1) < 1.2L or a Left ventricular ejection fraction (EF) < 0.4).

Surgical treatment:

- The type of surgical approach depends primarily on the anatomy and site of the oesophageal tumour.
- Ivor Lewis procedure (lower third oesophageal tumour): This entails an initial laparotomy to mobilise the stomach taking care to preserve the right gastro-epiploic arcade. In recent practice this part of the operation has been performed laparoscopically. The second part involves a right thoracotomy during which the tumour is resected and the stomach is brought up and an anastomosed to the remaining oesophagus.
- Trans-hiatal approach (upper to middle third oesophageal tumour): This involves an upper midline laparotomy and neck incision. The oesophagus is mobilised from above and below. A stomach conduit is brought up and an anastomosis is created with the cervical oesophagus.
- McKeown 3 stage procedure (upper third oesophageal tumour): This is similar to the Ivor Lewis procedure, but involves a third stage where a neck incision is made through which the stomach is brought up and anastomosed to the cervical oesophagus.

Palliative treatment:

- Stenting: self expanding metal stent is inserted under endoscopic guidance. This keeps the oesophageal lumen patent and improves the patient's swallowing. It is particular useful in the event of a tracheo-oesophageal fistula.
- Chemotherapy: particularly for AC
- Radiotherapy: particularly for SSC
- Laser therapy: neodymium-doped yttrium aluminium garnet (Nd:YAG) laser can debulk intrinsic tumours and improve swallowing.

Colon cancer

Epidemiology

Large bowel carcinomas are the second most common malignant cause of death in the UK. These tumours can occur at all ages with a peak incidence of 70–80 years. Females are affected more than males and the disease is more common in Western Europe than in developing countries. Approximately, 20% of cases present to the accident and emergency department with intestinal obstruction or peritonitis.

Aetiology

Conditions including polyps and ulcerative colitis (UC) are well known predisposing factors for the development of large bowel cancer. Inherited colorectal cancer syndromes such as familial adenomatous polyposis and hereditary non-polyposis colon cancer are also risk factors for developing cancer of the large bowel.

Familial adenomatous polyposis is rare autosomal dominant trait with a mutation in the familial adenomatous polyposis (FAP) gene. It commonly progresses to colon cancer, accounting for 0.5% of all cases. Polyps occur early resulting in symptoms such as rectal bleeding and diarrhoea in those less than 21 years old followed by progression to malignancy between the ages of 20 and 40 years.

Hereditary non-polyposis colon cancer (HNPCC) is an autosomal dominant trait where the deoxyribonucleic acid (DNA) mismatch repair occurs as a result of a gene mutation. It accounts for 5% of colorectal malignancy and presents before the age of 50. This condition has a strong association with ovarian, uterine, and gastric tumours too.

A high fat and low fibre diet can increase transit time of faeces prolonging gut exposure to potential carcinogens. Pelvic irradiation increases risk of developing recto-sigmoid carcinoma too.

Pathophysiology

Macroscopically the cancer is a colloid tumour that appears as a malignant ulcer with annular, infiltrating growth. Microscopically all tumours are adenocarcinomas (AC). The aggressiveness of the tumour normally correlates with the histological differentiation. (See Table 4.35).

Grade	Features
I	Well differentiated
II-III	Moderately differentiated
IV	Anaplastic

Table 4.35: Grading of colon cancers.

75% of the lesions are located in the rectum and sigmoid colon. Patients with FAP and HNPCC have a higher incidence of right sided tumours. The severity of the cancer can be determined by the spread and staging of the tumour. (see Table 4.36) Metastasis can occur via local spread, lymphatics, blood or trans-coelomic spread.

Local spread occurs when the tumour surrounds the wall of the bowel eventually moving to the adjacent viscera. If the cancer spreads via the lymphatics, it will first go to the regional lymph nodes and may continue through the thoracic duct eventually appearing at the supraclavicular nodes. Metastasis via the blood usually occurs via the portal vein to the liver (25–40%) and then to the lung (5% of cases).

Trans-coelomic spread results in malignant nodules deposited throughout the peritoneal cavity. If it spreads to the ovaries it is known as 'Krukenburg tumours'.

Stage	Features
A	The tumour is confined to the mucosa and submucosa of the bowel wall
B	The tumour has spread through the muscle layers and beyond the bowel wall
C	Regional lymph nodes are affected
D	Metastatic spread has occurred (e.g. to the liver or lungs)

Table 4.36: Staging of colon cancers according to the Dukes classification.

Key features in the history/examination

- Anorexia and weight loss
- Symptoms of anaemia: lethargy, malaise, shortness of breath, and light headedness.
- Change in bowel habit: constipation and diarrhoea
- Rectal bleeding and mucus production
- Symptoms of intestinal obstruction
- Abdominal pain associated with obstruction, mass and perforation of the tumour or bowel.
- Right-sided tumours tend to have a mass on palpation in the right iliac fossa. There may also be diarrhoea and lethargy secondary to anaemia.
- Left-sided tumours tend to present early with abdominal pain and change in bowel habit. Distension of the abdomen suggests intestinal obstruction.
- Signs of anaemia and weight loss (e.g. pallor and muscle wasting)
- A mass present on abdominal palpation or rectal examination
- Signs associated with metastatic spread (e.g. hepatomegaly, ascites, and jaundice)
- Tender and rigid abdomen in cases of perforation

Investigations

Blood Test:

- FBC: may reveal a low Hb in cases of anaemia
- Carcinoembyronic antigen (CEA): is a bowel tumour marker

Imaging:

- Erect chest X-ray (CXR): to exclude perforation and also to look for possible metastatic spread
- AXR: shows intestinal obstruction acutely and also to look for possible metastatic spread.
- CT: this is the investigation of choice in elderly patients who are unable to tolerate endoscopic investigation and those

presenting with acute intestinal obstruction. Colon tumours can be identified along with evidence of metastatic spread to the liver. A recent radiological technique called CT-colonography has demonstrated similar ability to colonoscopy in identifying bowel lesions.

- Ultrasound scan (USS): good for characterising of liver metastasis. Used pre-operatively and in following up post-colonic tumour resection patients. Trans-anal USS can be used in staging rectal tumours.

- Barium enema: a growth or stricture can be identified. A growth is seen as a filling defect (apple core stricture). Diverticula may also be identified which may hide smaller tumours of the bowel. A negative barium enema does not exclude a colonic tumour as small lesions can be missed.

Endoscopy:

- Sigmoidoscopy: can be used to identify rectal and sigmoid tumours and take a biopsy to confirm malignancy on histology.

- Colonoscopy: allows direct visualisation of the entire colon and biopsies to be taken of any masses seen.

Management

Pre-operative management:

➢ It is important to ensure the patients have had a complete pre-operative assessment, as it is likely that these patients will have other co-morbidities.

➢ Bowel prep. is important, for example 'Kleen prep' the day before the surgery and a phosphate enema on the morning of the surgery. All hospitals should have their own protocols, and it is important that you locate these early on your rotation.

➢ The stoma site is marked by the surgeon or the stoma nurse.

➢ Consent: It is important to discuss the possibility of a stoma being formed if an anastomosis is not possible or if a diversion is required.

Surgical management:

➢ The management of colon cancer consists of surgical removal of the tumour The bowel is emptied with oral laxatives and rectal enemas. If the Hb is low a blood transfusion may be required pre-operatively.

➢ It is important to define the extent of the tumour before deciding on the surgical procedure. Patients will require a staging CT scan and have tissue biopsies sent to histopathology. The results from these investigations are then discussed at the multi disciplinary team (MDT) meeting before advancing to surgery.

➢ The mainstay of treatment is to resect the tumour and its associated regional lymph nodes.

➢ In those cases without obstruction a primary resection is performed with an end to end anastomosis.

➢ In obstructed cases bowel preparation is contraindicated. The main aim of the surgery is to relieve the obstruction, ideally with a primary anastomosis. Obstructing tumours from the

right side of the colon can normally be resected and a primary anastomosis performed. However with left-side tumours an initial decompression or a Hartmann's procedure is usually performed.

➢ In some obstructed cases there is an increased risk of anastomotic breakdown due to the poor vascular supply to the area. In such cases a defunctioning colostomy or ileostomy may be constructed to protect the primary anastomosis.

➢ When resecting the tumour the surgeon must ensure that there is an adequate blood supply to the two cut ends of the bowel.

➢ The surgeon must also remove all of the bowel which has the same blood supply as the tumour.

➢ Post-operative chemotherapy may be an option to reduce the risk of recurrence. Radiotherapy has been shown to have no role in the management of bowel cancer.

Site of tumour	Operation
Right colon	Right hemicolectomy (see Figure 4.31)
Transverse colon	Extended right hemicolectomy
Descending colon	Left hemicolectomy
Rectum	Anterior resection is where the rectal tumour is resected and the colon above is anastomosed to the rectal stump. A temporary stoma (which can be later reversed) may be produced to allow the primary anastomosis to heel. Abdominoperineal excision is performed for low rectal tumours

Table 4.37: Type of operation required for the different locations of colon cancer.

In cases where metastatic spread has occurred, surgery is still an option for the palliative care of the patient. The obstruction is removed and a permanent colostomy may be required.

Prognosis:

The five-year survival rates vary according to the stage of the tumour. (See Table 4.38).

Stage of tumour	Five year survival rate
Dukes A	80–85%
Dukes B	60%
Dukes C	30%
Dukes D	5%

Table 4.38: The five year survival rate according to the tumour stage.

Stoma care:

➢ On the surgical wards the management of these patients will always involve a multidisciplinary approach. You will commonly see the stoma care nurses taking an active role in the management of the stoma.

4. Surgery

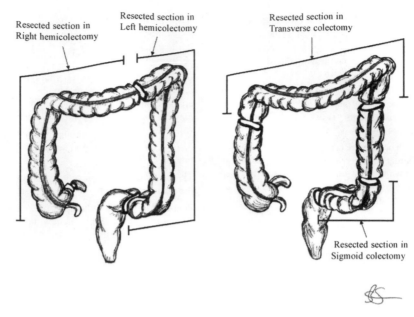

Figure 4.31: The common colectomies.

➤ Right lower quadrant stoma:

○ This is usually an ileostomy, which once constructed leaves a spout that has no contact with the skin.

○ The stoma can be an end ileostomy in which the patient has had a total colectomy, or a loop ileostomy in which the colonic resection has been difficult and the anastomosis is given time to heal before intestinal continuity is completed.

➤ Right upper quadrant stoma:

○ This is commonly a transverse colostomy, which once constructed leaves a stoma which is continuous with the skin.

○ This is usually a temporary stoma to allow the anastomosis to heal.

➤ Left Lower quadrant stoma:

○ These stomas can be end colostomies, loop colostomies, or double barrelled colostomies.

○ A temporary end colostomy is produced following resection of the sigmoid colon or rectum. (e.g. Hartman's procedure)

○ A permanent end colostomy is constructed after resection of the anus and rectum. This is often performed following an abdominoperineal excision for low rectal tumours.

○ A double barrelled colostomy is performed when an anastomosis cannot be performed and both ends of the colon are brought out to the surface, such as following a mid sigmoid gut volvulus.

○ A loop colostomy is constructed in cases where a resection has not occurred and the sigmoid colon has been brought

out to the surface. This is carried out in patients with inoperable rectal tumours which are likely to obstruct.

➤ Left upper quadrant stoma:

○ Stomas are not usually sited in this quadrant

○ If a stoma is found at this site, it is most likely a result of the technical practicality of the surgery.

Hepato-cellular carcinoma

Epidemiology

This is a common worldwide cancer (Africa and South-East Asia), but extremely rare in the UK.

Aetiology

80% of patients with Hepato-cellular carcinoma (HCC) have known liver cirrhosis. The common causes of liver cirrhosis progressing to cancer include hepatitis B virus (HBV) infection and hepatitis C virus (HCV) infection. In fact, HCC can develop 25 years after initial HCV infection. Alcoholic liver disease and haemachromatosis (iron overload) are also common causes of cirrhosis leading to HCC.

Other risk factors for HCC are drugs (e.g. steroids), aflatoxin exposure (fungal metabolite) and smoking.

Pathophysiology

Chronic inflammation within the liver, as a result of cirrhosis leads to development of HCC. Macroscopically, there is a large solitary tumour with multiple lesions throughout the liver. HCC commonly metastasises to the lungs and bones.

Key features in the history/examination

Patients will often be asymptomatic but can present with symptoms of chronic liver disease.

- Malaise and weakness
- Jaundice
- Upper gastrointestinal bleed
- Anorexia and weight loss
- Hepatomegaly
- Ascites
- Jaundice
- Decompensated liver disease leading to encephalopathy

Investigations

Blood tests:

- Serum α-fetoprotein (AFP): is raised in HCC and cirrhosis

Imaging:

- USS/CT/MRI: can easily identify large tumours. Small tumours (<1 cm) can be difficult to differentiate from nodules found in cirrhotic livers.
- Hepatic angiography: is performed to distinguish small HCCs from nodules.

Others:

- Liver biopsy: this will confirm the diagnosis. There is a 2% risk of tumour dissemination therefore this should be avoided if liver transplantation is a possibility.

Management

- ➢ Tumours not associated with cirrhosis and confined to a single lobe of the liver can be treated with a hemi-hepatectomy.
- ➢ Cirrhotic liver disease and HCC is difficult to treat as removal of liver substance will predispose the patient to postoperative liver decompensation and possible death.
- ➢ The final option is to undergo a liver transplant.
- ➢ Patients with cirrhosis and HCC have a median survival of 12 months.

Cholangiocarcinoma

Epidemiology

The incidence of this bile duct carcinoma is increasing, with the disease predominantly affecting adults over the age of 50 years.

Aetiology

Cholangiocarcinoma is associated with inflammatory bowel disease, sclerosing cholangitis, congenital hepatic fibrosis, and a polycystic liver.

Pathophysiology

Macroscopically, cholangiocarcinoma is seen within the liver substance and in the extra-hepatic bile ducts. Common sites include the point at which the right and left hepatic ducts meet, the common hepatic duct, and the cystic duct.

Microscopically, the tumour is typically slow growing and is a mucin secreting AC. Tumours at the right and left hepatic ducts invade the liver parenchyma, and become fibrous. This results in the development of duct strictures. Tumours at the distal end of the bile duct are polypoidal and commonly obstruct the bile duct lumen. They both invade the lymphatic system.

Key features in the history/examination

- Painless jaundice
- Dark urine and pale stools
- Weight loss
- Epigastric pain
- Steatorrhoea (foul smelling and difficult to flush away stool)
- Muscle wasting
- Pallor
- Clinically jaundiced (yellow discolouration of the skin and sclera of the eye)
- Abdominal pain on palpation
- Hepatomegaly

Investigations

Blood tests:

- Serum carcinoembryonic antigen (CEA) and carbohydrate antigen 19–9 (CA 19–9): are raised in approximately 20% of patients

Imaging:

- USS: dilated intra-hepatic ducts are present.
- MRCP: the biliary tree can be visualised.
- Percutaneous transhepatic cholangiography: may identify filling defects in the bile ducts but can often be mistaken for bile duct stones.
- CT guided needle biopsy: CT abdomen is only a sensitive tool if the tumour has infiltrated into the liver parenchyma. If a mass lesion is identified a needle biopsy can be performed.

Endoscopy:

- ERCP: the bile duct stone will be identified and potentially removed. Bile cytology and brushings of the stricture may be performed

Management

- ➢ Cholangiocarcinomas are rarely curable.

➢ Surgical treatment is radical resection of the liver parenchyma and the affected bile duct.

➢ Palliative management can include endoluminal stenting with ERCP or a surgical bypass.

➢ This tumour has a very poor prognosis with a one-year survival of < 20%.

Gallbladder cancer

Epidemiology

Gallbladder cancer is commonly found in Central and South America, northern India, Japan, and central and eastern Europe. It usually presents between the ages of 50–60 years, with women being affected more than men.

Aetiology

The aetiology is unknown however an association has been made to the presence of gallstones. It is thought that gallstones act as chronic irritants to the gallbladder mucosa. A calcified gallbladder, termed the 'porcelain' gallbladder has also been linked to the development of gallbladder cancer.

Pathophysiology

90% of tumours are AC whilst, 10% are SSC. The tumour usually spreads locally to the liver and its ducts.

Key features in the history/examination

• Right upper quadrant pain
• Nausea and vomiting
• Weight loss
• Jaundice
• Right upper quadrant tenderness on palpation
• Palpable mass

Investigations

Imaging:
• Spiral CT: is the investigation of choice to stage the tumour.
• Cholangiography: can aid with tumour staging.
• Hepatic angiography: can aid with tumour staging.

Management

➢ The tumour may be an incidental finding on performing a cholecystectomy for gallstones

➢ Radical surgical resection can include resection of the gallbladder, right lobe liver parenchyma, and the biliary tree.

➢ Chemotherapy does not have a role in gallbladder cancer.

➢ There is good prognosis in those patients with tumour confined

to the gallbladder mucosa. In advanced disease most patients are dead within a few months.

Pancreatic carcinoma

Epidemiology

Pancreatic carcinoma affects 10 per 100,000 of the population each year, and is the eighth commonest cause of death from cancer in the UK. Its incidence is increasing and usually affects the elderly population.

Aetiology

There are a few risk factors associated with pancreatic carcinoma. These include smoking, beta-naphthylamine (dye industry), benzidine, and an abnormality in drainage of the pancreas.

Pathophysiology

The majority (85%) of tumours are duct cell AC. Approximately 60% of tumours are found at the head of the pancreas, 25% in the body and 15% in the tail.

Macroscopically, the tumour appears irregular and hard. Microscopically, the cancers are usually undifferentiated. If an adenocarcinoma has been identified, it is typical to notice mucus secretion from the duct. However, an acinar cell carcinoma is a non-mucus secreting cancer, originating from the acinar cells.

Spread of the tumour can occur via direct invasion into the common bile duct, duodenum, portal vein, and the inferior vena cava or via lymphatic spread. Haematogenous spread can result in liver and lung metastasis whilst trans-coelomic spread results in peritoneal seeding and ascites.

Key features in the history/examination

Pancreatic cancer can have different presentations:

• Anorexia and weight loss
• Painless jaundice due to compression of the bile duct
• Continuous epigastric pain that is dull in character.
• Symptoms of diabetes (thirst, polyuria, polydipsia)
• Jaundice
• Epigastric mass on palpation
• Hepatomegaly and ascites suggestive of metastatic disease
• Courvoisier's law: 'Palpable painless mass in the presence of jaundice is unlikely to be a result of gallstones.' This law arises from the knowledge that recurrent gallstone attacks cause acute inflammation resulting in a thickened fibrosed gallbladder that does not distend easily.

Investigations

Blood tests:
• FBC
• U&Es

- LFTs
- Clotting
- Amylase
- Glucose

Imaging:

- USS: will identify bile duct dilatation.
- Spiral CT: the tumour can be identified and allows guidance for a needle biopsy. If the tumour is less than 4 cm, confined to the head of the pancreas, and without metastatic spread the patient should undergo surgical treatment. (See Figure 4.32)
- ERCP: may identify bile duct obstruction. During this procedure a stent may be inserted to relieve the obstruction.

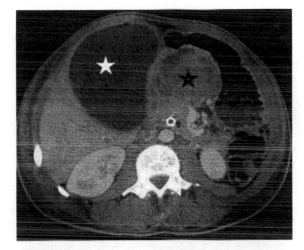

Figure 4.32: CT showing a large liver abscess (white star) in a patient with a big pancreatic malignant mass (black star).

Management

Pancreatic cancer usually presents late resulting in 90–95% of cases being unsuitable for operative management. Palliative treatment should be discussed with those inoperable cases.

Operative management:

- Patients with duct cell carcinomas (< 4 cm) and without metastatic spread should be offered surgical treatment. The operation of choice is a pancreato-duodenectomy (Whipple's procedure) with preservation of the pylorus.
- A cholecystectomy is initially performed
- The bile duct is dissected as well as removal of lymphatic tissue in the area.
- The common hepatic artery is identified and the gastroduodenal branch divided.
- This will expose the portal vein.
- The duodenum and right colon are mobilised, allowing

dissection of the fourth part of the duodenum. This results in the duodenum being released from the ligament of Treitz, (Ligament of Treitz is the anatomical demarcation of the duodenojejunal junction).

- The jejunum is dissected next, after which the proximal duodenum is divided.
- The pancreas is identified and divided.
- The surrounding structures and tissues are separated from the mesenteric artery and the vein, with continued separation until the bile duct is reached.
- The bile duct is then divided and the entire specimen is removed.
- Retroperitoneal lymph nodes are removed at the same time.
- A drain is placed in the subhepatic region.
- Reconstruction after removal of the specimen includes a choledochojejunostomy, pancreatojejunostomy, and gastrojejunostomy.
- The procedure can take up to six hours.
- Common postoperative complications include infection, bleeding and a pancreatic duct leak.

Palliative management:

- By inserting a stent the obstructive jaundice is relieved.
- If the duodenum becomes obstructed a gastrojejunostomy may be performed, however if the patient presents late, insertion of a metal stent is considered to be more appropriate.
- In those patients who have an inoperable tumour diagnosed at laparotomy, a palliative bypass is considered (cholecysto or choledochoduodenostomy with gastrojejunostomy).
- A biopsy is required for histological diagnosis. If this is not carried out at laparotomy, a percutaneous trucut biopsy should be performed.
- Chemotherapy has only shown a significant effect in certain tumours. Duct cell AC undergo remission in approximately 15–20% of patients. However, chemotherapy has not shown any benefit in the other tumours.
- Pain is controlled with opiate analgesia e.g. Morphine sulphate tablets (MST) or Oromorph.

Prognosis:

- Median survival is 20 weeks
- Less than 5% of patients will survive five years.

Prostate cancer

Epidemiology

Prostate carcinoma is the most common cancer in men. Its incidence increases with age, with 75% of cases found in those between the ages of 60–79 years.

Aetiology

The aetiology remains unknown however there are a few important predisposing factors associated with the disease. These include increasing age, changes in hormone levels such as oestrogen and testosterone, and exposure to carcinogens. A family history of prostate cancer in a first degree relative increases the risk by two-fold. The Afro-American population tend to have the highest risk of developing prostate cancer.

Pathophysiology

A layer of myoepithelial cells surround the prostate gland. Initially the basement membrane is lost and the cells appear less differentiated, but soon further layers of carcinoma cells are seen.

The cancer originates in the outer zone of the prostate gland, and later invades the entire gland. The carcinoma spreads initially to the peri-prostatic tissues, i.e. the bladder, urethra, and rectum. Further spread to the iliac and para-aortic nodes occurs via the lymphatic system.

Metastatic spread occurs through the blood stream via the vertebral venous plexus to the vertebra, skull, and pelvis. Macroscopically, the cancer appears hard, craggy, and pale. Microscopically, the cancer is an AC, and often moderately differentiated. The degree of differentiation is usually defined according to the Gleason grade of 2–10.

Staging:

The carcinoma is staged using the TNM system. (See Table 4.39)

TNM classification	Features
Tumour	TIS: Carcinoma *in situ*
	T1: Tumour found incidentally on needle biopsy or transurethral resection of the prostate (TURP)
	T2: Intracapsular palpable tumour
	T3: Tumour (mobile) spread beyond the capsule
	T4: Fixed tumour or locally invasive tumour
Nodes	N0: No lymph nodes
	N1–4: One or more lymph nodes
Metastasis	M0: No metastases
	M1: Metastatic spread

Table 4.39: The TNM classification for prostate cancer.

Key features in the history/examination

- Early stage of the disease can be asymptomatic whilst, advanced cases give rise to symptoms.
- Malaise and weight loss
- Pelvic pain
- Haematuria
- Symptoms of bladder outflow obstruction
- Bone pain
- The most important part of the examination is performing a digital rectal examination which may reveal:
  - A hard nodule
  - Enlarged and craggy prostate
  - The midline sulcus may have disappeared
  - There may be infiltration of the tumour on either side of the prostate into surrounding tissue.

Investigations

The initial investigations performed are the same as for benign prostatic hyperplasia (BPH).

Blood tests:

- PSA: is not a sensitive marker in early disease. It is elevated in prostatitis, post instrumentation and UTIs. A level of 10 ng/ml is suggestive of prostate cancer and values above 35 ng/ml are diagnostic. PSA can be further used to observe treatment response and recurrence.

Imaging:

- CXR/AXR: metastatic disease can be seen, on the ribs, lumbar vertebrae and pelvis.
- CT: of the abdomen and pelvis will help to stage the disease.
- MRI: information on capsular invasion.
- Transrectal USS (TRUS): can identify small tumours and it allows a needle-core biopsy to be taken from the prostate gland. However, there may be complications of infection or prostatic abscess formation.

Others:

- Trans-rectal biopsy: can be taken using an automated gun. The risk of sepsis increases, therefore antibiotic cover should be given.
- Trans-urethral resection of the prostate (TURP): can provide tissue for analysis as well as symptomatic relief.
- Isotope bone scan: will identify any 'hot spots' representing bony metastases

Management

Conservative management:

➢ Patients can be given the option to watch and wait as small well differentiated tumours have a ten-year survival rate without treatment.

➢ Patients are therefore not exposed to the adverse effects of treatment

➢ Patients must be followed up closely with regular rectal examinations and PSA levels.

Medical management:

Prostatic cancer is driven by androgens. Therefore, in locally invasive disease and metastatic disease the aim is to reduce androgen stimulation. This can be achieved with the following:

➤ Oestrogens e.g. Stilboesterol: Now rarely used due to adverse side-effects such as gynaecomastia, testicular atrophy, thrombosis and congestive cardiac failure (CCF).

➤ Luteinising-hormone releasing hormone (LHRH) analogues e.g. Goserelin (Zoladex):

  ○ These drugs down regulate the pituitary and therefore inhibit release of the luteinising hormone from the anterior pituitary.

  ○ This results in reduced production of testosterone.

  ○ At the start of treatment there may be a temporary acute rise in testosterone levels. A course of anti-androgens is given to counteract this.

  ○ LHRH analogues are administered as three-monthly subcutaneous injections.

➤ Anti-androgens (e.g. Cypreterone acetate, Flutamide): act by blocking dihydrotestosterone receptors.

➤ External beam radiotherapy: is the treatment of choice for bony metastases, providing symptomatic relief. It can supplement hormonal treatment to control disease progression.

Surgical management:

➤ Pre-operative counselling may be necessary to warn patients of the following:

  ○ Retrograde ejaculation occurs in 65% of men following the procedure.

  ○ 5% of men will suffer with erectile impotence.

  ○ 15% of patients will require a further procedure in 8–10 years.

  ○ Mortality rate is less than 0.5%.

  ○ Complications include urethral stricture, sepsis, haematuria, urinary incontinence, UTI and transurethral resection (TUR) syndrome.

➤ Trans-urethral resection of the prostate (TURP): should be performed if there are symptoms of bladder outflow obstruction.

➤ Radical Prostatectomy:

  ○ This procedure is only performed for stage T1 and T2 disease.

  ○ It involves the complete removal of the prostate, seminal vesicles, and pelvic lymph nodes.

  ○ The bladder neck is mobilised and anastomosed to the urethra distal to the prostate

➤ Bilateral orchidectomy: is used for stage T3, T4 and metastatic disease. Androgen ablation is achieved with this procedure. It is also suitable for patients not able to tolerate hormonal treatment.

➤ Brachytherapy: is a procedure involving the implantation of radioactive iodine or palladium seeds within the prostate. This allows a higher dose of radiation than with external beam radiotherapy.

Testicular cancer

Epidemiology

Testicular cancers are rare and account for only 2% of all malignancies affecting the male population. However, it is the commonest malignancy affecting young adult males.

Aetiology

Predisposing factors include a family history of testicular cancer, previous contralateral testicular cancer, undescended testis (cryptorchidism), trauma and mumps.

Pathophysiology

Approximately 95% of testicular tumours are of germ cell origin. Most of the remaining 5% are sex-cord gonadal stromal tumours derived from Leydig cells or Sertoli cells. There are two sub-categories for germ cell tumours of the testicles:

1 Seminomas account for 60% of testicular germ cell tumours. They typically occur in males aged 15–35 years with 10% of cases occurring in patients with undescended testes. Seminomas arise from the cells of the seminiferous tubules. Macroscopically, the tumour appears large, smooth, solid, and is often described as looking like a section of a cut potato. Microscopically, the cells appear as well differentiated spermatocytes or undifferentiated round cells. Seminomas spread through the lymphatic system (Para-aortic nodes) and rarely via the blood stream.

2 Non-seminomatous germ cell tumours (NSGCT) account for 40% of testicular germ cell tumours. They arise from primitive germ cells and contain embryonal stem cells. Therefore these tumours include embryonal carcinoma, teratoma (commonest), choriocarcinoma, and yolk sac tumour. Macroscopically the tumour has a cystic appearance and microscopically the cells differ greatly. The tumour can consist of bone, cartilage, fat, muscle and other tissue.

Key features in the history/examination

- Enlarging testicular lump
- Pain can occur in 30% of patients
- Patients may complain of a sensation of heaviness in the scrotum.
- The testis is smooth, enlarged, and heavy
- An associated hydrocele may be present
- Gynaecomastia is found in 5% of cases of testicular cancer.
- Shortness of breath suggests lung metastases
- Metastatic disease can present with abdominal lymph nodes and cervical lymphadenopathy, in particular supraclavicular lymphadenopathy. Table 4.40 describes the staging of testicular cancer.

Stage	Features
I	The tumour is confined to the testis
II	Abdominal lymph nodes are affected
III	Supra-diaphragmatic and infra-diaphragmatic lymph nodes are affected
IV	Other metastatic spread e.g. lungs and liver

Table 4.40: The Royal Marsden classification for testicular cancer.

Investigations

Blood tests:

- AFP: is raised in 50–70% of NSGCT. The only NSGCT not to secrete this is a true choriocarcinoma.
- Beta-HCG is raised in 5–10% of seminomas and 40–60% NSGCT.
- Lactate dehydrogenase (LDH) is a less specific marker for germ cell tumours but can be a gross marker of tumour burden.

Imaging:

- CXR: to look for metastatic disease. The classical picture of cannonball metastases may be identified.
- Scrotal USS: A solid tumour can be identified in the scrotum.
- CT of the abdomen: is used to stage the tumour.

Management

- ➢ An orchidectomy is performed to excise the primary tumour in all cases.
- ➢ A groin incision is performed and the spermatic cord is identified.
- ➢ To prevent spread of the tumour a soft clamp is placed over the cord.
- ➢ If a tumour has been identified or there is a strong suspicion, the cord is ligated at the inguinal ring and the testis is removed.
- ➢ It is sent for histological diagnosis.
- ➢ Seminomas:
  - o Stage I and II respond well to external beam radiotherapy
  - o Stage III and IV are treated with radiotherapy and chemotherapy (e.g. Cisplatin and Bleomycin).
  - o Five-year survival for stage I disease is 98% and stage II disease is 85%.
- ➢ Non-seminomas:
  - o Stage I is managed conservatively with monitoring of serum tumour markers.
  - o Stage II, III, and IV is treated with chemotherapy.
  - o 5-year survival of stage I and II disease is > 85%.

Further reading and references

- ➢ Steinert R, Nestler G, Sagynaliev E, et al. (2006). Laparoscopic cholecystectomy and gallbladder cancer. Journal of Surgical Oncology 93: 682–689.
- ➢ The UK testicular cancer incidence statistic: Cancer research UK.

HEAD INJURY

Differential diagnosis

Type of head injury	Differential diagnosis
Skull fracture	Simple linear fracture
	Depressed skull fracture
	Base of skull fracture
	Scalp laceration
Intracranial haemorrhage	Extradural haemorrhage
	Subdural haemorrhage
	Subarachnoid haemorrhage
	Intracerebral haemorrhage
Others	Cerebral concussion
	Diffuse axonal injury
	Seizure

It is estimated that approximately one million of the population present to the hospital with a head injury each year. It is one of the leading causes of mortality (40%) and morbidity in the UK.

Anatomy

The anatomy of the head can be divided into the following categories:

Scalp:

- The scalp is made up of skin, connective tissue, aponeurosis, loose areolar tissue and pericranium (SCALP itself is an acronym). (See Figure 4.33)
- The scalp is a vascular structure, and therefore a scalp laceration can result in significant blood loss.

Skull:

- The cranial vault (calvaria) and the base are the two main structures that form the skull.
- At the temporal regions the calvaria is found to be thin and as a result this area is protected by the temporalis muscle.
- The base of the skull has an irregular surface and therefore contributes to brain injury when there is movement of the brain during a head injury.
- The anterior, middle, and posterior cranial fossa make up the floor of the cranial cavity.

- In general the anterior fossa contains the frontal lobes, the middle fossa contains the temporal lobes, and the posterior fossa contains the brain stem, occipital lobe and the cerebellum.

Meninges:

- The meninges are a layer of coverings over the brain and spinal cord. It is composed of the dura mater, arachnoid mater, and pia mater. (See Figure 4.33)
- The dura mater is a membrane attached firmly to the internal surface of the skull.
- Meningeal arteries, found between the dura and the internal surface of the skull, are often injured in skull fractures. The middle meningeal artery in the temporal region can in particular be damaged in a head injury.
- The dura is composed of two layers namely the periosteal dura and the meningeal dura. It is between these layers that large venous sinuses are found. These sinuses are responsible for most of the venous drainage of the brain.
- The arachnoid lies beneath the dura mater. The space between these two structures is called the subdural space, which is a potential site for haemorrhage.
- The third layer is attached to the brain surface and is known as the pia mater.

Brain:

- The three main structures of the brain include the cerebrum, the brainstem and cerebellum.
- The cerebrum consists of a right and left hemisphere. These hemispheres are divided by a structure known as the falx cerebri.
- The brainstem consists of the midbrain, pons, and medulla. The essential cardio-respiratory centres are found within the

medulla. The medulla extends caudally to form the spinal cord.
- The cerebellum is found in the posterior fossa and forms links with the spinal cord and brainstem.

Cerebrospinal fluid (CSF):

- The choroid plexus in the roof of the ventricles produces CSF.
- CSF moves through the brain via a number of ventricles. The pathway starts at the lateral ventricles moving through the foramen of Monro into the third ventricle. From there the CSF flows through the aqueduct of Sylvius, and finally the fourth ventricle. Following flow through the ventricles, CSF enters the subarachnoid space and is eventually reabsorbed into the venous circulation.

Types of brain injury

With any head injury there is always a concern of underlying brain injury. Brain injury can be divided into primary and secondary.

Primary brain injury:

This occurs at the time of the head injury and can be a result of direct or indirect injury to the brain. The strength and varying features of the applied forces determine the severity of damage.

Secondary brain injury:

This type of damage occurs at any point after the primary injury. The common causes include hypoxia, hypercapnia, intracranial bleeding, hypotension, and increased intracranial pressure. If these problems are managed early this can prevent and reduce secondary brain injury.

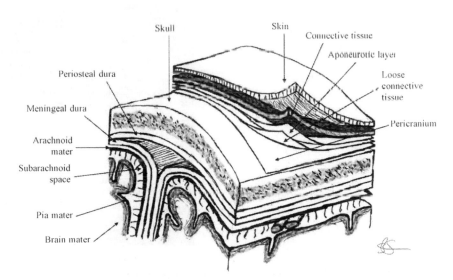

Figure 4.33: The scalp and meninges.

Physiological effects of head injury

The Monroe-Kelly doctrine:

The Monroe-Kelly doctrine assumes that the skull is a solid container in which the only contents are brain, CSF, and blood. It therefore follows that intracranial pressure (ICP) is proportional to the volume of these contents. The formula is as follows:

$$ICP = V_{CSF} + V_{Blood} + V_{Brain}$$

This formula is the basis of the Monroe-Kelly doctrine which states that the ICP will increase if the volume of any of the three components increases. This increase in ICP can only be compensated to a certain degree by changes in the volume of the other components. A space occupying lesion (SOL) of more than 100–150 ml exceeds the maximum compensation, resulting in a rise in the intracranial pressure.

A raised ICP has a number of consequences:

- Hydrocephalus: occurs when the circulation of CSF is occluded. Most commonly seen with posterior fossa lesions.
- Cerebral ischaemia: occurs due to a rise in ICP which eventually exceeds auto-regulation. The formula that describes the relationship between cerebral perfusion pressure, mean arterial pressure and ICP is as follows:

Cerebral perfusion pressure = mean arterial pressure − ICP

- Brain herniation: occurs when the ICP levels are high and therefore there is an increased risk of brain shift and resultant herniation. The herniation can occur through a number of sites. The commonly used term 'coning' actually refers to herniation of the mid brain through the tentorium.

Skull fracture

Simple linear fracture

- These appear as lucent lines on a skull X-ray (SXR).
- There is an increased risk of an intracranial bleed with skull fractures.
- Patients should therefore be admitted to hospital for neurological observations.

Depressed skull fracture

- This type of fracture is common following blunt trauma.
- This is where a segment of the skull can be pushed down onto the brain tissue, resulting in laceration of the brain.
- Management may consist of elevation of the depressed segment.
- Elevation is only performed is there are focal neurological signs on examination or if the segment is depressed more than the thickness of the skull.
- A course of IV antibiotics must be given if the wound has been contaminated.

Base of skull fracture

- This fracture is not identified on a SXR.
- If fluid is seen in the sphenoidal sinuses this fracture can be present.
- Other clinical signs include rhinorrhoea and otorrhoea (CSF leaking from the nose and ears).
- To test for the presence of blood in CSF, place a drop of the CSF onto filter paper; if blood is present, it remains in the centre and the CSF spreads out in a ring. This is known as the 'Halo' sign.
- Battle's sign (bruising around the mastoid process), haemotympanum, and Racoon eye sign (bruising around both eyes), may also be noted.
- This fracture is usually managed conservatively

Intracranial haemorrhage

Extradural haemorrhage

- This is a bleed between the skull and dura mater, i.e. in the extradural space. (See Figure 4.34)
- It usually arises as a result of damage to the middle meningeal artery following a temporal bone fracture.
- This injury is also associated with a parietal bone fracture.
- Patients initially have an episode of loss of consciousness, which is followed by a lucid interval.
- The haematoma continues to expand within the extradural space.
- The rise in ICP results in a second episode of reduced conscious levels.
- The pupil on the affected side initially constricts and then

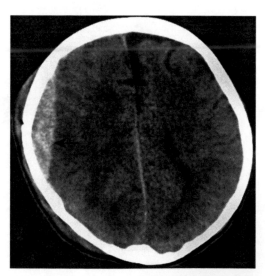

Figure 4.34: CT brain showing an area of increased density in the right parietal lobe (arrow), note the localised nature and internal convex border in keeping with an extradural haematoma.

later becomes fixed and dilated. A hemiparesis also develops on the same side.

- An urgent CT scan is performed and early neurosurgical intervention is required for possible surgical removal of the clot.

- If neurosurgical intervention is delayed the increase in ICP will eventually compress the brain and result in transtentorial herniation.

- There is a good prognosis with early treatment.

Subdural haemorrhage

- This is a result of a tear of the bridging veins between the dura and the cerebral cortex. (See Figure 4.35)

- Acute subdural haemorrhages are commonly seen following high velocity injuries.

- Chronic subdural haemorrhages can arise following trivial injuries. They are commonly seen in the elderly population, as a result of shrunken brains with veins that are under tension.

- A subdural haemorrhage presents similarly to that of an expansile cerebral mass and causes a decline in conscious levels.

- Treatment involves removal of the clot via a craniotomy.

- The prognosis with this type of bleed is poor as a result of extensive brain trauma.

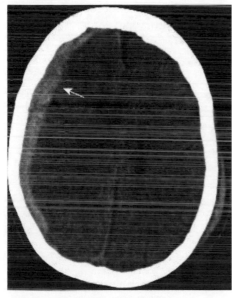

Figure 4.35: CT brain showing an area of increased density in the right parietal lobe (arrow), note the extension across the suture lines and concave internal border in keeping with a subdural haematoma.

Subarachnoid haemorrhage

- This type of bleed presents as a result of trauma or spontaneously following rupture of berry aneurysms and vascular malformations. (See Figure 4.36)

- Patients present with signs of meningism, i.e. headache, neck stiffness, nausea and vomiting.

- In 50–60% of cases, the patient dies immediately and one third suffer permanent disability due to hypoxic brain injury.

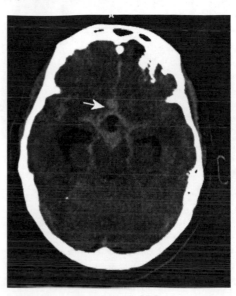

Figure 4.36: Non contrast enhanced CT brain showing increased density along the circle of Willis (arrow) in keeping with acute subarachnoid haemorrhage.

Intracerebral haemorrhage

- An expansile haematoma within the brain matter.

- These arise as a result of contusions joining to form a haematoma.

- Causes include hypertensive vascular disease (commonest), trauma and a bleeding tumour.

- These small haematomas are commonly seen in the frontal and temporal lobes.

- A CT scan will show lesions of increased density. (See Figure 4.37)

- Mass effect and a midline shift may also be seen, which may require evacuation of the haematoma.

Cerebral concussion

- If there is a temporary loss of neurological function following a head injury it can be defined as concussion.

- These signs are not permanent and will resolve, sometimes even before the patient arrives to hospital.

- The patient may complain of a headache, dizziness, and nausea.

- If the history is suspicious of loss of consciousness for greater than five minutes the patient should be admitted to hospital for observation.

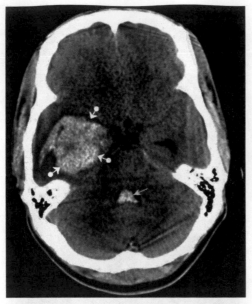

Figure 4.37: CT head showing a lesion with increased density in Right temporal lobe in keeping with intracerebral haematoma (round ended arrowd). Also note blood within the fourth ventricle (straight arrow).

Diffuse axonal injury

- This occurs following a deceleration injury, in which the axons are torn and disrupted.

- This is a severe injury often with patients presenting in a coma, lasting from days to weeks.

- Patients will also experience autonomic dysfunction and therefore experience raised temperatures, sweating, and hypertension.

- Macroscopically, punctuate haemorrhages can be seen.

- Microscopically within the white matter, axonal damage and clusters of microglia are seen.

- There is a high mortality rate with this type of head injury.

Clinical management of head injury

The Glasgow coma score (GCS) should be determined. Once the GCS has been calculated, the management pathway for patients is as stated in the NICE guidelines. (See Figure 4.38)

- In the accident and emergency department the patient should be assessed following the Advanced Trauma Live Support (ATLS) guidelines.

- Assess airway, breathing, circulation, disability and expose the patient (ABCDE).

Assessment in emergency department

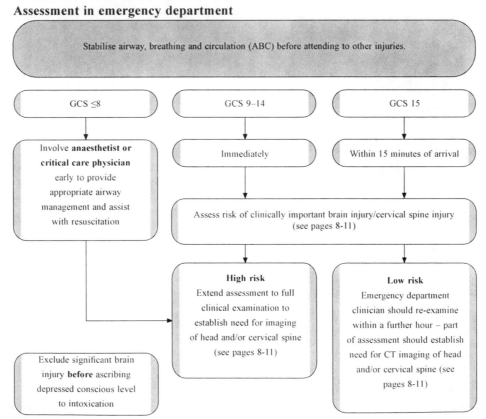

Figure 4.38: NICE guidelines showing the management pathway for patients with head injury. National Institute for Health and Clinical Excellence (2006) CG56 Head injury: triage, assessment, investigation and early management of head injury in infants, children and adults. London: NICE. Available from www.nice.org.uk/CG56. Reproduced with permission.

- GCS: is a quick and reliable method of initially determining the conscious state of a patient. (See Table 4.41)
  - GCS of 13–15 is a mild head injury
  - GCS of 9–12 is a moderate head injury
  - GCS of 3–8 is a severe head injury
  - GCS < 8 is a coma state
- Full neurological examination must be performed

Investigations

Imaging:

- Cervical spine X-rays: if the mechanism of injury involved a significant force these X-rays are important in identifying any other injuries. NICE guidelines for determining if patients require imaging of the cervical spine is shown in Figure 4.39
- CT: if the patient has a decreased level of consciousness or the neurological examination is abnormal, an urgent CT scan is required to exclude an intracranial bleed. NICE have clear guidelines on determining the need for a CT scan of patients with head trauma. (See Figure 4.40)
- SXR: are rarely performed.

	Response	Points
Eyes	Spontaneously	4
	Verbal command	3
	Pain	2
	No response	1
Verbal	Orientated	5
	Confused	4
	Inappropriate words	3
	Incomprehensible	2
	No response	1
Motor	Obeys commands	6
	Localises to pain	5
	Withdraws from pain	4
	Abnormal flexion	3
	Abnormal extension	2
	No response	1

Table 4.41: Calculating the GCS

Selection of adults and children (age 10+) for imaging of the cervical spine

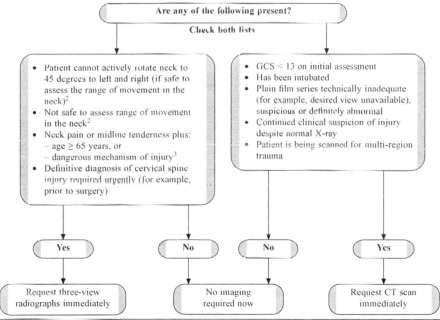

Figure 4.39: NICE guidelines for determining imaging of the cervical spine. National Institute for Health and Clinical Excellence (2006) CG56 Head injury: triage, assessment, investigation and early management of head injury in infants, children and adults. London: NICE. Available from www.nice.org.uk/CG56. Reproduced with permission.

Investigation for clinically important brain injury

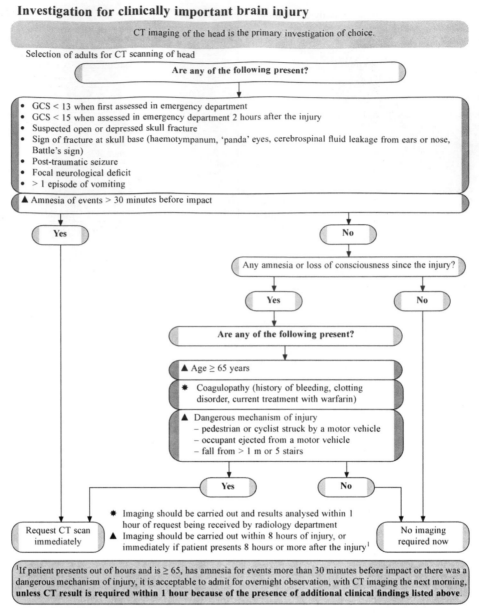

CT imaging of the head is the primary investigation of choice.

Selection of adults for CT scanning of head

Are any of the following present?

- GCS < 13 when first assessed in emergency department
- GCS < 15 when assessed in emergency department 2 hours after the injury
- Suspected open or depressed skull fracture
- Sign of fracture at skull base (haemotympanum, 'panda' eyes, cerebrospinal fluid leakage from ears or nose, Battle's sign)
- Post-traumatic seizure
- Focal neurological deficit
- > 1 episode of vomiting

▲ Amnesia of events > 30 minutes before impact

Yes | No

Any amnesia or loss of consciousness since the injury?

Yes | No

Are any of the following present?

▲ Age ≥ 65 years

✷ Coagulopathy (history of bleeding, clotting disorder, current treatment with warfarin)

▲ Dangerous mechanism of injury
– pedestrian or cyclist struck by a motor vehicle
– occupant ejected from a motor vehicle
– fall from > 1 m or 5 stairs

Yes | No

Request CT scan immediately

✷ Imaging should be carried out and results analysed within 1 hour of request being received by radiology department
▲ Imaging should be carried out within 8 hours of injury, or immediately if patient presents 8 hours or more after the injury[1]

No imaging required now

[1]If patient presents out of hours and is ≥ 65, has amnesia for events more than 30 minutes before impact or there was a dangerous mechanism of injury, it is acceptable to admit for overnight observation, with CT imaging the next morning, **unless CT result is required within 1 hour because of the presence of additional clinical findings listed above**.

Figure 4.40: NICE guidelines for determining the need for a CT scan of the head. National Institute for Health and Clinical Excellence (2006) CG56 Head injury: triage, assessment, investigation and early management of head injury in infants, children and adults. London: NICE. Available from www.nice.org.uk/CG56. Reproduced with permission.

Management

➤ A basic neurological examination is important to continually assess the patient.

➤ If the patient meets the criteria for a CT scan, it should be performed and the results discussed with the medical and neurosurgical teams. (See Figures 4.41 and 4.42)

➤ Patients, whom on clinical reassessment are fit to be discharged should be sent home with head injury advice and be accompanied by a reliable adult.

➤ The patient should be admitted to hospital if the following are present:

   o CT evidence of intracranial pathology

o Skull fracture

o Reduced conscious levels

o Neurological signs and symptoms

o Social circumstances, e.g. the patient lives alone

➤ Non-opiate analgesia is given to the patient in order to perform accurate regular neurological observations.

When to involve the neurosurgeon

- Discuss the care of all patients with new, surgically significant abnormalities on imaging with a neurosurgeon (definition of 'surgically significant' to be developed by local neurosurgical unit and agreed with referring hospitals).
- Regardless of imaging, other reasons for discussing a patient's care plan with a neurosurgeon include:
  - persisting coma (GCS ≤ 8) after initial resuscitation
  - unexplained confusion for more than 4 hours
  - deterioration in GCS after admission (pay greater attention to motor response deterioration)
  - progressive focal neurological signs
  - seizure without full recovery
  - definite or suspected penetrating injury
  - cerebrospinal fluid teak:

Figure 4.41: NICE guidelines on when to involve the neurosurgeon. National Institute for Health and Clinical Excellence (2006) CG56 Head injury: triage, assessment, investigation and early management of head injury in infants, children and adults. London: NICE. Available from www.nice.org.uk/CG56. Reproduced with permission.

Transfer from secondary setting to neuroscience unit

Follow local guidelines on patient transfer and transfer of responsibility for patient care – these should be drawn up by the referring hospital trusts, neuroscience unit and local ambulance service. They should recognise that transfer would benefit all patients with serious head injuries (GCS ≤ 8), irrespective of the need for neurosurgery, but if transfer of those who do not require neurosurgery is not possible, ongoing liaison with the neuroscience unit over clinical management is essential.

Figure 4.42: NICE guidelines on when to transfer patients to a neuroscience unit. National Institute for Health and Clinical Excellence (2006) CG56 Head injury: triage, assessment, investigation and early management of head injury in infants, children and adults. London: NICE. Available from www.nice.org.uk/CG56. Reproduced with permission.

Further reading and references

➤ Bulstrode CJK, Russell RCG, Williams NS (2000) Bailey & Love's Short Practice of Surgery (23 Ed.). Arnold.

➤ Calne R, Ellis H, Whatson C (2002). Lecture Notes on General Surgery. (10 Ed.) Blackwell Publishing.

➤ Goldberg A, Stansby G (2006). Surgical Talk: Revision in Surgery (2 Ed.). Imperial college press

➤ National Institute for Health and Clinical Excellence (2007). Head injury (CG56).

4. Surgery

INTRODUCTION

The information and algorithms in this chapter are correct at time of writing, but please note that the Resuscitation Council (UK) publishes new guidance in October 2010, when there may be some changes.

As a Foundation Year (FY) Doctor you will, at times, be reviewing critically unwell patients. You may be the first doctor to see the patient especially during ward cover shifts or on-call in the Emergency Department. At these times you will need to make a rapid assessment of the patient, formulate a problem list and initiate treatment, perhaps before senior support is able to reach you.

This can appear very daunting at first, but there are many training opportunities available to help in these situations. These include 'simulation training,' the ALERT Course and courses offered by the Resuscitation Council (UK). Many Foundation Schools sponsor FY1 doctors through an Immediate Life Support (ILS) course and FY2 doctors are expected to complete an Advanced Life Support (ALS) Provider course by the end of their year.

These courses teach a common approach to the assessment of the severely unwell patient. This is the 'A to E approach.' By using this, a comprehensive initial assessment can be made, initial interventions and potentially life-saving initial treatments can be put in place and then the patient can be reassessed using the same framework to check on progress.

THE A TO E APPROACH

Airway

Listening to noises made by the patient can give an indication of airway patency:

Talking normally:	Patent airway
Snoring, gurgling, stridor:	Partially occluded airway

Complete obstruction may be accompanied by a paradoxical movement of the chest and abdomen in a 'see-saw' pattern. If the airway is occluded then death will inevitably ensue within a few minutes. It is therefore critical that even non-anaesthetic doctors can assess and open the airway.

If airway obstruction is suspected, open the mouth and look for obstructions. Fluid matter can be suctioned using a Yankauer sucker under direct vision. Objects can be removed with forceps if safe to do so but close-fitting dentures should be left in situ. The airway can be maintained by using the simple manoeuvres of head-tilt/chin lift and jaw thrust. Adjuncts can be used to help keep it patent – the oropharyngeal and nasopharyngeal airways.

Breathing

Tachypnoea can be one of the first signs of illness, and is one of the most frequently missed vital signs from the observation chart! Looking at the pattern of breathing will show respiratory rate, symmetry, use of accessory muscles and cyanosis. The position of the trachea should be felt. Auscultation, percussion and assessment of vocal fremitus should follow.

Continuous pulse oximetry should be applied, a chest X-ray should be seen and an arterial blood gas (ABG) taken. High flow oxygen should be applied in the emergency situation as per British Thoracic Society (BTS, 2008) guidelines.

In the case of asthma or COPD a peak expiratory flow rate (PEFR) should be obtained, and initial management commenced – nebulised salbutamol and ipratropium and IV/oral steroids. The assessment and treatment of acute severe asthma should be governed by the BTS guidelines.

Circulation

Take the pulse and blood pressure (BP) and assess the capillary refill time by pressing for 5 seconds over the sternum (normal <2 seconds). The pulse should be palpated peripherally (at the radial artery) and centrally (at the carotid or femoral arteries). Look for rate, volume and quality. A barely palpable peripheral pulse may be indicative of a low blood pressure. Feel the skin and determine if the patient is vasodilated or peripherally shut down. Look at the veins in the neck and see if they are collapsed or well filled. Obtain intravenous (IV) access, preferably using a wide bore cannula. Take bloods as indicated and commence IV fluids. Take a 12-lead ECG and apply cardiac monitoring if available.

Disability

An assessment using the AVPU score is quicker than the full Glasgow coma scale (GCS).

A	Alert
V	Responds to your voice
P	Responds to painful stimulus
U	Unresponsive

Check the pupil reactivity, examine limb movements and power and take capillary blood glucose (CBG).

Exposure

Fully expose the patient whilst being mindful of dignity and warmth. Inspect fully, in particular checking for signs of haemorrhage, oedema, rash or any other injury. Take the temperature.

At the end of the assessment the same framework can be used to re-assess at a later point, particularly if treatments have been instigated, as well as to document the findings.

The FY doctor should expect to receive a high level of support when dealing with critically unwell patients. It is important to know who to ask for help, and if in doubt always ask for help early. More senior doctors are an obvious choice and in particular the on-call medical Registrar. However, care for the critically unwell is a multidisciplinary skill. Many hospitals have outreach teams, which may consist of ICU staff, specialist outreach nurses or resuscitation officers. They can often be contacted using 'triggers' such as Early Warning Scores (commonly the Modified Early Warning Score MEWS).

Cardiac arrest

Cardiac arrests can and do happen anywhere within a hospital. No matter what the situation, the Resuscitation Council (UK) guidelines should be followed. These guarantee a standardised approach to treating a cardiac arrest and are taught on the ILS and ALS courses. It is important for you to be up-to-date with the current guidelines.

The FY doctor would be expected to identify and confirm cardiac arrest, call for help and ensure the cardiac arrest team is called by dialling 2222 in hospitals and initiate resuscitation in the absence of a more senior experienced member of clinical staff. The chain of survival is important to know. (See Figure 5.1).

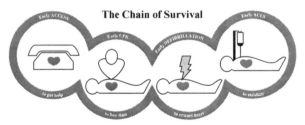

The Chain of Survival

Figure 5.1: Chain of Survival highlighting the four important factors in reducing mortality during a cardiac arrest. *Courtesy of Laerdal Medical Ltd. Reproduced with permission.*

The FY doctor can have a big impact in this chain, certainly in the first two links, but also by ensuring rapid connection of the defibrillator and even giving early defibrillation (if competent to do so) even before the arrival of the cardiac arrest team.

The Resuscitation Team

Cardiac arrests require a team to work together to provide the patient with the best possible chances of survival. The team should comprise a variety of people with a number of specific skills including advanced airway management, defibrillation, chest compressions and drug administration. In addition it is usual to have a scribe who should also monitor timings and if required to explain to any observers such as family or students what is happening.

The team should be clearly led by a team leader, who is often the medical Registrar but may be the Emergency Department Consultant/Registrar or Resuscitation Officer. Typically the FY

doctor will be a team member and will directed by the team leader to perform tasks such as inserting cannulae, taking bloods and blood gases and performing chest compressions. Hence the FY doctor should ensure their basic life support training is up-to-date. Evidence shows that good quality chest compressions are important to maintain coronary perfusion pressure and maximise the chances of survival. Therefore one should ensure that they are being performed correctly – a rate of 100 per minute and at a depth of 4–5 cm. Care should be taken to minimise interruptions in chest compressions.

The Universal Algorithm

The Universal Algorithm (see Figure 5.2) is the standard approach to a cardiac arrest and the one taught on Resuscitation Council (UK) courses. This is the standard approach used in the event of all cardiac arrests and so all junior doctors should be familiar with it.

The initial action to be taken is to open the airway and confirm cardiac arrest, by *looking*, *listening* and *feeling* for respiratory effort and pulse for not more than 10 seconds. On confirmation of cardiac arrest, basic life support should begin whilst the cardiac arrest team is called. A defibrillator should be obtained as soon as possible.

Once the patient is connected to the defibrillator the rhythm must be analysed to ensure that the correct pathway of the algorithm is followed. The rhythm can be analysed by an automated external defibrillator or manually by a person competent to do so. There are only four possible rhythms associated with cardiac arrest and as an FY doctor you would be expected to be able to identify these rhythms and initiate the appropriate treatment.

Shockable rhythms:

Shockable rhythms (those that require defibrillation) are:

* **Ventricular fibrillation** - identified by the absence of pulse and the presence of chaotic electrical activity on the monitor.
* **Pulseless ventricular tachycardia** - identified by organised broad complex (QRS greater than 3 small squares or 0.12 seconds) tachycardia and the absence of a pulse.

Once these rhythms are identified the patient should be defibrillated followed by immediate chest compressions as specified in Figure 5.2. The following drugs should also be administered.

Adrenaline 1mg 1:10,000 should be given before the third shock and then every other cycle.

Amiodarone 300mg should be given before the fourth shock.

Non-shockable rhythms:

Non-shockable rhythms consist of:

* **Asystole:** identified by the absence of pulse and no discernable electrical activity on the monitor.
* **Pulseless electrical activity (PEA):** identified by the absence of a pulse with any other rhythm.

The treatment on this side of the algorithm is effective chest compressions and the administration of the following drugs:

> Adrenaline 1mg 1:10,000 every other cycle of chest compressions
>
> Add atropine 3mg ONCE ONLY for asystole and PEA with a heart rate less than 60

As an FY doctor it is your responsibility to ensure that you are familiar with the defibrillators that are used in the clinical areas that you work. Different makes of defibrillator use different energy levels and it is not uncommon to have more than one type of defibrillator in use within the hospital. All Resuscitation Officers offer induction training to new staff and you should ensure that you attend to familiarise yourself with the equipment and energy levels used.

Adult Advanced Life Support Algorithm

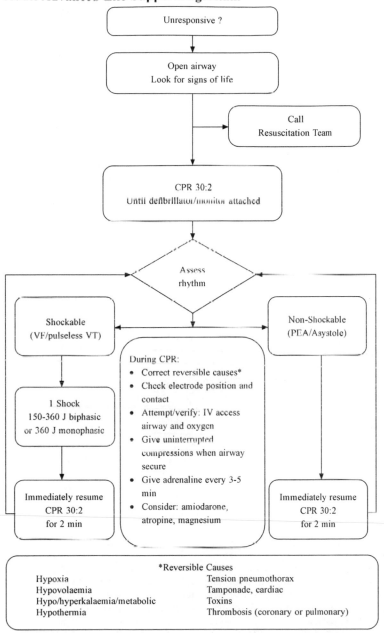

Figure 5.2: The Adult Advanced Life Support Algorithm. *Courtesy of the Resuscitation Council UK. Reproduced with permission.*

5. Resuscitation

Reversible causes (4H's and 4T's)

Whilst resuscitation is underway the team should be considering interventions that may treat a possible cause of the cardiac arrest – the reversible causes. There are eight recognised reversible causes; the four H's and four T's. The most obvious cause should be treated first, for example hypovolaemia for the patient with a gastro-intestinal bleed. The history of the presenting complaint, past medical history, observation charts and physical assessment of the patient may provide the resuscitation team with information about which of the reversible causes is the most relevant. However all of the reversible causes should be considered to avoid missing an intervention. It should be noted that more than one reversible cause might be present in the same patient.

Hypoxia:

Hypoxia should be considered in all patients experiencing cardiac arrest and as soon as practical the patient should have a definitive airway inserted (laryngeal mask, oropharangeal airway or endotracheal intubation depending on the skills available.) Until such time as advanced help arrives 15 litres of oxygen should be administered using a bag valve mask. One should actively bag valve mask at a rate of two breaths every cycle of 30 chest compressions, and involve two people – one to ensure the mask makes a good seal on the face and one to squeeze the bag. It is worth taking an arterial blood gas (ABG) but it should be remembered that patients in cardiac arrest will be hypoxic due to lack of spontaneous respiration unless adequate artificial ventilation is provided.

Hypovolaemia:

Hypovolaemia should be considered in patients where there is a suspicion of fluid loss. Note that a patient in cardiac arrest will not have a blood pressure so other means will need to be used in order to establish whether the patient may be hypovolaemic. The patient should be examined for signs of active bleeding and previous vital signs and fluid balance charts should be checked. Intravenous access should be obtained with a large bore cannula in both antecubital fossae and a rapid infusion of fluids given.

Hyper/hypokalaemia:

Hyper/hypokalaemia and other metabolic disorders should be considered in patients with relevant past medical history. Recent blood results should be reviewed and a sample should be sent for rapid analysis. Many ABGs provide results of important electrolytes. Any identified electrolyte disturbance should be corrected. Hypokalaemia should be treated by the administration of intravenous potassium at a maximum rate of 2 mmol/min for 10 minutes followed by 10 mmol over 5–10 minutes. Hyperkalaemia involves a three-stage treatment approach during cardiac arrest, the first of which is to protect the myocardium by giving 10ml of 10% calcium chloride. This is followed by shifting the potassium out of the circulatory system into the cells using a rapid dextrose/insulin infusion (usually 10 units of actrapid with 50 mls of 50% dextrose). The final step is to remove the potassium from the body and in cardiac arrest this can be achieved by haemodialysis, but this is unlikely to be available unless the patient is in an intensive

care setting. Should the patient have a severe acidosis or renal failure, then 50 mmol of sodium bicarbonate can be given by rapid infusion.

Hypothermia:

Hypothermia should be particularly considered in patients who have sustained out-of-hospital cardiac arrests. In theory patients should not become hypothermic whilst in hospital. A core temperature should be taken. Patients can be warmed during cardiac arrest by the administration of warmed fluids intravenously, warmed oxygen and lavage of the major body cavities with warmed fluids.

Tension pneumothorax:

Tension pneumothorax should be considered in patients who have sustained trauma or who have respiratory conditions such as asthma and COPD. Identification of a tension pneumothorax is through clinical examination. Signs are hyper-resonance on percussion and reduced air entry on the affected side; a much later sign is tracheal deviation away from the pneumothorax. Treatment is through needle decompression using a wide bore cannula on the affected side in the second intercostal space in the mid clavicular line. Should resuscitation be successful, a chest drain should be inserted.

Toxic:

Toxic causes should be considered for patients that are in hospital in receipt of medications as well as for out-of-hospital arrests, particularly those in which the collapse was un-witnessed. Ambulance crews who attended the scene should examine the patient for signs of drug use such as track marks and for any packages or articles that may provide clues as to the drugs that may have been involved. For inpatients the patient's hospital drug charts should be reviewed. If it is possible that a toxin may have led to the cardiac arrest then any appropriate antidote should be given.

Tamponade:

Tamponade should only be considered where there is reasonable suspicion that fluid (such as blood) has accumulated in the pericardial space either through cardiothoracic surgery, trauma to the chest or more rarely post myocardial infarction. There is no way of diagnosing tamponade in cardiac arrest unless you have immediate access to a portable ultrasound machine. Treatment is pericardiocentisis; a pericardiocentesis needle should be inserted to the left of the xiphisternum at an angle of 45 degrees pointed towards the left scapula. This should be done by seniors only!

Thromboembolic:

Thromboembolism should be considered in all patients with relevant history, such as ischaemic heart disease, previous stroke, recent prolonged period of immobility, previous thromboembolism or hypercoagulability. Occasionally during a cardiac arrest it is possible to see a demarcation line across the chest with profound cyanosis above the line suggesting the patient has had a massive Pulmonary Embolus. There may be evidence to suggest a thromboembolic cause in the events preceding the cardiac arrest - for example chest pain. The treatment for thromboembolic causes of cardiac arrest is thrombolysis. If thrombolysis is given during cardiac arrest the arrest must be continued for sufficient time to allow the thrombolysis to work. This may mean continuing the resuscitation for a period of up to 90 minutes.

Post-resuscitation care

Resuscitation does not stop on return of spontaneous circulation (ROSC). At the point of ROSC the patient is likely to be very unstable and requires a full examination and stabilisation of their condition. It is important to use the systematic A to E approach to assess the patient and guide ongoing treatment. Almost all patients require intensive support following cardiac arrest with many requiring ventilation and inotrope support and some may require definitive treatment such as surgery. To achieve this invasive monitoring needs inserting in the form of a central venous catheter, an arterial line and urinary catheter. Full and regular observations should be recorded and bloods sent including FBC, U&Es, LFTs and serial ABGs. An ECG and Chest X-ray should be performed. Prior to transfer, patients should be stabilised and lines secured.

Therapeutic induced hypothermia should be considered for patients that have sustained out of hospital VF cardiac arrests. Therapeutic induced hypothermia has been demonstrated to have a neuroprotective effect and improve outcomes. The patient's core temperature is reduced to 32–34°C for 24 hours post arrest. There are a number of methods that can be utilised to achieve this from cooling jackets and helmets to the use of cooled fluids – the exact method will depend on the local Intensive Care Unit policy.

Documentation and audit

During a resuscitation attempt it is important to ensure that there is a member of the team keeping a written record of what has occurred. Resuscitation attempts may be prolonged and it may not be possible to recall exactly what occurred afterwards. Remember that many patients undergoing resuscitation will need to be referred to the Coroner's Officer and be the subject of a post mortem examination. Therefore it is useful for the Coroner to be able to identify easily drugs and procedures that the patient had during the arrest. Most hospitals will have an audit form on which a record of the resuscitation is made. These forms can be used during the resuscitation to create a written record and used after to assist documentation in the multidisciplinary notes. After completion the audit forms are usually sent to the Resuscitation Officer. They allow identification of good practice and can highlight issues within local services as well as being used nationally and internationally for research and comparisons into the outcomes of cardiac arrest.

Decision to stop resuscitation

The majority of resuscitation attempts are unsuccessful and a decision to stop will have to be made. The decision to stop should be a team decision and all members of the team have a right to have their say. As an FY doctor you will have an opportunity to express an opinion. When the team is in agreement for the attempt to be stopped, resuscitation is terminated and the time recorded. If the team is not in agreement the team leader should lead a discussion to explore the underlying reasons and to reach an agreement. During this discussion resuscitation should continue.

Relatives witnessing resuscitation

Relatives observing resuscitation remains a contentious issue for many healthcare professionals. It is common practice for parents to be present during the resuscitation of their child yet frequently relatives of adult patients are excluded from the resuscitation. Relatives may have been present when their loved one collapsed, are likely to be the first person to have attempted to resuscitate the patient and to have witnessed pre-hospital resuscitation attempts. The public are generally aware of what happens during hospital resuscitation attempts due to both hospital dramas and reality television programmes that follow hospital and emergency service staff. A large body of evidence has demonstrated that relatives who witness the resuscitation of their loved ones find it easier to accept the outcome and generally have fewer concerns regarding alternative treatment that could have been attempted to save their relative.

People who have witnessed the resuscitation of their relatives report that they could see how hard the Resuscitation Team had tried to revive their relative. It is important that relatives that are witnessing resuscitation attempts should be supported by a member of staff who is able to explain to them exactly what is happening. This person should be experienced in resuscitation. It is important that certain ground rules are established early in the resuscitation process. The relative should agree that they stand back and allow the team to work on the patient and that if the team request the relative should leave the room. At anytime should the relative wish to leave they must be accompanied by a staff member. Many find the presence of a relative a stressful experience for a variety of reasons. Resuscitations can be very stressful for the team and members may feel their skills are under scrutiny particularly if they are not very experienced. For this reason all members of the team should be happy with the relative being present. It is an issue that is worth considering during your Foundation Years and exploring with Senior Members of staff as well as the hospital's Resuscitation Officers.

Breaking bad news

Cardiac arrests often end in a patient's death and this news must be broken to the next of kin and family members in a compassionate manner. The best person to break bad news is someone who had some prior interaction with the next of kin. This may not always be possible and in that case someone who knows exactly what happened, often the team leader, should break the news. The FY doctor should not routinely be expected to inform the next of kin that their relative has died. However, you may be presented with the situation in which you may wish to observe a colleague breaking the news or wish to break the news yourself because you knew the patient and their family well.

Whenever bad news is being broken there are specific principles that should be followed to ensure that the message is communicated sensitively and effectively. The setting must be appropriate. Ensure privacy, provide comfortable seating, make sure that the room is well lit and have access to a telephone and tissues. It is important that whoever is breaking the news ensures that they are not going to be disturbed; this may mean handing a bleep to another member of staff and ensuring that mobile phones are switched to silent. No one should break bad news alone; reactions to upsetting news can range from stunned silence, through to uncontrollable crying, through to violent and aggressive outbursts. Consequently, you should ensure that you are able to exit the room easily should you need to. The language used should be clear and unambiguous. Phrases such as 'gone to a better place' and 'gone to rest' should be avoided and words such as 'died' and 'dead' should be used as early as possible. It is important to explain what will happen next and wherever possible provide the information in a written format including relevant contact details such as the hospital bereavement office, local support networks and the Coroner's Office. Many hospitals have this information pre-printed in a booklet. Finally, it is important to allow the family and next of kin to ask any questions and give them the opportunity to view their deceased relative if they so wish.

Aftermath

Cardiac arrests and resuscitation attempts are stressful for all those involved. Other patients may ask you questions about what happened and it is important that you are honest with them without breaching patient confidentiality. Student nurses and medical students may not have witnessed a resuscitation attempt before and it is important that they have an opportunity to ask questions and discuss how they are feeling. Treating a patient in cardiac arrest or being with a patient as they arrest can be very traumatic. This is especially the case for allied health care professions such as therapy or administration staff who are not generally exposed to critically unwell patient. You can never predict how a resuscitation may affect you and it may depend on the circumstances of the arrest and your own personal circumstances. Debriefs with the team can be useful, allowing a review of what happened and understanding areas that could be improved upon. These can either be informal, shortly after the event or more formal at a later stage. Hospital chaplains are good resources when there has been a traumatic resuscitation and many hospitals provide counselling services through the Occupational Health department.

Decisions not to attempt resuscitation

There are some patients who are not suitable for resuscitation as attempts would be futile. This decision ultimately lies with the Consultant responsible for the patient's care. A decision not to attempt resuscitation (DNAR) should be discussed with the patient (where possible), their next of kin, members of the medical team and the nursing staff. The discussion and subsequent decision should be clearly documented in the medical notes and communicated to all parties following Resuscitation Council Guidelines issued in 2009. Hospitals will have local policies regarding DNAR forms and FY doctors should be familiar with them.

A DNAR decision does not mean that the patient should not be actively treated if their condition deteriorates. It only stipulates that in the event of cardio-respiratory arrest no treatment should be instigated.

Advance directives and Capacity

There are some patients who are very clear about the treatment that they do or do not wish to receive, should their condition deteriorate. A competent person may not wish to be resuscitated, and this is a reason for completing a DNAR form. Alternatively, under the Mental Capacity Act (2005), a nominated person with lasting power of attorney can make medical decisions on behalf of those now lacking capacity to decide on resuscitation.

Legally binding advance directives are becoming more common and generally these are used by patients in the terminal stages of a disease process. A valid legally binding advance directive has to be made whilst a person is deemed to have capacity to give consent.

As an FY doctor you would not be expected to make a decision about whether a patient has capacity, nor to judge whether an advance directive is valid. However you would be expected to alert others to the existence of a directive, or to issues relating to capacity.

Further reading and references

➢ A Joint Statement from the British Medical Association, the Resuscitation Council (UK), and the Royal College of Nursing (2007). *Decisions relating to Cardiopulmonary Resuscitation.*

➢ Adams S, Whitlock M, Bloomfield P, et al., *Should relatives watch resuscitation?* BMJ 1994, **308**: 1687-9

➢ Awoonor-Renner S (1991). I desperately need to see my son. *BMJ* 302: 351.

➢ British Thoracic Society (2008). *Guideline for emergency use of oxygen in adult patients.*

➢ British Thoracic Society and Scottish Intercollegiate Guidelines Network (2008). *British Guideline on the management of asthma.*

➢ Hanson C, Strawser D (1992). Family presence during cardio-pulmonary resuscitation: Foote Hospital ED nine year perspective. *Journal of Emergency Nursing* 18:104-106.

➢ Martin J (1991). Rethinking traditional thoughts. *Journal of Emergency Nursing* 17: 67–8.

➢ Resuscitation Council (UK) (2008). *Advanced Life Support* (5 Ed.).

➢ Resuscitation Council (UK) (2006). *Should Relatives Witness Resuscitation?*

➢ Royal College of Nurses (2002). *Witnessing Resuscitation. Guidance for nurses.*

INTRODUCTION

The radiology department occupies a pivotal role in every medical institution. The majority of patients attending the outpatient or inpatient services of a hospital utilise the facilities of the radiology department. Radiologists not only aid with a diagnosis but also offer valuable therapeutic services. For these simple reasons, it is paramount that you foster a congenial relationship with the radiology department.

DIFFERENT IMAGING TECHNIQUES

A radiologist has different imaging techniques in his/her armoury to answer a relevant clinical question. The selection of the appropriate technique is guided by multiple factors, some of which are:

- The clinical question
- Age of the patient
- Patient mobility
- Amount of radiation exposure
- Availability of facilities

In the UK, clinical radiation exposure of patients is guided by the basic principle of keeping all radiation exposures 'As Low As Reasonably Practical' (ALARP).

Plain film (X-ray/radiographs)

Plain films tend to be the first line investigation of many common clinical presentations. Radiographs are performed relatively quickly and are available 24 hours in a day and can even be done by the bedside of the patient in emergencies. These are useful in imaging patients presenting with cardiothoracic, musculoskeletal and gastrointestinal problems.

Fluoroscopy

Fluoroscopy is based on the same principles of radiographs and allows continuous, i.e. live, monitoring of the area of interest. Common procedures utilising fluoroscopy include:

- Contrast examinations such as barium swallow/enema, intravenous pyelogram (IVP), etc. (See Figure 6.1).
- Interventional procedures such as angiography, hepato-biliary or colonic stenting, etc.

Some of the contrast examinations are either being complemented or supplemented by other imaging techniques for example IVP or urinary tract and barium enema being complemented by computed tomography (CT).

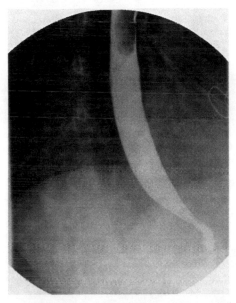

Figure 6.1: Static image from a barium swallow examination showing a normal distal oesophagus.

Ultrasound scans (USS)

Ultrasound is perhaps the safest and most widely available imaging modality. USS does not involve any ionising radiation so it can be used for imaging pregnant women, children and young adults. USS works on the same principal as sonar used by submarines, i.e. sound waves are reflected back by tissues to form an image. As a Foundation Year (FY) doctor, you would be expected to organise a multitude of ultrasound scans in your day-to-day practice. The current clinical utilities of USS include:

- Imaging abdominal viscera
- Imaging chest/thorax for pleural effusions.
- Visualising vascular abnormalities in deep vein thrombosis (DVT) and strokes.
- Imaging of soft tissues such as breasts
- Imaging of joints such as the shoulder, wrist, etc.

USS guided interventions are also available such as biopsies and drains. Recent British Thoracic Society (BTS) and National Institute for Health and Clinical Excellence (NICE) guidelines advocate the use of ultrasound imaging for inserting all central venous catheters and chest drains.

Computed tomography

Recent technological advances in CT have revolutionised the world of medical imaging. The current generation multi-detector

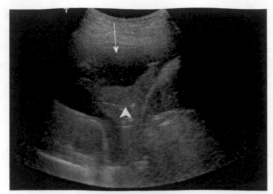

Figure 6.2: USS image of right chest showing a moderate sized effusion (arrow) and the underlying collapsed lung (arrowhead).

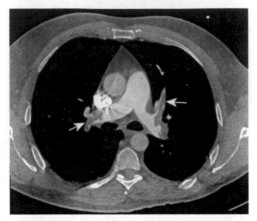

Figure 6.3: Computer tomography pulmonary angiogram (CTPA) showing filling defects (arrows) that can be seen as dark areas in the pulmonary arteries in keeping with pulmonary embolus.

computer tomography (MDCT) allows rapid acquisition of a significant amount of data in a single breath hold. MDCT imparts a relatively higher dose of radiation than plain films and fluoroscopy, hence extra care should be taken prior to requesting an MDCT examination. MDCT is commonly used for diagnosing pathologies of the chest, abdomen, pelvis and brain. (See Figure 6.3).

Magnetic resonance imaging (MRI)

MRI is another modality that has come on in leaps and bounds in the last decade due to technical advances. MRI is based on magnetic properties of the hydrogen nuclei found within the hydrogen atom. Given that the majority of the body consists of fluid, which is made of hydrogen atoms and nuclei, nearly every part of the body can be imaged with MRI. The relative advantages and disadvantages of MRI are shown in Table 6.1.

MRI is widely used for imaging brain, heart, liver and musculoskeletal pathologies. Although no further MRI knowledge would be expected of an FY doctor, it might be prudent to know that MRI has two basic imaging sequences, namely T1 and T2. In T2 sequence fluids (cerebrospinal fluid (CSF), effusion,

Advantages	Disadvantages
Lack of exposure to ionising radiation	Longer scan times
High quality detailed images	Expensive equipment
Ability to produce images in all 3 planes (axial, coronal and sagittal)	Significant contraindications including defibrillators/ some pacemakers, metallic neurosurgical clips

Table 6.1: The advantages and disadvantages of MRI.

ascites etc) appear bright and it appears dark on T1 sequence. T1 sequences are good at depicting the anatomy while T2 are good at highlighting areas of inflammation. (See Figure 6.4).

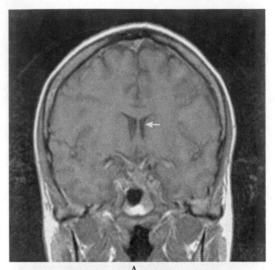

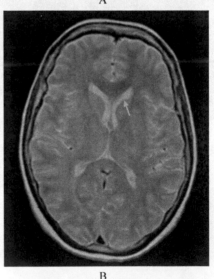

Figure 6.4: (A) MRI of the brain in coronal plane showing dark CSF (arrow) in keeping with T1-weighted image. (B) MRI of the brain in axial plane pointing at CSF (arrow) that is bright, in other words T2-weighted image.

Radionuclide imaging

Radionuclide imaging makes use of radioactive isotopes for the diagnosis of diseases. The radiation dose from isotope studies can vary depending on the isotope used and the part of the body imaged. Most common nuclear studies that you might come across are shown in the Table 6.2.

Radionuclide imaging technique	Indication
Ventilation Perfusion (V/Q)	Detecting pulmonary embolism for patients who cannot have CT
Bone Scan	Detect metastasis
Renal isotope study	Assess function and anatomy
Cardiac and oncology imaging (See Figure 6.6)	Analyse molecular and functional data

Table 6.2: Types of radionuclide imaging techniques and their indications.

Radiation dosage

All clinicians should aspire to keep radiation exposures as low as reasonably practical in accordance with 'ALARP'. This is

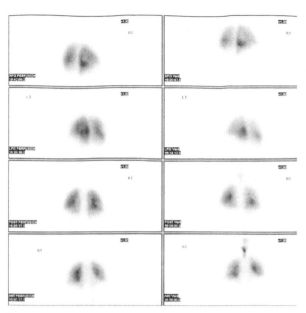

Figure 6.5: Normal V/Q scan of the chest. Images on the left depict the perfusion of lungs while the ones on the right depict ventilation.

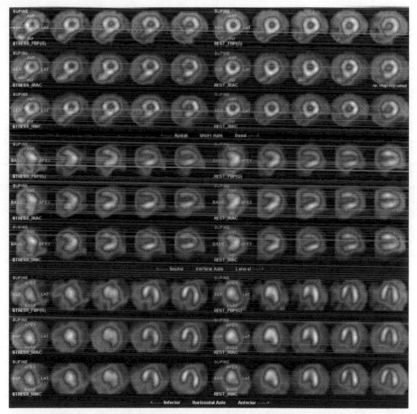

Figure 6.6: Image of a normal myocardial radionuclide perfusion study. The lighter areas denote the uptake of tracer material by viable myocardium implying adequate perfusion. Images can be reconstructed in different planes (short, vertical and horizontal axis) and are acquired at both rest and stress to demonstrate stress induced perfusion defect.

6. Radiology

important as excessive radiation exposure can cause serious physical and genetic damage. Table 6.3 outlines the commonly used imaging studies with their respective equivalent radiation dose compared to the natural background radiation. This information should help you in weighing the risk/benefit ratio of each test prior to requesting it.

Modality	Equivalent period of natural background radiation
X-ray/radiography	Days to months
Chest X-ray (CXR)	3 days
Abdominal X-ray (AXR)	4 months
Fluoroscopy/angiography	Months to years
Barium swallow	8 months
Barium enema	3.2 years
CT	Months to years
CT head	10 months
CT chest	3.6 years
CT abdomen or pelvis	4.5 years
Radionuclide imaging	Month to years
V/Q	7 months
Cardiac perfusion	2.7 years
Positron emission tomography (PET) of the head	2.3 years

Table 6.3: Different imaging techniques with respective equivalent background natural radiation. (RCR 2007) (Hart & Wall 2002).

HOW TO READ

Chest X-ray

This is perhaps the most common investigation that an FY doctor will be exposed to in their work. Without adequate attention to detail and training, a CXR can be a nemesis for the FY doctor. However, to avoid making unnecessary errors of interpretation, especially in the early days of your career, emphasis should be on 'things not to miss' rather than 'what is the diagnosis'. To successfully achieve this, a systematic approach is suggested for reviewing a CXR. (See Table 6.4).

	Reviewing CXRs:
1.	Confirm the identity of the patient
2.	The date of examination
3.	Identify which side is the right and left
4.	State if the film is anterio-posterior (AP) or postero-anterior (PA)
5.	Assess the position of lines and drains
6.	Study the lungs
7.	Study the mediastinum
8.	Review all other areas of soft tissue

Table 6.4: A systematic approach to reviewing a CXR.

AP or PA:

A CXR can be acquired by passing the X-ray beam from front to back (AP), from back to front (PA), or from side to side (lateral). Patients who are bedbound tend to have AP films while patients who are mobile have a PA films taken. An AP film will usually have an annotation (supine, AP), which should make it easier to decide. (See Figure 6.7).

Assessing the position of lines and drains:

Endotracheal (ET) tube tip should be about 2 inches above the carina, nasogastric (NG) tubes should be below the level of diaphragm, and Central venous catheter (subclavian or internal jugular) tip should be at the level of 2nd costo-chondral junction i.e. superior vena cava. (See Figures 6.7, 6.8 and 6.9).

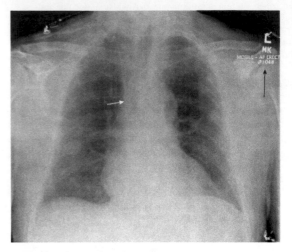

Figure 6.7: An AP CXR film (black arrow) with right internal jugular line (white arrow) tip at the level of the second costo-chondral junction.

The location of the chest drain will vary depending on the clinical indication for drainage. For example the tip of the drain should ideally be at the base for pleural effusions. It is important to ensure that the draining holes are within the thoracic cavity rather than subcutaneous tissue; the latter can lead to extensive surgical emphysema. (See Figure 6.10).

Lungs:

Spend time looking at each lung from the apex to the base. In a pneumothorax, you would see the pleural margin and there will be lack of vascular markings beyond this margin. Tension pneumothorax is a medical emergency whereby there is contralateral mediastinal shift due to increasing pressure, i.e. size of pneumothorax. (See Figure 6.9).

Pleural effusions will appear different depending on how the film was taken. On an erect CXR, the effusion gravitates to the lung bases and therefore it is seen as a white opacity with a meniscus. (See Figure 6.11). On the other hand, if the patient was in a supine position during the CXR, then the fluid gravitates to the posterior

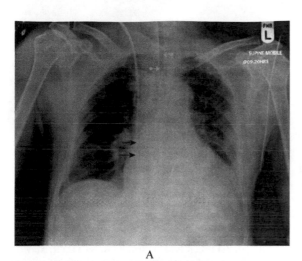

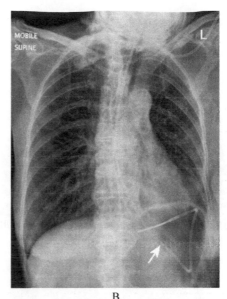

A   B

Figure 6.8: (A) Supine CXR with an Endo Tracheal tube (white arrow with ball) and a Swan Ganz catheter (black arrow) with its tip in the pulmonary artery. In the background you can also see a prosthetic valve and mediastinal drain. (B) CXR showing a NG tube coiled in the stomach below the diaphragm (white arrow).

5. Radiology

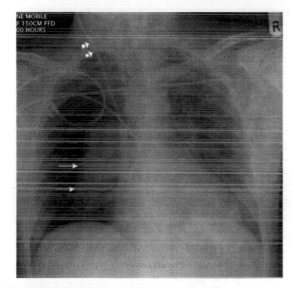

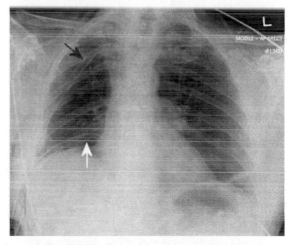

Figure 6.10: AP CXR of a patient with an apical (black arrow) and basal (white arrow) chest drain.

Figure 6.9: CXR showing the collapsed lung edge (white arrow) in a large right tension pneumothorax following an internal jugular line insertion (arrow with ball).

help of clinical history and the CXR as the latter tends to be more focal and well defined. (See Figure 6.13).

Lobar collapse is seen as increased opacity in a lung with loss of volume and ipsilateral shift of the mediastinum. The affected lobe can be localised by simple silhouette principles, for example: if the opacity obscures the right heart border then the involved lobe is the middle lobe of the right lung, whereas if the left heart border is obscured it is the lingula part of the left upper lobe that is involved. In a similar fashion if the diaphragm is obscured by the opacity then the affected lobe is the lower lobe. (See Figure 6.14).

lung and the lung would appear hazy and whiter compared to the other side with no obvious meniscus. (See Figure 6.12).

Consolidation on a CXR is essentially pulmonary opacification caused by replacement of air in the distal air spaces by fluid (transudate, exudate or blood) or tissue (carcinoma, lymphoma). In most cases, consolidation secondary to fluid replacement can be differentiated from that due to tissue replacement with the

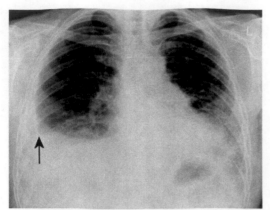

Figure 6.11: Moderate sized right pleural effusion with the meniscus sign (arrow) on an erect CXR.

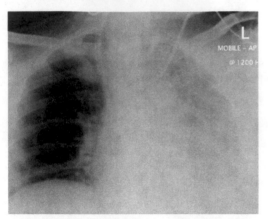

Figure 6.12: Mobile AP supine CXR, note the diffuse increased opacification of left lung compared to the right due to underlying pleural effusion.

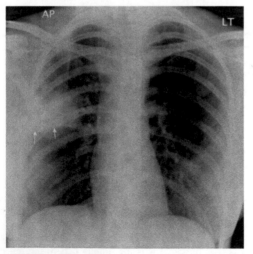

Figure 6.13: AP CXR with increased opacity in the right mid zone in keeping with consolidation. The horizontal fissure is clearly visible (arrows) confirming the involvement of the right upper lobe.

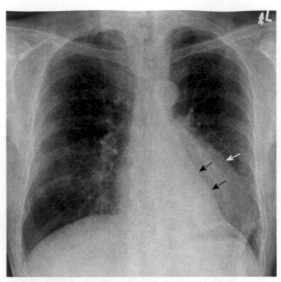

Figure 6.14: Left lower lobe collapse on a CXR. Note the obscured medial aspect of the left hemidiaphragm due to collapsed lung (black arrow), which is projected behind the heart (white arrow).

Mediastinum:

Ensure trachea is central and does not have any foreign bodies. The size of the heart will vary depending on the type of acquisition of the CXR, i.e. AP or PA. As a rule of thumb, the heart is enlarged when the maximum width of the cardiac shadow is more than 50% of the width of thorax on a PA film. (See Figure 6.15).

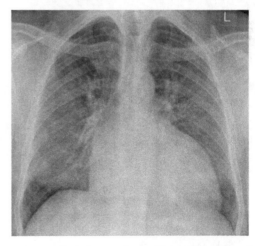

Figure 6.15: PA CXR in a patient with cardiomegaly where cardiac shadow is more than 50% of the thoracic width. This is secondary to dilated cardiomyopathy.

Pneumo-mediastinum is seen as streaks of air or free air along the mediastinal margins. This can be seen secondary to oesophageal rupture, abdominal viscera perforation and alveolar rupture in acute asthma. (See Figure 6.16).

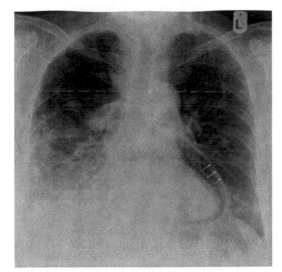

Figure 6.16: CXR following right pleura resection shows opacification in the right lower zone in keeping with recent surgery and extensive air outlining the pericardial surface (arrows) in keeping with pneumo-mediastinum.

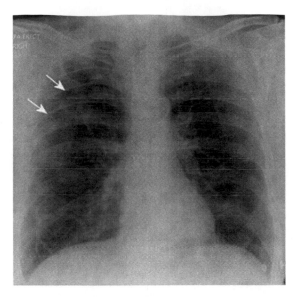

Figure 6.18: Erect CXR of a patient who presented at the chest out-patient department with cough. A small right apical pneumothorax (arrows) is seen but this can be easily missed if not reviewed thoroughly.

Review areas:

Review the area under the diaphragm. In particular, it is important to ensure that there is no free air under the diaphragm secondary to hollow viscera perforation. (See Figure 6.17).

Review behind the heart to make sure there is no mass behind the heart. Inparticular, look at the shoulder areas. (See Figure 6.19).

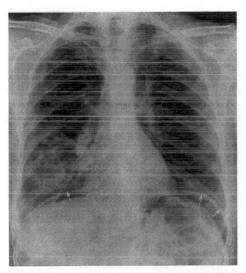

Figure 6.17: CXR of a 55-year-old man who presented with central chest pain. Note extensive free intra-peritoneal air under the diaphragm (arrows) in keeping with abdominal viscera perforation.

Review the lung apices as it is very easy to miss a small pneumothorax or a mass in this area due to overcrowding of ribs and clavicle. Extra attention should be paid to the apices to prevent errors. (See Figure 6.18).

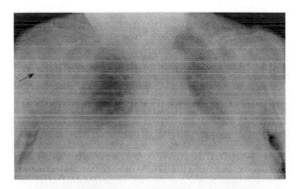

Figure 6.19: CXR of an elderly lady who came to the emergency department with chest pain. There is a fracture of the right neck of humerus (arrow) with significant displacement.

Abdominal X-ray

The most common indications for AXRs are suspected small bowel obstructions or suspected large bowel obstructions.

AXR is not the investigation of choice if a hollow viscera perforation is suspected. An erect CXR is more likely to pick up free air than an AXR. In a normal AXR, air is within the stomach, in two to three loops of small bowel and the distal large bowel (sigmoid and rectum). (See Figure 6.20).

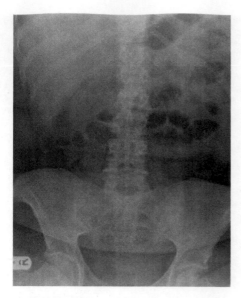

Figure 6.20: A normal AXR of a young female patient showing normal small and large bowel loops.

Small bowel obstruction:

Central distended loops of bowel with very little gas in the colon, especially rectum is suggestive of small bowel obstruction. The valvulae (intra-luminal markings) extend from one end of the lumen to the other. (See Figure 6.21)

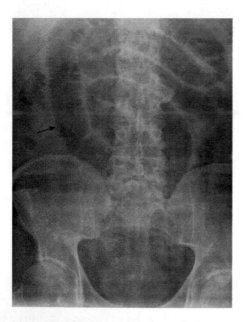

Figure 6.21: AXR of a 70-year-old man who presented with abdominal pain, vomiting and distension. There is extensive dilatation of central small bowel loops (arrow) with very little air in distal large bowel, in keeping with small bowel obstruction.

Large bowel obstruction:

Peripheral distended loops of bowel where haustral markings do not extend from wall to wall is suggestive of large bowel obstruction. (See Figure 6.22). The rectum and sigmoid colon might not have any air if the obstruction is proximal to the sigmoid colon. The central small bowel loops may or may not be dilated depending on the competency of the ilio-caecal valve. Sigmoid and caecal volvulus appear as extensively distended loops of large bowel.

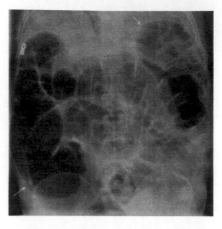

Figure 6.22: AXR of an 80-year-old woman who presented with abdominal distension and constipation. Note dilated peripheral loops of bowel (arrows) with a lack of complete haustral markings in keeping with large bowel obstruction.

Ileus:

An ileus is commonly seen in patients with reduced mobility during the post-operative period or in intensive care patients. There is distension with air in both small and large bowel including the rectum. (See Figure 6.23). This is a clinico-radiological diagnosis and correlation with biochemical profile, especially potassium, levels are necessary.

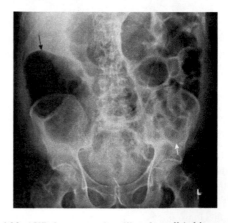

Figure 6.23: AXR demonstrating dilated small (white arrow) and large bowel (black arrow) loops with some air in the rectum in a patient post sternotomy.

Hollow viscera perforation:

Free intra-peritoneal air can be difficult to detect on an AXR. When present, you will be able to see a clear outline of the bowel wall due to the presence of air on either side of it (Rigler sign). This is a surgical emergency. (See Figure 6.24).

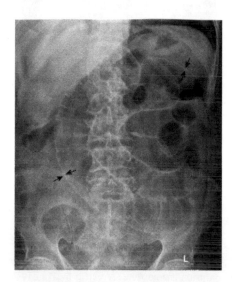

Figure 6.24: AXR demonstrating central small bowel obstruction in a patient who presented with abdominal pain. In this film it is possible to delineate both sides of the bowel wall (arrow), compared to Figure 6.21 where only the internal aspect of the wall is clearly seen, in keeping with free intra peritoneal air (Rigler sign).

Renal calculi:

Renal calculi can be present either in the kidney, bladder or along the ureters and are seen as high-density foci. Non-contrast CT has a better sensitivity and specificity, compared to plain film, in detecting renal stones but may not be the first line investigation in your centre. (See Figure 6.25).

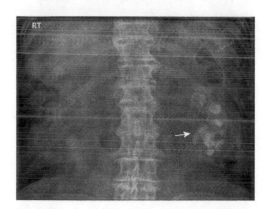

Figure 6.25: Focused AXR of the kidneys demonstrating extensive calcification filling the pelvic calyceal system of the left kidney (arrow) in keeping with a Staghorn calculus.

CT head

In line with the NICE guidelines, a significant numbers of patients with head injury are investigated with a CT scan of the head. As an FY doctor you might be quizzed or asked to review a CT head scan but in routine practice a radiologist reports these. Some examples of common acute pathologies found in such scans have been described.

Stroke:

The different types of stroke and their appearance on CT are summarised in Table 6.5.

Type of stroke	Appearance on CT
Ischaemic	Usually seen as area of hypo density (dark) in one cerebral hemisphere (See Figure 6.26)
Haemorrhagic	Haemorrhage is seen as an area of hyper-density (bright). (See Figure 6.27). Haemorrhagic stroke has areas of both hyper and hypodensity and is one of the main contraindications for thrombolysis.

Table 6.5: The different types of stroke and their imaging appearance.

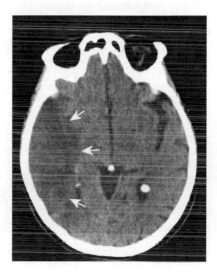

Figure 6.26: Non-contrast CT head showing a large area of hypo-density in the right temporo-parietal lobe (arrows) in keeping with an acute ischaemic infarct in the middle cerebral artery territory.

Extradural haemorrhage:

Extradural haemorrhage is usually due to an arterial bleed secondary to trauma. It is seen as a localised peripheral area of hyper-density (blood) that has a convex internal margin and does not cross suture lines. This is a surgical emergency as there is usually associated midline shift to the contralateral side with increasing risk of coning/brain herniation. (See Figure 6.28).

6. Radiology

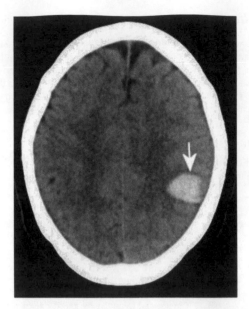

Figure 6.27: CT head showing focal area of increased density (arrow) in the left parietal lobe with minimal surrounding hypo density.

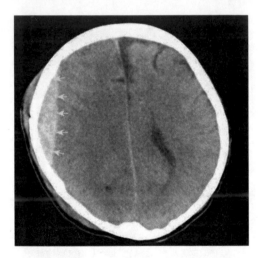

Figure 6.28: Non-contrast CT head showing a peripheral hyper-dense area in the right cerebral hemisphere. Note the convex internal outline (arrows) in keeping with an acute extradural haemorrhage.

Subdural haemorrhage:

Subdural haemorrhage is secondary to a venous bleed and is commonly seen in elderly patients. In the acute phase it is seen as a hyper-dense peripheral area that has concave internal margins. The management can either be conservative or surgical depending on the size of the haemorrhage and the patient's clinical condition. In subacute and chronic stages the haemorrhage tends to decrease in density and become isodense to the brain parenchyma. (See Figure 6.29).

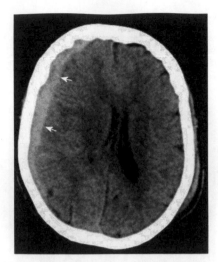

Figure 6.29: Non-contrast CT head showing the relatively hyper-dense region outlining the right cerebral cortex, this has an internal concave outline (arrows) in keeping with an acute subdural haemorrhage.

Cerebral contusion/haemorrhage:

Cerebral contusion/haemorrhage is seen as focal area of increased density. These are usually seen secondary to head injury, underlying brain malignancy or coagulopathy. (See Figure 6.27).

Hydrocephalus:

Hydrocephalus is secondary to blockage of CSF outflow in the ventricles. It can be secondary to multiple pathologies and is usually seen as dilated ventricles especially the temporal horn of the lateral ventricles. (See Figure 6.30).

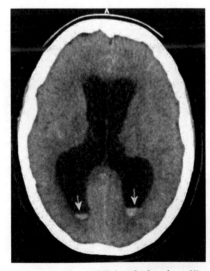

Figure 6.30: Non-contrast CT head showing dilated lateral ventricles with layering of hyper-dense blood in the occipital horns (arrows). This patient had a subarachnoid haemorrhage with intra-ventricular spread and secondary hydrocephalus.

Skull fractures:

CT is the investigation of choice as skull X-rays are no longer used to diagnose skull fractures.

COMMUNICATING WITH THE RADIOLOGIST

An FY doctor is responsible for the organisation and co-ordination of essential imaging investigations for in-patients. Many of these investigations will be performed on the basis of the clinical information you provide either on the request card or during your discussion with the radiologist. Some of the points you should consider while requesting a radiological investigation are described in Table 6.6.

Head-to-toe case-based imaging

Knowing what radiological test to do and when to do them will not only aid patient care but will also reduce unnecessary time wasting for all. Table 6.7 gives examples of the most appropriate imaging techniques for the patient's presenting symptoms.

Has this test been done already? Every attempt should be made to avoid repeating tests by getting previous images and reports.

Do I need it? The results of some tests are unlikely to affect patient management either because they are unexpected or they are irrelevant.

Do I need it now?

Is this the best investigation? If in doubt discuss with a radiologist. Prior to any discussion with a radiologist ensure that you have gone through the clinical notes and are aware of the differential diagnosis. If you have not been involved in day-to-day care of the patient, it might be best to carry the notes with you.

Have I explained the problem? Make sure your handwriting is legible and all the relevant clinical details are provided and relevant questions asked. If irrelevant clinical details are provided the reports are likely to be clinically irrelevant. In other words, 'garbage in, garbage out'.

Are all these investigations needed?

Table 6.6: Points to consider when requesting radiological investigations.

Clinical presentation	Primary imaging test	Secondary/definitive imaging test
Head injury (vomiting, focal neuralgia, headache, etc)	CT head	–
Headache, vomiting, visual disturbance (query subarachnoid haemorrhage)	CT head	Lumbar puncture
Acute stroke, transient ischaemic attack (TIA)	CT head	MRI
Neck pain (road traffic accident (RTA))	Cervical spine X-Ray	CT cervical spine
Chest pain (pulmonary emboli (PE), aortic dissection, acute coronary syndrome (ACS))	CXR	CT, MRI, V/Q
Cough, fever (pyrexia of unknown origin (PUO))	CXR	CT chest
Haemoptysis, weight loss (malignancy)	CXR	CT chest
Upper abdominal pain (gall stones, pancreatitis)	Erect CXR	USS, CT, MRI
Loin to groin pain (renal colic)	X-Ray kidneys-ureters-bladder (KUB)	USS, CT KUB
Acute loin pain, hypotension (abdominal aortic aneurysm)	USS	CT abdomen and pelvis
Abdominal pain, distension and constipation (small or large bowel obstruction)	Erect CXR, AXR	CT abdomen and pelvis
Change in bowel habit, weight loss (large bowel malignancy)	Colonoscopy	CT abdomen and pelvis
Acute limb ischaemia	CXR	Angiography
Swollen calf (query DVT)	USS	CT, venography

Table 6.7: Appropriate imaging techniques for the patient's presenting symptoms.

Further reading and references

➢ Agramunt M, Coronel B, Errando J, et al (2004). Suspected ureteral colic: plain film and sonography vs. unenhanced helical CT. A prospective study in 66 patients. *European radiology*, 14: 129–36.

➢ Bankier AA, Hansell DM, MacMahon H, et al (2008). Fleischner Society: glossary of terms for thoracic imaging, *Radiology* 246(3): 697–722.

➢ Duffy J, Laws D, Neville E, Pleural Diseases Group, Standards of Care Committee, British Thoracic Society (2003). BTS guidelines for the insertion of a chest drain, *Thorax*, 58 Suppl 2: ii53–9.

➢ Hart DH, Wall BFW (2002). Radiation exposure of the UK population from medical and dental X-ray examinations, *Didcot: National Radiological Protection Board.*

➢ Health and Safety Executive (1999). *Ionising Radiations Regulations, Statutory Instrument 1999 No. 3232.*

➢ Khoo TK, Lin MB, Teh HS (2001). Flank pain: is Intravenous Urogram necessary? *Singapore medical journal*, 42(9): 425–7.

➢ Ly JQ (2003). The Rigler sign, *Radiology*, 228(3): 706–7.

➢ National Institute for Health and Clinical Excellence (2002). *Guidance on the use of ultrasound locating devices for placing central venous catheters, Technology Appraisal Guidance No. 49.*

➢ National Institute for Health and Clinical Excellence (2007). *Head injury. Triage, assessment, investigation and early management of head injury in infants, children and adults, Guideline 56.*

➢ RCR (2007). *Making the best use of clinical radiology services-Referral Guidelines. (6 Ed.)* Royal College of Radiologists.

FLUID MANAGEMENT

On your first day as a Foundation Year One doctor you will definitely be asked to write up intravenous fluids onto a patient's fluid/drug chart. As a result it is important to have an in-depth knowledge of fluid balance in the body.

Compartments of the human body

The human body consists of approximately two thirds (60%) water. Body water is divided into two physiological compartments. They are known as intracellular fluid (ICF) and extracellular fluid (ECF). In addition there is a pathological area known as the third space which arises due to a mismatch in the normal homeostatic mechanisms within the two physiological compartments.

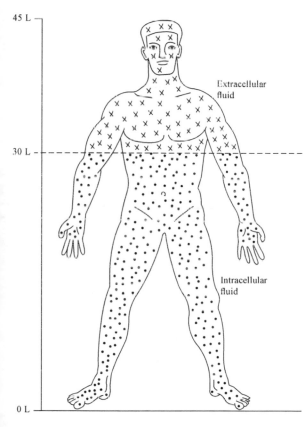

Figure 7.1: The physiological fluid compartment of the average 70 kg man

For the average 70 kilogram man:

Physiological		Pathological
Intracellular fluid (30 litres)	**Extracellular fluid (15 litres)**	**Third Space**
• Consists of two thirds of total body water	• Consists of a third of total body water. • This compartment is subdivided into plasma (3.5 L), interstitial fluid (8.5 L), lymph (1.5 L) and transcellular fluid (1.5 L) (Defined as being separated by a layer of epithelium; CSF, synovial, digestive secretions)	• Fluid accumulates in this space in disease. • Fluid in this compartment *is not* readily exchangeable with the rest of ECF • This leads to dehydration

Table 7.1: Fluid distribution for an average 70 kg male.

Fluid can move between each compartment as a result of osmotic pressure. This pressure reverses osmosis through a semi-permeable membrane, i.e. allowing a solute to attract water. Proteins, however, exert a pressure known as oncotic pressure, which allows water to be drawn back in to the cell.

Osmolality is the total particle concentration, which is the same in all body compartments.

The fluid distribution between ICF and ECF compartments is determined by osmotic pressure changes. Isotonic fluid has the same osmolality as plasma, therefore when placed in plasma this fluid will not enter the ICF compartment as the osmolalities are equal. Fluid distribution between the plasma and interstitial fluid (within the ECF compartment) is determined by Starling's forces. Starling's forces involve hydrostatic pressure (forcing fluid out of a blood vessel) and oncotic pressure (drawing fluid back into the vessel).

The distribution of extra-cellular fluid between plasma and the interstitial space is regulated by the capillary and lymphatic system.

ECF_d = [Capillary hydrostatic pressure + Tissue oncotic pressure] − [Tissue hydrostatic pressure + Capillary oncotic pressure]

Electrolyte distribution within each compartment differs:

- ICF: K^+ and Mg^{2+} main cations, Phosphate and proteins, main anions
- ECF: Na^+ main cation, Chloride and Bicarbonate main anions

Each individual patient requires 2 mmol/kg/24 hrs of Sodium (approximately 140 mmol), and 1.0 mmol/kg/24 hrs of Potassium (approximately 60 mmol).

Normal fluid input and output:

INPUT (ml)		OUTPUT (ml)	
Oral Fluid	1500	Urine	1500
Water content of food	750–1000	Faeces	300
Water of oxidation	300	Lungs	500
		Skin	500
Total (ml)	2800	Total	2800

Table 7.2: Normal fluid input and output for an average 70 kg male.

There are specific circumstances in which intravenous fluids must be prescribed including:

- Replacement of abnormal fluid losses e.g. diarrhoea and vomiting, burns
- Normal fluid requirements for a patient who is NBM
- Pre-operative resuscitation
- Post operative resuscitation
- Electrolyte imbalance

Types of fluid

There are three different classes of fluid commonly used. As an FY you will soon become familiar with these when having to prescribe them on both surgical and medical wards.

Crystalloids:

- This is an electrolyte solution in water
- These fluids can move through a semi-permeable membrane
- They include normal saline, dextrose saline and Hartmann's solution.
- They are typically used as maintenance fluids on the general surgical wards.

Colloids:

- This is a type of fluid that contains high molecular weight molecules, therefore cannot move through a semi-permeable membrane.
- Colloids therefore stay in the vascular compartment for longer.
- Albumin is a natural colloid
- Gelofusin and haemaccel are synthetic types of colloid.

Blood:

- Cross-matched is the ideal type of blood replacement, and usually takes one hour to produce.
- Type specific blood (e.g. ABO and Rh) can be produced in ten minutes
- O negative blood is used in an emergency with extensive haemorrhage.

Prescribing fluids

It is your responsibility as an FY doctor to prescribe fluids on the wards. You will be managing the patient's fluid balance on a daily basis. The average adult daily requirements are 2–3 litres of water, 100 mmol sodium and 60 mmol potassium.

An example of a normal fluid prescription is shown below;

Intravenous treatment							
Date	Route	Solution	Vol.	Additives	Dose	Duration	Signature
10/06/09	IV	Normal Saline	1L	KCL	20 mmol	8 hours	MKK
10/06/09	IV	5% Dextrose	1L	KCL	20 mmol	8 hours	MKK
10/06/09	IV	5% Dextrose	1L	KCL	20 mmol	8 hours	MKK

Figure 7.2: An example of a normal fluid prescription chart.

or

Intravenous treatment							
Date	Route	Solution	Vol.	Additives	Dose	Duration	Signature
10/06/09	IV	Dextrose Saline	1L	KCL	20 mmol	8 hours	MKK
10/06/09	IV	Dextrose Saline	1L	KCL	20 mmol	8 hours	MKK
10/06/09	IV	Dextrose Saline	1L	KCL	20 mmol	8 hours	MKK

Figure 7.3: An example of a normal fluid prescription chart.

If the patient is losing additional fluid (e.g. vomiting, diarrhoea or has an NG tube), they will require extra fluid replacement. An input/output chart should be started and additional losses should be replaced with normal saline.

Fluid balance

When prescribing any fluid it is important to assess the fluid status of a patient through clinical examination, urine output and CVP.

Clinical examination:

- Look for signs of dehydration. These include dry mucous membranes, sunken eyes, low BP and postural hypotension, raised pulse rate, low JVP, and the patient may be confused.

- Fluid overload can also occur. This presents as pulmonary oedema, and peripheral oedema.

Urine output:

- Urine output is a useful guide when assessing a patient's fluid status

- A patient should have a urine output of at least 0.5 ml/kg/hr

CVP:

- This is only a possibility if a patient has a central venous catheter

- The changes/trend in CVP pressures over time in response to fluid are more important than the absolute values.

Fluid challenge:

- This is another useful tool in assessing fluid status.

- A 250 ml colloid bolus is given to the patient STAT.

- Positive response should be seen in the urine output and CVP within minutes.

Top tips before giving a fluid challenge

- Check to see if the catheter is still in place and has not fallen out

- Check to see if the catheter is not blocked. Flushing the catheter (50 ml bladder syringe and sterile water) will identify this.

- Palpate the bladder to identify or rule out urinary retention.

Post-operative fluid therapy

Post operatively a number of hormones (catecholamines, ADH, cortisol, and aldosterone) increase as a result of the stress involved in surgery. Over 24–48 hours postoperatively, this results in the conservation of salt and water, and increased losses of potassium and hydrogen ions by the kidneys. With this water retention it is sensible to reduce the daily intake of water to 2L 24 hours postoperatively. Potassium supplements are often not given due to the increased release of potassium following tissue injury during surgery.

In patients who have undergone abdominal surgery a bowel ileus may develop (from mechanical handling or general anaesthetic), resulting in third space losses, as fluid in the bowel is not reabsorbed. These patients require additional fluid replacement which is prescribed according to urine output/Nasogastric tube aspirates. On day 2 or 3 postoperatively the patient will experience a sudden diuresis, which signifies recovery of the bowel. Fluid therapy can also be guided by checking serum electrolytes.

SHOCK

'Shock is inadequate perfusion of vital organs and tissue oxygenation'.

Classification of shock

- Hypovolaemic:

7. Fluids & Shock

- o Haemorrhagic shock is the most common cause after injury
- o Diarrhoea and vomiting
- Septic
- Anaphylactic
- Cardiogenic:
  - o Blunt injury
  - o Cardiac infarct
  - o Cardiac tamponade
- Neurogenic
  - o Spinal injuries

Stages of hypovolaemic shock

- There are four important stages of hypovolaemic shock, which are classified according to the percentage of blood loss. These percentages are similar to the system used for scoring tennis.
- Table 7.3 illustrates the stages of hypovolaemic shock;

Management

- ➢ A standard ABC assessment should be performed initially and appropriate initial resuscitation undertaken.
- ➢ All patients require fluid resuscitation
- ➢ Inform your senior colleague early
- ➢ Two large bore cannulas should be inserted into the Antecubital Fossae.
- ➢ Bloods are sent for FBC, U&E's, cross-match, glucose, pregnancy test, and toxicology tests.
- ➢ Hourly urine output
- ➢ ECG
- ➢ A central line can be inserted to monitor fluid replacement.
- ➢ ATLS guidelines recommend 2 litres of crystalloid replacement for all major trauma patients.

Response to fluid resuscitation

Initial fluid resuscitation can lead to three different types of response;

Rapid response:

- There is usually < 20% of fluid loss
- Patients respond rapidly to fluid replacement
- Patients remain haemodynamically stable when the fluids are slowed or stopped.

Transient response:

- There is usually 20–40% of fluid loss
- A small initial response to fluid therapy may be seen
- However if the fluids are slowed they rapidly deteriorate and become haemodynamically unstable.
- This indicates inadequate fluid resuscitation or continuous haemorrhage.
- These patients may require surgical management.

No response:

- There is usually > 40% of fluid loss.
- There is little or no response to fluid resuscitation
- This indicates severe haemorrhage which requires urgent blood replacement. Typically type-specific blood is used, which takes about ten minutes to prepare.
- Urgent surgical intervention is usually needed to control the haemorrhage.
- It is important to remember the non-haemorrhagic causes of shock such as cardiac tamponade, as this will not respond to fluid resuscitation.
- Depending on the severity of shock and the degree of organ ischaemia, high level input (i.e. inotropic support and close monitoring (arterial line and CVP pressures), may be required on the HDU or ITU.

Stage	Blood Loss (%)	Blood Loss (ml)	Heart Rate	BP	RR	Conscious State	Urine Output	Fluid Replacement
I	0–15	750	Normal	Normal	Normal	Mild anxiety	Normal	Crystalloid
II	15–30	750–1500	> 100	Normal	20–30	Agitated	20–30	Colloid
III	30–40	1500–2000	> 120	Decreased	30–40	Confused	5–15	Colloid +/- Blood
IV	> 40	> 2000	> 140	Decreased	> 35	Drowsy/ lethargic	0	Colloid +/- Blood

Table 7.3: The stage of hypovolaemic shock and their consequences.

Further reading and references

- ➢ Bulstrode CJK, Russell RCG, Williams NS (2000) *Bailey & Love's Short Practice of Surgery* (23 Ed.). Arnold.

- ➢ Calne R, Ellis H, Whatson C (2002). *Lecture Notes on General Surgery*. (10 Ed.) Blackwell Publishing.
- ➢ Goldberg A, Stansby G (2006). *Surgical Talk: Revision in Surgery* (2 Ed.). Imperial college press.

INTRODUCTION

This chapter aims to cover the theoretical aspects behind the procedures that should be learnt during the Foundation Programme. It will not replace practical experience on the wards but will address the indications, contraindications, relevant anatomy and complications of each Direct Observation of Procedural Skills (DOPS). In addition it will include a brief description of each DOPS and helpful tips to achieve success. Issues regarding consent, post procedure care, and professionalism will also be included. Where appropriate there will be a brief guide to the interpretation of results gained from performing the procedure.

Direct Observation of Procedural Skills covered

Foundation Year 1	Foundation Year 2
1. Venepuncture	14. Lumbar puncture
2. IV cannulation	15. Aspiration of pleural fluid or air
3. Arterial puncture and interpretation of arterial blood gases (ABG)	16. Chest drain
4. Blood cultures from peripheral and central sites	17. Aspiration of ascitic fluid
5. Subcutaneous, Intra-dermal & Intra-muscular Injections	18. Insertion of a central venous line
6. Administration of IV medications and IV fluid	19. Aspiration of a joint effusion
7. Prescription and administration of blood products	20. Skin suturing
8. Local anaesthetics	
9. Performing and interpretating an electrocardiogram (ECG)	
10. Performing and interpretating spirometry	
11. Airway care	
12. Nasogastric tube insertion	
13. Urethral catheterisation	

DOPS ASSESSMENTS

DOPS assessments require completion of paper or web based assessment forms by an assessor. These assess an individual on a range of aspects from knowledge, technical ability to communication skills and professionalism. This chapter concentrates on the knowledge aspects.

Common themes

Primo non nocere: A cardinal rule in medicine is to 'first do no harm'. In all cases procedures should only be performed when you have sufficient competency, or with sufficient support.

Preparation:

Preparation is frequently the key to success in all DOPS. Correct identification of the patient is clearly important. Consent should be gained and consideration given to where the procedure should be carried out. In addition one has to be aware of the need for extra monitoring and the need for assistance from nursing or allied medical staff, especially if the procedure is likely to be difficult.

Be sure to obtain all of the necessary equipment required before beginning the procedure. Spend time palpating/percussing the patient if required to familiarise yourself with the local anatomy before proceeding. Consider in advance the need for adequate analgesia and/or sedation prior to the procedure.

Sterility:

Most invasive procedures either use an aseptic ('as clean as possible') non touch technique ('avoiding touching key parts') or sterile technique (creating a sterile field and using sterile gloves and gowns). The specifics are highlighted for each DOPS, as always do not forget to wash your hands!

Consent:

Undertaking a procedure without consent is legally known as 'battery'. Consider what form of consent is required (implied/verbal/written). Some trusts may require formal consent forms to be completed for certain procedures. For consent to be valid the patient must be adequately informed; meaning the indication, the procedure and the complications (common and rare) have been explained to them. Does the patient have capacity? This means are they able to understand and retain the information, weigh up the pros and cons and communicate their decision. If the patient lacks capacity, the doctor can proceed if acting in the patient's best interests. If a second party holds lasting power of attorney, consent will need to be obtained from them. In any case, if a patient lacks capacity it is considered good practice to discuss the procedure with a relative, especially if there are potentially serious implications. When explaining potential complications consider the circumstances specific to the patient i.e. risk of bruising when taking blood.

Post procedure management:

Clear up sharps and dispose of biological waste promptly and appropriately. Arrange for follow-up of results and for further management. See individual procedures for specific details.

Documentation:

The use of documentation is vital for completion of any DOPS. This is particularly important when undertaking invasive procedures. Some trusts may require completion of specific proformas. When documenting, consider the need to document all aspects of the procedure including; consent, sterility, details of equipment (e.g. size), important stages that prevent or limit complications (e.g. replacement of foreskin after urethral catheterisation), any complications encountered and ongoing management issues.

Communication skills:

Good communication with patients and relatives, is vital to the success of any DOPS and helps to ensure ongoing co-operation throughout the procedure. Prior to the procedure, and as part of consent, explain to the patient what will happen, what to expect during and after the procedure. Take time to address their ideas concerns and expectations. In addition, remember to communicate effectively with other professionals, be it professionals involved in the procedure itself or those who will manage the patient's post procedural care. For example, explain to nursing staff clearly on how to care for a patient's chest drain and what parameters would warrant a cause for concern.

Professionalism:

As with all aspects of medicine, a professional approach is essential. In addition to the points outlined previously, patient dignity should be maintained at all times. All doctors should recognise their own limitations in performing a particular procedure and should not be afraid to seek senior assistance when concerned.

1. VENEPUNCTURE

Indications

- Diagnostic testing of blood
- Monitoring of physiological or pharmacological parameters

Contraindications

- Limbs post local/regional lymph node dissection

Relevant anatomy

Common sites of venepuncture include the Antecubital Fossa, small veins of the hand, forearm and the Femoral vein

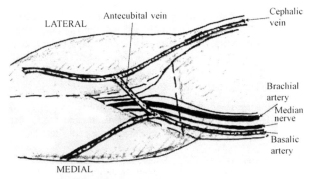

Figure 8.1: Anatomy of the antecubetal fossa.

Locating the Femoral vein:

The Femoral vein lies just medial to the Femoral artery which can be identified immediately inferior of the mid-inguinal point (midway from anterior superior iliac spine (ASIS) and pubic symphysis).

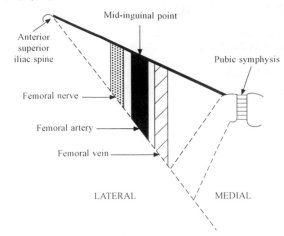

Figure 8.2: Anatomical landmarks for the Femoral triangle.

Equipment required

Tourniquet, gloves, chlorhexidine/alcohol swab, needle, syringe/vacutainer, cotton wool/gauze, tape, connectors and appropriate blood bottles.

Procedure

Venepuncture can be performed with a needle and syringe or, using closed vacutainer systems.

An aseptic non-touch technique should be used:

1. Apply tourniquet and identify suitable vein
2. Prepare skin: wipe with chlorhexidine/alcohol swab
3. Fix vein (using a spare finger)
4. Warn patient of a 'sharp scratch'
5. Insert the needle at a 30–45° angle into vein, always pointing away from yourself
6. Take sample:
   a. When using a needle and syringe a flashback of blood will be seen as the needle enters the vein, once this is seen draw back the syringe to collect the sample.
   b. When using a vacutainer system no flashback will be seen: connect a sample bottle into the vacutainer and the vacuum will result in blood being collected. If needed adjust the position of the needle beneath the skin. Once the vacuum has been lost the sample bottle cannot be used again.
7. Remove tourniquet
8. Remove needle and syringe/vacutainer (removing tourniquet first may reduce bruising)

9. Apply cotton wool/gauze to puncture site with pressure. If appropriate, tape in place

10. Dispose of any sharps in the sharps bin

11. Label blood bottles immediately as per trust guidelines

12. Document in the notes

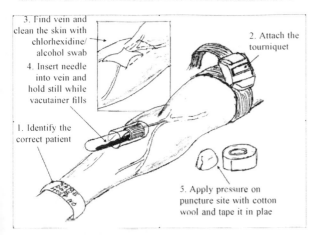

3. Find vein and clean the skin with chlorhexidine/ alcohol swab

4. Insert needle into vein and hold still while vacutainer fills

1. Identify the correct patient

2. Attach the tourniquet

5. Apply pressure on puncture site with cotton wool and tape it in plae

Figure 8.3: Venepuncture at the Antecubetal Fossa.

Post procedure management

Check site for bleeding, infection risk and excessive bruising

Complications

- Bleeding, bruising, haematoma (minimised by applying pressure immediately after venepuncture)

- Inadvertent arterial puncture (if this occurs be prepared to apply prolonged pressure over the site after removal of the needle)

- Damage to local structures, including nerves

Top tips
- A comfortable position for both patient and doctor is essential for success

- Spend plenty of time examining sites to find the most appropriate vein

- Ensure vein is adequately fixed, failure to do this may result in it being pushed away, rather than punctured by the needle

2. INTRAVENOUS CANNULATION

Indications

- Administration of intravenous (IV) fluids, medications and blood products

Contraindications

- Localised skin infection
- Limbs post local/regional lymph node dissection

Relevant anatomy

Common sites of IV cannulation include the Antecubital Fossa, small veins of the hand and forearm and in patients who are difficult to cannulate consider the long Saphenous vein and foot veins.

When deciding on an appropriate site, consider the patient's comfort, avoiding crossing joints and the risk of inadvertent or deliberate removal by the patient.

Equipment required

Tourniquet, gloves, chlorhexidine/alcohol swab, cannula, 10ml syringe, 10ml normal saline, cannula site dressing and gauze

Procedure

This procedure should be performed with an aseptic, non-touch technique:

1. Apply tourniquet

2. Identify suitable vein

3. Prepare skin – wipe with chlorhexidine/alcohol swab

4. Fix vein (using a spare finger)

5. Warn patient of a 'sharp scratch'

6. Insert cannula at a 10–15° angle into vein

7. When flashback is observed flatten the cannula

8. Advance cannula further into vein, whilst slowly withdrawing needle

9. Remove tourniquet

10. Depress vein to prevent bleeding

11. Remove needle completely and dispose in sharps bin

12. Place cap on to end of cannula

13. Flush with 5–10 ml normal saline

14. Fix cannula in place with cannula site dressing

15. If blood sampling is also required connect syringe to cannula and remove sample prior to flushing

16. Label date of insertion on cannula dressing

17. Document completion of procedure appropriately in patient's medical notes

Post procedure management

Regularly review the need to re-site cannulae. Review the site for evidence of infection

8. DOPS

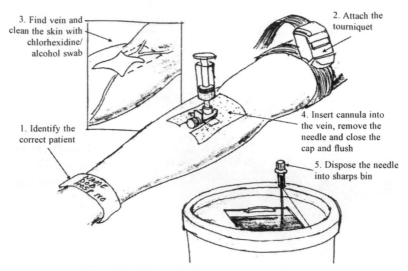

3. Find vein and
clean the skin with
chlorhexidine/
alcohol swab

1. Identify the
correct patient

2. Attach the
tourniquet

4. Insert cannula into
the vein, remove the
needle and close the
cap and flush

5. Dispose the needle
into sharps bin

Figure 8.4: IV cannulation at Antecubetal Fossa site

Complications

- Infection – cellulitis, bacteraemia and septicaemia
- Bleeding, bruising, haematoma
- Damage to local structures, including nerves

Top tips

- A comfortable position for both patient and doctor is essential for success
- Spend plenty of time examining sites to find the most appropriate vein
- Ensure vein is adequately fixed, failure to do this may result in it being pushed away, rather than punctured by the needle
- If the vein is peripherally shut down, consider immersing arm in warm water to bring out veins

3. ARTERIAL PUNCTURE AND INTERPRETATION OF ARTERIAL BLOOD GASES (ABG)

Indications

- To assess respiratory and/or metabolic status, in particular pH, PaO_2, $PaCO_2$, HCO_3^-, base excess (BE), and lactate
- It may also be used to gain rapid electrolyte information including glucose

Contraindications

- No collateral circulation through Ulnar artery, as determined by Allen's test (lack of spontaneous return of circulation to hand on release of ulnar artery when radial and ulnar arteries have been occluded with digital pressure)
- History of severe artery spasm following previous puncture

Relevant anatomy

Sites for ABG sampling are the *Radial artery* (most common, just lateral to tendon of Flexor Carpi Radialis), *Brachial artery* (beneath the bicipital aponeurosis and medial to biceps tendon).

Equipment required

Chlorhexidine/alcohol swab, gloves, specialised heparinised ABG syringe, cotton wool/gauze, tape and needle (25 gauge orange needle). You may want to consider the need for a longer needle (21 gauge green needle) for Femoral puncture.

Procedure

This procedure should be performed using an aseptic non-touch technique:

1. Locate artery and identify area of maximum pulsation
2. Do Allen's test to show if there is adequate collateral circulation through ulnar artery, if using the radial artery
3. Clean skin with alcohol swab
4. Ensure syringe plunger is partially retracted
5. Warn patient that it may hurt
6. Insert needle perpendicular to skin into the artery
7. Observe for pulsation of blood into syringe
8. If needed adjust position of needle beneath skin
9. Remove needle and dispose in sharps bin
10. Apply cotton wool/gauze with pressure and hold for 3–5 minutes
11. Take sample rapidly for analysis
12. Document results and procedure in the notes

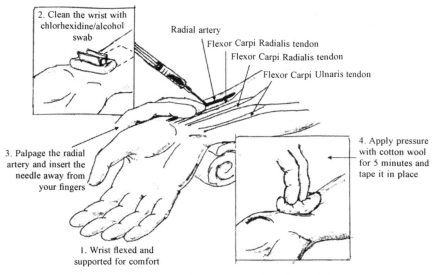

Figure 8.5: Arterial blood gas sampling from the radial artery.

It is also possible to make a small 'skin bleb' above the artery using local anaesthetic prior to inserting the ABG syringe into the artery

Post procedure management

Review site for any evidence of on going bleeding

Complications

- Bleeding, bruising, haematoma
- False aneurysm
- Prolonged arterial spasm (may result in pain/numbness)
- Arterial occlusion
- Damage to local structures, including nerves

Interpretation

The following is a brief guide on how to interpretate ABGs, covering normal ranges and the results in common medical situations. It is important to know the FIO2 (concentration of inspired oxygen) to meaningfully interpret results.

Normal ranges

pH	7.35 – 7.45
pO_2	Depends on F_1O_2 (approx F_1O_2 – 10%)
CO_2	4.5 – 6.0 kPa
HCO_3^-	22 – 28 mmol/L
B.E.	–2 to +2

Table 8.1: Ranges required for interpretation of ABG.

Definitions of respiratory failure

Type I: PaO_2 <8kPa on air

Type II: PaO_2 <8kPa on air AND $PaCO_2$ >6kPa

Common acid-base disturbances

Disorder	pH	pCO_2	HCO_3^-	B.E.
Acute respiratory acidosis	Low	High	Normal	Normal
Chronic compensated respiratory acidosis	Normal	High	High	Positive
Acute on chronic respiratory acidosis	Low	High	High	Positive
Acute respiratory alkalosis	High	Low	Normal	Normal
Acute metabolic acidosis	Low	Normal or Low (Respiratory compensation)	Low	Negative
Acute metabolic alkalosis	High	Normal or high (Respiratory compensation)	High	Positive
Mixed respiratory and metabolic acidosis	Low	High	Low	Negative

Table 8.2: Common acid-base disturbances and their effect on various ranges.

8. DOPS

For metabolic acidosis the anion gap should be calculated, so as to elucidate the diagnosis. The anion gap is calculated by following:

$$\text{Anion gap} = [Na^+ + K^+] - [Cl^- + HCO_3^-]$$

$$\text{Normal anion gap} = 10–18$$

Causes of a raised anion gap are: Lactic acidosis, ketones (DKA, starvation or alcohol), urate (renal failure), exogenous acids (salicylates, ethylene glycol and methanol) and biguanides (metformin).

Causes of metabolic acidosis with normal anion gap (due to loss of bicarbonate or ingestion of acid with retained chloride): Diarrhoea, Renal Tubular Acidosis, drugs (e.g. acetazolamide), Addison's disease and pancreatic fistulae.

Top tips

- Inserting the needle whilst palpating proximally and distally to the puncture site. This can help to determine direction of the artery and guide angulation of the needle
- Rapidly take sample to machine for interpretation to avoid clotting and distorted results
- Remember to record the flow rate, concentration of O_2, settings of invasive or non-invasive ventilators to allow accurate interpretation

4. BLOOD CULTURES FROM PERIPHERAL AND CENTRAL SITES

Indications

- Patients with features of suspected infection
- Blood cultures should ideally be taken before administration of antibiotics, or if already given, prior to the next dose

Contraindications

- Limbs post local/regional lymph node dissection

Relevant anatomy

Peripheral blood cultures are normally taken from the same site as venepunctures, or wherever access is possible

Equipment required

Tourniquet, gloves, Chlorhexidine/alcohol swab, needle, 20 ml syringes or vacutainer (and connectors), cotton wool/gauze, tape, aerobic and anaerobic blood culture sets (two to three sets depending on condition)

Procedure for peripheral blood cultures

1. Blood cultures should be taken in the same way as one would take blood during venepuncture
2. Blood cultures should be taken from a fresh venepuncture and not from IV cannulae
3. If possible avoid Femoral puncture due to increased risk of contamination
4. The Department of Health recommends the use of 2% Chlorhexidine in 70% isopropyl alcohol impregnated swabs for disinfecting the skin
5. Clean skin with chlorhexidine/alcohol wipe for 30 seconds and allow to dry by evaporation. Do not re-touch the skin over the vein as this will contaminate the site
6. Remove the tops from the culture bottles and clean with chlorhexidine/alcohol wipe for 30 seconds and allow to dry by evaporation
7. Take blood cultures, filling the aerobic bottle first
8. Dispose of any sharps in the sharps bin
9. Once taken blood cultures should be stored in an incubator or sent to microbiology quickly
10. Remember to document in the notes, including the site and indication

Procedure for blood cultures from central lines

The following applies for taking any samples from central venous lines:

1. Remove the tops from the culture bottles and clean with chlorhexidine/alcohol wipe for 30 seconds and allow to dry by evaporation
2. Put on sterile gloves
3. Remove the cap of the central line port
4. Wipe with Chlorhexidine/alcohol swab
5. Connect 10 ml syringe and aspirate 5–10 mls
6. Discard this syringe
7. Connect another new syringe and aspirate a further 5–10 mls
8. This is your sample. Empty it into the culture bottles (anaerobic first), which should then be sent to microbiology quickly or stored in an incubator
9. Dispose of any sharps in the sharps bin
10. Flush the line with 10 ml normal saline
11. Replace the cap
12. Remember to document in the notes, including site and indication
13. Always consider the need for paired peripheral samples (ideally take before)

Post procedure management

Ensure microbiology team are aware of the status of the patient. Discuss with nursing staff the duration of the central line.

Complications

- Bleeding, bruising, haematoma (minimised by applying pressure immediately after venepuncture)

- Inadvertent arterial puncture (if this occurs be prepared to apply prolonged pressure over the site after removal of the needle)

- Damage to local structures, including nerves

Top tips

- In unwell patients, do not delay prescribing antibiotics whilst awaiting to take blood cultures

- The more blood you inoculate into each bottle the more likely you are to identify an infection through successful culture. Aim for at least 5 mls per bottle

- To increase the chance of identifying an organism blood cultures are best done when patients spike a temperature. However, in the elderly sepsis can often occur without spikes in temperature

5. SUBCUTANEOUS, INTRA-DERMAL & INTRA-MUSCULAR INJECTIONS

Subcutaneous injections

Indications

- Where IV access is difficult or would pose unnecessary trauma to the patient (palliative patients). For example insulin, Low Molecular Weight Heparins (LMWH), morphine, antibiotics and some vaccines

Contraindications

- Cellulitis
- Surgical emphysema
- Obesity (as this would greatly reduce the bioavailability of the drug due to poor absorption)

Relevant anatomy

The most common sites for subcutaneous injections are the deltoid area of the arm, abdomen and thigh

Equipment required

Needle, gloves, syringe, alcohol swab and appropriate medication

Procedure

1. Draw up the medication into a syringe (or use a specifically designed injector pen)
2. Clean skin with alcohol swab
3. Pinch and raise up a small area of the skin and subcutaneous tissue between your fingers
4. Inject the medication into the subcutaneous tissue using a 25–27 gauge needle
5. Once the medication has been injected, dispose of the needle and syringe into the sharps bin
6. Ensure documentation of the site, time and drug injected is done

Post procedure management

Check for signs of localised redness, swelling, bleeding, or inflammation at the injection site

Complications

- Long term use of the subcutaneous route, e.g. in diabetics, can result in lipodystrophy. Therefore rotation of the injection site is important.

- Skin irritation can occur. Therefore only use 0.9% saline, and not 5% dextrose if injecting fluids.

Intra-dermal Injections

Indications

- Where IV access is not necessary and will provide least infection risk for diagnostic testing. For example Mantoux test and RAS allergen testing.

Contraindications

- Cellulitis
- Surgical emphysema
- Obesity (as this would greatly reduce the bioavailability of the drug due to poor absorption)

Relevant anatomy

The most common sites is usually the upper limb

Equipment required

Needle, gloves, syringe, alcohol swab and appropriate medication/allergen

Procedure

1. Draw up substance into syringe
2. Clean skin with alcohol steret
3. Inject using a 25–27 gauge needle advancing it parallel to the skin, into the epidermal dermal junction

8. DOPS

4. Injection will result in slight separation of the different layers of the skin

5. Once the medication has been injected, dispose the needle and syringe into the sharps bin

6. Ensure documentation of the site, time and drug injected is done

Post procedure management

Check for signs of localised redness, swelling, bleeding, or inflammation at the injection site. Be aware some people may have a localised reaction to the allergen and so should consult medical help if this should occur.

Complications

- Localised infection

Intra-muscular Injections

Indications

- Where IV access is difficult or would pose unnecessary trauma to the patient (palliative patients). For example Adrenaline, some vaccines, analgesics (e.g. tramadol), anti-emetics (e.g. Cyclizine), sedative medications (e.g. Lorazepam, Haloperidol).
- Allows rapid bolus of medication without the need for IV access.

Advantages	Disadvantages
• Sites easily accessible • No need for venous access • Relatively fast action • Larger volumes can be injected than for subcutaneous injections	• Pain • Risk to damage of local structures, especially nerves • If severely hypotensive systemic absorption is slowed

Table 8.3: Advantages and disadvantages of intra-muscular injections.

Contraindications

- Thrombocytopenia
- Coagulation disorders

Relevant anatomy

There are five potential sites for IM injection:

- **Deltoid**: In an inverted equilateral triangle with the acromion process as its base, which avoids the axillary nerve. See Figure 8.6.
- **Dorsogluteal**: In the upper outer quadrant of the buttock, so as to avoid the sciatic nerve in the lower medial quadrant.
- **Ventrogluteal**: This is now the favoured site. The palm of a hand is placed on the greater trochanter of the femur with

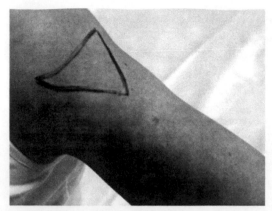

Figure 8.6: The deltoid site for intra-muscular injections.

the second finger extending along the iliac crest. The middle finger is placed medially creating a triangle within which the injection should be performed. See Figure 8.7.

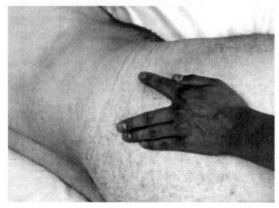

Figure 8.7: The ventrogluteal site for intra-muscular injections.

- **Vastus lateralis and Rectus femoris** – Lateral and medial thigh respectively.

The exact absorption properties differ between the sites, with absorption being fastest in the arm and slowest in the buttock.

Equipment required

Needle, gloves, syringe, alcohol swab and appropriate medication

Procedure

1. Draw up the medication into a syringe.
2. Select a needle long enough to reach the muscle
3. Wipe skin with an alcohol swab
4. Slide the skin and subcutaneous 2–3 cm in any direction and hold taut
5. Insert the needle perpendicular into the skin

6. Aspirate for blood, alter position of needle if blood aspirated
7. Inject medication (<1 ml/10 seconds)
8. Release skin
9. Remove needle and dispose of sharps in the sharps bin
10. Ensure documentation of the site, time and drug injected is done

Post procedure management

Check for signs of localised redness, swelling, bleeding, or inflammation at the injection site.

Complications

- Pain
- Haematoma
- Damage to local structures – including arterial puncture, reversible and irreversible damage to nerves, tissue necrosis, fibrosis

Adrenaline auto-injectors

Adrenaline auto-injectors (Epipen® or Anapen®) are prescribed to patients who have had a previous severe allergic reaction i.e. anaphylaxis, severe reaction involving the airway. These devices are designed to be easy to use, allowing rapid self-administration of intra-muscular adrenaline during a severe allergic reaction.

It is important that patients given adrenaline auto-injectors are educated in their correct administration with regular review of their technique.

Procedure for Epipen® auto-injector

1. Remove device from plastic container
2. Remove grey safety-cap
3. Place black tip of pen perpendicular to the lateral aspect of thigh
4. Push pen into thigh until click is heard (releases needle) and hold against thigh for 10 seconds
5. Remove pen and rub skin area for several seconds
6. Place pen back into plastic container and dispose of device safely in the sharps bin

Procedure for Anapen® auto-injector

1. Remove black needle cap
2. Take care not to place fingers over this end of device
3. Remove the black safety cap
4. Press needle end perpendicular to the lateral aspect of thigh
5. Push red firing button and hold for 10 seconds.
6. Remove device and rub skin area for several seconds.
7. Dispose of device safely in the sharps bin

Top tips

- Be aware how to effectively use Epipen® and Anapen® auto-injectors
- Epipens® are often found in the resuscitation trolley
- Take time to adequately document all sites and types of injections in the patient's notes
- Always be aware of the local anatomy of the site you are injecting, so to avoid the neurovascular bundle

6. ADMINISTRATION OF INTRAVENOUS MEDICATIONS AND FLUIDS

Indications

- For rapid administration of medication and/or fluids in an acute scenario
- If patient unable to take oral medications or fluid

Contraindications

- None

Relevant anatomy

IV medications and fluids are administered via the cannula. Common sites of IV cannulation include the Antecubital Fossa, small veins of the hand and forearm and in patients who are difficult to cannulate consider the long Saphenous vein and foot veins.

Equipment required

Saline, gloves, appropriate medication, 10ml syringe, 10 ml 0.9% saline and alcohol swab

Procedure for administrating Intravenous medication

IV injections can be given directly through a needle and syringe, or more commonly through a cannula. This is an aseptic procedure:

1. Identify the correct patient
2. Cross check details of prescription with the medication especially identity of drug, dose and expiry date
3. Check for allergies with patient
4. Wear gloves
5. Examine cannula for signs of infection, or patency of cannula

8. DOPS

6. Clean port with alcohol swab

7. Ensure cannula is patent through flushing with 10 ml normal saline

8. Administer drug as directed by prescription

9. Re-flush cannula with 10 ml normal saline

10. Document that drug has been administered (sign prescription with date and time)

11. Be vigilant for any reactions post administration

Procedure for setting up an Intravenous Infusion

1. Unwrap IV bag and check for any leaks or loss of integrity of bag

2. Unwrap giving set, and close adjustable valve

3. Insert giving set into the bag outlet

4. Hang bag on drip stand

5. Prime the giving set by half filling the giving set chamber

6. Slowly open the valve and allow fluid to drip/flow to the distal end of the giving set

7. Close valve

8. Check for air bubbles in the giving set. If present run them out

9. Connect the giving set to the cannula

10. Adjust position of the valve to set the flow rate

Determining the flow rate of the infusion:

The flow rate of infusion is determined by adjusting the number of drips per minute into the giving set chamber.

For a standard giving set: 20 drops = 1 ml

For a blood giving set: 35 drops = 1 ml

This formula can be used to calculate the drip flow rate:

$$\text{Flow rate (drops/min)} = \frac{\text{Volume of fluid (ml)} \times \text{Drops (drops)}}{\text{Number of hours (hr)} \times 60 \text{ (mins)}}$$

E.g. for a 8hr bag of 0.9% Saline

$$\text{Flow rate (drops/min)} = \frac{1000 \text{ ml} \times 20 \text{ drops}}{8 \text{ hr} \times 60 \text{ mins}}$$

Flow rate (drops/min) approximately 42 drops per minute

Maximum Flow rates for common cannula sizes:

Cannula Gauge	Maximum flow rate (ml/min)	Minimum time to infuse 1L (min)
Blue (22G)	31	32
Pink (20G)	55	18
Green (18G)	90	11
Grey (16G)	170	6

Table 8.4: The maximum flow rate and the minimum times to infuse 1 litre of saline according to the cannula gauge.

Post procedure management

Regularly review the need to re-site cannulae. Review the site for evidence of infection

Complications

- Phlebitis
- Infection: cellulitis, bacteraemia and septicaemia
- Extravasation: oedema, local toxic effects of drugs
- Embolism

Top tips

- Cytotoxics should never be prescribed or administered by anyone without specialist cytotoxic training
- Liaise with nursing staff about how you can help administer IV medication/fluids
- Always use aseptic techniques and always cross check the expiry date of all IV medications/fluids

7. PRESCRIPTION AND ADMINISTRATION OF BLOOD PRODUCTS

Indications

- Acute blood loss: to keep Hb>7g/dL in otherwise fit patients, >9g/dL in elderly and those with known cardiovascular disease
- Perioperative transfusion
- Critical care: Hb >8g/dL
- Post chemotherapy: Usually threshold of 8–9g/dL
- Radiotherapy: to keep Hb >10–12g/dL
- Chronic anaemia: to keep Hb just above level so as not to become symptomatic
- Prescribing of platelets and Fresh Frozen Plasma (FFP) should be done in consultation with seniors at all times

See the UK blood transfusion services website (www.transfusionguidelines.org.uk) for full details and guidelines for other blood products.

Contraindications

- Be aware of autoimmune haemolytic anaemias

Relevant anatomy

Blood product transfusions are administered via the cannula. Common sites of IV cannulation include the Antecubital Fossa, small veins of the hand and forearm. In addition blood can be given through central venous access if peripheral access is difficult.

Equipment required

Tourniquet, gloves, alcohol swab, needle, syringe/vacutainer (and connectors), appropriate blood bottles, 10 ml syringe, 10 ml normal saline, cannula dressing, gauze and sterile blood giving set.

Procedure

Individual trusts will have their own protocols regarding transfusion, but will include the following processes:

Requesting blood transfusions:

This should include the following information:

1. Full identification of the patient – surname, first name, date of birth (DOB), sex, patient identification number
2. Location of the patient
3. Number and type of blood components
4. Past obstetric and transfusion history where possible
5. Diagnosis and reason for the request
6. Special requirements, if in doubt seek expert opinion

CMV negative:	HIV infection
	Many bone marrow/stem cell transplant patients*
Gamma Irradiated	Hodgkin's disease
	Congenital immunodeficient states*
	Patients treated with purine analogues e.g. fludarabine*
	Many bone marrow/stem cell recipients*
	Bone marrow donors over time of harvest*
*Seek expert advice	

Table 8.5: Special transfusion requirements

Procedure for prescribing:

Should include the following details:

1. Patient identification details
2. Blood component to be administered
3. Quantity
4. Special requirements
5. Duration of transfusion
6. Any special instructions. E.g. concomitant furosemide bolus

Procedure for collection of samples:

1. Positive identification – ask the patient their name, DOB and verify the patient's wristband
2. Only perform venepuncture on one patient at a time
3. Label sample tubes immediately after the sample has been taken
4. Label the sample with name, DOB, gender, identification number, signed by person taking sample

Procedure for collection of blood products:

1. This must be completed using the correct documentation (collection slip, prescription chart, medical notes or electronic tagging systems) of the patient identification details
2. Check details on the blood unit with correct documentation
3. Document removal from the fridge and arrival at the site of transfusion

Procedure for administration:

1. Ensure the hospital guidelines are followed and all relevant documentation is completed
2. Perform bedside checks: positively identify the patient, check full patient details on the patient's wristband, blood transfusion compatibility form, compatibility label attached to blood pack, prescription chart and the medical notes
3. Check blood group and unit number are the same on the unit on the compatibility form
4. Check details of blood units are compatible with patient's blood group
5. Check for compliance with special requirements
6. Check expiry date
7. Administer product as described in 'giving IV medications' through a sterile blood giving set; avoid infusion pumps due to damage of cells
8. Sign compatibility report form and or transfusion prescription sheet

Monitoring during transfusion:

Vital signs should be recorded, before beginning transfusion, after 15 minutes, and at the end. Additional observations should be made if the patient is unconscious or if there are any concerns.

8. DOPS

Complications and management

Complication	Clinical Features	Management
Acute haemolytic transfusion reaction *Cause: ABO incompatibility resulting in intravascular haemolysis mediated by IgM and complement activation.*	Symptoms occur within minutes of starting transfusion: fever, rigors, anxiety, flushing, chest/lumbar pain, dyspnoea, hypotension haemoglobinuria and renal failure. Disseminated Intravascular Coagulopathy (DIC)	Stop transfusion. Return donor units to lab. Take new blood sample from patient for cross-matching. Transfuse compatible RBCs. Maintain blood pressure and renal function with IV fluids.
Delayed haemolytic transfusion reaction *Cause: Allo-immunisation by previous transfusions/pregnancies results in IgG-mediated extravascular haemolysis.*	Jaundice, fever and symptoms of anaemia develop 1 week after transfusion. Patient may be asymptomatic.	Take new blood sample for direct antiglobulin test (positive). Monitor Hb. Give further transfusions for symptomatic anaemia.
Febrile non haemolytic reaction *Cause: Anti-leucocyte antibodies in allo-immunised recipients reacting against leucocytes in transfused blood. Cytokines released from donor leucocytes in platelet concentrates.*	Symptoms tend to develop towards end of infusion: fever, rigors, flushing, tachycardia. Becoming less common with use of leucocyte-depleted blood products.	Mild: slow transfusion, give Paracetamol, increase observations. Severe: stop transfusion, seek advice from transfusion laboratory. Call haematologist.
Urticaria *Cause: Auto-antibodies in recipient reacting with donor plasma proteins.*	More common during transfusion of platelets or plasma than red cells. Symptoms occur during transfusion and include urticaria and itch.	Slow transfusion, give 10mg Chlorpheniramine IV, increase observations.
Anaphylaxis *Cause: tends to occur in patients lacking IgA. Anti-IgA reacts with IgA in transfused blood.*	Life-threatening features of anaphyaxis including airway compromise and circulatory collapse.	Stop transfusion immediately. Maintain airway (call anaesthestist and consider endotracheal intubation). Give 0.5mg 1:1000 Adrenaline IM and repeat every 10 mins until improvement occurs. Give 10 mg chlorpheniramine IV. Prevent recurrence by using washed red cells or blood from IgA deficient donors.
Infective Shock *Cause: bacterial contamination of blood products e.g. Yersinia, S.aureus.*	Symptoms usually develop during infusion of first 100ml. Fever, rigors, tachycardia, hypotension, DIC. Very high mortality.	Manage septic shock with IV antibiotics and fluids (maintain BP and urine output)
Transfusion-related acute lung injury (TRALI) *Cause: reaction antibody in donor plasma with leucocytes of recipient.*	Symptoms develop during or soon after blood transfusion: fever, shortness of breath. Typical appearances on chest x-ray. Can be life-threatening.	Maintain airway. Manage as for acute respiratory distress syndrome. Give ventilatory support if necessary.

Table 8.6: An outline of the clinical features and management of common and serious complications of blood transfusion.

Top tips
- Always verify the patient
- Check and cross check with a colleague any blood products prior to administration
- Consult senior help in any signs of complications during or post transfusion

8. LOCAL ANAESTHETICS

Indications

- To provide local anaesthetic so as to gain access for structures, vessels and excision

Contraindications

- Refer to previous history of hypersensitivity reactions to local anaesthetics
- Hypovolaemia during procedure

Relevant anatomy

Local anaesthetics can be administered topically or via injection. If an injection is required, take into consideration the site and the depth of injection required. If injecting into digits do not use adrenaline.

Equipment required

Local anaesthetic, gloves, needle, syringe, and alcohol swab

Procedure

Local injection:

Field block (infiltration into tissue surrounding a given area). This should be done under supervision

1. Draw up local anaesthetic into a syringe
2. Warn patient of stinging sensation
3. Use a small 25G (Orange) needle to raise a bleb under the skin
4. Before injecting any local anaesthetic always try to aspirate to prevent inadvertent intravascular injection
5. Should you aspirate blood, alter the position of the needle, and re-aspirate until satisfied you are no longer in a vessel
6. Having raised a bleb in the skin remove the syringe and change to a larger needle
7. Using the original site of the injection one can anaesthetise deeper structures
8. Test an area by lightly applying pressure before inserting larger needles/scalpels to ensure adequate analgesia has been achieved.

For example:

• Peripheral nerve blocks - where a specific nerve is blocked:
• Epidural or Spinal anaesthesia
• Local injections into other structures i.e. joints

Topically:

Creams- e.g. EMLA ® for cannulation/venepuncture

Gel e.g. Instillagel for urethral catheterisation

Mouth spray e.g. Lidocaine for pre-endoscopy/trans-oesophageal echocardiography

Some local anaesthetics also have other uses, e.g. Lidocaine as an anti-dysrhythmic drug.

Properties of different local anaesthetics

Doses of local anaesthetics are usually stated in percentages, where 1% = 10 mg/ml, 2% = 20 mg/ml etc. For example adrenaline must NEVER be used on appendages or digits as vasoconstriction can result in ischaemic necrosis. The dose of adrenaline with the local anaesthetic should be no more than 1:200,000 (5mcg/ml) and the total dose should not exceed 500 mcg.

Preparations containing adrenaline prolong the duration of action of the local anaesthetic, increase the maximal dose and reduce bleeding.

When using any of these be sure to check:
• Name of drug
• With or without adrenaline?
• Concentration

Name of Local Anaesthetic	Onset of Action	Duration of Action	Maximum Dosage
Lidocaine	Fast: 1–2 mins	Medium 30–60 minutes	3 mg/kg or 200 mg 7 mg/kg or 500 mg if given with Adrenaline
Bupivucaine	Medium: 5–10 mins	Long 4–6 hrs	2 mg/kg, or 150 mg

Table 8.7: Properties and maximal doses of commonly used anaesthetics.

• Expiry date
• Maximum dose for patient
• Allergies

Post procedure management

Observe the patient carefully during procedure and have monitoring equipment to hand such as ECG.

Complications

Inadvertent intravascular administration can cause the following:

• Hypersensitivity reactions: mainly with esterified local anaesthetics (benzocaine, cocaine, procaine, tetracaine)
• Cardiovascular side effects (hypotension, conduction defects, arrhythmias, and asystole)
• CNS effects (light-headedness, sedation, twitching, and if severe seizures and coma)
• Symptoms of mild toxicity include peri-oral tingling, metallic taste, tinnitus, visual disturbance and slurred speech

Top tips
• Local anaesthetic administration should be done under strict supervision
• Seek senior help early when there are any signs of complication

9. PERFORMING AND INTERPRETING AN ELECTROCARDIOGRAM (ECG)

Indications

• Patients with active chest pain, syncope, palpitations, shortness of breath etc
• Provide baseline measurements pre-operatively

Contraindications

• Chest wall trauma

8. DOPS

Relevant anatomy

An ECG provides a 3D representation of the electrical activity of the heart. Consequently, accurate lead placement is essential in enabling interpretation and subsequent management. An example of correct lead placement is shown in Table 8.8 and Figure 8.9.

Lead	Electrode placement
V1	4th intercostal space just right of the sternum
V2	4th intercostal space just left of the sternum
V3	Between V2 and V4
V4	5th intercostal space mid-clavicular line
V5	5th intercostal space anterior axillary line
V6	5th intercostal space mid-axillary line
Limb leads	1 electrode is placed on each of R wrist, L wrist, L ankle and R ankle (on bony points)

Table 8.8: Sites for ECG electrode attachment

Procedure

1. Expose patient's chest and if necessary shave any excessive hair
2. Apply ECG electrodes and connect leads as described in Table 8.8
3. Ensure machine is calibrated – (speed – 25 mm/sec, voltage 1mV/cm)
4. Ask the patient to lie still. Make sure all mobile phones are switched off around the machine
5. Record the trace

Post-procedure management

This is based on the results of the ECG. Consider the need for subsequent treatment; serial ECGs and discussion with senior colleagues.

Complications

- None

Interpretation

The following is a brief system for interpreting an ECG. This is one of many such systems but all should include the following:

Ask yourself:	Is this the right ECG?
	Right patient: name, DOB, hospital number?
	Right ECG: date, time?
	What is the clinical setting?
	With or without chest pain? Palpitations? Syncope?
Check:	Calibration
	Speed (25 mm/sec)
	Amplitude (1mV/cm)

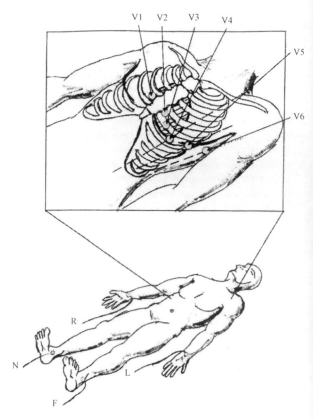

Figure 8.8: Sites for ECG electrode attachment.

Rate:	Normal, bradycardia, tachycardia?
Rhythm:	Regular, regularly irregular or irregularly irregular?
P waves:	Present? Morphology? Relation of P waves to QRS?
PR interval?	Pacing spikes?
Axis:	Normal, left, right?
QRS complexes:	Pathological Q waves? (>2 mm depth >1 mm width) Narrow or wide? (< or > than 3 mm (0.12sec)) Pattern? e.g. LBBB/RBBB Size? e.g. LVH/RVH
ST segment	Isoelectric, depressed, elevated Pattern of depression/elevation Site in relation to coronary artery territory Shape (saddle, high take off, reverse tick, etc...)
T waves	Inversion? site? associated changes?
Corrected QT interval	Causes of elongation?
Anything else?	Any particular patterns synonymous with a particular syndrome? i.e. Brugada syndrome.
Comparison with old ECGs	Old vs. new/dynamic changes.

Table 8.9: A systematic guide to interpreting ECGs.

Normal values:

PR interval, 0.12–0.2 ms

QRS complex <0.12 ms

QT interval: The QT interval depends on the heart rate, a corrected QT (QTc) can be calculated using the following formula. The normal QT is 0.30 – 0.44 (0.45 in women) seconds.

$$QTc = \frac{QT}{\sqrt{RR}}$$

Table 8.10: Normal ECG values.

Top tips

• p waves are normally negative in AVR, if they are positive this should raise suspicion of inaccurate lead placement or dextrocardia

• 'Ride your green bike' (Red, Yellow, Green, Black) is a mnemonic that can be used to remember the colour for the limb lead wires (starting right upper limb lead and working clockwise)

10. PERFORMING AND INTERPRETING SPIROMETRY

Indications

Use for the diagnosis of:

• Obstructive airways disease

  o COPD

  o Asthma (demonstrating reversibility of airways obstruction)

• Restrictive lung disease

• Monitoring disease progression/response to treatment

Spirometry is used to assess the mechanical function of the lung by measuring the total volume of air expelled from a fully-inflated lung during expiration. The forced vital capacity (FVC), forced expiratory volume in one second (FEV$_1$) and the ratio of FVC to FEV$_1$ reflect the combined function of the lung, chest wall and respiratory muscles.

Contraindications

• Pneumothorax

• Recent cerebral/abdominal aneurysm

• Recent ocular, thoracic or abdominal surgery

• Acute illness/exacerbation of obstructive airways disease can lead to misleading results

Relevant anatomy

Not applicable

Equipment required

There are a number of different types of spirometers. There are hand-held devices that generally have no graphical display but calculate FEV$_1$ and FVC and larger, fixed devices that, in addition, print out a graph (spirogram) including flow-volume loops.

Procedure

1. The patient can be sitting or standing (standing may provide better results but sitting is safer for elderly patients)

2. Ask the patient to take a deep breath in

3. Instruct the patient to seal their lips around the mouthpiece of the spirometer

4. Then ask them to blow into the mouthpiece as hard and as fast as possible, whilst continuing to exhale until they feel their lungs are empty

5. Ask the patient to repeat this process 2 or 3 times and take the best values for interpretation

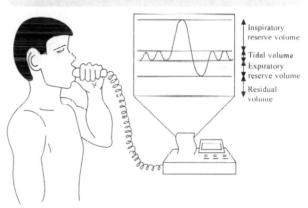

Figure 8.9: Using a spirometer and the spirograph obtained.

If reversibility of airways obstruction with bronchodilators is being tested, baseline spirometry should be first and then repeated 15 minutes after a bronchodilator is administered. Prior to testing, short-acting bronchodilators should be stopped for 6 hours, long-acting bronchodilators for 12 hours and theophylline for 24 hours.

Post procedure management

Be aware that some patients, especially the elderly may be acutely short of breath. Therefore it is important to have oxygen close to hand in such situations.

Complications

• Not applicable

Interpretation

Abnormal spirometry reflects a mechanical dysfunction of

8. DOPS

ventilation due to abnormalities in the lung, chest wall or respiratory musculature. There are two types of abnormality:

Parameter	Obstructive airways disease	Restrictive airways disease
FEV_1	• Decreased • (<80% predicted)	• Decreased
FVC	• Normal	• Decreased • (<80% predicted)
Forced expiratory ratio (FER) = (FEV_1/FVC) x 100	• < 70%	• > 70%
Examples	• COPD • Asthma • Extensive bronchiectasis • Lung tumours	• Lung parenchymal pathology e.g. fibrotic lung disease. • Chest wall deformities e.g. kyphosis, scoliosis. • Abnormalities in respiratory musculature.

Table 8.11: The difference in obstructive and restrictive airways disease.

FEV_1 is reliable and reproducible and a good predictor of morbidity and mortality. Serial measurement of FEV_1 is used to monitor disease progression.

Normal values for each of the above parameters are dependent on the patient's age, sex, height and race.

Peak Flow

Spirometry is preferred to peak expiratory flow (PEF) to confirm the diagnosis of obstructive airways disease in asthma and COPD.

However, in acute asthma exacerbations, the guidelines (*British Thoracic Society, 2008*) recommend the use of PEF to assess the severity of the exacerbation and to monitor response to treatment. PEF is most useful in this clinical situation when expressed as a percentage of the patient's previous best value. If the patient's usual PEF is not known, it can be expressed as a percentage of the patient's predicted value based on their age, sex, height and race.

> **Top tips**
> • In the acute setting, peak flow compared to the normal value for the patient is more useful than the absolute value
> • Beware of over-interpreting data if technique is poor and vice versa

11. AIRWAY CARE

Indication

• Reduced conscious level (of any cause) due to obstruction by tongue and other soft tissues
• Intra-luminal obstruction. e.g. Vomit, blood, foreign body
• Swelling of airway. e.g. Anaphylaxis, angio-oedema, epiglottitis
• Laryngospasm. e.g. epiglottitis
• Exogenous compression. e.g. tumour
• Trauma

Airway compromise is a medical emergency and if complete can rapidly result in death. When suspected, seek senior help immediately. However, foundation doctors should be familiar with simple manoeuvres and adjuncts for maintaining an airway.

When managing an acutely compromised airway give high flow oxygen, continually reassess the patient's airway after implementing any of the following manoeuvres/adjuncts, or if there is any change in the patient's condition.

Recognising a compromised airway

Look:

For chest wall movements, cyanosis, signs of respiratory distress

Listen:

For breath sounds, stridor, choking, gurgling, snoring, inability to speak in sentences

Feel:

For air movement.

If complete, you may see paradoxical respiration. A see-saw pattern of breathing, with abdominal distension and in-drawing of chest and intercostal muscles on inspiration can be seen. Whilst the reverse can be seen on expiration due to the movement of the diaphragm.

The airway should be assumed to be compromised, or potentially compromised in patients with a Glasgow Coma Scale score <8.

Procedures

Simple manoeuvres
Open mouth:

1. Look for any obstructions. If any obstructions are found they should be removed under direct vision
2. McGill's forceps can be used to remove defined objects
3. A wide bore, rigid (Yankauer) sucker is useful in removing liquids e.g. blood and vomit
4. Narrow bore, flexible suction tubes can also be used in some circumstances
5. If found carefully remove obstruction if it can be seen at all times

Head tilt/chin lift: (Figure 8.10)

1. Tilt the head back, extending the airway and reducing compression by anterior structures
2. With fingertips beneath the anterior mandible, lift the chin forward

Jaw thrust: (Figure 8.10)

1. With index and other fingers behind the angle of the mandible, lift ('thrust') the mandible anteriorly and support it with sustained pressure

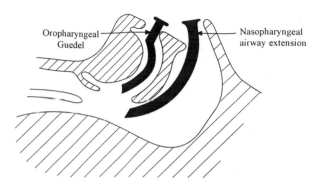

Figure 8.11: A cross section diagram of the nasopharynx demonstrating how far an oropharyngeal and a nasopharyngeal airway extends when fully inserted.

Oropharyngeal (Guedel®) airway

This is a curved flattened tube that can be inserted to lie between the tongue and hard palate.

Indications

- Useful in unconscious patients in protecting them from posterior displacement of the tongue

Contraindications

- Patients with an intact gag reflex; may lead to vomiting or laryngospasm
- Maxillofacial injuries

Relevant anatomy

Identify that there are no obstructions within the mouth

Procedure (figure 8.12)

1. Estimate the size of the guedel® required by holding different sizes parallel to head. The correct size should reach from the incisors to the angle of the jaw. (Sizes 2, 3, 4 are the most commonly used for adults)
2. Open the mouth and remove any foreign material as above
3. Initially insert the guedel® upside down. As it hits the palate rotate it 180° so that the curve is lying over the curve of the tongue
4. Reassess the patient

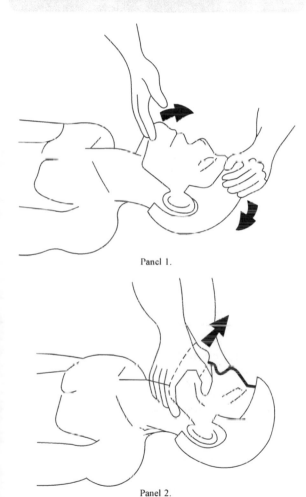

Panel 1.

Panel 2.

Figure 8.10: (Panel 1) The head tilt/chin lift manoeuvre. (Panel 2) showing the jaw thrust manoeuvre.

Adjuncts

When considering using adjuncts consider where within the airway the obstruction is and which parts of the airway the adjunct will support.

Nasopharyngeal airway

This is a flexible tube that is inserted through the nose to the oropharynx.

8. DOPS

Indications

- Useful in patients with reduced levels of consciousness but with intact gag reflexes.

Contraindications

- Known or suspected base of skull fractures
- Grossly abnormal nasal anatomy
- Severe maxillofacial injuries

Relevant anatomy

Identify that there are no obstructions or clots in the nasopharynx prior to the procedure. Examine the nasal bridges and ethmoid sinuses to rule out any inflammation of trauma

Procedure (figure 8.12)

1. Estimate the size required by holding different sized nasopharyngeal airways parallel to head. The diameter has traditionally been estimated by using a size correlating to the size of the patient's little finger. (6–8 mm are the most commonly used in adults)

2. In older models place a safety pin should be inserted across the end to prevent the airway slipping further into the nose

3. Lubricate the end of the tube, without obstructing the lumen

4. Examine both nares to look for obstruction (e.g. septal deviation, polyps) and insert on the right for preference and insert into the larger one

5. Advance directly posteriorly, (not superiorly) until the flange lies against the nares

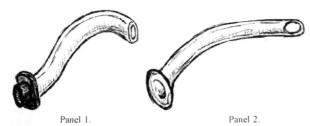

Panel 1.   Panel 2.

Figure 8.12: (Panel 1.) Oropharyngeal (Guedel®) airway. (Panel 2.) nasopharyngeal airway.

Advanced airways

A number of more advanced airways are available, including laryngeal mask airways, Combi-tube®, iGel and laryngeal tubes. These should only be used when one is adequately trained. A cufffed endo-tracheal tube is the only definitive airway.

Tracheostomy tubes:

A tracheostomy is a procedure that creates a direct opening into the trachea, creating a surgical airway. The patency of this surgical opening is maintained by the placement of a tracheostomy tube, creating a stoma.

Tracheostomy tubes come in a variety of different sizes. When first inserted, a tube with a lumen roughly ¾ the size of the patient's tracheal lumen should be used. As the patient is weaned off their tracheostomy, the size of the tube is gradually decreased to allow greater movement of air around the tube through the upper airways when the tracheostomy lumen has finally plugged.

Indications

- Ventilation in the presence of any obstruction of the upper airways is an emergency case
- Prolonged mechanical ventilation in patients with respiratory failure
- Severe trauma and/or burns around the head and neck area
- Subcutaneous emphysema

Contraindications

- None

Relevant anatomy

Identify the position of the cricoid cartilage, which is located inferiorly to the thyroid cartilage.

Tracheostomy care:

Aspects of tracheostomy care include:

- Care of stoma site and changing tracheostomy dressings
- Monitoring cuff pressures
- Suctioning
- Changing a tracheostomy tube

There are many different types of tracheostomy tube, which serve a variety of different functions as highlighted in Table 8.12:

Care of tracheostomy site and changing dressings:

The stoma site should be cleaned daily to prevent build-up of secretions and debris, so as to maintain healthy skin around stoma and to prevent infection.

- Prior to cleaning, be sure to wash hands and wear gloves.
- Using an aseptic technique, remove the old dressing and examine the site carefully for evidence of any skin irritation and infection.
- Carefully clean the skin around the tracheostomy with sterile saline and gauze
- Dry the skin and replace with a new tracheostomy dressing.

Older tracheostomies may not require dressings so long as the skin appears intact.

Monitoring cuff pressures:

Patients with cuffed tracheostomies often require careful

Tracheostomy tube	Description
Cuffed	• Allows positive pressure mechanical ventilation and protects against aspiration of gastric contents. • Cuff pressures should be monitored meticulously and cuffs deflated regularly to reduce risk of tracheal stenosis.
Uncuffed	• Should be used in preference to cuffed tubes if the cuff is not necessary. • Allows movement of air around tracheostomy tube to facilitate speaking and weaning.
Fenestrated	• Additional opening in body of tube to allow air to pass through tube when external opening is plugged i.e. for speaking and weaning. • Fenestrations are often not in the correct place and can cause irritation and granulation of the tracheal mucosa.
Double-cannula tube	• This consists of an outer (permanent) tube and an inner tube which can be removed for short periods of time to be cleaned (or replaced). • It maintains patency of tracheostomy lumen for longer.
Single-cannula tube	• Single-lumen tube without an inner cannula. • They need to be changed more frequently to maintain patency of airway.

Table 8.12: The different types of tracheostomy tubes.

monitoring of their cuff pressures and regular cuff deflation is required, so as to reduce the risk of tracheal stenosis. Cuff pressures should be checked twice daily using a manometer. Cuff pressures should be kept within the range 15–20 mmHg. Daily cuff deflation also allows for the removal of secretions that may accumulate above the cuff.

Suctioning:

Suctioning of tracheostomy tubes is required when build-up of respiratory secretions within the tube lumen occurs. The frequency of suctioning varies with the ability of the patient to clear their secretions through expectorating. Luminal obstruction increases the work of breathing and causes respiratory distress e.g. tachypnoea, stridor, sweating, tachycardia, and decreased oxygen saturations.

Procedure for suction of tracheotomy tube

1. Prior to suctioning, be sure to wash your hands and wear gloves
2. Open sterile suctioning catheter and attach to the suction tubing using non-touch technique
3. Insert suction catheter gently into tracheostomy tube to approximately one-third of the catheter length
4. Start suctioning as catheter is removed by placing thumb over suction port
5. Suction should not be applied for longer than 10 seconds to avoid hypoxia
6. If further suctioning is required, a fresh suction catheter should be used.
7. Repeat suctioning until airway is clear
8. Observe and document the amount of secretions, colour and consistency and document this in the notes

Changing a tracheostomy tube

Tracheostomy tubes need to be changed when the lumen becomes blocked with secretions in order to maintain airway patency. When single-cannula tracheostomies become blocked with secretions, the whole tube needs to be removed and a new tracheostomy placed through the stoma. This should be done with two people present; one to change the tracheostomy, the other to provide suction.

Double-cannula tracheostomies have an inner tube which can be removed and, either cleaned, or replaced with a new inner tube, whilst the outer tube remains in situ. The inner tube should be removed during exhalation and replaced within 15 minutes.

Procedure for changing a tracheotomy tube

1. Wash hands and wear gloves
2. Prepare trolley with new tracheostomy tubes (1 tube same size as tube being replaced, 1 a size smaller), lubricant gel, sterile saline, gauze, tracheal dilators, suction equipment
3. Lubricate the new tube with plenty of gel
4. Position patient in upright or semi-recumbent position with neck slightly extended (place rolled towel under shoulders if necessary to help extend neck)
5. Remove old tracheostomy tube while asking patient to breathe out
6. Insert new, clean the tracheostomy tube using 'up and over' action
7. Remove introducer from the tracheostomy tube (to allow patient to breathe).
8. Replacing a tracheostomy tube will cause patient to cough which may dislodge the tube – **do not let go of tube until secured in place**
9. If replacing a double-cannula tracheostomy, place an inner tube in position once an outer tube has been inserted
10. Secure the tracheostomy tube in place with tapes
11. Administer suction through tracheostomy tube if required
12. If replacing the cuffed tube, inflate the cuff to pressure of 15–20 mmHg (check with manometer)
13. Always clean around the tracheostomy site with normal saline and gauze and apply the tracheostomy dressing if required

8. DOPS

Post procedure management

Always ensure thorough suction and cleaning of the tracheostomy site is done regularly. It is important to liaise with the nursing staff with regards to the ongoing management of such patients on a daily basis. Such patients are often better monitored in a High Dependency Unit (HDU)/Intensive Care Unit (ICU) setting.

Complications

- Mucus plugging can often occur in patients with a tracheostomy. This may cause acute respiratory distress for the patient.

Top tips

- Always regularly use suction and clean the tracheostomy sites
- Consult senior help from other specialities such as Ear, Nose and Throat (ENT) at an early stage for such patients

12. NASOGASTRIC TUBE (NGT) INSERTION

Indications

- Feeding (Ryle's tube)
- Decompression of stomach during bowel obstruction
- Patients who have an increased risk of aspirating
- Gastric lavage

Contraindications

- Known or suspected base of skull or facial fractures
- Suspected oesophageal perforation
- Grossly abnormal nasal anatomy; patients with large nasal polyps or adenoids

Relevant anatomy

The nasal cavity extends directly posteriorly from the nares to the nasopharynx. The tube should be inserted directly posteriorly and not superiorly. The approximate distance from the nares to the stomach is 45 cm.

Equipment required

NG tube, gloves, lubricant, glass of water, 50 ml syringe and litmus paper to confirm correct positioning

Procedure

1. Sit the patient up, slightly extending the neck
2. Inspect the nares for deviation of septum/asymmetry
3. Estimate the length from the nares to the stomach by holding the tube along its course externally

4. Lubricate the tip and the first few centimetres of the tube, avoiding blocking the lumen
5. Insert into the nostril and advance directly posteriorly
6. Whilst advancing, ask the patient to take sip of water and to hold it in their mouth
7. Request the patient to swallow and, as the patient swallows, advance the tube down oesophagus
8. Continue to advance the tube until 10–20 cm beyond estimated distance to the stomach (usually ~ 60–70 cm total)
9. Remove guide-wire if present
10. Either place cap onto the end of NG tube (if being used for feeding) or attach a drainage bag (if being used to decompress stomach)
11. Secure the tube in place by taping to nose +/- face

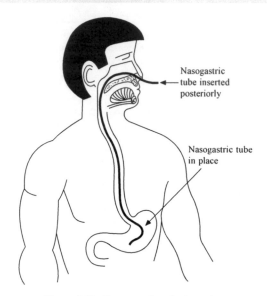

Nasogastric tube inserted posteriorly

Nasogastric tube in place

Figure 8.13: Nasogastric tube insertion.

Post-procedure management

Confirm correct positioning:

- Connect syringe, attempt aspiration, and test aspirate pH with a litmus paper.
  - Acidic pH is generally confirmatory of correct positioning.
  - If unable to aspirate consider advancing the NG tube by 1–2 cm whilst simultaneously withdrawing the syringe and retrying.
- If unsure obtain a Chest X-ray (CXR) with a view of the stomach.
  - The tips of the narrow bore tubes may not be visible on CXR and a new tube should be placed, leaving the guide-wire in situ.

o Do not attempt to re-insert a guide wire due to the risk of perforation.
- Although commonly done on the wards. Injecting 5–10 ml of air into the tube whilst auscultating for bubbling with stethoscope placed over stomach is not generally considered adequate for confirmation of position.

Complications

- Discomfort, pain, gagging
- Bleeding (at any site, but particularly nose)
- Failure to correctly place tube e.g. placement in trachea or bronchi
- Perforation of oesophagus and/or stomach
- Electrolyte imbalance if rapid decompression of stomach
- Oesophagitis
- Nasal or retropharyngeal necrosis

Top tips

- Keeping the patient calm, informed and reassured is essential in maintaining patient co-operation during this procedure
- Ensuring the patient is in an upright position aids insertion
- Place the tube in the fridge before hand as this helps maintain the curvature of the tube
- Advance the tube slowly, allowing the patient to get used to the sensation
- If the tube will not advance through the nasal cavity, the nostril is probably blocked. Stop and try the other side
- Beware of patients with a reduced conscious level as they may lack gag responses that usually prevent tracheal intubation
- If in doubt about placement ask for a CXR

13. URETHRAL CATHETERISATION

Indications

- To relieve urinary retention
- To accurately monitor urine output

Urethral catheterisation involves passing a flexible tube per urethra into the urinary bladder allowing drainage of urine.

Contraindications

- Established or suspected urethral trauma

Relevant anatomy

The anatomy of the male urethra is shown in Figure 8.14. The female urethra is shorter and straight. The external urethral meatus is immediately anterior to the vagina within the vestibule.

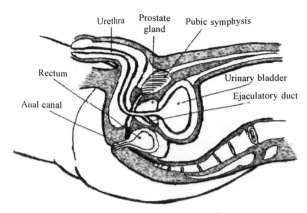

Figure 8.14: Anatomy of the male urethra.

Equipment required

Sterile gloves (x2), catheter pack (sterile drape, galli pot, cotton wool, gauze, kidney dish-exact contents vary between trusts), sterile normal saline, foley catheter, Lidocaine/local anaesthetic gel, 10 ml syringe, 10 ml sterile water) and catheter bag (urometer, day/leg/night bags).

Catheter types:

Male catheters are longer than female catheters due to the greater length of the urethra. Catheter sizes are quoted in Ch/French gauge, with the larger the number, the larger the diameter of the catheter. In most cases a 12–14G is appropriate for males. Catheters used for intermittent self catheterisation are usually narrower and do not have a balloon.

Short term catheters are latex with or without Polytetrafluroethylene (PTFE) coating and should be removed or changed after two weeks. However, long term catheters can remain in situ for up to 12 weeks. In particular, patients with, or who are at risk of clot retention (e.g. post urological surgery, gross haematuria) should have a triple lumen/three way catheter inserted, the third lumen allowing irrigation. The minimal size is 18Ch.

Other types of urethral catheter include, Caudé catheters (angled tip) and Teeman catheters (tapered end) useful for negotiating enlarged prostates.

Procedure

This is a sterile procedure; the following describes a two gloved technique.

1. Prepare equipment on clean trolley
2. Expose the patient
3. Put on two pairs of sterile gloves
4. Place drape over the area
5. Place gauze around shaft of the penis
6. Whilst holding penis in one hand, retract foreskin, clean glans with sterile normal saline starting centrally and working around

8. DOPS

7. Insert local anaesthetic gel into the external urethral meatus

8. Hold penis upright so as to limit leak of gel and wait for 1–2 mins

9. Remove outer pair of gloves

10. Insert Foley catheter into urethra to bi/trifurcation whilst holding the penis taut, perpendicular to the body

11. Once inserted urine should start to drain from the catheter

12. Inflate balloon with 10 ml sterile water, whilst observing patients face for evidence of pain

13. Withdraw catheter until resistance felt

14. Connect to catheter bag

15. **Replace foreskin**

Female catheters can be directly inserted, after cleansing of the meatus, with simple lubrication of the catheter.

Post-procedure management

Document the procedure, note details regarding the catheter (size, type) and describe the sterile nature of the technique. Also note the volume of sterile water instilled into the balloon, foreskin replacement and any complications e.g. bleeding. Remember to note and document the residual volume of urine upon insertion of the catheter. Be aware of your local trust policy in regards to prophylactic antibiotic cover during this procedure, especially in the elderly who are at a higher risk of developing urinary tract infection/sepsis.

Complications

• Infection: urethritis, cystitis, pyelonephritis, bacteraemia, septicaemia

• Bleeding

• Paraphimosis

• Urethral perforation

• Creation of a false passage

• Urethral stricture – with long term use

Top tips

• Place kidney dish on bed between the patient's legs so as to catch urine prior to connecting catheter to bag

• If unable to pass catheter try again with a larger catheter, and adjust the positioning of penis

• If struggling to identify the urethral meatus in females, warn the patient, insert index finger into vagina elevating the anterior vulva. Guide the catheter along the finger into the urethra

---

14. LUMBAR PUNCTURE

Indications

• A diagnostic test for pathology affecting the central nervous system e.g. meningitis and multiple sclerosis.

• Provides therapy e.g. in benign intracranial hypertension.

Contraindications

• Raised CSF pressure associated with 'brain shift' e.g. secondary to focal lesion (due to risk of cerebral herniation). Detected by CT brain.

• Localised sepsis

• Bleeding diathesis (due to increased risk of epidural haematoma (check and document platelets, PT, INR/APTT. Avoid if INR>1.5)

• Cardio-respiratory compromise if positioning is likely to worsen this

• Previous spinal surgery/spinal deformity (relative contraindication)

Relevant anatomy

Lumbar puncture is typically performed at the level of L3/4 or L4/5 well below the termination of the spinal cord at L1. (See Figure 8.15). The needle is inserted through the ligaments of the spine into the subarachnoid space as shown in the Figure 8.16.

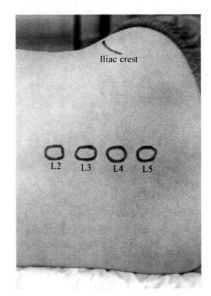

Figure 8.15: Surface anatomy landmarks for lumbar puncture.

Equipment

Sterile gloves, sterile gown, sterile dressing pack, sterile cleaning solution, lidocaine 1%, 10 ml syringe, 25G (orange) and 21G

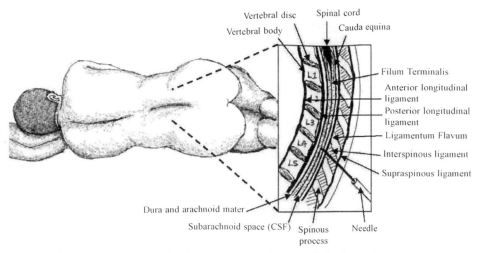

Figure 8.16: Insertion of lumbar puncture needle through the interspinous space.

(green) needles (for local anaesthesia), spinal needle, manometer, sample pots (label 1, 2, 3), fluoride oxalate (grey) sample tube (for glucose), sterile dressing.

Procedure

This is a sterile procedure

1. Position the patient in a lateral position with hips and knees flexed in the foetal position
2. Identify the landmarks as stated previously
3. Clean the skin with a preparation solution e.g. iodine, Chlorhexidine
4. Inject local anaesthetic initially subcutaneously, then deeper
5. Insert lumbar puncture needle into interspinous space, aiming towards umbilicus
6. Advance needle until it 'gives' once is passes through the ligamentum flavum
7. Remove stylet and observe for drainage of CSF
8. Attach manometer and wait for CSF to reach a steady level
9. Fill sample bottles
10. Replace stylet into needle
11. Remove needle and apply dressing
12. Send samples for analysis (MC+S, glucose, protein, others e.g. oligoclonal bands, AFB....)
13. Consider the need for matched serum samples, e.g. glucose, oligoclonal bands

Post-procedure management

Ensure the patient is kept under supervision as complications can occur within 48 hours.

Complications

- Headache often occurs (approximately one third of all patients) within 48 hours post lumbar puncture
- Bleeding: local, epidural haematoma
- Infection: epidural abscess
- Pain: local or referred
- Damage to local structures e.g. nerves, in particular nerve root, cauda equina, and spinal cord
- Cerebral herniation
- Subarachnoid epidermal cysts as a result of introducing a skin plug

Management for post-lumbar puncture headache:

- Advise the patient to lie on their backs for a few hours post-procedure and keep well hydrated
- Caffeine may be of benefit but further studies are required before it can be recommended as a routine treatment for post-lumbar puncture headache
- A blood patch can be performed by the anaesthetist for severe cases
- Remember to consider other causes of headache

Interpretation

This will depend on the clinical context, e.g. suspected meningitis vs. suspected multiple sclerosis. Table 8.13 below provides an example on how to interpret CSF results.

8. DOPS

Parameters	Normal	Bacterial	Viral	TB
Appearance	Clear	Cloudy/purulent	Clear	Clear/turbid
Opening pressure	7-20cm	High	-	-
Protein	<0.4g/L	>1.0g/L	0.5-0.9g/L	>1.0g/L (often much higher)
Glucose	>70% of plasma glucose	Very low	>70% plasma glucose	<50% plasma glucose
White Cells	<4x109/L	5-2000x109 Neutrophils	5-1000x109 Lymphocytes	5-500x109 Lymphocytes
Other useful tests	-	Gram stain/Culture	Viral PCR	AFB staining/culture/PCR

Table 8.13: How to interpretate a CSF result

The immuno-compromised patient:

Immuno-compromised patients, such as HIV patients, can develop CNS infections caused by organisms which are not commonly pathogenic in the disease process. These include:

- *Cryptococcus neoformans*: can be cultured from the CSF or visualised directly using the Indian ink stain. Antigen can also be detected in CSF using latex agglutination techniques.
- *Toxoplasmosis gondii* and *Aspergillus:* tend to cause intracerebral abscess/cyst formation which can be detected using CT / MRI scanning of the brain.

Space-occupying lesions such as abscesses can cause localised cerebral oedema, which can later promote mid-line shift of the brain. Hence, a CT brain is of paramount importance prior to performing an LP.

Top tips

- Position is the key to success. Ensure the iliac spines are level and perpendicular to the bed and the knees are flexed as much as possible. Where identification of landmarks is difficult consider performing the LP with the patient sat upright, leant forward over a pillow
- Pain being felt to shoot down each leg indicates you likely to be very close to a nerve, therefore withdraw needle slightly and subtly alter the angulation prior to reinsertion
- Always continue to reassure the patient
- Injecting large quantities of local anaesthetic can distort the anatomy and make the procedure more difficult
- 500 red cells per 1 white cell is suggestive of a bloody tap

15. ASPIRATION OF PLEURAL FLUID OR AIR

Aspiration of pleural fluid

Indications

- Diagnostic testing
- Therapeutic removal of fluid

Contraindications

- Localised skin infection
- Development of pneumothorax/tension pneumothorax

Relevant anatomy

The recommended site for a pleural aspiration is approximately 1–2 intercostal spaces below the upper limit of the pleural effusion, which is determined by percussion and/or ausculation within the mid-clavicular line. The needle should always be inserted above the upper edge of the rib to avoid damaging the neurovascular bundle.

Current NICE guidelines actively encourage the use of ultrasound guidance to mark the site for or guide aspiration for small or loculated pleural effusions.

Equipment required

Sterile dressing pack (gallipot, cotton wool, sterile drape), sterile cleansing solution, sterile gloves, gauze, 1% lidocaine, syringes (10 ml, 20 ml), orange needle (25G), green needle (21G), universal sample pots, fluoride oxalate (grey) sample tube, heparinised (ABG) syringe, dressing

Procedure

This is a sterile procedure:

1. Prepare the equipment on a clean trolley
2. Position the patient
3. Percuss and auscultate the chest to identify suitable site for aspiration, which can be marked
4. Put on the sterile gloves
5. Clean the skin with a preparation solution e.g. iodine, Chlorhexidine
6. Inject local anaesthetic, initially subcutaneously using a 25 gauge (orange) needle, then deeper down to the parietal pleura using a 21 gauge (green) needle
7. Attach the green needle (21G) onto the 20 ml syringe, then advance the needle through anaesthetised skin; always pulling back on plunger whilst advancing

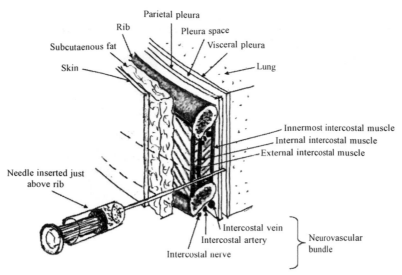

Figure 8.17: Rib and neurovascular bundle.

7. Attach the green needle (21G) onto the 20 ml syringe, then advance the needle through anaesthetised skin; always pulling back on plunger whilst advancing

8. Stop advancing the needle when pleural fluid is aspirated into the syringe

9. Aspirate 20 ml of pleural fluid into the syringe

10. Remove the needle and the syringe and dispose of them in the sharps bin

11. Apply the sterile dressing

12. Distribute the pleural fluid into the sterile sample pots, fluoride oxalate (grey) sample tube for measuring glucose and heparinised (ABG) syringe for measuring pH

13. Document in the notes

If a therapeutic aspiration is required, insert 14G IV cannula (rather than 21G needle) into the intercostal space. Withdraw the stylet (or use 17 gauge (white) needle) and attach a 3-way tap, closing the pleural aspiration kit (consisting of tubing attached to bag for collection of fluid). Attach a 50ml syringe to the 3-way tap and aspirate 50ml of pleural fluid at a time into the bag.

Post-procedure management

Document the procedure, noting the gross appearance of pleural fluid, pH and if further tests were requested.

Send the pleural fluid aspirates for analysis, including:

- Biochemistry: protein and Lactate Dehdyrogenase (LDH)
- Microbiology (Gram stain, M,C&S and AAFB)
- Cytology
- pH (in heparinised (ABG) syringe) if empyema suspected
- Glucose (in fluoride oxalate (grey-top) sample tube)

Send matched serum samples for LDH, protein and glucose. Request a post-procedural CXR.

Complications

- Pneumothorax
- Haemothorax
- Damage to local structures (including intercostal neurovascular bundle)
- Infection e.g. empyema
- Removal of excessive volumes of pleural fluid can result in large fluid shifts, causing haemodynamic instability or (re-expansion +/- neurogenic) pulmonary oedema. This risk is reduced if fluid is removed slowly and if a maximum of 1.5L is removed at any one time.

Interpretation

Exudate vs. transudate:

Pleural effusions can be divided into exudates and transudates based on biochemical testing

- Pleural fluid protein > 35g/L = Exudate
- Pleural fluid protein < 25g/L = Transudate

If pleural fluid protein is between 25–35g/L, *Light's* criteria should be applied to more accurately distinguish between an exudate and a transudate:

- **Light's criteria consists of:**

  A pleural fluid is an exudate if 1 of the following 3 criteria are met:

  ○ Pleural fluid:serum total protein ratio ≥ 0.5

  ○ Pleural fluid:serum LDH ratio ≥ 0.6

  ○ Pleural fluid LDH ≥ two thirds upper limit normal for serum LDH

8. DOPS

Causes of Transudative pleural effusions include:

(result of high venous pressures, hypo-albuminaemia, 'failures')

- Cardiac Failure
- Liver failure
- Nephrotic syndrome (renal failure)
- Protein losing enteropathy (gut failure)
- Meig's syndrome (R pleural effusion, ovarian fibroma)
- Hypothyroidism
- If milky – Chylothorax

Causes of Exudative pleural effusions include:

(result of increased capillary leakage)

- Neoplasia: Primary, secondary, haematological
- Infection: Parapneumonic effusion, empyema, Tuberculosis (TB), other
- Infarction: Pulmonary Embolus(PE) and Tuberculosis
- Inflammation: Connective tissue diseases e.g. Rheumatoid Arthritis (RA), SLE

Empyema:

An empyema is the accumulation of pus in the pleural cavity

The criteria for an empyema consists of the following:

- Grossly purulent pleural fluid
- Fluid pH <7.2
- Fluid glucose <2.2 mmol/L
- Fluid LDH >1000 IU/l

Top tips
- Correct positioning of patient is the key to successful pleural aspiration
- The patient must be comfortable
- Ideally, the patient should be sitting, leaning forwards over a table (resting on a pillow for comfort) with his/her arms folded in front of them
- Inform nursing staff to monitor patient's oxygen saturations post procedure
- Always remember to review your patient half an hour to one hour post procedure

Aspiration of air

Indications

- Small pneumothorax

The following applies for aspiration of a spontaneous primary small pneumothorax (occurring in a patient without underlying lung disease with no apparent precipitating event). A primary spontaneous pneumothorax should be aspirated only if the patient

is symptomatic with respiratory comprise and/or a rim of air >2 cm as demonstrated on chest radiograph. See Figure 8.18.

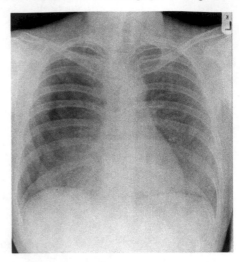

Figure 8.18: A CXR of a right pneumothorax

A spontaneous secondary pneumothorax (occurring in a patient with underlying lung disease) is usually managed with an intercostal drain insertion, unless the pneumothorax is very small and the patient is asymptomatic and under the age of 50; in which case a single attempt at simple aspiration is appropriate.

Contraindications

- If the patient is asymptomatic and has a rim of air <2 cm on chest radiograph, aspiration should not be attempted. These patients should be considered for discharge with early outpatient review. (See BTS guidelines for management of spontaneous pneumothorax, Thorax 2003).

Relevant anatomy

Attempt to identify the areas to be aspirated through auscultating and percussing the lung fields. However no procedure should be attempted until a CXR has been seen.

Equipment required

A dressing pack, alcohol/chlorhexidine, gown and sterile gloves, local anaesthetic, large gauge venflon, 50 ml syringe and three way tap.

Procedure

1. Locate the site to be aspirated, which is the 2nd or 3rd intercostal space at the mid-clavicular line or the 4th or 5th intercostal space anterior axillary line
2. Put on sterile gloves
3. Clean the skin with the cleansing solution
4. Insert the 16 gauge (grey) cannula over superior rib margin into the pleural space

5. Remove needle and connect to a three-way tap and a 50 ml syringe

6. Slowly aspirate the air

7. Stop when resistance is felt or when the patient coughs excessively

8. Repeat a CXR following the procedure, so as to confirm successful aspiration of air

9. Document in the notes

Post-procedure management

Document the procedure. Attach a oxygen saturation probe to the patient during and post procedure.

Complications

- Thoracic organ injury
- Wing scapula due to long thoracic nerve of Bell damage
- Chylothorax due to lymphatic damage

> **Top tips**
> - Take time to carefully identify the area for aspiration on the CXR, if in doubt seek help
> - Prepare all equipment prior to positioning the patient
> - Attach oxygen saturation probe during and post procedure
> - Liaise with nursing staff on when to be alerted if patient's saturations drop or there is any change in the patient's condition

16. CHEST DRAIN INSERTION

Indications

- Pneumothorax
- Haemothorax
- Empyema
- Symptomatic large pleural effusions

Contraindications

- Localised skin infection
- Uncorrected bleeding diathesis/anticoagulation
- Uncertainty over diagnosis or site (e.g. bullous disease vs. pneumothorax, unable to aspirate fluid).

Relevant anatomy

The preferred site for the insertion of a chest drain is in the mid-axillary line, within the 'safe triangle' (see Figure 8.19). This is a triangle bordered by the anterior border of Latissimus dorsi, the lateral border of pectoralis major, a line just above the horizontal level of the nipple with the apex below the axilla. This position minimises risk to underlying structures and avoids excessive scarring.

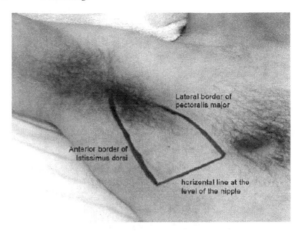

Figure 8.19: Triangle of safety.

Ultrasound guidance:

Ultrasound can be useful in guiding chest drain insertion if the pleural effusion cannot be confidently localised using chest x-rays and clinical examination (see Figure 8.20). This is particularly useful for empyemas and loculated pleural effusions as the diaphragm can be easily visualised and fluid loculi and areas of pleural thickening clearly defined.

Radiologists can mark the site for drain insertion. Alternatively, it can be used by physicians at the time of the chest drain insertion, through using a portable scanning machine. This increases the positional accuracy of drain placement and reduces the risk of complications such as pneumothorax.

The British Thoracic Society guidelines recommend the use of ultrasound for chest drain insertion if air or fluid cannot be aspirated at the time of blind insertion or if the effusion is very small.

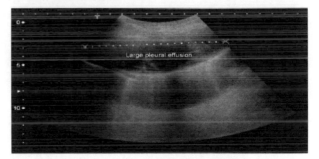

Figure 8.20: An ultrasound image of a large right pleural effusion (marked between two crosses.) *Courtesy of Dr Raj Vimal*

Equipment required

Chest drain pack (containing gallipot, gauze, sterile drapes, forceps, scissors), Seldinger chest drain kit (containing Seldinger needle, guide-wire, dilator(s), chest drain, 3-way tap and connectors), bottle with underwater seal, sterile gloves, sterile cleansing solution, 1% lidocaine, syringes (5 ml, 10 ml), orange needle (25G), green needle (21G), suture, scalpel, sterile dressings, plenty of gauze.

Procedure

The following describes the Seldinger technique for chest drain insertion. In trauma and some other instances 'surgical' insertion technique may be required/used. For full details see BTS guidelines for insertion.

This is a sterile procedure and should ideally be performed with an assistant present:

1. Give pre-medication to prevent/reduce patient stress (Benzodiazepines are particularly useful in this scenario unless contraindicated)
2. Prepare all equipment on a clean trolley
3. Position the patient
4. Confirm location of the pleural effusion by auscultating and percussing. Remember to check the CXR.
5. Identify the anatomical landmarks (see relevant anatomy) to determine the site for the chest drain insertion
6. Put on sterile gloves
7. Clean the skin with a sterile preparation solution e.g. iodine, Chlorhexidine
8. Use sterile drapes to create a sterile field
9. Infiltrate the skin with local anaesthetic, initially subcutaneously using a orange (25G) needle, then deeper down to the parietal pleura using a green (21G) needle
10. Attach the Seldinger needle to a 10 ml syringe; insert needle into intercostal space and advance slowly through the anaesthetised skin, pulling back on plunger all the time
11. Stop advancing the needle when the pleural fluid or air is aspirated into the syringe
12. Whilst keeping the needle still, remove the syringe and pass the guide-wire through the needle
13. Always keep hold of the guide wire
14. When half the guide-wire has been inserted into pleural space, remove needle
15. Using a scalpel, make a small skin incision immediately adjacent to the guide-wire
16. Pass the dilator along the guide-wire and advance through the skin into pleural space
17. Remove the dilator (and repeat above step with the larger dilators if necessary), leaving the guide-wire in place in the end
18. Pass the chest drain over the guide-wire and advance through the skin into the pleural space
19. Remove the guide-wire
20. Attach a 3-way tap to end of chest drain so that it is turned 'off' towards the chest
21. Suture the drain to the skin; further local anaesthetic may be required for this
22. Connect the bottle with the underwater seal to the 3-way tap
23. Open the 3-way tap such that pleural space communicates directly with the under-water seal
24. Confirm functioning of the chest drain by observing water in the bottle to be swinging/bubbling +/- fluid draining.
25. Furthermore secure the chest drain insertion site with gauze and sterile dressing
26. Document in the notes

1. Clean the skin with Chlorhexidine and inject local anaesthetic all the way up to the parietal pleura.

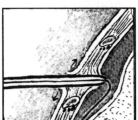

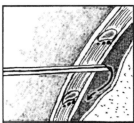

2. Using a Seldinger needle enter the pleural space and insert a guide wire in place.

3. Use a dilator along the guide wire to make the hole larger. This may follow the use of a scalpel to make a larger incision first.

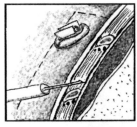

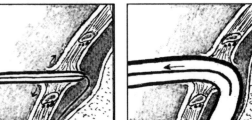

4. When the hole is large enough insert the chest drain and then remove the guide wire. Ensure that fluid is draining before doing this.

Figure 8.21: Chest drain insertion.

Procedure for flushing chest drains

1. Wearing sterile gloves clean the ports of the three-way tap
2. Connect a syringe containing 20–50 mls of sterile 0.9% saline
3. Turn 3-way tap to allowing flushing into the drain
4. Slowly inject saline into pleural cavity (minimal resistance and no pain should be felt)
5. Aspirate the same amount of fluid injected into the cavity
6. Close the tap prior to disconnecting the syringe
7. Document in the notes

Procedure for the removal of a chest drain

1. Chest drains should be removed during expiration
2. Wearing sterile gloves remove the dressings around the drain
3. Cut the suture and whilst asking the patient to exhale firmly pull the chest drain out
4. With your other hand, apply sterile gauze to the wound and secure in place with sterile dressings
5. Arrange a follow-up CXR to rule out pneumothorax or surgical emphysema
6. If the wound is large or there is considerable bleeding consider the need for sutures
7. Document in the notes

Pigtail drains:

Pigtail catheters are typically inserted under radiological guidance e.g. ultrasound. They can be used to drain loculated pleural effusions or empyemas. Once inserted, there is a string, which is pulled tight and wrapped around the catheter to lock it in position. This draws the tip of the catheter into a loose coil, resembling a pig-tail (hence the catheter's name), which helps to keep the drain in the correct position and prevents accidental dislodgement. Before removing this type of drain, it is important to remember to release the string lock so that the catheter resumes its original linear shape as it is removed. Failure to do this will result in trauma to surrounding tissues as the catheter is removed.

Complications

- Pneumothorax/tension pnemothorax
- Haemothorax
- Damage to local structures (intercostal neurovascular bundle, liver, spleen, visceral puncture)
- Infection e.g. local or pleural (empyema)

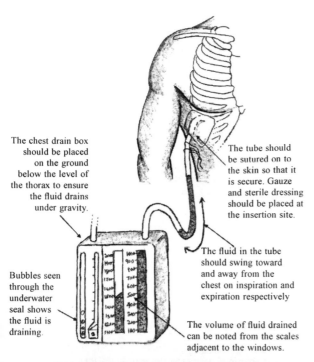

Figure 8.22: Chest drain with drainage bottle.

The chest drain box should be placed on the ground below the level of the thorax to ensure the fluid drains under gravity.

The tube should be sutured on to the skin so that it is secure. Gauze and sterile dressing should be placed at the insertion site.

Bubbles seen through the underwater seal shows the fluid is draining.

The fluid in the tube should swing toward and away from the chest on inspiration and expiration respectively

The volume of fluid drained can be noted from the scales adjacent to the windows.

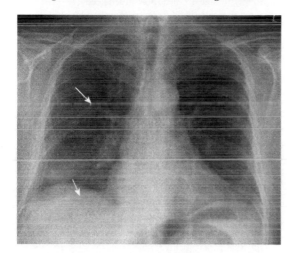

Figure 8.23: Correctly inserted left chest drain.

Post-procedure management

Confirm correct positioning of chest drain:

- Observe water in bottle for swinging/bubbling
- Determine whether the fluid or air is draining from the pleural space
- Obtain post-procedure CXR

Document the procedure, noting size of chest drain inserted and any complications encountered e.g. multiple passes, pneumothorax, bleeding etc.

8. DOPS

- Removal of excessive volumes of pleural fluid can result in large fluid shifts, causing haemodynamic instability or re-expansion +/- neurogenic pulmonary oedema. This risk is reduced if a maximum of 1.5L is removed at any one time

Top tips

- Correct positioning of patient is the key to successful insertion of a chest drain
- Two positions are commonly used: The patient can be sitting, leaning forwards over a table with his/her arms folded in front of him/her. Alternatively, they can be supine, lying at an angle of about 45° with their ipsilateral arm above and behind their head
- Infiltrate the skin and pleura with an adequate amount of local anaesthetic to minimise discomfort during the procedure
- For pneumothoraces the bevel should be angled up and for effusions it should be angled down
- Do not try to advance guide-wire if resistance is felt as it may not be in the pleural space. Remove wire, re-position needle and try again

17. ASPIRATION OF ASCITIC FLUID

Indications

- Diagnosis of new-onset ascites
- Diagnosis of suspected spontaneous bacterial peritonitis

Contraindications

- Localised skin infection
- Uncorrected bleeding diathesis/anticoagulation
- Acute abdomen
- Bowel obstruction
- Pregnancy
- Urinary retention with distended bladder

Relevant anatomy

The patient's abdomen should be examined to confirm the presence of ascites (shifting dullness +/- fluid thrill). Aspiration should be performed at an area of dullness ideally at the level of the umbilicus, 3–4 cm lateral to the mid-inguinal line. This avoids intra-abdominal organs such as the liver and spleen as well as more mid-line structures such as the bladder and abdominal wall vessels (superior and inferior epigastric vessels).

Avoid inserting a needle close to old abdominal wall scars as adhesions of bowel to abdominal wall are more likely at these sites.

If a portable ultrasound is available, this can be useful to confirm the presence of a pocket of ascitic fluid directly below proposed site for aspiration and to rule out the presence of small bowel

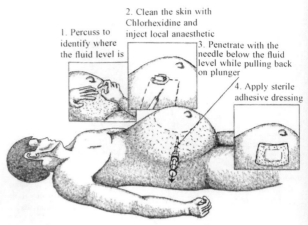

Figure 8.24: A diagrammatic representation of ascitic fluid aspiration.

adhesions at this site. If concerned a formal ultrasound guided aspiration should be arranged.

Equipment required

Sterile dressing pack (gallipot, cotton wool, sterile drape), sterile cleansing solution, sterile gloves, gauze, 1% lidocaine, syringes (10 ml, 20 ml), orange needle (25G), green needle (21G), universal sample pots, fluoride oxalate (grey) sample tube, dressing.

Procedure

This is a sterile procedure:

1. Prepare equipment on a clean trolley
2. Percuss the abdomen to identify location of the ascites and determine a suitable site for aspiration, which can be marked
3. Position patient lying flat on their back with the bed tilted slightly towards the side of the aspiration
4. Put on sterile gloves
5. Clean the skin with a preparation solution e.g. iodine, Chlorhexidine
6. Inject local anaesthetic (see details above), initially subcutaneously using orange (25G) needle, then deeper towards the peritoneum using green (21G) needle
7. Using a green needle (21G) attached to a 20 ml syringe, advance the needle through the anaesthetised skin, perpendicular to the abdominal wall, pulling back on the plunger all the time
8. Stop advancing the needle when ascitic fluid is aspirated into the syringe
9. Aspirate 20 ml of ascitic fluid
10. Remove the needle and dispose in the sharps bin
11. Apply the sterile, adhesive dressing
12. Separate the ascitic fluid into sterile sample pots
13. Document in the notes

Post-procedure management

Document the procedure, noting the gross appearance of the ascitic fluid (straw-coloured, blood-stained, turbulent, purulent), further tests requested (see below) and any complications encountered e.g. multiple passes, bleeding etc.

Send ascitic fluid samples for analysis including:

- Biochemistry (total protein, albumin, LDH, amylase)
- Microbiology (Gram stain, M,C&S and AAFB)
- Cytology
- Glucose (in fluoride oxalate (grey-top) sample tube)

Send matched serum samples for total protein, albumin and glucose.

Complications

- Perforation of intra-abdominal viscus (bowel, bladder, liver, spleen (rare))
- Bleeding
- Infection (of puncture site, peritonitis)
- Persistent leak of ascitic fluid from puncture site
- Failure to obtain ascitic fluid sample

Interpretation

Gross inspection of ascitic fluid

Normal ascitic fluid appears clear and straw-coloured. Blood-stained fluid can be caused by a traumatic tap or malignancy. A neutrophil count of >50,000/μl results in turbulent, purulent-appearing ascites this suggests infection.

Serum-ascites albumin gradient:

The preferred means of categorising ascites is based on the serum-ascitic albumin gradient (SAAG). This is calculated by subtracting the ascitic albumin concentration from the serum albumin concentration (a serum sample should be taken at the same time as the ascitic tap). The SAAG correlates directly with portal pressure and allows ascites to be categorised into those that are caused by portal hypertension (SAAG >1.1g/dL) and those that are not (SAAG <1.1g/dL).

The terms 'high-albumin gradient' and 'low-albumin gradient' are now preferred to 'transudate' and 'exudate' in the categorisation of ascites.

Cell count:

Normal ascitic fluid contains fewer than 500 leukocytes/μl and fewer than 250 neutrophils (polymorphonuclear leukocytes) per microliter. A neutrophil count of more than 250 cells/μl is suggestive of bacterial peritonitis. An elevated lymphocyte count is suggestive of tuberculous or malignant ascites.

Causes of ascites:

Causes of ascites can be divided into those associated with a diseased peritoneum and those associated with a normal peritoneum.

Normal peritoneum	Diseased peritoneum
Portal hypertension (SAAG >1.1g/dL): - Liver disease: cirrhosis, hepatic metastases. - Liver congestion: congestive cardiac failure, constrictive pericarditis, tricuspid regurgitation, Budd-Chiari syndrome.	Infection: - Bacterial peritonitis - Tuberculous peritonitis Malignancy: - Peritoneal carcinomatosis - Hepatocellular carcinoma - Primary mesothelioma
Hypoalbuminaemia (SAAG <1.1g/dL): - Nephrotic syndrome - Protein-losing enteropathy - Severe malnutrition - Synthetic Liver failure	
Miscellaneous: - Chylous ascites - Ovarian disease - Hypothyroidism - Pancreatic ascites	

Table 8.14: Causes of ascites.

Large volume paracentesis:

Large-volume paracentesis (LVP) – otherwise known as therapeutic paracentesis - is a therapeutic procedure performed to relieve the symptoms of large volume or tense ascites. The technique is the same as that described above for diagnostic paracentesis except that a larger-bore cannula is inserted into the peritoneal space rather than a green (21G) needle.

Bonanno® catheters, large-bore IV cannulas, Caldwell cannulas or Angiocath needles are commonly used to perform this procedure. The needle is advanced into the peritoneal space as described above until peritoneal fluid is aspirated into the syringe. The catheter is then advanced over the needle further into the peritoneal space and the needle removed. The catheter is attached to the vacuum bottles to allow the peritoneal fluid to drain fully.

Draining large volume ascites using this technique can cause significant haemodynamic changes which may result in severe hypotension. There is evidence that for therapeutic paracentesis of more than 5L, an infusion of albumin (8–10g for every litre of fluid removed) should be considered to expand plasma volume to counteract these large fluid shifts. However, there is controversy over whether albumin should be administered routinely in this situation and it is not recommended if volumes of less than 5L are being removed. Always seek senior advice in this regard.

Once all the ascitic fluid has been drained, the catheter can be removed and a sterile dressing applied over puncture site to prevent leakage of any residual ascitic fluid and the introduction of any infection.

8. DOPS

Top tips

- To minimise leak of ascitic fluid following the procedure, create a 'Z-track' during insertion of the needle. This is created by pulling the skin taught while the needle is inserted perpendicular to abdominal wall. When the needle is removed and the abdominal skin is released, a 'Z-track' is formed which prevents direct communication of the peritoneal space with the abdominal surface

18. INSERTION OF CENTRAL VENOUS LINE

Indications

- Monitoring of central venous pressure (CVP) to guide fluid administration
- IV access if peripheral IV access is not possible
- Administration of certain drugs (inotropes, potassium chloride, TPN)
- Urgent haemodialysis

Contraindications

Relative contraindications include:

- Local skin infection
- Uncorrected bleeding diathesis
- Uncooperative patient (likely to pull it out)

Relevant anatomy

Central lines can be inserted into the Internal Jugular, Subclavian (right side for these is preferred due to a more direct course) or the Femoral vein. The Internal Jugular and Subclavian sites are cleaner than the Femoral site and are generally preferred. The Internal Jugular site is also associated with a higher risk of arterial puncture (Common Carotid artery) whereas the subclavian site is associated with a higher incidence of pneumothorax.

Internal jugular site:

NICE guidelines actively encourage the use of ultrasound guidance when inserting central lines into the Internal Jugular vein due to the proximity of the Common Carotid artery, which can be easily punctured. However, it is also important to have an understanding of the anatomy in the neck related to the Internal Jugular vein.

The Right Internal Jugular vein lies in the neck within a triangle formed by the medial and lateral heads of the sternocleidomastoid muscle and the clavicle (the clavicle forms the base of the triangle). This triangle can be more easily visualised if the patient's head is turned towards the left. The vein runs from the apex of the triangle towards its base and lies superficial and lateral to the Common Carotid artery, which can be easily palpated. When inserting a central line at this site, the operator should be positioned at the head of the bed. The skin is usually punctured at the apex of the triangle with the needle angled at 45°, aiming towards the ipsilateral nipple as it is advanced to avoid puncturing the Common Carotid artery.

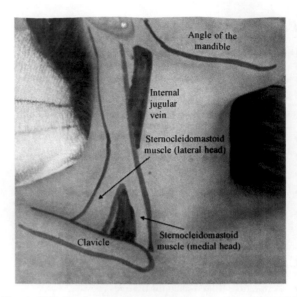

Figure 8.25: Surface anatomy illustrating the location of the Internal Juglar vein.

Equipment required

Central line insertion is optimally done if there is assistance. Sterile drapes, sterile gauze, 2 sterile gallipots, sterile cleansing solution, sterile saline, sterile gloves, sterile gown, mask, 1% lidocaine, syringes (5 ml, 10 ml), orange needle (25G), central line pack (introducer needle, guide-wire, dilator(s), central venous catheter), scalpel, suture, sterile dressings, portable ultrasound machine, sterile gel for ultrasound.

Procedure

This is a sterile procedure and should ideally be performed with an assistant present and with cardiac monitoring if the internal jugular or subclavian sites are being used.

The preferred technique for central line insertion into the internal jugular vein using the Seldinger technique will be described in detail here:

1. Prepare all equipment on a clean trolley
2. Position the patient lying flat with the bed tilted head-down and patient's head turned to the left
3. Stand at the head of the bed
4. Identify the anatomical landmarks to determine the site for central line insertion
5. Use ultrasound probe to confirm position of the Internal Jugular vein in the neck making sure that the probe head is immersed in a sterile glove containing the ultrasound gel
6. The vein is differentiated from the Common Carotid artery by its ability to be compressed. However, the artery is not compressible
7. Put on sterile gloves

8. Fill 10 ml syringe with saline, attach it to each port of central line in turn, flush each port with saline to verify patency within each port. Clamp each of the ports
9. Clean the skin with a sterile preparation solution e.g. Iodine, Chlorhexidine
10. Use sterile drapes to create sterile field
11. Infiltrate the skin around the proposed site of the line insertion with local anaesthetic, using a 25G orange needle
12. With the aid of an assistant, place some ultrasound gel on the tip of the probe and cover it with a sterile sheath
13. Use the ultrasound probe to confirm position of the Internal Jugular vein in the neck
14. Attach the Seldinger needle to 5 ml syringe and advance needle, bevel up, through subcutaneous tissues into Internal Jugular vein under direct ultrasound guidance, pulling back on the plunger at all times
15. Stop advancing the needle when venous blood is aspirated into syringe.
16. Stabilise the needle with one hand, remove the syringe and pass the guide-wire through the needle (looking at cardiac monitor as the wire is advanced, as arrhythmias may occur at this stage)
17. At this point, it is important to keep hold of the guide-wire at all times
18. Remove needle, keeping hold of the guide-wire
19. Use the scalpel to make a small skin incision immediately adjacent to the guide-wire
20. Pass the dilator along the guide-wire and advance through the skin into the vein
21. Remove the dilator, leaving the guide-wire in place
22. Pass the central line over the guide-wire and advance it through the skin into the vein to a suitable depth (see top tips)
23. Remove the guide-wire
24. Fill 10 ml syringe with saline, attach it to each port of central line in turn, ensure blood can be aspirated freely and then flush with saline to prevent blockage of the ports with clotted blood
25. Ensure that all the ports of the central line are clamped after they have been flushed
26. Secure the central line to the skin with the sutures
27. Place sterile dressing over central line at point of insertion
28. Dispose of all sharps in the sharps bin
29. Document in notes

Types of central venous catheter:

Type of central line	Description	Uses
Standard triple lumen catheter	Standard central line with three lumens inserted into central vein (Subclavian, Internal Jugular or Femoral vein).	Inserted for temporary central venous access e.g. in ITU for IV access, administration of inotropes and potassium, measurement of CVP etc.
Hickman line	Multi-lumen catheter inserted into large central vein (usually Subclavian or Internal Jugular) with tip lying at junction between Superior Vena Cava (SVC) and right atrium. A section of the line is tunnelled subcutaneously to separate the venous entry site from the skin surface (reduces risk of line infection). A cuff in the tunnelled section of the line encourages growth of subcutaneous tissue around line which helps prevent tracking of micro-organisms along the line, causing infection.	Provides more long-term IV access e.g. for administration of antibiotics or chemotherapy.
PICC line	Inserted in a peripheral vein (usually cephalic vein in Antecubital Fossa under ultrasound guidance) and advanced into a central vein (Subclavian vein/SVC).	Provides medium-term venous access up to several months. Prolonged antibiotic courses, chemotherapy administration.
Midline	Shorter than a PICC line (7 inches long) Inserted into a peripheral vein in antecubital region and advanced so that tip lies in the Axillary vein (i.e. does not enter central vein).	Can be used for up to 4 weeks to administer prolonged antibiotic courses Not suitable for TPN or chemotherapy.
Temporary dual-lumen haemodialysis catheters	Shorter lines than standard central venous catheters with larger lumens to provide high flow rates required by haemodialysis machines. Inserted into central vein (internal jugular, subclavian or (less commonly) Femoral vein) Cuffed, tunnelled haemodialysis catheters are used for longer-term access in certain patients. There are 3 main types.	Provides short term vascular access for haemodialysis (prior to creation of AV fistula or AV graft). Cuffed, tunnelled catheters provide longer-term vascular access suitable for certain patients.

Table 8.15: Types of central venous catheter.

8. DOPS

Subclavian site:

To insert a central line into the Right Subclavian vein, the operator should be positioned on the right-hand site of the patient. The skin is punctured just below the junction between the medial and middle thirds of the clavicle. The angle of the needle should be kept as flat as possible as it is advanced just below the clavicle, directed towards the sternal notch, to puncture the right subclavian vein.

The angle of the needle must not dip below the horizontal plane as this risks pleural puncture resulting in a pneumothorax.

Femoral site:

The Femoral vein lies just medial to the Femoral artery, which can be palpated just below the inguinal ligament at the mid-inguinal point (half way between the anterior superior iliac spine and the pubic tubercle). See Figure 8.2.

To insert a central line into the Femoral vein, the operator should be positioned at the side of the bed. The patient should be lying flat with their legs straight. The Femoral artery is palpated and the skin punctured 1–2 cm below the inguinal ligament and approximately 1cm medial to the Femoral pulse. The needle should be angled at 45° and advanced towards the patient's head to puncture the Femoral vein.

Post-procedure management

Request CXR to confirm correct position of line (just above junction between SVC and right atrium) and to rule out complications e.g. pneumothorax.

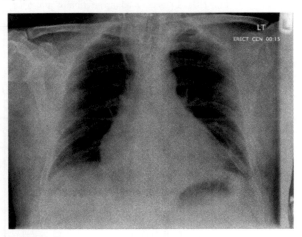

Figure 8.26: A CXR showing a right central line correctly inserted into the right internal jugular vein.

Handling the external parts of a central line:

An aseptic non-touch technique should be used whenever the external parts of an *in situ* central venous catheter are handled to reduce the risk of line infection. Gloves must be worn.

Each port of the catheter should be capped with a needleless IV access connector with a luer lock (e.g. Bionector®). This allows access to the line (for administration of fluids or medications, or to take blood samples) without having to remove the port cap, which would disrupt the closed system and increase the risk of air embolisation and introduction of infection.

If the port extensions of a central line have an integral clamp, these should be used whenever the port is not being used e.g. for fluid administration. This helps to prevent bleeding, air embolisation or introduction of infection if the port cap becomes accidentally dislodged.

Preventing air embolisation:

To prevent air embolism, great care must be taken to ensure that air bubbles are absent from port extensions and giving sets before fluids or medications are administered through a central line.

Giving sets should be carefully primed before attaching them to the line. If air bubbles are present in the port extensions of a line, attach a syringe to the relevant port and aspirate until the bubbles are removed.

Taking blood from a central line:

The following applies for taking any samples from central venous lines:

- Wear sterile gloves
- Wipe luer lock connector with Chlorhexidine/alcohol swab
- Connect 10 ml syringe and aspirate 5–10 mls
- Discard this syringe
- Connect another new syringe and aspirate a further 5–10 mls
- This is your sample
- Flush the line with normal saline
- Replace the integral clamp on the port extension if present

Flushing central lines:

Central lines should always be flushed following administration of IV medications or blood sampling. The choice of flush solution depends on the catheter type, its frequency of use and local policy.

In general, 0.9% saline is used to flush a line in between infusions and following blood sampling. If the same lumen is due to be accessed again with 1 day, it can be locked with 10 mls of 0.9% saline. If the lumen is unlikely to be used again for the next 24 hours, some recommend locking it with 5mls of Hepsal (10IU/ml) to reduce to the risk of luminal obstruction with thrombus.

Unused lumens should be flushed once a week with 10 ml 0.9% saline (and then locked with 5 mls Hepsal (10IU/ml)) to maintain patency of lumen.

Complications

- Pneumothorax
- Cardiac arrhythmia
- Arterial puncture
- Bleeding, including haematoma formation
- Infection (cellulitis, line infection, bacteraemia and septicaemia)

- Venous thrombosis
- Air embolism

Interpretation

Central lines are often used to monitor central CVP in acutely unwell patients. CVP refers to the pressure within the right atrium and is influenced by right heart function and the pressure of venous blood within the superior vena cava. It can be used to estimate circulating blood volume and therefore guide IV fluid administration in critical care. A low CVP may suggest hypovolaemia requiring fluid resuscitation and/or inotropic support.

CVP is measured by attaching a lumen of the central line to a manometer filled with IV infusion fluid (or electronic transducer in intensive care units). A patient breathing spontaneously usually has a CVP between 5–10 cmH$_2$O. Patients receiving mechanical ventilation have a CVP 3–5 cmH$_2$O higher.

However, it must be remembered that CVP is not a direct measure of circulating blood volume and is affected by right heart function, pulmonary arterial pressure, right heart compliance and venous return. It should be used in conjunction with other parameters such as heart rate, blood pressure, urine output and peripheral perfusion (assessed by capillary refill time) to estimate circulating blood volume and guide further management.

Top tips

- Positioning the patient appropriately
- Placing a rolled up towel under the neck can enable extension of the neck enhancing better demonstration of anatomy
- Prepare the central line by 'priming' it with sterile saline, which should be injected into each port in turn to displace air in each lumen and ensures patency. Then ensure that all ports excluding the distal port (which communicates with the end lumen through which the guide-wire will be passed) are clamped
- All patients should be attached to a cardiac monitor during central line insertion and the monitor should be watched carefully while guide-wire is advanced
- The risk of central line infection is reduced by ensuring that lines are inserted under strict sterile conditions with full sterile barrier protection (sterile drapes, gown, mask, gloves etc.). Lines should be removed as soon as they are no longer needed to reduce complications such as vein thrombosis and line infection

19. ASPIRATION OF A JOINT EFFUSION

Indications

- Unexplained joint effusion
- Suspected septic arthritis
- Suspected gout and haemarthrosis.
- Aspirating large joint effusions

Contraindications

- Prosthetic joint
- Bacteraemia
- Severe uncorrected coagulopathy (risk of haemarthrosis)

Relevant anatomy

The knee joint is the most common and easiest joint to aspirate and will be covered in detail here.

Aspiration of other joints should ideally be performed by a specialist (i.e. rheumatologist or orthopaedic surgeon) or by individuals that have received training and have experience of aspirating effusions at other sites.

An effusion in the knee usually produces a visible supra-patella swelling. A positive 'bulge test' is confirmed when fluid is 'milked' out of the supra-patellar pouch with one hand and pushed from the medial side of the knee to the lateral side and back again, with the other hand. Large knee effusions may allow the patella to be balloted.

Equipment required

Sterile drapes, sterile gauze, sterile gallipot, sterile cleansing solution, sterile gloves, 1% lidocaine, syringes (5 ml, 20 ml), orange needle (25G), green needle (21G), sterile dressing, sterile universal sample pots.

Procedure

This is a sterile procedure:
1. Prepare all equipment on clean trolley
2. Position the patient supine with a rolled towel placed below the knee to hold the joint in a slightly flexed position
3. Identify the anatomical landmarks and palpate the patella to determine the site for insertion
4. Put on sterile gloves
5. Clean the skin surrounding proposed site for needle insertion using sterile preparation solution e.g. Iodine, Chlorhexidine
6. Use sterile drapes to create sterile field around needle insertion site.
7. Infiltrate local anaesthetic into subcutaneous tissue surrounding proposed needle insertion site using orange (25G) needle
8. Attach green (21G) needle to 20 ml syringe and advance into joint space pulling back on plunger as needle is advanced
9. Stop advancing needle when synovial fluid is aspirated into syringe
10. Remove 20 ml of fluid in syringe

11. If large effusion is present, syringe can be detached from needle (while needle is held in place with other hand) and replaced with another syringe to remove further fluid
12. Remove the needle and dispose in the sharps bin
13. Apply a sterile dressing
14. Fill sample pots with aspirated fluid
15. Document in notes

Fluid can also be aspirated from the knee using a medial or lateral approach. The parapatellar approach will be described here.

1. Identify the midpoint of the medial or lateral border of the patella
2. Palpate the space beneath the patella at this point with the non-dominant hand
3. With the dominant hand, insert the needle into this space (about 3–4 mm below the midpoint)
4. Direct the needle perpendicular to the long axis of the femur and advance it into the synovial space until synovial fluid is aspirated
5. Apply a sterile dressing
6. Dispose of all sharps in the sharps bin
7. Document in the notes

Post-procedure management

Request the patient not to apply any pressure to the aspirated knee half an hour post procedure. Document the procedure, noting the gross appearance of the aspirated joint fluid and state any complications encountered (e.g. multiple passes) and state details of the tests ordered on the aspirates.

Send fluid samples for analysis including:

- Microbiology (Gram stain, M,C & S, AAFB)
- Polarised light microscopy (to assess for negatively bi-refringent monosodium urate crystals)
- Biochemistry (glucose, protein and LDH)

Complications

- Introduction of infection causing septic arthritis
- Haemarthrosis
- Damage to joint structures e.g. cartilage
- Failure to obtain synovial fluid

Interpretation

Synovial fluid is normally straw-coloured, clear and slightly viscous. Cloudy fluid suggests infection indicating septic arthritis.

Analysis of the cellular and biochemical composition of synovial fluid can help diagnose the underlying cause of a joint effusion. The composition of synovial fluid in different types of joint effusion is summarised in Table 8.16.

Top tips
- Position knee in slightly flexed position by resting it on a rolled-up towel. This relaxes the quadriceps muscles and opens up the joint space making access to joint space easier
- Ensure familiarity with local joint anatomy before attempting procedure as this increases the chances of success and reduces the risk of damage to joint structures e.g. tendons and cartilage

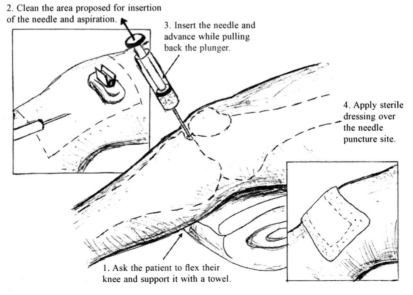

2. Clean the area proposed for insertion of the needle and aspiration.

3. Insert the needle and advance while pulling back the plunger.

4. Apply sterile dressing over the needle puncture site.

1. Ask the patient to flex their knee and support it with a towel.

Figure 8.27: Aspiration of a knee joint.

Cause of joint effusion	Appearance	Cells (cells/µl) Protein (g/dL) Glucose (mg/dL)	Other
Normal	Straw-coloured, clear	WBC: <200 Neutrophils: <25% Protein: 1–2 Glucose: Serum glucose	–
Non-inflammatory	Clear or slightly turbulent	WBC 0–2000 Neutrophils <30% Protein: 2–3 Glucose: Serum glucose	–
Inflammatory joint disease e.g. RA, SLE	Cloudy	WBC 2000–100,000 Neutrophils >50% Protein: >3–4 Glucose: <25	–
Septic arthritis	Purulent	WBC 50,000–200,000 Neutrophils >90% Protein: >3–4 Glucose: <25	Gram stain may reveal organisms in fluid
Crystal arthropathy	Cloudy	WBC 500–100,000 Neutrophils <90%	Polarised light microscopy reveals crystals

Table 8.16: Summarising the different types of joint effusions and their compositions.

20. SKIN SUTURING

Indications

- To close the skin of surgical and accidental wounds
- Securing lines and drains to the skin

For a wound to successfully heal there should be:

- Absence of haematoma and infection
- Accurate skin apposition
- Tension free apposition
- Adequate blood supply

Contraindications

- If the wound is contaminated it may be better to leave open. Consider other forms of closure, dependent on the anatomical position of the wound e.g. glue for superficial scalp wounds

Relevant anatomy

This is dependent on the wound.

Equipment required

Types of Suture:

Sutures can be divided into.

Absorbable vs. non absorbable:

- Absorbable sutures provide temporary support whilst healing occurs.
- Non-absorbable sutures are used when healing is expected to be poor, where they are subject to higher loads, or where breakdown could be disastrous e.g. vascular anastomosis

Mono-filament vs. braided/multi-filament:

- Mono-filament consists of a single strand and have a lower rate of infections though they are harder to handle than braided sutures.

Suture	Absorbable vs. non-absorbable	Mono-filament vs. Braided
Vicryl	Absorbable	Braided
PDS (polydioxanone)	Absorbable	Monofilament
Mersilk	Non absorbable	Braided
Prolene	Non absorbable	Monofilament

Table 8.17: The characteristics of common suture materials.

Suture sizes are referred to as fractions of gauge zero. For example for 3.0, 3 sutures would equal the width of one gauge 0 suture. **The higher the first number the finer the suture.**

Types of Needle:

Needles are described by type and shape.

Type refers to the cross directional shape of the needle – this may be a taper cut, cutting or reversed cutting. These are selected against the properties of the tissues through which they will be inserted. The shape may be straight or curved.

Straight needles can be used without needle holders and are useful for sub-cuticular stitches and for sutures used to fix lines and drains.

Basic suture procedure

The following is a brief description of inserting and tying a simple suture using a curved needle.

After gaining consent, wearing sterile glove, cleaning the skin, injecting local anaesthetic and determining appropriate alignment and apposition of the skin:

1. Select an appropriate suture and needle and hold with needle holders – hold the needle at the junction of the distal third to the proximal (sharp) two thirds. This area is often flattened
2. Lifting the skin with toothed forceps, the needle should be inserted perpendicular to the skin

3. Advance the needle along its curve by supinating the hand

4. When the tip of the needle is once again visible continue to advance, remove the suture holders and use it to extract the needle, again drawing the needle out along its curve

5. Repeat on the other side of the wound

6. Remove the suture holders and pull the suture through, leaving a short end on the side of the initial insertion

7. Wrap the long end of the suture twice around the needle holders

8. Take hold of the short end of the suture with the needle holders and pull through the half stitch formed around the instrument

9. Pull tight ensuring the edges of the wound are accurately drawn together

10. Repeat twice more, though each time only wrap the long end once round the needle holders

11. Cut off the remaining long and short ends

12. Dispose of sharps in the sharps bin

13. Clean the skin and apply a dressing

14. Document in notes

Types of stitch

Type of stitch	Description
Simple interrupted	Single sutures as described above individually placed along a wound
Vertical mattress	A second more superficial suture is placed in the opposite direction. This helps prevent inversion of the wound promoting healing.
Continuous	A single suture placed over and over before tying. Breakage leads to complete wound breakdown.
Subcuticular	Here the sutures are inserted into the epidermal/dermal junction. They are used when tension in deeper structures has been relieved and give a good cosmetic result.
Blanket/ locking continuous	This type of technique allows controlled tension on the flap margin as the wound is closed. It requires less stitches thus reduces irritation of underlying tissue. It also requires fewer knots thus reduces irritation of the underlying tissue.

Table 8.18: Types of stitch and their description.

Post procedural management

Non absorbable sutures require removal. The timing of the removal should be determined by the site and the time of insertion; as a rough guide:

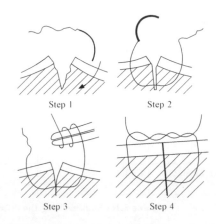

Figure 8.28: A step-by-step pictorial guide to performing a basic suture.

- Face: 3–5 days
- Abdomen 7–10 days
- High Tension areas: 10–14 days

Complications

- Infection
- Wound dehiscence

Top tips

- Ensure adequate and firm apposition prior to suturing
- Inform nursing staff and patient in regards to when sutures need to be taken out
- Leave sufficient length of the suture to allow easy removal
- Align all knots to one particular side of the wound

Further Reading and References

➢ 57th British National Formulary

➢ British Thoracic Society (2008). *Guideline for emergency use of oxygen in adult patients.*

➢ British Thoracic Society and Scottish Intercollegiate Guidelines Network (2008). *British Guideline on the management of asthma.*

➢ Duffy J, Laws D, Neville E (2003), Guidelines for the insertion of a Chest Drain *Thorax*; 58 (suppl II: ii53-59).

➢ www.bcshguidelines.com

➢ www.clean-safe-care.nhs.uk

➢ www.transfusionguidelines.org.uk

INTRODUCTION

Prescribing mishaps make a major contribution to hospital adverse events and medico-legal activities. It is estimated that about 7% of hospital admissions are related to medication problems, though this may rise to 30% in the typical elderly medical intake, and these account for 4,000 to 7,000 deaths per year in the UK. The financial implications of this for the National Health Service (NHS) are also great. It has been reported that the leading cause of medical injury in hospital practice is adverse drug events, about half of which are the result of errors. Reports from independent insurers continue to show that injuries caused by drugs are the most common reason for procedure-related malpractice claims.

Many of these mishaps are blamed on Foundation Year (FY) doctors even though the chain of events usually includes someone else, perhaps a nurse, a general practitioner (GP) or a carer. Adverse events, a term officially used to describe any kind of mishap without attributing blame, nearly always involves several people, each of whom could have prevented the event if they had been on top form that day. It is therefore essential that when prescribing you do not assume someone else will cover for any of your errors.

Naturally, prescribing is not just about avoiding errors but is about achieving the best for patients. This chapter seeks to outline some important features of prescribing in general and then gives some detail on a few specific areas that are known to trouble new prescribers.

PRESCRIBING IS ABOUT COMMUNICATING

It may sound obvious, but the act of prescribing is to communicate the prescriber's intentions for a patient to the persons who will dispense or administer the drugs. For this to work properly, the very minimum information required is the drug name, form (liquid, cream, patch, etc), dose, route, and frequency of administration.

There are also legalities such as signature, date and additional instructions which might include duration of treatment, precautions or limitations such as 'only if diastolic blood pressure >60 mmHg', or other notes.

In surveys in Thames Valley hospitals, 21% of inpatient drug prescriptions lacked even the basic information and 32% were endorsed by a pharmacist to provide the necessary warnings and advice for the nurses to administer the drug safely. (See Figure 9.1). 80% of patients had their charts endorsed by pharmacists.

Remember that you are not the only person who gets tired on duty. Even nurses can lose concentration or fail to read your mind accurately in the absence of a clear prescription!

Avoiding errors

1. Complete every box.

2. Write in BLOCK CAPITALS. Once you get into the habit it does not slow you down too much and it does prevent a lot of confusion. There are numerous cases of poor handwriting leading to the wrong drug being given and the patient suffering.

3. Do not use unorthodox abbreviations. Patients who should have had zidovudine have been given azathioprine because someone wrote 'AZT' on a chart, thinking everyone would know what it meant.

4. The dose should be specified clearly in appropriate units. Never abbreviate the word 'units' to 'U' because it looks too much like an extra zero and many patients have had a ten-fold overdose of insulin or heparin as a result. 'Micrograms' and 'nanograms' should never be abbreviated. Doses less than 1mg are more likely to be given correctly if written as micrograms e.g. DIGOXIN 125 micrograms rather than 0.125 mg.

5. Do not write several routes down e.g. IV/IM/oral, unless the dose is the same for each route. If you do want to give nurses the option, make it clear which is the preferred route.

6. Make sure the dosing frequency and times of administration match (it is surprising how often a twice-daily drug is given

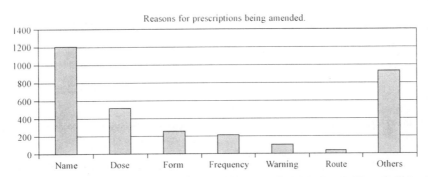

Reasons for prescriptions being amended.

Figure 9.1: Endorsements made by pharmacists in 10,155 in-patient prescriptions in Thames Valley hospitals.

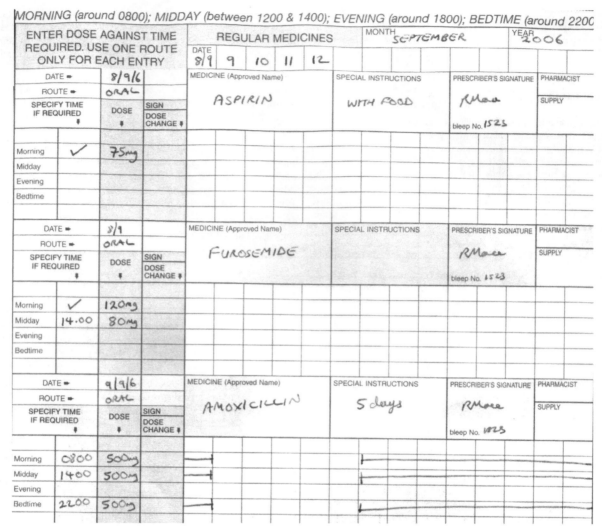

MORNING (around 0800); MIDDAY (between 1200 & 1400); EVENING (around 1800); BEDTIME (around 2200

ENTER DOSE AGAINST TIME REQUIRED. USE ONE ROUTE ONLY FOR EACH ENTRY			REGULAR MEDICINES		MONTH SEPTEMBER		YEAR 2006	
		DATE	8/9	9	10	11	12	
DATE → 8/9/6			MEDICINE (Approved Name)		SPECIAL INSTRUCTIONS		PRESCRIBER'S SIGNATURE	PHARMACIST
ROUTE → ORAL			ASPIRIN		WITH FOOD		RMoa	SUPPLY
SPECIFY TIME IF REQUIRED ↓	DOSE ↓	SIGN DOSE CHANGE ↓					bleep No. 1523	
Morning	✓	75mg						
Midday								
Evening								
Bedtime								
DATE → 8/9			MEDICINE (Approved Name)		SPECIAL INSTRUCTIONS		PRESCRIBER'S SIGNATURE	PHARMACIST
ROUTE → ORAL			FUROSEMIDE				RMoa	SUPPLY
SPECIFY TIME IF REQUIRED ↓	DOSE ↓	SIGN DOSE CHANGE ↓					bleep No. 1523	
Morning	✓	120mg						
Midday	14.00	80mg						
Evening								
Bedtime								
DATE → 9/9/6			MEDICINE (Approved Name)		SPECIAL INSTRUCTIONS		PRESCRIBER'S SIGNATURE	PHARMACIST
ROUTE → ORAL			AMOXICILLIN		5 days		RMoa	SUPPLY
SPECIFY TIME IF REQUIRED ↓	DOSE ↓	SIGN DOSE CHANGE ↓					bleep No. 1523	
Morning	0800	500mg						
Midday	1400	500mg						
Evening								
Bedtime	2200	500mg						

Figure 9.2: A typical in-patient prescription form.

once daily) and the times suit the nursing procedures as well as the patient's needs. A quick enquiry of the nurses on your ward about the best times to administer drugs will save you a lot of hassle later.

7. If writing a *prn* drug make the indication clear, for example when prescribing Codeine make sure to indicate whether it is for pain or diarrhoea. If prescribing two *prn* analgesics, which one should the nurse give and in what circumstances?

8. Specify any restrictions very clearly. Heart failure drugs may be required even if the blood pressure is low whereas the same drug given for hypertension is contraindicated when the pressure drops. Consider what you write in the patient's notes as well as on the chart; will a cover doctor know what to do when the nurse calls them on the weekend?

9. The differences between brands of the same medication are closely controlled by the licensing authorities and are not often important; the pharmacy will buy and supply the best deal, which may not be the cheapest brand. The ease of administration and other practical issues would have been taken into account. Therefore you should use generic (non-proprietary) names for most prescribing. In some cases, however, the differences between brands can matter and the British National Formulary (BNF) advises the use of brand names for some drugs including anti-epileptic and transplant medication. When patients bring in their own medication, make sure you do not duplicate items by prescribing some with brand names and some with generic names; analgesics are a particular problem in this respect.

There is good advice on prescribing at the front of the BNF and it is worth reminding yourself from time to time. The rules for writing controlled drug prescriptions can also be complicated but the BNF offers some good advice and your hospital should have a procedure for doing this. Your ward pharmacist will also guide you if asked.

COMMUNICATION ISSUES

When a patient arrives

Good communication is not only important when a patient is in the hospital, it is vital when the patient moves from community into hospital and back again.

Getting an accurate drug history when a patient arrives is notoriously difficult. There are national moves to have a system of 'green bags' for patients and ambulance crew to transport their medicines and most GPs can provide a list of what has been prescribed. The problem may be, however, that the patient is not taking what the GP prescribed; they may take too much or too little. This non-adherence is widespread for all sorts of good and bad reasons. Treatment strategies must be agreed with patients (concordance) or they are doomed to failure.

In most hospitals, medical admissions will be checked by a pharmacist within the first day or so of their stay and several sources of information will be used to create an accurate drug history. Surgical patients will often have been seen in a pre-admission clinic where medicine-taking can be checked.

If in doubt about a patient's medication when they arrive, follow the principle of 'first do no harm'. Many medications can be stopped safely for a period while checks are made or progress is observed. Some of these problems are due to non-adherence but some are due to adverse reactions. However, stopping medications without careful consideration would not be wise, for anti-epileptic medications, many cardiac medications, transplant immunosuppression medication, anti-psychotic drugs, and bronchodilators.

When a patient leaves

When a patient leaves your care they may be cared-for by a lay carer or relative, a residential home assistant or no-one. It is essential that your intentions are clear to all.

If prescribing antibiotics or other short courses, including steroids for asthma or post acute coronary syndrome (ACS) anti-platelet agents, make sure the stop date is clear.

A number of discharge situations require advance planning on your part. Try to insist that your seniors give you a clear plan for each patient so that you are not taken by surprise when they say 'the patient can go now'! All drugs need to be dispensed or checked for discharge and this will inevitably take time. The patient will also need to have their final counselling on their medication and this too cannot be done at the drop of a hat. If the patient is not clear on what to do, or is not happy with it, you will be seeing them again, all too soon. The British Thoracic Society (BTS) guidelines recommend that patients on respiratory medication should use their exact discharge prescription for 24 hours in hospital before discharge to establish that it is indeed the appropriate prescription.

If the patient needs a special administration system, e.g. a Dossette box, to help them adhere to their prescription the pharmacy will need advance notice to make arrangements with a community pharmacy and the GP to continue the supply without interruption. A carer may need to be instructed on how to deal with such devices. Therefore, try to predict the discharge prescription well before the patient goes home. Some medications are a part of a shared-care agreement between primary and secondary care organisations and there are protocols for this that must be followed.

Some common issues

A chapter like this cannot cover all the issues that will arise in prescribing. The BNF and the 'BNF for children' have deserved world-wide reputations for their detailed guidance and should be consulted frequently. The NHS has set up a 'one-stop' web site for accessing guidelines on all sorts of medical issues from organisations such as the National Institute for Health and Clinical Excellence (NICE), the Scottish Inter-collegiate Guidelines Network (SIGN). What follows are some brief hints on a few areas known to give concern to FY doctors.

ADVERSE DRUG REACTIONS

All drugs cause adverse reactions and it is illegal in the UK to advertise a medicine as safe. Some adverse effects are consequence of their intended action, known as Type A, e.g. hypotension from an angiotensin converting enzyme (ACE) inhibitor. Others are due to a different mechanism, known as Type B, e.g. hepatotoxicity with isoniazid. Yet, others are immune-mediated, known as anaphylaxis.

Type A reactions are relatively straightforward to detect and to deal with, i.e. reduce the dose or stop the drug.

Type B reactions are more difficult to deal with. They include rashes (but due to which drug?), headaches (is it due to any drug?), abnormal hepatic enzyme tests (which drug or which underlying condition?), decreased renal function, cough and many other reactions.

Dealing with a possible reaction

1. Take a very thorough history. Note all the drugs the patient has consumed (suspect or not, prescribed or not, conventional or alternative, legal or illicit) in the relevant period. Check at what times they were taken and check whether they were actually consumed and not just prescribed by using the nurses' administration chart. Ask if the patient has ever had a similar reaction; what caused/alleviated/resolved it? Has anything else changed recently e.g. diet, cosmetics, food supplements or minor illnesses?

2. Write a thorough description of the reaction: time and nature of onset, progression, relieving or aggravating factors.

3. Consider any relevant laboratory tests that should be done e.g. renal and hepatic function tests. Consider spirometry for a wheeze and photograph any rash to help describe it in dermatology-speak.

4. Consult pharmacy's medicines information department on the likelihood of this reaction being attributable to any of the listed drugs. The temporal link will be crucial to attributing blame; some reactions occur immediately on exposure, some

take a standard period e.g. a few days or a few weeks, and some require a long exposure.

5. Stop the most likely drug (or several drugs if safe to do so) and observe the patient. However, do not forget to deal with the condition for which the drug was prescribed originally.

6. Do not make a re-challenge without senior support; some reactions are much more intense, even life-threatening, on re-challenge.

COMMONLY PRESCRIBED MEDICATIONS

Cardiology

Cardiology is an expanding area, with a strong evidence base for many of the interventions used. When prescribing for patients with cardiovascular disease, it is essential to check the diagnosis since several drugs can be used for multiple indications but will be dosed differently and to check on the patient's drug history. When doing this, do not rely upon a previous discharge letter alone, nor on a GP letter alone; always use the documents available but also ask the patient what they are actually taking. They may have varied their dosage, with or without medical advice, and it is crucial to know this to make appropriate adjustments.

Hypertensive emergencies require senior management. There is a need to balance the dangers of acute hypertension with those of lowering pressures rapidly in patients who have adjusted to high pressures; rapid changes may induce cerebral hypoperfusion and thus stroke.

Patients who present with a stroke and have raised blood pressure should have their previous medications continued but new medications should not be started until the acute phase (7–10 days) is over unless a senior review indicates that there is immediate danger from the raised pressure. Blood pressure is often volatile in acute stroke patients and hypoperfusion may be induced by over-zealous treatment.

Arrhythmias are commonly present in sick or elderly patients, mostly as atrial fibrillation (AF), but the management of many arrhythmias is much less dependent on drugs and is more dependent on electrical intervention e.g. pacing, cardioversion, and ablation in specialist units. Electrolyte disturbances, especially hypokalaemia, predispose to arrhythmias and checking and correcting levels is one of the most important roles for an FY doctor.

The drug list should also be checked for precipitating causes including beta-blockers, diuretics, antidepressants and anti-histamines. The latter are amongst many drugs that can cause a prolongation of the corrected QT interval and render the patient at risk of the dangerous ventricular arrhythmia, Torsade de Pointes. This is most often a problem when they are combined with an anti-arrhythmic such as Amiodarone or with a cytochrome enzyme inhibitor such as Erythromycin.

It should be remembered that all anti-arrhythmic drugs are also pro-arrhythmic. Beta-blockers are widely used because they reduce the sympathetic drive that underlies many tachy arrhythmias and are well known and relatively safe agents. Amiodarone is also widely used because it is highly effective in many arrhythmias,

hence it has been called 'cardiological Domestos', but it has many long-term adverse effects too.

ACE inhibitors and angiotensin receptor blockers are used in lower doses in heart failure than in hypertension. They must be initiated much more cautiously in heart failure to avoid first dose hypotension, especially in elderly patients. Patients should be appropriately counselled regarding hypotensive risks when initiating and increasing dose. It may be appropriate to give initial doses at bedtime if the patient is unlikely to need to get out of bed until normal waking hours. Anti-hypertensive therapy should revert to morning dosing once treatment is stabilised.

Beta-blockers are now less commonly used as first-line anti-hypertensives but are still widely used in ischaemic heart disease (IHD). Abrupt withdrawal can lead to rebound ischaemia and caution should be exercised in diabetes and in respiratory disease.

Nitrate treatments for angina necessitate asymmetric dosing to prevent the development of tolerance. A 'nitrate free' period each day (at least 14 hours between doses of isosorbide mononitrate tablets) should be arranged, e.g. by dosing at 8am and 2pm. Tolerance can develop quickly and lead to not only withdrawal/rebound symptoms in the absence of the drug, but a loss of beneficial response.

Anti-platelet agents, most notably aspirin, should be kept to a minimum effective dose to reduce the risk of gastrointestinal bleeding. Vulnerable patients such as the elderly, patients with prior history of bleeding or dyspepsia, or patients with concomitant use of steroids should be given a proton-pump inhibitor (PPI).

Anti-coagulants cause more avoidable mishaps than any other agents. Prescribers' minds tend to focus on avoiding over-dosing but it is equally important not to under-dose. The most common error is to fail to monitor the bleeding tendency, i.e. the international normalized ratio INR or activated partial thromboplastin time (APTT), as often as is required. Interacting drugs, including those that inhibit hepatic metabolism of warfarin, and those which may predispose to bleeding e.g. non-steroidal anti-inflammatory drugs (NSAID) should be ruthlessly avoided. The BNF gives lists of interacting drugs and of target values for INR and APTT in various clinical circumstances.

Diabetes mellitus

Diabetics are particularly vulnerable to changes in prescribing, especially on arrival at hospital or around surgery when a nil-by-mouth regimen is used.

Sliding scales for insulin are common and every hospital has a local version in which insulin is diluted in normal saline and infused at a rate determined by frequent blood glucose measurements. The prescriber must ensure that the scale is written clearly and in the units which the nurse will use when adjusting rates. For example, if the infusion device is calibrated in ml/hour then the prescription must be in ml/hour with the concentration of the insulin solution specified. The nurse should not be expected to convert the rate from units/hour or units/kg/hour or anything else. Such mental conversions are a major source of error.

A sliding scale should be set up for all diabetics who are undergoing surgery even if they are not normally insulin-dependent. However, well-controlled patients undergoing short procedures may not need any insulin. Diet-controlled diabetes patients do not usually need any specific intervention before surgery.

Patients on short-acting sulphonylureas should omit the morning dose on the day of operation but longer-acting sulphonylureas should only be stopped 2-3 days before surgery to prevent peri-operative hypoglycaemia. Patients may be converted to a short-acting sulphonylurea or insulin.

Metformin should be stopped at least 48 hours before elective surgery and not restarted for at least 48 hours post-operatively to prevent lactic acidosis. For radiological studies metformin should be discontinued, preferably, 24 hours before the time of the test and for three days after the procedure.

Thiazolidinediones should be omitted on the morning of surgery and restarted once patient is eating and drinking post-operatively.

Regular insulin is given by a variety of regimens but most include a fast-acting insulin and a medium or long-acting insulin. Brand-name prescribing is essential because of the variation in effect due to subtle changes in insulin preparations.

Infections

Increasing bacterial resistance, 'super-bug' outbreaks and treatment failure have been widely blamed on poor prescribing. Government action has strengthened microbial surveillance and is backed strong measures to control antibiotic prescribing. Such measures emphasise avoiding unnecessary prescribing and selecting the right drug and route for the severity of illness. Therefore, you should familiarise yourself with your hospital's antibiotic policy. This will be in place to reduce the incidence of resistance and hospital acquired infection and will take local resistance patterns into account.

Always take samples for microbiology before starting treatment. The presence of any antibiotic reduces the likelihood of growing organisms in the lab.

Monitor the duration of antibiotic course. In simple infections such as acute cystitis, specify the full course on the prescription chart so the course is not unnecessarily prolonged.

Review intravenous (IV) antibiotics regularly to avoid the risks associated with IV cannulae

Always record the time and date of sampling on laboratory request forms for drug levels. Take the sample in the morning if possible to enable results to be back the same day.

Severe infections such as sepsis, require a regime of high-intensity treatment followed by a step-down to more specific drugs when the infecting organism is identified. This is contrary to previous practice and may require permission from a senior or a microbiologist. Do not hesitate to seek that permission; it can save lives.

Analgesia

Analgesia has classically been under-prescribed and patients have been brushed off with words like 'discomfort'. How different when we are the ones in pain!

To promote the proper use of opiate analgesia, the World Health Organisation (WHO) published an Analgesic Ladder in 1996. It is applicable to chronic pain where it builds up from Paracetamol to Morphine. For acute pain, including surgical pain, the ladder is reversed and prescriptions start with major analgesics and step down as time permits.

Paracetamol is the starting point for treating all chronic pain and should continue through all stages of management at the maximum dose, i.e. 1g qds in adults. There is no danger of acute toxicity with this dose and analgesic nephropathy, if it occurs at all, will take years to develop. IV Paracetamol is available but it is not popular because of expense. Rectal Paracetamol is available for patients who cannot take it by mouth.

NSAIDs may be used instead, or in addition, but these all have risks of gastrointestinal damage and bleeding as well as renal impairment in dehydrated patients, heart failure patients or patients taking ACE inhibitors.

The second step is to add an oral mild opiate such as Dihydrocodeine (30mg qds in adults). Codeine is not metabolised to the active metabolite (morphine) in some patients and is best avoided. Laxatives, e.g. Lactulose, should automatically be prescribed prophylactically and not after constipation is evident.

The third step is to use Morphine instead of Dihydrocodeine. Morphine does not have a dose-ceiling, unlike Dihydrocodeine, and may be increased as required. Laxatives are essential and anti-nauseants may be required whenever the dose is increased. The UK is one of only two countries in the world to license diamorphine but apart from increased solubility, which makes it easier to use in a small portable syringe, it has no advantage over morphine. In fact it is less stable than morphine when mixed with other IV solutions. Other opiates are only useful if their formulation is particularly convenient or if Morphine supplies are low.

When prescribing opiates, ensure that they are given regularly at intervals that suit the formulation e.g. 12-hourly for modified release tablets. In addition, always make provision for break-through pain. If using tablets or intermittent injections, prescribe a *prn* dose that is one-sixth of the daily dose in current use; if using a continuous infusion allow for boluses to be given at the equivalent of 30-60 minutes infusion.

Review opiate prescriptions at least once a day to adjust up or down according to the patient's use of break-through medication.

Top tips

- Communicate clearly and fully
- Abbreviation is a shortcut to disaster
- Do not assume others will cover your deficiencies
- Asking for help is a sign of strength and not a weakness

FURTHER READING AND REFERENCES

➤ Barber N, Dean B, Schachter M, et al. (2002). Causes of prescribing errors in hospital inpatients: a prospective study. *Lancet* 359: 1373–8.

➤ Brennan TA, Laird NM, Leape LL, et al. (1991). Incidence of adverse events and negligence in hospitalized patients: results of the Harvard Medical Practice Study I. *NEJM* 324: 370–6.

➤ Karch FE, Lasagna L (1975). Adverse drug reactions: a critical review. *JAMA* 234: 1236–41.

➤ Peyriere H, Cassan S, Floutard E, et al. (2003). Adverse drug events associated with hospital admission. *Ann Pharmacother* 37: 5–11.

➤ Pirmohamed M, James S, Meakin S, et al. (2004). Adverse drug reactions as cause of admission to hospital: prospective analysis of 18820 patients. *BMJ* 329: 15–19.

➤ Shakur R, Scott D (2008). The art of prescribing. *Br J Hosp Med (Lond)* 69(5): M72–3.

➤ www.evidnce.nhs.uk

INTRODUCTION

Mini-CEX assessments assess a doctor's performance in a given clinical encounter. These encounters can vary from taking a history, performing specific examinations, to discussing diagnosis and/or management plans with patients or their relatives.

This chapter aims to cover the basic structures of history taking, common examinations and a simple guide to basic communication skills. Further aspects specific to certain cases and conditions are discussed in the CBD chapters.

	Activity
Communication Skills	Basic communication skills
	Communication in Mini-CEX assessments
	Special cases
History Taking	Basic structure and concepts
Medical Examinations	Cardiovascular system examination
	Respiratory system examination
	Gastrointestinal system examination
	Peripheral nervous system examination
	Cranial nerve examination
	(Examination of Speech)
	(Parkinson Disease - Examination of Extra-pyramidal system)
	(Examination of Cerebellum)
	Musculoskeletal system screening examination
	Locomotor system examination
Pre-operative history	Basic Format and Structure
Surgical Examinations	Pre-operative examination
	Lump examination
	Hernia examination
	Thyroid examination
	Varicose vein examination
	Peripheral vascular examination

Mini-CEX assessments

Mini-CEX assessments require completion of web based assessment forms by an assessor. The assessments can range from history taking to clinical judgement, professionalism, organisation and efficiency. The exact content of the assessment will depend on the nature of the encounter.

COMMUNICATION SKILLS

Basic communication skills

How to talk to people

Most of your time as a junior doctor will be spent communicating with patients, relatives, nurses, fellow colleagues, and other health care professionals. Remember that most complaints about doctors are not about mistakes, but about communication failure. Modern medical schools place a huge emphasis on communication skills, so you may be feeling confident about your ability to deal with communication problems. This confidence may evaporate the second you are faced with an angry relative, or when having to break bad news to a patient or relative. More often these intense communication situations occur when the ward is busy, or when there are a number of people present. Relatives will want to know 'what is going on with mum', without telling you who 'mum' is, or without allowing you time to collect your thoughts. They will expect you to know all of the medical information with regards to their family member, and it is in these pressured situations where you are in danger of forgetting your training and making communication errors.

As with all skills, communication is something that you will improve on over time, and with practice. There is no substitute for this, however this does not mean your communication skills will be poor! Some people are natural when it comes to communicating, others are less so. The most effective communicators are those that are able to explore the patient's knowledge, thoughts and expectations, and at the same time obtain the information required to complete the assessment. Listening to the patient, asking both open and closed questions and ensuring the conversation is a two way process, will almost inevitably lead to a positive outcome. Communication skills are part of Mini-CEX assessments, and a description of how they fit in is included later. The following are some useful tips that will help you whilst communicating:

- Be prepared
- Get off to a good start
- Find the agenda
- Be polite and caring
- Be clear
- End your conversation
- Have an exit strategy

Mini-Clinical Evaluation Exercise (CEX)

F1

Please complete the questions using a cross: ☒   Please use black ink and CAPITAL LETTERS

Doctor's   Surname: [ ]

            Forename: [ ]

GMC Number: [ ][ ][ ][ ][ ][ ][ ]   **YOUR GMC NUMBER MUST BE COMPLETED**

Clinical setting:	A&E ☐		OPD ☐	In-patient ☐	Acute Admission ☐	GP Surgery ☐	Other [ ]

Clinical problem category:	Airway/ Breathing ☐	CVS/ Circulation ☐	Gastro ☐	Neuro ☐	Pain ☐	Psych/ Behaviour ☐	Other [ ]

New or FU:	New ☐	FU ☐	Focus of clinical encounter:	History ☐	Diagnosis ☐	Management ☐	Explanation ☐

Number of times patient seen before by trainee:	0 ☐	1-4 ☐	5-9 ☐	>10 ☐	Complexity of case:	Low ☐	Average ☐	High ☐

Assessor's position:	Consultant ☐	GP ☐	SpR ☐	SASG ☐	SHO ☐	Other [ ]

Number of previous mini-CEXs observed by assessor with any trainee:	0 ☐	1 ☐	2 ☐	3 ☐	4 ☐	5-9 ☐	>9 ☐

Please grade the following areas using the scale below	Below expectations for F1 completion		Borderline for F1 completion	Meets expectations for F1 completion	Above expectations for F1 completion		U/C*
	1	2	3	4	5	6	
1 History Taking	☐	☐	☐	☐	☐	☐	☐
2 Physical Examination Skills	☐	☐	☐	☐	☐	☐	☐
3 Communication Skills	☐	☐	☐	☐	☐	☐	☐
4 Critical Judgement	☐	☐	☐	☐	☐	☐	☐
5 Professionalism	☐	☐	☐	☐	☐	☐	☐
6 Organisation / Efficiency	☐	☐	☐	☐	☐	☐	☐
7 Overall clinical care	☐	☐	☐	☐	☐	☐	☐

*U/C Please mark this if you have not observed the behaviour and therefore feel unable to comment.

Anything especially good?   **Suggestions for development:**

Agreed action:

Have you had training in the use of this assessment tool?   ☐ Face-to-Face   ☐ Have Read Guidelines   ☐ Web / CD-rom

Assessor's Signature:

Date (mm/yy):   Time taken for observation: (in minutes) [ ][ ]
M M Y Y
[ ][ ] / [ ][ ]   Time taken for feedback: (in minutes) [ ][ ]

Assessor's Surname: [ ]

Assessor's registration number*: [ ][ ][ ][ ][ ][ ][ ][ ][ ][ ][ ][ ][ ][ ]

Please note: Failure of return of all completed forms to your administrator is a probity issue.

Figure 10.1: The assessment form for Mini-CEX. *Courtesy of United Kingdom Foundation Programme Office.*

Be prepared:

If you have time before initiating a conversation, always try to have all of the information to hand. An appropriate setting ensuring privacy with a chaperone is important, for example a private room, or often on the ward drawing the curtains of the cubicle.

Read the notes, look at any reports and blood tests, and ensure you are clear about the management plan. By having all of this information you will avoid the embarrassing situation of seeming to know very little about the patient in question, or worse, giving inaccurate information. Common questions often asked by patients include, do you have a firm diagnosis? If you do not, how are you planning on reaching one? What is my prognosis? How long will I stay in hospital? If you are prepared and have the answers to these questions, you will more likely be taken seriously.

Have an exit strategy:

Never start a conversation that you are unable to finish. Always know what your intended outcomes are: do you want to give the family some information, or do you want some information from them? Usually it will be a mixture of these.

You must also consider if you have sufficient time to continue a particular conversation. For example if you are being approached for a 'quick word' on a hospital ward, and you are in the middle of looking after an acutely unwell patient, politely explain that this is not the best time and try to arrange a specific time, or for another member of the team to talk to the person in question. Consideration should also be given to whether you are the right person to be talking to this patient or relative.

Get off to a good start:

Make an effort to look smart, and dress appropriately. The rest is simple: introduce yourself, make direct eye-contact with everyone involved in the conversation and ensure you know who you are talking to. Smile if it is appropriate.

Find the agenda:

Rarely do people just want to have "a chat." Usually there is another motive to people wanting to speak with you. It is your job to find out what the other issues are, in order for you to address any of their concerns. There is no fixed method to achieve this, but there are some ways to make the situation easy for you. Start the conversation with the patients or relatives with an open statement inviting them to express their expectations. Try:

'How may I help you?'

or

'Is there anything you would like to know?'

Let the person you are talking to do most of the talking to start with. This will allow you to get a feel for what they want out of the conversation. Sometimes agendas are hidden, and will take all of your skill, and potentially more than one conversation, to elicit. People have to trust you before they tell you their deepest secrets and concerns, so give them time and space to talk.

Be polite and caring:

Again, this sounds obvious, and something you would normally do, but there is a special sort of politeness that helps with communicating with patients and relatives. Your aim should be to actively listen and ensure the patient feels they have your complete attention. Making people feel like they are your number one priority will make them feel their concerns are valued, and that you genuinely care for them. Try not to break off from a conversation until it is obviously finished. In situations where you are explaining delicate and potentially difficult information, make sure you handover your bleep to a colleague, and ensure you have a nurse present.

Be clear:

Always say exactly what you mean, in a manner that your audience will understand. Avoid medical jargon, abbreviations or technical terms. People will remember only a fraction of what you are saying, so do not be afraid to repeat the important facts. If you have any doubts as to whether you are being clear, ask the person directly: "Does that make sense?" or "Am I being clear?" Ask them to summarise or repeat back to you what you have said, therefore confirming that they have understood the information.

End your conversation:

Ending the conversation can sometimes be difficult, however there are a number of ways to do this; the easiest way is to summarise the conversation and then ask the other person if they agree. Finally thank them for their time and leave. Other, more subtle, techniques are just as effective. Try listening for a while whilst crouching or kneeling at the bedside, and then standing up when you want to end the conversation. Your actions can be interpreted as 'stretching your legs', but it gives a sense of movement to the conversation. Always ensure the patient is happy to end the conversation, and that they have been able to ask all their questions.

Communication in Mini-CEX assessments

Mini Clinical Evaluation Exercises (Mini-CEX) are observed encounters with patients. They may take the form of any interaction of the doctor and the patient, but are often stereotyped encounters, where a senior watches you take a history from a patient or perform a clinical examination. There are separate sections for history taking and communication skills, although these are often closely linked in the actual clinical event.

Treat the assessment as you would any simple interaction with a patient. There should be nothing different done just because someone is watching you, and the following is good practice for any clinical encounter.

Generic history

Introduce yourself and explain who you are in the team. Apologise for the presence of your assessor and explain that they are watching to make sure that you are doing the right things. Confirm with the patient they consent to this.

Find out who anyone else around the patient might be (partner, friend, or taxi driver) and check if the patient wants them to stay whilst you talk to them, or if they would rather be on their own.

Start with some open questions; find out what the patient is worried about most, why they are in hospital/your office. Try to spend the first third of the conversation saying as little as possible.

Then move on to asking some closed questions. By now you should have a good idea about which system is troubling the patient. If you don't, you haven't let the patient say enough early on. Focus on a system and ask the patient some specific questions. These questions are covered in the history taking mini-cex below.

Ideas, concerns and expectations

Explain what you are going to do next (examine patient, take blood etc.) and ask the patient if they have any questions they might like to ask. Use specific signpost questions, so your assessor can tick this box:

- 'Tell me about what you think is causing your symptoms?'
- 'What do you think might be happening?'
- 'What are your main concerns?'
- 'Is there anything particular or specific that you are concerned about?'
- 'What do you think might be the best plan of action?'
- 'How might I best help you with this?'

Closing the encounter

When you have finished your clinical encounter, thank the patient for their time, and ask them again if they have any questions. Tell them what your plan is and ensure they understand what will happen next. Try to give them a feel for how long they might have to wait, and what sorts of outcomes they might expect. Give them a way of getting hold of you again, even if it is just telling them that the nurses can bleep you if needed.

Special cases

There are a few special situations where all your skills will be tested, and it is a good idea to have a strategy for dealing with them. Here we will discuss dealing with an angry person, and breaking bad news.

Talking to angry people

People get angry because they cannot control the situation they are in. They might be afraid, or in pain, or have unrealistic expectations that have not been met. They have resorted to anger because they cannot get what they want through more peaceful means. Different people resort to anger at different times, but the basic formula is the same.

Usually you will be called to see an angry patient or relative because they are angry, for example at the nursing staff, and they have decided they need your help to deal with it. Alternatively the person themselves have demanded to see a doctor, because they think you will be able to give them what they want. Sometimes they will approach you directly.

Remember when dealing with angry people if they are verbally or physically threatening or abusive, you simply do not have to talk to them. Warn them that they are overstepping the mark, and if they continue to be aggressive, walk away stating they

are being hostile, therefore you will not discuss anything further and will call security.

Usually, people are angry within the limits of social acceptability. In these cases, your aim should be to diffuse the situation, and then identify with them exactly what it is making them angry. The following may assist you in achieving this;

1. Diffuse the situation by remaining calm yourself.
2. Never lose your composure.
3. Use 'open' body language; do not fold your arms or stand over people's beds.
4. Use slow, deliberate and open gestures.
5. Ensure appropriate eye contact and tone of voice.
6. Simply listening to an angry person for a few minutes is usually enough to calm the situation.
7. If it is possible to apologise for the problem, do so. This is not an admission of guilt or fault, but it will help placate the person and show that you are trying to be constructive and not defensive. For example, 'I am really sorry that you feel that the nurse/doctor did not get your mother the analgesia when she asked. I can see that this has really upset you'.
8. Once the situation has become calm, enquire about the exact nature of why the person is angry.
9. They may have lots of different complaints, and therefore may not seem all that focused; in which case try to get them to tell you what is mostly upsetting them.
10. Ask them for their opinion on how the problem can be resolved. If this is possible, go ahead and do it. However if it is not possible, calmly explain the reason why this is, and offer an alternative solution.
11. Sometimes, people will be directly angry at you, or at something you have done. Again, if they are threatening or abusive, walk away from the situation. If they are willing to listen and remain calm, try to explain your reasoning and thoughts with regards to the incident they are angry about.
12. If you are genuinely to blame for an incident, then apologise and take their criticism on board.
13. Patients and relatives should be made aware of the Patient Liason Service (PALS) if they wish to lodge an official complaint.
14. After the situation has resolved, speak to your consultant to discuss the event and acknowledge any important learning points from the incident. At the same time write a short piece known as reflective practice to insert into your learning portfolio, which again will help you to identify both positive and negative aspects about the incident, and help you to identify areas to improve on when faced with similar situations in the future.

If during the interaction you feel out of your depth, request a senior to deal with the problem. Remember the NHS has a zero tolerance policy on violence or abuse of any of its staff.

Breaking bad news

Telling someone bad news is always difficult. There are a number of different methods used, and you may have heard of some of these strategies before. This is simply a general guide to the sorts of things that you will need to consider when breaking bad news.

Placement:

1. Explain that you want to have an important discussion, and ask the patient if there is anyone they would like to have around when this discussion takes place.
2. If there is, you can arrange a time for you to meet them.
3. Try to meet in a quiet place where there is a low chance of being interrupted.
4. Take a nurse with you.
5. Ideally the person breaking the bad news should be a senior doctor, but this is not always the case.
6. Hand your bleep to a colleague to ensure you will not be disturbed.

Information:

1. Again, enter this encounter armed with as much information as you can.
2. Usually, patients will want not only to know the piece of bad news, but what this means for them.
3. You should aim to know the prognosis for the condition in question, and what the immediate management will be.
4. Talk to your seniors about this if you have the chance.

Prior knowledge:

1. Ask directly what the patient knows, and what sort of news they are expecting.
2. They may tell you that they are worried about the specific piece of bad news you are bearing.
3. They may have completely unrealistic expectations, in which case you can explain that their understanding is not quite accurate, and slowly introduce a more realistic view.

Be direct:

1. When the time comes to tell your patient the news, do so clearly and without medical jargon or euphemism.
2. Allow this information to sink in, and answer any questions to the best of your ability.
3. If there is information that you do not have – admit it, and promise to find out.
4. Offer the services of the hospital counsellors or the bereavement team.
5. Leave the way open to talk to a senior doctor at a later time.

Prognosis:

1. Patients will want a prognosis.
2. You can never provide an exact answer.
3. Describe prognosis if your seniors have mentioned one, or explain that more tests will be required before a prognosis can be made.

Documentation:

1. Record in the multidisciplinary notes what was discussed and who was present at the meeting.
2. Document what the patient wanted to know, what their expectations were, as well as a description of their reaction.
3. Ensure that the date, time, signature, name and designation are clearly documented.

Confidentiality

Breaking confidentiality is illegal and unprofessional. Confidentiality is often broken through carelessness, rather than malice, so be on your guard. Simple measures, like refraining from discussing patients in public (including the corridors of the hospital, lifts, on the bus etc.) should ensure you never breach confidentiality. Never leave your 'patient ward list' lying around. Always be careful about carrying patient data around on electronic devices such as USB memory sticks. Ensure these are encrypted if you do use them.

Relatives:

Relatives have no absolute right to information. They can only be told about your patient's condition if your patient agrees to this. The 2005 mental capacity act has been put in place to protect those individuals who do not have the capacity to make decisions for themselves, (e.g. patients with dementia, head injuries and learning disabilities). Sometimes this can lead to difficulties with relatives, especially those of elderly people. If someone is not deemed capable of giving consent for this, then talking to their relatives can be done under the 'doctrine of necessity', if you determine that the conversation is in the patients best interest.

Telephone conversations are often difficult, as you are never quite sure who you are talking to. Best practice is to ask the person on the phone to come in and speak to you in person, and at the same time take the patient's consent to speak about them with this person.

Children:

Talking to parents is not considered to be a breach of confidentiality unless the child is 'Gillick' or 'Fraser' competent and expresses the wish that his or her parents are not informed. Children under the age of 16 are considered to be 'Gillick' or 'Fraser' competent if they have the ability to sufficiently understand the information given to them, and fully understand what is being proposed. Obviously, this requires a judgement to be made, so if you identify any potential problems, call a senior early on.

HISTORY TAKING

A good, well structured, and accurate history is often the key to successful diagnosis, and consequently management. All histories should follow a basic common structure, though certain aspects may be moved depending on the clinical setting. The following section will outline the basic structure of a history, for further case specific aspects please see the CBD chapters.

10. Mini-CEX

Good communication skills are important to ensuring success in history taking and are discussed in more detail below. Always consider why you are asking the questions and what you aim to gain from the history. This allows you to target your questions to the clinical questions you are asking and allows you to interpret the significance of the answers. For instance, the significance of smoking is different for a patient being assessed pre-operatively, to a patient presenting with possible lung cancer. The typical format and structure of a history is as follows:

1. **Presenting complaint:** Why has the patient presented, and what is the main problem?

2. **History of presenting complaint:**
   a. Detailed questioning of the presenting complaint
   b. What/Where/When
   c. Events before/during/after
   d. Can include details from any of the below sections

3. **Past medical history:**
   a. Detailed questions of the patients past medical, surgical and if appropriate psychiatric, and obstetric history. This should include previous hospital admissions and operations.
   b. Screen for common conditions e.g. diabetes, epilepsy, asthma, etc. Often remembered through the mnemonic MJTHREADS, (MI/IHD, Jaundice, TB, Hypertension, Rheumatic fever, Epilepsy, Asthma, Diabetes, Strokes/TIAs,) with DVT/PE and Cancer added to the end. A number of different mnemonics exist therefore choose one which is best suited to you.

4. **Drug history:**
   a. Regular medications
      i. Name
      ii. Dose
      iii. Time of administration
      iv. Indication
      v. PRN Medications
      vi. Over the counter (OTC) medications
      vii. Herbal remedies
   b. Drug Allergies
      i. What happens, timing in relation to drug, how it was treated
      ii. Previous medications that have been tried

5. **Family history:** Define specific details for example, age, relation, and the outcome of relevant conditions.

6. **Social history:**
   a. Where the patient lives and with whom?
   b. Any extra support form family or carers?
   c. Occupation(s): current and past
   d. Activities of daily living
   e. Other activities/hobbies
   f. Pets
   g. Smoking history:
      i. Define what is/has been smoked

ii. If possible define in pack years

$$1 \text{ pack year} = 20 \text{ cigarettes/day for 1 year}$$

   h. Alcohol history:
      i. Volume
      ii. Type of alcohol – classify in Units

$$\frac{\text{Volume of drink (ml)} \times \text{Alcoholic strength (\%)}}{1,000}$$
$$= \text{Number of units}$$

      iii. Pattern of drinking: regular, binge
      iv. Features of alcoholism: Formal CAGE criteria.
   i. Illicit drugs: ask directly

7. **Systemic enquiry:**
   a. Systematically ask about any other symptoms
   b. Cardiovascular system: Chest pain, palpitations, dyspnoea, orthopnoea, paroxysmal nocturnal dyspnoea, syncope
   c. Respiratory system: SOB, cough, sputum, haemoptysis, pleuritic chest pain
   d. Gastrointestinal system: Constipation, diarrhoea, rectal bleeding, nausea and vomiting, jaundice, haematemesis, change in appetite, abdominal pain or lump, change in bowel habit.
   e. Musculoskeletal: Joint pain or stiffness, rash
   f. Central and peripheral nervous system: Headache, collapse, seizure, dizziness, limb weakness or numbness
   g. Genitourinary system – frequency, dysuria, nocturia
   h. General: Fatigue, weight loss, lethargy

Once the history has been taken, this naturally progresses to performing a clinical examination after obtaining consent from the patient.

MEDICAL EXAMINATIONS

Common principles

Structure overview:

- Inspection
- Palpation
- Percussion
- Auscultation

This section will describe the suggested structure for each of the common clinical examinations. Further details of the examination findings will be highlighted. Important points to emphasise include the overall inspection of the patient, good communication with the patient throughout the examination, the need for a chaperone, and succinct and logical presentation of your findings.

Cardiovascular system examination

1. Wash your hands/clean hands with alcohol hand wash

2. Introduce yourself appropriately (full name and role)

3. Explain the examination and gain verbal consent

4. Expose the patient as required ensuring privacy and dignity is maintained

5. Ensure the patient is comfortable, and encourage them to ask questions at any point during the consultation. Reiterate to the patient if they feel uncomfortable at any point or have any concerns you will be happy to stop the examination

6. When examining females it is always best to have a chaperone

7. Ensure the patient is lying at 45 degrees

8. *Perform adequate examination:*

   a. Inspect general appearance (ill/well, in pain, pale, obvious scars, mitral facies, marfanoid features)

   b. Examine the hands for signs of clubbing, stigmata of infective endocarditis (splinter haemorrhages, Osler's nodes, Janeway lesions)

   c. Measure capillary refill after pressing on a nailbed for 5 seconds

   d. Palpate both the radial pulses noting the rate, rhythm, and radio-radio delay

   e. Palpate for a collapsing pulse

   f. Measure blood pressure accurately

   g. Examine the JVP, including examining for hepatojugular reflux if required

   h. Palpate the carotid pulse for character

   i. Examine the conjunctival membrane for anaemia and sclera for jaundice

   j. Examine the mouth for cyanosis, dentition, high arched palate (Marfan's syndrome)

   k. Expose the chest and examine precordium, including axilla for thoracotomy scars

   l. Palpate and show understanding of the apex beat (most lateral and inferior pulsation)

   m. Palpate for heaves and thrills

   n. Auscultate the heart in all 4 areas, the left axilla and over the carotids

   o. Roll the patient to the left to accentuate mitral murmurs and listen in the mitral area and axilla

   p. Sit the patient up to accentuate aortic murmurs and listen at the left sternal edge in expiration

   q. Auscultate, and if necessary percuss, the lungs

   r. Examine for peripheral (ankle &/or sacral) oedema

   s. Examine for scars over the lower legs consistent with venous harvesting

   t. Complete the examination by examining the observation chart, available ECGs and offering to examine for an abdominal aortic aneurysm, the peripheral vascular system, and other features relevant to any positive findings.

9. Reposition the patient to ensure dignity and comfort. Thank the patient

10. Attend to the patient's dignity and privacy throughout the examination

11. Communicate well with the patient throughout

12. Present findings in a logical and appropriate manner

Characterising murmurs

The following features of any murmur should be noted:

Character	Ejection vs Pansystolic
Timing	systolic/diastolic, early/mid/late
Loudness	Grading • 1/6: very soft • 2/6: soft but detectable immediately • 3/6: clearly audible, no thrill • 4/6: palpable thrill • 5/6: audible with stethoscope only partially touching chest • 6/6: audible without placing stethoscope on chest
Area where loudest	Site where the murmur can be heard the loudest. E.g. Apex, left sternal edge, or aortic and pulmonary areas.
Radiation	Note if the murmur radiates to the axilla or carotids.
Accentuating manoeuvres	Inspiration: increases flow to right side of the heart enhancing murmurs from right sided valvular lesions. Expiration: conversely enhances left sided murmurs

Table 10.1: How to note a heart murmur.

Respiratory system examination

1. Wash your hands/clean hands with alcohol hand wash

2. Introduce yourself appropriately (full name and role)

3. Explain the examination and gain verbal consent

4. Expose the patient as required ensuring privacy and dignity is maintained

5. Ensure the patient is comfortable, and encourage them to ask questions at any point during the consultation. Reiterate to the patient if they feel uncomfortable at any point or have any concerns you will be happy to stop the examination

6. When examining females it is always best to have a chaperone

7. Ensure the patient is lying at 45 degrees

8. *Perform adequate examination:*

   a. Inspect general appearance (ill/well, in pain, pale, obvious

Disease	Features
Aortic stenosis	*Causes:* rheumatic heart disease, congenital bicuspid valve. *Pulse:* low volume pulse, slow rising *Apex:* heaving/Pressure overloaded, non displaced *Auscultation:* ejection systolic murmur over aortic area radiating to carotids, loss of P2 if severe. *Other features:* narrow pulse pressure
Mitral Regurgitation	*Causes:* rheumatic heart disease, prolapsing mitral valve, infective endocarditis *Pulse:* AF *Apex:* displaced thrusting/volume overloaded *Auscultation:* pansystolic murmur over mitral area radiating to axilla
Aortic Regurgitation	*Causes:* rheumatic fever, infective endocarditis *Pulse:* collapsing (water-hammer) pulse *Apex:* displaced, thrusting *Auscultation:* early diastolic murmur at the left sternal edge fourth intercostals space. Mid-diastolic murmur (Austin flint) over the apex. *Other features:* wide pulse pressure, Corrigan's sign (visible carotid pulsations), De Musset sign (head bobbing) and Quincke's sign (visible pulsations in the nail-bed).
Mitral Stenosis	*Causes:* rheumatic heart disease *Pulse:* low volume pulse, AF *Apex:* tapping *Auscultation:* loud first heart sound, an opening snap followed by a mid-diastolic (rumbling) murmur *Other features:* mitral facies

Table 10.2: Features of common valvular heart conditions.

scars, signs of respiratory distress such as accessory muscle use, nasal flaring, cyanosis and use of oxygen)

b. Count the respiratory rate

c. Examine the hands for signs of clubbing, tar stains, wasting of the small muscles, CO_2 retention flap and tremor

d. Palpate the radial pulse

e. Examine the JVP

f. Examine the eyes for Horner's syndrome (miosis, ipsilateral partial ptosis, enophthalmos, and ipsilateral anhydrosis)

g. Examine the conjunctival membrane for anaemia

h. Examine the mouth for central cyanosis

i. Palpate for tracheal position and apex beat

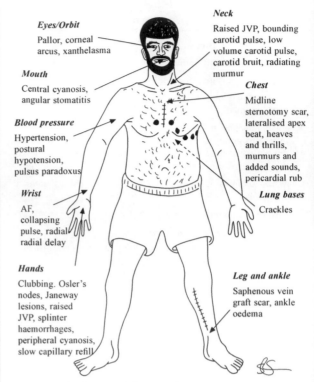

Figure 10.2: Common findings in a cardiovascular system examination.

j. Examine the cervical, supraclavicular, and axilliary lymph glands for lymphadenopathy

k. Expose the chest and examine the precordium, including axilla for thoracotomy scars

l. Measure chest expansion, assessing for symmetry

m. Percuss anterior chest, identifying hypo- or hyper-resonance

n. Palpate for tactile focal fremitus (NB this gives the same information as auscultation for vocal resonance)

o. Auscultate the anterior chest in the same areas which have been percussed, asking the patient to take deep breaths in and out.

p. Auscultate for vocal resonance/whispering pectoriloquy

q. Repeat steps k-p on the posterior chest

r. Examine for peripheral (ankle &/or sacral) oedema

s. Cover the patient and ensure they are comfortable.

t. Complete the examination by examining the observation chart, drug chart, peak flow readings and looking in the sputum pot.

9. Reposition the patient to ensure dignity and comfort. Thank the patient

10. Attend to the patient's dignity and privacy throughout the examination

11. Communicate well with the patient throughout

12. Present findings in a logical and appropriate manner

Disease	Features
Consolidation	*Mediastinum:* central
	Ipsilateral chest wall movement: decreased
	Percussion: dull
	Auscultation: bronchial breathing, reduced breath sounds, coarse crackles
	Vocal Resonance/Whispering Pectoriloquy/Tactile Vocal Fremitus: increased
Collapse	*Mediastinum:* shifted towards collapse
	Ipsilateral chest wall movement: decreased
	Percussion: decreased
	Auscultation: reduced breath sounds
Effusion	*Mediastinum:* shifted away from effusion
	Ipsilateral chest wall movement: decreased
	Percussion: stony dull
	Auscultation: reduced breath sounds Crackles &/or bronchial breathing just above the effusion.
	Vocal Resonance /Tactile Vocal Fremitus: reduced
Simple Pneumothorax	*Mediastinum:* central
	Ipsilateral chest wall movement: decreased on affected side
	Percussion: resonant
	Auscultation: reduced breath sounds
Tension Pneumothorax	*Mediastinum:* shifted away from affected side
	Ipsilateral chest wall movement: decreased on affected side
	Percussion: hyper-resonant
	Auscultation: reduced breath sounds

Table 10.3: Examination findings of common respiratory conditions.

Gastrointestinal system examination

1. Wash your hands/clean hands with alcohol hand wash

2. Introduction yourself appropriately (full name and role)

3. Explain the examination and gain verbal consent

4. Expose the patient as required ensuring privacy and dignity is maintained

5. Ensure the patient is comfortable, and encourage them to ask questions at any point during the consultation. Reiterate to the patient if they feel uncomfortable at any point or have

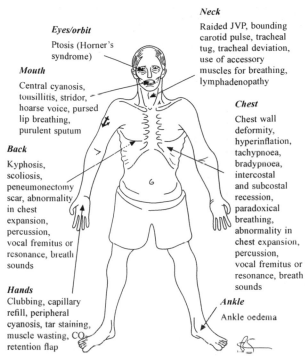

Eyes/orbit
Ptosis (Horner's syndrome)

Mouth
Central cyanosis, tonsillitis, stridor, hoarse voice, pursed lip breathing, purulent sputum

Neck
Raided JVP, bounding carotid pulse, tracheal tug, tracheal deviation, use of accessory muscles for breathing, lymphadenopathy

Back
Kyphosis, scoliosis, peneumonectomy scar, abnormality in chest expansion, percussion, vocal fremitus or resonance, breath sounds

Chest
Chest wall deformity, hyperinflation, tachypnoea, bradypnoea, intercostal and subcostal recession, paradoxical breathing, abnormality in chest expansion, percussion, vocal fremitus or resonance, breath sounds

Hands
Clubbing, capillary refill, peripheral cyanosis, tar staining, muscle wasting, CO₂ retention flap

Ankle
Ankle oedema

Figure 10.3: Common findings in a respiratory system examination.

any concerns you will be happy to stop the examination

6. When examining females it is always best to have a chaperone

7. *Perform adequate examination:*

   a. Inspect general appearance (ill/well, in pain, pale, jaundice, dehydrated etc)

   b. Examine the hands for signs of chronic liver disease (clubbing, leukconychia, koilonychia, palmar erythema, dupytren's contracture)

   c. Check for liver flap (ideally for 20–30 seconds)

   d. Examine the radial pulse and comments on the rate and rhythm of pulse

   e. Examine the arms for tattoos, needle marks, scars/ intravenous drug marks and dialysis fistulae

   f. Examine the eyes for anaemia, jaundice and xanthelasma

   g. Look around the mouth for angular stomatitis (iron deficiency)

   h. Look inside the mouth for smooth tongue, and ulcers (Crohn's disease).

   i. Check for ketotic breath

   j. Palpate the supraclavicular lymph nodes (Virchow's node)

   k. Inspect the chest for spider naevi, gynaecomastia, loss of axillary hair

   l. Inspect the abdomen for abdominal striae, scars, body

10. Mini-CEX

hair distribution, dilated veins, shape, and obvious swellings/masses/hernias

m. Ask the patient to breathe in (to exaggerate masses/organomegaly) and to cough (to exaggerate hernias)

n. Kneel down to the level of the patient's abdomen – check for visible pulsations (aneurysms) and visible peristalsis (small bowel obstruction)

o. Ask the patient if there is any pain in abdomen and look at the face throughout the examination

p. Palpate gently all four quadrants of the abdomen (starting away from pain)

q. Check for tenderness (percussion/rebound), guarding, masses/lumps and bumps

r. Palpate deeply for the above

s. Palpates the liver, starting at the right iliac fossa (RIF) and asking patient to breathe in/out

t. Percuss the liver, from the nipple line down to the RIF

u. If enlarged, assess size, tenderness, regularity and pulsatility

v. Palpate for the spleen, starting at the RIF and asking pt to breath in/out

w. If enlarged, assess size and surface

x. Percuss the spleen in correct manner

y. Balott for both kidneys

z. If enlarged, assess size, surface and consistency

aa. Palpate for an abdominal aortic aneurysm

ab. If there is generalised abdominal swelling, check for shifting dullness

ac. Listen for bowel sounds (ideally for 30s and in 3 places)

ad. Complete the examination by asking to: listen for aortic and renal bruits, perform a digital rectal examination, dipstick the urine (urinalysis), examine for hernias and examining the external genitalia (in a male)

8. Reposition the patient to ensure dignity and comfort, thanks patient

9. Attend to the patient's dignity and privacy throughout the examination

10. Communicate well with the patient throughout

11. Present findings in a logical and appropriate manner

Peripheral nervous system examination

It is important to remember that you will be asking a patient to perform some 'strange' and complicated manoeuvres during this examination, so knowing what you are going to say to describe the movements, and having some back-up descriptions, is of paramount importance.

Always remember to compare one side to the other.

Upper limb

1. Wash your hands/clean hands with alcohol hand wash

2. Introduce yourself appropriately (full name and role)

3. Explain the examination and gain verbal consent

4. Expose the patient as required ensuring privacy and dignity is maintained

5. Ensure the patient is comfortable, and encourage them to ask questions at any point during the consultation. Reiterate to the patient if they feel uncomfortable at any point or have any concerns you will be happy to stop the examination

6. Expose the upper limb

7. Ensure the patient is comfortable and has no pain in the upper limbs

8. General inspection: look for obvious deformities, wasting, fasciculations and resting tremor

9. Ask the patient to stretch their arms out in front of them, palms upward and eyes closed. Look for pronator (or parietal) drift where one hand drifting downwards and beginning to pronate

10. Tone:

   a. Ensure the patient is relaxed and not trying to 'help' you. Flex and extend the elbow and pronate and supinate at the wrist looking for hypotonia or rigidity – 'clasp-knife' or 'leadpipe'. Look for 'cogwheeling' at the wrist. If it is suspected ask the patient to move their opposite arm up and down to reinforce the cogwheel effect.

11. Power:

   a. Shoulder abduction and adduction: ' Make wings with

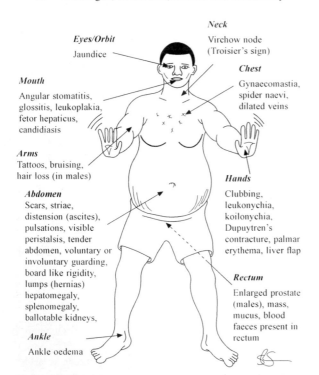

Neck
Virchow node
(Troisier's sign)

Eyes/Orbit
Jaundice

Chest
Gynaecomastia,
spider naevi,
dilated veins

Mouth
Angular stomatitis,
glossitis, leukoplakia,
fetor hepaticus,
candidiasis

Arms
Tattoos, bruising,
hair loss (in males)

Abdomen
Scars, striae,
distension (ascites),
pulsations, visible
peristalsis, tender
abdomen, voluntary or
involuntary guarding,
board like rigidity,
lumps (hernias)
hepatomegaly,
splenomegaly,
ballotable kidneys,

Ankle
Ankle oedema

Hands
Clubbing,
leukonychia,
koilonychia,
Dupuytren's
contracture, palmar
erythema, liver flap

Rectum
Enlarged prostate
(males), mass,
mucus, blood
faeces present in
rectum

Figure 10.4: Common findings in a gastrointestinal system examination.

your arms and don't let me push them up or down.' (Note that although supraspinatus is responsible for the initial 60 degrees of abduction, this will not be examined by this test).

b. Elbow flexion and extension: 'Hold your arms in front of you with the elbows bent. Pull me towards you. Push me away.'

c. Wrist flexion and extension: 'Hold your fists out in front of you. Don't let me push them down. Don't let me push them up.'

d. Grip strength (long and short finger flexors): 'Squeeze my fingers as hard as you can'.

e. Thumb abduction: 'Hold your hands out, palm upwards and thumbs to the sky. Don't let me push it down'.

f. Finger abduction: 'Spread your fingers. Don't let me push them together'.

12. Additional possible tests of power in the hand include

a. Finger extension: 'Hold your fingers out straight, don't let me bend them'

b. Finger adduction: 'put this paper between 2 fingers and don't let me pull it out'.

Movement/action	Muscle	Innervation
Shoulder abduction (first 60)	Supraspinatus	C5
Shoulder abduction	Deltoid	C5
Shoulder adduction	Pectoralis muscles	C5-C8
Elbow flexion	Biceps	C5/C6
Elbow extension	Triceps	C7
Wrist flexion	Flexor Carpi Radialis	Median nerve
	Flexor Carpi Ulnaris	Ulnar nerve
Wrist extension	Long extensors	Radial nerve
Power grip (finger flexion)	Long and short flexors	C8–T1
Thumb abduction	Abductor Pollicis Brevis	Median nerve
Finger abduction	Dorsal Interossei	Ulnar nerve/T1
Finger extension	Long extensors	Radial nerve/C8
Finger adduction	Palmar Interossei	Ulnar nerve/T1

Table 10.4: Movements/actions of the upper limb and the muscle and nerves involved.

13. Reflexes

a. Note: if reflexes are absent use re-inforcement (ask patient to clench teeth immediately before testing reflex)

b. Biceps (C5/6)

c. Triceps (C7)

d. Supinator (C5/6)

e. Finger – positive Hoffmann's sign in upper motor neurone (UMN) lesions

14. Co-ordination

a. Past-pointing with the 'finger-nose' test

b. Dysdiadochokinesis

15. Joint position sense:

a. Gripping the thumb by the sides ask the patient to close their eyes and demonstrate an up movement and a down movement. Then move the thumb up or down and ask the patient which direction you have moved it. If unable to tell reliably, move up a joint and test the wrist.

16. Sensation:

a. Light touch. Ask the patient to close their eyes and demonstrate light touch with some cotton wool over the upper part of the sternum. Take care not to stroke. Then, with the upper limbs in the anatomical position, randomly touch them asking the patient to say 'yes' whenever you do so. Check that the touch feels the same in each place. Ensure every dermatome (C5-T2) is touched and that the radial, median and ulnar nerves are checked (anatomical snuffbox, lateral side of the index finger and medial side of the little finger respectively).

b. Pin-prick.

c. Vibration. Use a 128 Hz tuning fork. After demonstrating on the sternum, start on the thumb and if unable to distinguish the vibration work proximally on bony prominences on the wrist and elbow.

17. Reposition the patient to ensure dignity and comfort, thank the patient

18 Attend to the patient's dignity and privacy throughout the examination

19. Communicate well with the patient throughout

20. Present findings in a logical and appropriate manner

Lower limb

1. Wash your hands/clean hands with alcohol hand wash

2. Introduce yourself appropriately (full name and role)

3. Explain the examination and gain verbal consent

4. Expose the patient as required ensuring privacy and dignity is maintained

5. Ensure the patient is comfortable, and encourage them to ask questions at any point during the consultation. Reiterate to the patient if they feel uncomfortable at any point or have any concerns you will be happy to stop the examination

6. Expose the lower limb

7. Ensure the patient is comfortable and has no pain in the lower limbs

8. General inspection – look for obvious deformities, wasting, fasciculations and resting tremor

9. If they are able, ask the patient to stand and walk

a. Examine their gait.

b. Check tandem walking.

10. Mini-CEX

c. Romberg's test 'Stand with your feet together. Now close your eyes.' Ensure you reassure the patient that they won't fall and that you lightly support them at the shoulders.

10. Tone

a. Ensure the patient is relaxed and not trying to 'help' you. Roll the leg from side to side, looking at the toes to help decide on abnormal tone. Quickly lift under the knee and release.

b. Check for ankle clonus (up to 4 beats is normal)

11. Power

a. Hip flexion/extension: 'keep your leg straight and lift it off the bed. Do not let me push it down. Now push down against my hand'.

b. Knee flexion and extension: 'bend your legs. Pull your ankle towards your bottom. Now push out against my hand'.

c. Ankle dorsiflexion and plantar flexion: 'stop me pushing your foot down. Now push down against my hand'.

Movement/action	Muscle	Innervation
Hip flexion	Iliopsoas	L1/L2
Hip extension	Gluteal muscles	L4/L5
Knee flexion	Hamstring muscles	L5/S1
Knee extension	Quadriceps	L3/L4
Dorsiflexion of the ankle	Tibialis anterior and long flexors	L4/L5
Plantar flexion of the ankle	Gastronemius	S1
Extension of the great toe	Extensor Hallucis Longus	L5

Table 10.5: Movements/actions of the lower limb and the muscle and nerves involved.

12. Reflexes

a. Note: if reflexes are absent use re-inforcement (The Jendrassik manoeuvre - ask patient to clasp hands together and try to pull apart immediately before testing the reflex)

b. Knee (L3/4)

c. Ankle (S1)

d. Plantar – Babinski sign (upgoing in upper motor neurone lesions)

13. Co-ordination: heel-shin test

14. Joint position sense:

a. Gripping the great toe by the sides ask the patient to close their eyes and demonstrate an up movement and a down movement. Then move the toe up or down and ask the patient which direction you have moved it. If unable to tell reliably, move up a joint and rest the ankle.

15. Sensation

a. Light touch. Ask the patient to close their eyes and demonstrate light touch with some cotton wool over the upper part of the sternum. Take care not to stroke. Then randomly touch the lower limbs asking the patient to say 'yes' whenever you do so. Check that the touch feels the same in each place. Ensure every dermatome (L1-S1) is touched.

b. Pin-prick.

c. Vibration. Use a 128 Hz tuning fork. After demonstrating on the sternum, start on the great toe then, if absent there, move proximally to the medial malleolus, knee and iliac crest.

d. Remember that sensory loss may be in a dermatomal pattern, but much more commonly it will be in a 'stocking' distribution. If this is the case, delineate the level by touching up and down the leg and asking where the sensation changes.

16. Reposition the patient to ensure dignity and comfort, thank the patient

17. Attend to the patient's dignity and privacy throughout the examination

18. Communicate well with the patient throughout

19. Present findings in a logical and appropriate manner

Power should be graded using the Medical Research Council (MRC) power scale:

0	Complete absence of movement
1	Flicker of movement
2	Movement when gravity eliminated
3	Movement against gravity but not against resistance
4	Movement against resistance but not full power
5	Normal power

Table 10.6: MRC power scale.

Reflexes are conventionally graded:

–	No response. Abnormal
+	Slight response. May be normal
++	Brisk response. Normal
+++	Very brisk response. May be abnormal
++++	Clonus or abnormal

Table 10.7: Reflex grading scale.

Tract	Ascending or Descending	Site of decussation	Function
Corticospinal Tracts	Descending	Medulla	Motor
Dorsal Columns	Ascending	Brainstem	Proprioception Vibration 2 point discrimination
Spinothalamic Tracts	Ascending	On entry in spinal cord	Pain Temperature

Table 10.8: Summary of the spinal column tracts.

Patterns of peripheral weakness

Upper motor neuron (UMN):

- Increased tone/spasticity (NB acute stroke may have hypotonia)
- Pyramidal pattern of weakness: all muscles are weaker but the arm flexors are stronger than the extensors and the leg extensors are stronger than the flexors
- Hyper-reflexia
- Up-going plantars
- Typical causes: stroke, demyelination, and spinal cord damage

Lower motor neuron (LMN):

- Wasting and fasciculations
- Flaccid tone
- Weakness
- Hypo-reflexia
- Typical causes: radiculopathy, mononeuropathy, and damage to a peripheral nerve

Neuromuscular junction:

- Symmetrical weakness
- Fatigability: muscles become weaker with ongoing activity
- Typical cause: myasthenia gravis

Muscle weakness:

- Symmetrical weakness
- Usually proximal
- No other neurological signs
- Typical causes: muscular dystrophy, Cushing's syndrome, paraneoplastic, polymyositis
- NB: Myotonic dystrophy is atypical and causes distal weakness. Polymyalgia rheumatica causes pain and stiffness but not weakness

Types of abnormal gait

Spastic:

- Foot turned inward
- Hip tilts upwards to lift the affected foot off the floor
- Look for hemiplegia and UMN lesion

Cerebellar:

- Foot turned outwards
- Wide based, and unsteady
- Lurching from side to side
- Look for other cerebellar signs

Ataxic:

- Wide based
- Stamping
- Patient looks at the floor to see where their feet are
- Check Romberg's sign and proprioception

High stepping:

- Knee lifted high to lift the forefoot from the ground
- Foot drop
- Common peroneal nerve palsy

Parkinsonian:

- Difficulty instigating movement
- Short and shuffling steps ('festinant gait')
- Loss of arm swing
- Look for other signs of Parkinson's disease

Waddling:

- Wide gait
- Weight shifted from side to side
- Look for proximal neuropathy

Nerve palsies

Median nerve:

Motor	Sensory
Motor to 4 muscles – 'LOAF' • Lateral 2 lumbricals • Opponens pollicis • Abductor pollicis brevis • Flexor pollicis brevis	Sensation to thumb and lateral 2 ½ fingers

Table 10.9: Motor and sensory innervations of the median nerve.

Causes of median nerve lesions:

- Carpal tunnel syndrome: idiopathic, rheumatoid arthritis, pregnancy, hypothyroidism, and acromegaly
- Trauma to the wrist
- Supracondylar humeral fracture
- Mononeuropathies

Clinical features:

- Thenar wasting
- Tinel's and Phalen's signs
- Test with thumb abduction and opposition
- Sensory loss to the area supplied
- Should have nerve conduction studies prior to any surgical decompression of the carpal tunnel

Ulnar nerve:

Motor	Sensory
Motor to all the other intrinsic muscles of the hand.	Sensation to the little and medial border of the ring finger.

Table 10.10: Motor and sensory innervations of the ulnar nerve.

Causes of ulnar nerve lesions:

- Trauma or arthritis at the medial epicondyle of the elbow
- Wrist trauma
- Compression against the pisiform and hamate bones of the hand. This is commonly seen in occupations with prolonged pressure to the outer part of the palm such as road workers using vibrating drills
- Mononeuropathies

Clinical features:

- Generalised wasting of the hand with sparing of the thenar eminence
- Dorsal guttering
- Froment's sign
- Low lesion (at the wrist): claw hand is paralysis of the lumbricals causing hyperextension of the metacarpophalangeal joints. At the same time, the intact flexor digitorum profundus (FDP) flexes the distal interphalangeal joints.
- High lesion (at the elbow): the less pronounced claw hand (the ulnar paradox) as the FDPs are also paralysed.
- Sensory loss to the area supplied

Radial nerve

Motor	Sensory
Motor to the forearm extensors (extends the wrist)	Sensation to the anatomical snuff-box

Table 10.11: Motor and sensory innervations of the radial nerve.

Causes of radial nerve lesions:

- Fracture of humeral shaft: the nerve runs along the radial groove on the lateral border
- Saturday night palsy: sleeping with the arm over the back of a chair
- Trauma to brachial plexus
- Mononeuropathies

Clinical features

- Wrist drop: test power of wrist extension
- Grip strength is reduced as wrist extension is required for full strength

- Finger ab/adduction is unaffected but must be tested with the palm of the hand flat on the table
- Sensory impairment in the area supplied

Central nervous system examination

1. Wash your hands/clean hands with alcohol hand wash
2. Introduce yourself appropriately (full name and role)
3. Explain the examination and gain verbal consent
4. Ensure the patient is comfortable, and encourage them to ask questions at any point during the consultation. Reiterate to the patient if they feel uncomfortable at any point or have any concerns you will be happy to stop the examination
5. Examination is best carried out seated, facing the patient.
6. Look at the face for obvious abnormalities
7. Cranial Nerve 1 (Olfactory)
   a. This is not routinely fully examined
   b. Ask about any changes in taste or smell
8. Cranial Nerve 2 (Optic)
   a. Visual acuity: Use a Snellen chart if possible if not, ask the patient to read from a book or newspaper. If acuity is too poor to read, use finger movement, hand movement or test the ability to detect light
   b. Visual fields:
      i. Using the 'confrontation' approach with about 1 metre separation between you and the patient. Classically performed using a white hatpin but usually a wiggling finger is used.
      ii. Scotoma can be tested for with a red pin. The blind spot is found at 30 degrees in the temporal field
   c. Accommodation: ask the patient to look at a near and far object
   d. Light response:
      i. Shine light into the eye from an angle (to avoid triggering the accommodation reflex) and check both direct and consensual reflexes.
      ii. Swinging light reflex: test for relative afferent papillary defect
   e. Fundoscopy
9. Cranial Nerves 3, 4 and 6 (oculomotor, trochlear and abducens)
   a. Cranial nerve 3 lesion will result in the pupil appearing 'down and out' There will be ptosis with or without papillary involvement
   b. Cranial nerve 6 lesion will result in the eye being unable to abduct on the affected side.
   c. Ask the patient to keep their head still and follow your finger as you initially move from side to side. Once satisfied pursuit movement is intact and nystagmus is not observed, move the finger up and down, classically in the 'H' shape to test all directions of movement.
   d. Remember to ask the patient to tell you if they see double at any point. If diplopia is found, cover each eye in turn

(the outer image will disappear when the abnormal eye is occluded).

 e. Test saccadic movement and look for internuclear opthalmoplegia.

 f. Look for nystagmus

10. Cranial Nerve 5 (Trigeminal)

 a. Trigeminal nerve has 3 divisions: optic, maxillary and mandibular

 b. Test light touch sensation bilaterally in all 3 divisions using cotton wool.

 c. Feel the masseters once you have asked the patient 'Clench your jaw'

 d. 'Open your mouth' (pterygoids): look for deviation (towards the lesion)

 e. Offer, but do not perform the corneal reflex unless necessary

 f. Jaw jerk. Positive in UMN lesions.

11. Cranial Nerve 7 (Facial). See Facial nerve palsy on next page.

 a. Predominantly motor. More detailed information is given below

 b. Always remember the distinguishing feature of forehead involvement as being, forehead sparing in upper motor neurone lesions. With lower motor neurone lesions the forehead is affected.

 c. Inspect for unilateral loss of the nasolabial fold

 d. Ask the patient to: Frown, screw eyes tightly shut (and endeavour to open them), puff cheeks out and smile.

12. Cranial Nerve 8 (vestibulocochlear)

 a. A brief test of hearing involves whispering a number in each ear whilst occluding the other.

 b. Perform the Rinne and Weber tests using a 512Hz tuning fork

  i. Rinne's test: Place the tuning fork both behind the ear on the mastoid bone and in the air next to the ear. Ask which is loudest. Air conduction is better than bone conduction normally but this pattern is also seen with sensorineural hearing loss. In conductive hearing loss, bone conduction is better.

  ii. Weber's test: Place the tuning fork on the centre of the forehead. Sound will localise to the deaf ear in conductive deafness, but will localise to the contralateral ear in sensorineural loss.

13. Cranial Nerve 9 and 10 (Glossopharyngeal and Vagus)

 a. Ask to look in the mouth and ask the patient to say 'AAAIIIIIIII'. Observe palatial movement and look for deviation of the uvula (towards the lesion)

 b. Offer, but do not perform the gag reflex unless necessary

14. Cranial Nerve 11 (Accessory)

 a. Ask the patient to shrug their shoulders whilst testing power by pushing down on them.

 b. Ask the patient to turn their head and test sternocleido-mastoid power (palpate the contralateral muscle)

15. Cranial Nerve 12 (Hypoglossal)

 a. Inspect the tongue for wasting or fasciculations

 b. 'Stick your tongue out' and look for deviation (away from the lesion)

16. Reposition the patient to ensure dignity and comfort, thank the patient

17. Attend to the patient's dignity and privacy throughout the examination

18. Communicate well with the patient throughout

19. Present findings in a logical and appropriate manner

Pupils

Causes of Mydriatic (large) pupil:

- Third nerve palsy
- Holmes-Adie pupil. Classically reacting to accommodation but slowly to light.
- Traumatic iridoplegia
- Drugs: Tropicamide, cocaine and amphetamines

Causes of Miotic (small) pupil:

- Horner's Syndrome
- Argyll Robertson pupil. Classically bilateral, reacting to accommodation but not to light.
- Age related and are bilateral
- Anisocoria: asymmetric pupil size

Ptosis

- Horner's syndrome: there is usually partial ptosis.
- Third nerve palsy: usually complete ptosis. The eye is 'down and out' with a large pupil.
- Myasthenia gravis: may be unilateral or bilateral. The pupils are normal. It is associated with fatigability and complex opthalmoplegia
- Myotonic dystrophy: usually bilateral. The pupils are normal. It is associated with cataracts, frontal balding and myotonia

Visual field defects

Site of lesion	Visual field defect
Optic Nerve	Unilateral Blindness
Optic Chiasm	Bitemporal hemianopia
Optic Tract	Contralateral homonymous hemianopia
Optic Radiation – parietal lobe	Contralateral homonymous quadrantanopia (inferior)
Optic Radiation – temporal lobe	Contralateral homonymous quadrantanopia (superior)
Occipital Cortex	Cortical Blindness

Table 10.12: Summary of visual field defects.

10. Mini-CEX

Internuclear opthalmoplegia

- The abducting eye is seen to move smoothly but the adducting eye is slow to move. A brief nystagmus is seen in the abducting eye.
- This results from damage to the medial longitudinal facsiculus which co-ordinates uniform horizontal gaze movements.
- Most commonly from demyelination as seen in Multiple Sclerosis
- If found, look for the five signs of optic nerve damage
  - Central scotoma
  - Decreased visual acuity
  - Decreased colour vision
  - Relative afferent papillary defect
  - Optic atrophy

Horner's syndrome

Underlying pathology involves a lesion in the sympathetic chain.

Causes of Horner's syndrome:

- Interruption to the supply from the hypothalamus to the synapse in the spinal cord
  - Stroke
  - Demyelination
  - Syrinx
  - Space occupying lesion
  - Spinal cord trauma
- Interruption to preganglionic neurones running from the cord to the superior cervical ganglion
  - Pancoast's tumour
  - Cervical rib
  - Post neck surgery
- Interruption to post ganglionic neurones running to the pupil
  - Carotid artery dissection or aneurysm

Clinical features (all ipsilateral)

- Miosis (reduced innervation to pupillodilators)
- Partial ptosis (levator palpabrae supplied both by the sympathetic but also the parasympathetic chain)
- Anhydrosis
- Enophthalmosis

Facial nerve palsy

Course of the facial nerve:

- Leaves the brainstem from the pons at the cerebellopontine angle.
- Enters the internal auditory meatus

- Gives off the Greater Petrosal Nerve which is secretomotor to the lacrimal gland.
- Enters the facial canal
- Gives off the nerve to the Stapedius
- Gives off the Chorda Tympani which gives parasympathetic innervation to the submandibular and sublingual glands as well as supplying taste to the anterior 2/3 of the tongue.
- Exits via the stylomastoid foramen
- Splits as it transverses the parotid gland

Causes of facial nerve palsy:

- Bell's palsy
- Ramsay Hunt syndrome
- Parotid swelling/tumour
- Stroke
- Demyelination
- Cerebellopontine angle tumour
- Bilateral Facial Nerve palsy: neurosarcoid, lyme disease, Guillain-Barré syndrome.

Clinical features:

- Unilateral facial weakness
- Inability to completely close the eye
- Bell's phenomenon: eyeball rolls upwards on attempted eye closure
- Loss of naso-labial fold
- Mouth droop

Bulbar and pseudobulbar palsies

Bulbar:

- LMN lesion
- Flaccid, nasal speech
- Feels as if the tongue is too big and keeps getting in the way
- Salivary pooling
- Caused by a unilateral lesion

Pseudobulbar:

- UMN lesion
- Spastic speech: 'Donald duck,' 'hot potato,' 'high pitched.'
- Tongue feels tight and moves very little from the floor of the mouth
- Caused by bilateral lesions: demyelination or bilateral internal capsule strokes

Cerebellar examination

There are two classical mnemonics for remembering the main clinical features of cerebellar disease:

Face

Lack of sensation, loss of nasolabial fold and wrinkles on forehead

Eyes

Ptosis, miosis (Horner's syndrome), Bell's phenomenon, ophthalmoplegia, squint

Mouth

Hoarse voice, dysphonia, dysphagia, dysphasia, fasciculation and wasting of tongue, deviation to one side of tongue on protrusion

Upper limbs

Muscle wasting, fasciculations, flaccid or spastic paralysis, abnormality in power and reflexes, dysmetria, loss of sensation

Lower limbs

Abnormality in tone (clonus), power and reflexes and co-ordination, Romberg's test, ataxia, abnormal gait

Hands

Intentional tremor, resting tremor

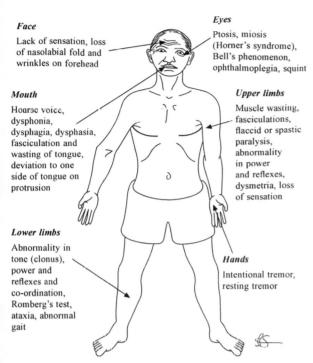

Figure 10.5: Common findings in a neurological examination.

DANISH	**DASHING**
• Dysdiadochokinesis	• Dysdiadochokinesis
• Ataxia	• Ataxia
• Nystagmus	• Slurred speech
• Intention tremor	• Heel-shin incoordination
• Shin-heel incoordination	• Intention tremor
	• Nystagmus
	• Gait: wide-based

However there are other signs which should be elicited and the examination should appear systematic.

1. Wash your hands/clean hands with alcohol hand wash
2. Introduce yourself appropriately (full name and role)
3. Explain the examination and gain verbal consent
4. Ensure the patient is comfortable, and encourage them to ask questions at any point during the consultation. Reiterate to the patient if they feel uncomfortable at any point or have any concerns you will be happy to stop the examination
5. General inspection at rest
6. Upper Limb:
   a. Dysdiadochokinesis is the inability to execute rapidly alternating movements, particularly of the limbs. It is most readily demonstrated by asking the patient to pronate and supinate an arm at speed.
   b. Intention tremor can be abolished with the hand at rest in the patient's lap. It is readily demonstrated with past-pointing when the patient is asked to repeatedly place the tip of their index finger on the tip of their nose and then on the tip of your finger. The effect is emphasised if the patient is forced to stretch the arm out fully to reach your finger-tip. If the patient is weak in the arm there will be apparent past-pointing (a false positive)

7. Lower limb: the heel-shin test
8. Head:
   a. Nystagmus
   b. Fundoscopy: look for pale discs indicative of optic atrophy in multiple sclerosis
9. Trunk: ask the patient to sit upright in the chair or bed. A significant midline (vermis) lesion of the cerebellum will result in truncal ataxia. Therefore the patient will be unable to sit up without steadying themselves.
10. Gait:
    a. Romberg's Test is where the patient may be unable to stand without aid, even with their eyes open (NB Romberg's test is strictly a test of proprioception, so the ataxia seen in cerebellar lesions cannot accurately be described as a positive Romberg's test)
    b. Ask the patient to walk. The gait will be wide-based and the patient will not be able to perform tandem walking
11. Speech: ask the patient to talk. Speech is characteristically dysarthric with either 'scanning speech' where the words are spoken carefully and slowly, or 'staccato speech' where the words are spoken in bursts.
12. Further examination if appropriate, can look for signs suggestive of an underlying pathology, especially in conditions such as multiple sclerosis, stroke or a posterior fossa space-occupying lesion
13. Reposition the patient to ensure dignity and comfort, thank the patient
14. Attend to the patient's dignity and privacy throughout the examination
15. Communicate well with the patient throughout
16. Present findings in a logical and appropriate manner

Speech examination

Disordered speech is not an uncommon finding. There is a temptation to label such a patient as 'confused.' An examination of speech will be able to distinguish the 'confused' from those with an underlying pathology causing the problem.

The testing of speech is also dependent on language. The details below rely on the ability of the patient to understand and speak English. Some modifications will be required if this is not the case.

1. Wash your hands/clean hands with alcohol hand wash
2. Introduction yourself appropriately (full name and role)
3. Explain the examination and gain verbal consent
4. Ensure the patient is comfortable, and encourage them to ask questions at any point during the consultation. Reiterate to the patient if they feel uncomfortable at any point or have

any concerns you will be happy to stop the examination

5. Ask a few general questions to get the feel of the speech e.g. what the patient had for breakfast

6. Test comprehension

   a. Stick your tongue out

   b. Close your eyes

   c. Can increase complexity to 2-step commands such as touch your left ear with your right hand

7. Test expression

   a. Name

   b. Age

   c. Address

8. Test naming

   a. Watch

   b. Pen

   c. Tie

9. Test articulation

   a. British constitution

   b. West register street

   c. Baby hippopotamus

Speech problem	Lesion	Features
Expressive Dysphasia	CNS lesion in Broca's area in the inferior part of the dominant frontal lobe	Inability to verbally express despite adequate comprehension. Patient knows what they want to say but are unable to so. This can be very frustrating
Receptive Dysphasia	CNS lesion in Wernicke's area in the superior temporal lobe	Inability to understand speech. Fluent speech but not related to the conversation
Nominal Dysphasia	CNS lesion in posterior part of the dominant superior temporal gyrus	Inability to name objects. Usually part of a wider dysphasia
Global Dysphasia	CNS lesion in Wernicke's area and Broca's area	Inability to comprehend or express
Dysarthria	Cerebellar disease, extrapyramidal lesions including Parkinson's disease and dystonias, bulbar palsy, pseudobulbar palsy, myasthenia, oral ulceration or severe oral candidiasis	Inability to articulate but no underlying disorder of speech content. See individual sections for further detail

Table 10.13: The different types of speech disorders and the features and lesion associated with them.

10. Test specific structures responsible for articulation

    a. Lips: 'me me me'

    b. Tongue: 'la la la'

    c. Palate: 'k k k'

11. Reposition the patient to ensure dignity and comfort, thank the patient

12. Attend to the patient's dignity and privacy throughout the examination

13. Communicate well with the patient throughout

14. Present findings in a logical and appropriate manner

Parkinson's disease

The classical triad of symptoms are:

- Hypokinesia (poverty of movement)

- Bradykinesia (slowness of movement)

- Rigidity

Other symptoms:

- Are usually asymmetrical

- Are usually seen first in the upper body

- May fluctuate a little with some days worse than others

1. Wash hands/clean hands with alcohol hand wash

2. Introduce yourself appropriately (full name and role)

3. Explain the examination and gain verbal consent

4. Ensure the patient is comfortable, and encourage them to ask questions at any point during the consultation. Reiterate to the patient if they feel uncomfortable at any point or have any concerns you will be happy to stop the examination

5. General inspection at rest

6. Look at the hands, lying at rest in the lap. Examine for 'pill-rolling' tremor:

   a. Typically 4–6 Hz

   b. Intensified by stress

7. Rotate the hand at the wrist, testing for tone and cog-wheel rigidity. If none present ask the patient to repeatedly abduct and adduct the contralateral arm. This 'distraction' will act to re-inforce the cogwheel rigidity.

8. Ask the patient to perform a rhythmic or repetitive movement and look for a gradual deduction in amplitude.

9. Test for 'lead-pipe' rigidity in the upper limbs.

   a. Increased resistance which does not change when passively flexing and extending the elbow joint

   b. Ensure you ask about any pain in the upper limb/shoulder before testing.

10. Look carefully at the face for

    a. Expressionless facies

    b. Drooling of saliva

11. Examine the eye movements looking for impaired vertical gaze and evidence of a progressive supra-nuclear palsy.

12. Test postural blood pressure looking for postural hypotension and evidence of multi-system atrophy

13. Ask the patient to walk and look for:

    a. Difficulty in initiating movement

    b. Short stride length

    c. Shuffling, 'festinant' gait

    d. Stooped posture

    e. Reduction/absence of arm swing

    f. Inability to walk 'heel-to-toe'

    g. Difficulty when turning

    h. Instability, especially on performing the 'retropulsion test.' Stand behind the patient and push them forwards or pull them backwards. Sufferers of Parkinson's disease have difficulty remaining upright, so be prepared to catch and support them!

14. Ask the patient to write: this may reveal micrographia.

15. Ask the patient to talk

    a. Dysarthria caused by bradykinesia and rigidity of orolingual and laryngeal muscles

    b. Low volume, monotone voice

    c. Slurring of words

    d. Reduced gesticulations

16. Perform a mini mental state examination (MMSE): Lewy body dementia may be a feature

17. Reposition the patient to ensure dignity and comfort, thank the patient

18. Attend to the patient's dignity and privacy throughout the examination

19. Communicate well with the patient throughout

20. Present findings in a logical and appropriate manner

Musculoskeletal system screening examination

The musculoskeletal system can be assessed using a screening history and examination. This screening system is known as the GALS assessment, (gait, arms, legs, and spine).

Screening questions

A screening history is comprised of asking three important questions:

1. Do you have any pain/stiffness in your joints or muscles?

2. Are you able to walk up and down stairs without any problems?

3. Can you undress/dress yourself without any difficulty?

The screening examination

1. Wash your hands/clean hands with alcohol hand wash

2. Introduce yourself appropriately (full name and role)

3. Explain the examination and gain verbal consent

4. Expose the patient as required ensuring privacy and dignity is maintained

5. Ensure the patient is comfortable, and encourage them to ask questions at any point during the consultation. Reiterate to the patient if they feel uncomfortable at any point or have any concerns you will be happy to stop the examination

6. When examining females it is always best to have a chaperone

7. *Perform adequate examination*:

    a. Gait

        i. Inspect the patient as they get up from a sitting position

        ii. Inspect the patient as they walk.

        iii. Inspect the patient as they turn whilst walking

    b. Spine

        i. Inspect the spine from the back and each side of the patient

        ii. Ask the patient to bend and touch their toes

        iii. Ask the patient to flex their neck laterally (touch each ear to each shoulder)

    c. Arms

        i. Ask the patient to stand with both hands by their sides

        ii. Ask the patient to hold both hands out in front of them with there palms down and there fingers straight

        iii. Ask the patient to turn both there hands over

        iv. Ask the patient to make a fist with both hands

        v. Ask the patient to touch the tip of each finger with the thumb

        vi. Press across the second and fifth metacarpals. This will identify any pain

        vii. Ask the patient to put both hands behind the head

    d. Legs

        i. Inspect the legs from the front and back with the patient standing

        ii. With the patient lying flat inspect the legs closer

        iii. Flex each hip and knee whilst holding the knee

        iv. Passively perform internal and external hip rotation

        v. Whilst straightening each leg feel for crepitus

        vi. Palpate the knee for tenderness and any swelling

        vii. Press across the metatarsal joints to identify any tenderness

        viii. Inspect the soles of the feet for any callosities.

8. Reposition the patient to ensure dignity and comfort, thank the patient

9. Attend to the patient's dignity and privacy throughout the examination

10. Communicate well with the patient throughout

11. Present findings in a logical and appropriate manner
12. If any abnormalities are identified the joint involved should be examined in more detail

Locomotor system examination

When examining a joint it is important to perform a systematic examination including inspection, palpation, and assessment of joint movement. Always compare each joint with the opposite limb.

1. Wash your hands/clean hands with alcohol hand wash
2. Introduce yourself appropriately (full name and role)
3. Explain the examination and gain verbal consent
4. Expose the patient as required ensuring privacy and dignity is maintained
5. Ensure patient is comfortable, and encourage them to ask questions at any point during the consultation. Reiterate to the patient if they feel uncomfortable at any point or have any concerns you will be happy to stop the examination
6. When examining females it is always best to have a chaperone
7. *Perform adequate examination*:
   a. Inspection
      i. Look for swelling of the joint
      ii. Deformity of the joint, if identified may be fixed or mobile. Examples include trauma, metacarpophalangeal (MCP) and interphalangeal (ICP) joint deformities.
      iii. Skin changes such as redness can indicate joint inflammation.
      iv. Adjacent structures may be affected, such as muscle wasting.
   b. Palpation
      i. Assess the joint for swelling. It is important to identify the consistency of the swelling. A hard swelling suggests deformity of the bone (e.g. osteoarthritis). A boggy swelling can be seen with synovial thickening associated with rheumatoid arthritis. Fluctuant swellings indicated enlargement of joint bursae.
      ii. Palpate the joint margins and surrounding structures (bones, tendons, and ligaments). By palpating the joint identify whether there is tenderness within the joint or outside the joint.
      iii. Assess the temperature of the joint by feeling above and below the joint with the back of your hand. Compare the temperature of the contralateral joint.
   c. Joint movement
      i. The range of movement is assessed. Joint movement may be affected if there is pain or if there is instability.
      ii. Active movement of the joint is where the patient moves the joint, and passive movement is when the joint is moved by the examiner.
      iii. Note the degree of movement (flexion, extension, abduction, adduction, internal and external rotation), of the joint from the neutral position.

8. Shoulder examination
   a. Inspection
      i. Inspect the shoulder from the front, side and back of the patient
      ii. Look for redness, deformity and swelling.
      iii. Identify the muscles (deltoid, supraspinatous, infraspinatous) of the shoulder and note any wasting.
   b. Palpation
      i. Palpate the shoulder and sternoclavicular joints, noting any deformities and tenderness.
      ii. An effusion or swelling may be easily palpated.
      iii. Forward and downward displacement of the joint is known as an anterior dislocation.
      iv. Posterior dislocation of the joint is often more noticeable.
   c. Joint movement
      i. The shoulder joint is assessed by testing flexion, extension, abduction, adduction and internal and external rotation.
      ii. Both active and passive movement must be performed.
      iii. Ask the patient to abduct the arm/shoulder (arc). A painful arc occurs with inflammation of the rotator cuff muscles. The typical sequence is of no initial pain, followed by pain occurring as the muscles come into contact with the acromium. During the final part of abduction the pain disappears.

9. Examination of the hand
   a. Inspection
      i. Inspect the hands of the patient on a flat surface in front of you.
      ii. Look for swelling, deformity, skin changes, and nail changes.
      iii. Ask the patient to turn over their hands to allow inspection of the palms. Look for any tendon thickening or callosities.
      iv. Identify any muscle wasting.
   b. Palpation
      i. There are three important joints to palpate; the wrist, MCP and ICP joints.
      ii. Identify if the patient has any pain in the hands
      iii. Identify any swelling, nodules, and deformities.
      iv. In osteoarthritis you may identify heberden's nodes on the distal ICP joints and bouchard's nodes over the proximal ICP joints.
   c. Joint movement
      i. Movement of the thumb and fingers must be assessed.

ii. Ask the patient to adduct and abduct the fingers

iii. Assess function of the hands by asking the patient to open and 'do up' a button on their shirt.

10. Reposition the patient to ensure dignity and comfort, thank the patient

11. Attend to the patient's dignity and privacy throughout the examination

12. Communicate well with the patient throughout

13. Present findings in a logical and appropriate manner

PRE-OPERATIVE HISTORY

1. Introduce yourself appropriately (full name and role)

2. Inform the patient that a number of questions will be asked to obtain an accurate history.

3. Gain verbal consent for the interview

4. Ensure the patient is comfortable, and encourage them to ask questions at any point during the consultation. Reiterate to the patient if they feel uncomfortable at any point or have any concerns you will be happy to stop

5. Brief history of presenting complaint

    a. Ask the patient what operation they are due to undergo

    b. What symptoms the patient is experiencing?

    c. Take a pain history

        i. Remember the mnemonics SOCRATES: site, onset, character, radiation, alleviating factors, time (duration of pain), exacerbating factors and the severity of the pain.

    d. How was their condition diagnosed?

    e. Have they had any investigations or undergone any procedures to assist with the diagnosis?

6. Past medical history

    a. A mnemonics MJTHREADS can be used to identify any pre-existing conditions; MI, Jaundice, TB, Hypertension, Rheumatic fever, Epilepsy, Asthma, Diabetes mellitus, Sickel cell disease.

7. Past surgical history

    a. Any previous operations?

    b. If yes, what procedure have they undergone?

    c. Were there any previous operative and/or post operative complications?

    d. Did they have a general anaesthetic?

    e. Did they require ITU admission?

    f. How many days did the patient stay in hospital?

8. Drug history

    a. Prescribed medication (e.g. anticoagulants, and steroids)

    b. OTC drugs.

    c. Previous illicit drugs use?

    d. Allergies (e.g. antibiotics or anaesthetic drugs)

    e. Previous blood transfusion

9. Family history

    a. Identify any familial condition such as clotting disorders.

10. Social history

    a. A detailed social history will assist with post operative rehabilitation and discharge planning.

    b. Identify the normal functioning level of the patient by enquiring about activities of daily living (ADLs), such as bathing, cooking, and cleaning.

    c. Ask about current housing and living conditions. For example the number of stairs, shower or bath, and the presence of handrails within there residence. This will help to predict how well the patient will cope in their own home post operatively.

    d. Ask about the patient's support network, which will be invaluable in the patients recovery.

    e. Elderly patients may be receiving support from carers and social services

    f. Enquire about the patient's alcohol consumption for one week in units.

    g. Ensure a smoking history is taken and patients are encouraged to stop at least 4 weeks prior to surgery.

11. Review of systems

    a. It is important to identify and rule out any other potential problems as a result of undergoing the operation

    b. Asks about the following:

        i. Head: headaches, dizziness, visual problems, faints, fits or falls

        ii. Neck: dysphagia, and stiffness

        iii. Chest: dyspnoea, chest pain, palpatations, wheeze, haemoptysis, PND, and orthopnoea

        iv. Abdomen: haematemesis, bowel habit, tenesmus, malaena, and pain

        v. Urinary: dymptoms of UTI, retention, frequency, urgency, nocturia, and dribbling

        vi. Joints: pain, stiffness, swelling, and back pain.

        vii. Constitutional symptoms: weight loss, fatigue, and change in appetite

12. Summary

    a. Ask if the patient has any questions

    b. Provide information to the patient including any useful leaflets

    c. Attemp to alleviate all of the patient's concerns

    d. Inform the patient of the plan for the day of admission

SURGICAL EXAMINATIONS

Common principles:

Structure overview:

- Inspection

- Palpation
- Percussion
- Auscultation

This section will describe the suggested structure for each of the common clinical examinations. Further details of the examination findings will be highlighted. Important points to emphasise include the overall inspection of the patient, good communication with the patient throughout the examination, the need for a chaperone, and succinct and logical presentation of your findings.

Pre-operative examination

1. Wash hands/clean hands with alcohol hand wash
2. Introduce yourself appropriately (full name and role)
3. Explain the examination and gain verbal consent
4. Expose the patient as required ensuring privacy and dignity is maintained
5. Ensure patient is comfortable, and encourage them to ask questions at any point during the consultation. Reiterate to the patient if they feel uncomfortable at any point or have any concerns you will be happy to stop the examination
6. When examining females it is always best to have a chaperone
7. *Cardiovascular examination:*
    a. This examination is performed as described in the cardiovascular system examination. There are specific features which are important to identify if present.
    b. What is the rate and rhythm of the pulse?
    c. Atrial fibrillation (AF) is very common and should be identified and treated prior to surgery.
    d. Is there a murmur present?
        i. It may be necessary to perform an echocardiogram prior to surgery.
    e. Are there signs of heart failure?
        i. Pitting oedema, raised JVP, displaced apex beat.
        ii. An echocardiogram should be performed.
    f. Are there any carotid bruits present?
        i. The risk of stroke increases if the operation is carried out.
        ii. A carotid doppler may be required pre-operatively
    g. Is there a pulsatile mass in the abdomen?
        i. Ask the patient if they have a history of an abdominal aneurysm
        ii. An abdominal ultrasound should be performed urgently.
    h. Is the patient a known hypertensive?
        i. Blood pressure readings must be optimised prior to surgery.
        ii. This involves working closely with the GP.
8. *Respiratory examination:*
    a. This examination is performed as described in the respiratory system examination. There are specific features which are important to identify if present.
    b. Is there a history and clinical signs of underlying lung disease
    c. Pre-operative investigations may therefore include CXR, formal pulmonary lung function tests and a baseline arterial blood gas.
9. *Abdominal examination:*
    a. Identify important signs such as hepatomegaly, splenomegaly, and any abdominal masses.
    b. Any new findings will need further pre-operative investigation.
10. *Neurological examination:*
    a. A baseline abbreviated mental test score should be documented for all elderly patients. The test is marked out of ten and consists of the following questions:
        i. Date of birth
        ii. Age
        iii. Year
        iv. Recognition
        v. Place
        vi. Address recall
        vii. Year of WW2
        viii. Prime Minister
        ix. Time
        x. Count backwards from 20 down to 1

    A score of 8 or less should warrant further MMSE
    Score < 7/10 = suggests cognitive impairment
    Score < 6/10 = possible dementia, delirium

11. *Neck examination:*
    a. Can the patient completely flex and extend the neck?
    b. Does the patient have a history of arthritis in the neck?
    c. This can result in difficulty when managing the airway, and therefore the patient should be discussed with the anaesthetist.
12. *Airway examination:*
    a. This is important to inform the anaesthetist of potential difficulties when managing the patients airway.
    b. The Mallampati classification is commonly used. Each class is determined by what features are seen when the mouth is opened:
        - Class I: Soft palate, fauces, uvula and pillars
        - Class II: Soft palate, fauces, portion of the uvula
        - Class III: Soft palate, base of uvula
        - Class IV: Hard palate only
13. Maintain an orderly manner throughout the examination

14. Attend to the patient's dignity and privacy throughout the examination

15. Communicate well with the patient throughout

16. Allow the patient to dress in private

17. Baseline Measurements should be documented

    a. BP, Pulse rate and peak flow

    b. BMI should be calculated

    c. A baseline ECG should be performed

    d. Baseline blood tests

        i. FBC – look for anaemia, infection, and platelet level

        ii. U&E's – look for impaired renal function

        iii. LFT's – deranged LFT's may require further investigation

        iv. Coagulation screen – patients taking anticoagulants.

        v. Group and save – if there is a likelihood of the patient requiring a blood transfusion.

18. Summary

    a. Ask if the patient has any questions.

    b. Discuss the need for any further investigations.

    c. If any problems have been identified discuss this with the anaesthetist and consultant surgeon.

Top tips

- Do not rush through the examination; be thorough and systematic in your approach.
- Try to arrive to the clinic early as they are often busy and run late behind schedule.
- Individual hospitals may have pre-assessment pro formas, which you should familiarise yourself with.

Lump examination

When examining any lump or mass it is important to have a systematic approach and ensure a thorough assessment is performed. Document the following:

- Site
- Size
- Shape
- Surface
- Colour
- Contour (edge)
- Consistency
- Temperature
- Tenderness
- Transilluminance
- Mobility
- Pulsatility
- Auscultation sounds

These findings will aid in the diagnosis of any lump. See lump section in Surgery chapter.

Hernia examination

1. Wash your hands/clean hands with alcohol hand wash

2. Introduce the yourself appropriately (full name and role)

3. Explain the examination and gain verbal consent

4. Expose the patient as required ensuring privacy and dignity is maintained

5. Ensure the patient is comfortable, and encourage them to ask questions at any point during the consultation. Reiterate to the patient if they feel uncomfortable at any point or have any concerns you will be happy to stop the examination

6. Take a brief history of the lump

    a. Is there a lump in the groin?

    b. Is it tender to touch?

    c. Can the patient reduce the lump?

    d. Has the lump increased in size?

    e. Are there any associated symptoms e.g. nausea and vomiting?

7. Ensure a chaperone is present

8. Expose the patient (waist down)

9. ***Perform adequate examination:***

    a. Ask the patient to stand (hernias are best visualised like this)

    b. Inspect the groin area looking for

        i. Swellings (site, size, shape and format)

        ii. Scars

        iii. Discolouration

    c. Examine the swelling

        i. Inspect the groin looking for scars, signs of infection or hernia strangulation

        ii. The swelling should be palpated and its consistency, temperature, tenderness, pulsations, and colour should be documented

        iii. Determine the size and shape of the lump

        iv. Ask the patient to attempt to reduce the swelling themselves, as this is usually less painful

        v. Observe and identify the site at which the hernia is reduced

        vi. With the hernia reduced performs the cough test by placing a hand over the swelling and asking the patient to cough, feeling for a positive cough impulse.

        vii. Determine the type of hernia by placing a finger at the pubic tubercle and asking the patient to cough. Inguinal hernias are found superior and medial to the pubic tubercle. Femoral hernias are found inferior and lateral to the pubic tubercle

        viii. To distinguish between a direct and indirect inguinal hernia, the hernia is reduced and pressure is applied over the deep inguinal ring (mid-point of the inguinal ligament). The patient is then asked to cough. If the hernia is controlled this is an indirect hernia, and if the hernia is revealed it is a direct hernia. This is clinically accurate in only 20–30% of cases

        ix. In male patients examine the scrotum to identify

hernia extension. If a mass in the scrotum is present and you cannot get above it, then the likely diagnosis is a hernia.

   x. An attempt should be made to transilluminate the lump. If this is positive a hydrocele in the scrotum is a possible diagnosis

   xi. Examine the opposite site for other or similar swellings

   xii. Palpate for other swellings such as lymph nodes

   xiii. Repeat palpation of the groin area with the patient lying down on the couch

   xiv. Auscultate the swelling to identify bowel sounds.

   d. Abdominal examination should be performed to complete the examination

10. Reposition the patient to ensure dignity and comfort, thank the patient

11. Attend to the patient's dignity and privacy throughout the examination

12. Communicate well with the patient throughout

13. Present findings in a logical and appropriate manner

Thyroid examination

Examination of the neck includes examination of all swellings, lymph nodes and the thyroid gland. It is important to understand the possible aetiologies of neck swellings, as this will assist you in performing a focused examination. Here we will concentrate on the thyroid gland, however it is important to observe the patient for other stigmata of thyroid disease.

1. Wash your hands/clean hands with alcohol hand wash

2. Introduce the yourself appropriately (full name and role)

3. Explain the examination and gain verbal consent

4. Expose the patient as required ensuring privacy and dignity is maintained

5. Ensure the patient is comfortable, and encourage them to ask questions at any point during the consultation. Reiterate to the patient if they feel uncomfortable at any point or have any concerns you will be happy to stop the examination

6. Take a brief history of the presenting complaint:

   a. When did the patient first notice the lump?

   b. Has the lump changed over time?

   c. Any there any associated symptoms?

   d. Is there any pain, dyspnoea or dysphagia associated with the lump?

   e. Is there any family history of thyroid problems or neck lumps?

7. ***Perform adequate examination***

   a. Adequately expose the patient this will require unbuttoning the top of shirt as both neck triangles and supraclavicular fossae should be clearly visible.

   b. Carry out a general inspection of the patient:

      i.   Is the patient comfortable at rest

      ii. Agitated (hyperthyroidism)

      iii. Restless (hyperthyroidism/pain)

      iv. Sweating (hyperthyroidism)

      v.   Underweight (hyperthyroidism/malignancy)

      vi. Overweight (myxoedema)

      vii. Peaches and cream complexion (hypothyroidism)

      viii. Pretibial myxodema (myxodema)

      ix. Dry skin/hair (hypothyroidism)

   c. Examine the neck from the front and the side of the patient looking for:

      i.   Lump position

      ii. Number of lumps

      iii. Overlying skin (tethering in malignancy, erythema with inflammation)

      iv. Asymmetry

      v.   Scars

   d. Ask the patient to swallow some water. If the lump ascends on swallowing then it is associated with the thyroid gland.

   e. Ask the patient to open their mouth and protrude the tongue. A thyroglossal cyst is likely if the lump moves up on tongue protrusion.

   f. Inspect the hands for:

      i.   Sweating

      ii. Pulse rate (tachycardia, bradycardia and atrial fribillation)

      iii. Palmar erythema

      iv. Thyroid acropachy

      v.   Ask the patient to hold their arms/hands out in front of them in a straight position. A fine tremor is seen in thyrotoxicosis.

   g. Inspect the eyes from all angles looking for:

      i.   Exophthalmos/proptosis (abnormal projection of the eyeball)

      ii. Ophthamoplegia (limited eye movement), or chemosis (oedema of the conjunctiva)

      iii. Looks for lid lag (the patient follows your finger with their eyes resulting in the eyelids lagging behind the eyeball)

      iv. Look for lid retraction, (wherby the sclera visible between the iris and upper eyelid)

      v.   Lid lag and lid retraction are a result of overactivity of the levator palpebrae superioris which is due to increased activity of the sympathetic pathway.

   h. Palpate the lump

      i.   Ask if there is any pain prior to and on palpation.

      ii. A visible lump is examined from the front and from behind the patient.

      iii. Ensure trachea is central as thyroid enlargement can displace the trachea.

iv. When examining the neck from behind stand behind the patient and inform them of what you are about to do.

v. Rest the fingers of both hands on each side of the neck.

vi. Palpate the isthmus, lateral lobes of thyroid gland and any other swellings. (a normal thyroid gland is not palpable).

vii. Ask the patient to swallow again whilst palpating to confirm if the lump ascends on swallowing.

viii. Examine for the presence of lymph nodes (anterior and posterior cervical chains, submandibular, submental, pre-auricular, post-auricular and occipital nodes).

i. Percuss the lump

   i. Percuss over the clavicles, upper sternum and the anterior chest wall to identify the presence of retrosternal extension of the swelling/thyroid gland.

j. Auscultate the lump

   i. Listen for any bruits over the swelling as a result of increased vascularity

8. Request the patient to get up from his/her chair without using one's arms (looking for proximal myopathy)

9. Reposition the patient to ensure dignity and comfort, thank the patient

10. Attend to the patient's dignity and privacy throughout the examination

11. Communicate well with the patient throughout

12. Present findings in a logical and appropriate manner

Top tips

- Inspect the oral cavity, as oral malignancy can present with neck lymphadenopathy.

- Large retrosternal goitres will elicit facial flushing, distended neck veins and stridor on elevation of both arms above patients head. This is called Pemberton's signs and occurs due to superior vena caval compression by a mediastinal mass.

- Possible further investigations include thyroid function tests, ultrasound scan of thyroid gland/neck, a radionuclide scan of thyroid or a lymph node biopsy.

Varicose vein examination

1. Wash your hands/clean hands with alcohol hand wash

2. Introduce yourself appropriately (full name and role)

3. Explain the examination and gain verbal consent

4 Expose the patient as required ensuring privacy and dignity is maintained

5. Ensure the patient is comfortable, and encourage them to ask questions at any point during the consultation. Reiterate to the patient if they feel uncomfortable at any point or have any concerns you will be happy to stop the examination

6. When examining females it is always best to have a chaperone

7. Take a brief history of the presenting complaint:

a. How long have the varicose veins been present?

b. Are there any associate risk factors? (Obesity, pregnancy, abdominal mass).

c. Are there are associated symptoms? (Ulcers, pain, pruritis, discolouration)

d. Have the veins changed over time?

e. Any previous varicose vein or vascular surgery?

8. ***Perform adequate examination:***

a. Adequately expose the patient

   i. Expose the patient from the groin down (it is not necessary to remove the underwear).

   ii. Stands the patient up to examine the legs

b. Inspect the legs

   i. Look for dilated tortuous veins.

   ii. Document the site, severity and size of the veins. A diagram of the limbs can be drawn to achieve this.

   iii. Press the veins gently and observe the varicosities refill. This confirms the vascularity of the affected areas.

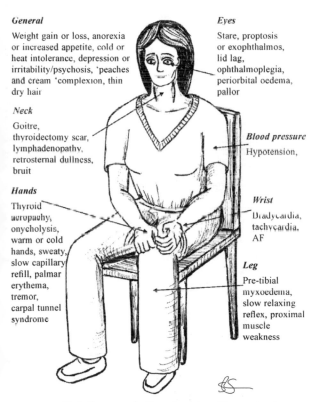

General

Weight gain or loss, anorexia or increased appetite, cold or heat intolerance, depression or irritability/psychosis, 'peaches and cream' complexion, thin dry hair

Neck

Goitre, thyroidectomy scar, lymphadenopathy, retrosternal dullness, bruit

Hands

Thyroid acropachy, onycholysis, warm or cold hands, sweaty, slow capillary refill, palmar erythema, tremor, carpal tunnel syndrome

Eyes

Stare, proptosis or exophthalmos, lid lag, ophthalmoplegia, periorbital oedema, pallor

Blood pressure

Hypotension,

Wrist

Bradycardia, tachycardia, AF

Leg

Pre-tibial myxoedema, slow relaxing reflex, proximal muscle weakness

Figure 10.6: Common findings in a thyroid examination.

10. Mini-CEX

iv. Identify any ulcers, eczema, haemosiderin deposits (brown pigmentation) and scars.

v. Identify short and long saphenous vein involvement. Long saphenous varicosities are seen along the medial aspect of the entire leg, and the short saphenous along the posterolateral lower leg

vi. Make a point of looking at the front and back of both legs

c. Palpate the legs

i. Assess the temperature of the affected areas and the associated surrounding skin

ii. Feel for skin and subcutaneous tissue texture of the lower limb

iii. Identify lipodermatosclerosis (progressive sclerosis of the skin) with pain, pitting oedema and erythema

iv. Palpate the sapheno-femoral junction (SFJ) located 3 cm below and lateral to the pubic tubercle. In particular feel for a saphena varix. This presents as a lump in the groin that is a dilatation of the the long saphenous vein at its origin. It should empty on minimal pressure and refills on release

v. Whilst palpating the SFJ get the patient to cough and feel for a cough impulse. A positive result indicates an incompetent SFJ

d. Trendelenburg test

i. This is a tourniquet test to assess the site of valve incompetence in the superficial veins of the legs

ii. Examines each leg independently

iii. Lie the patient down on their back and raise the leg to empty the veins.

iv. Apply a tourniquet just below the saphenous opening (upper thigh) and asks the patient to stand up

v. If the veins remain empty the sapheno-femoral junction is incompetent and is the cause of the superficial venous reflux

vi. If the tourniquet does not control the varicose veins and allows the vein to fill with blood, the test can be repeated with the tourniquet placed lower down the leg until the point of control is reached

e. Perthes test assesses the patency of the deep venous system.

i. With the tourniquet still on ask the patient to walk around and stand up and down on their tiptoes. If the veins improve the deep system is intact. If the calf veins become engorged and there is increasing calf discomfort the deep venous system is occluded

f. Tap test

i. The visible vein at the upper end is tapped, with a finger placed on the lower end of the vein

ii. This is best performed just below the SFJ

iii. A percussion wave may be felt if an incompetent valve is present

iv. The stronger the percussion wave, the larger the vein and fewer competent valves

v. This is a particularly unreliable test that has been replaced by doppler ultrasound testing, but be aware of it!

g. Check all foot pulses before moving onto auscultation. One of the treatments for varicose veins is compression stockings but this is contraindiacted if there is evidence of lower limb arterial insufficiency.

h. Auscultate the vein

i. Auscultate over the veins for bruits.

ii. A bruit is suggestive of an arteriovenous fistula, which is often mistaken for varicosities.

9. Reposition the patient to ensure dignity and comfort, thank the patient

10. Attend to the patient's dignity and privacy throughout the examination

11. Communicate well with the patient throughout

12. Present findings in a logical and appropriate manner

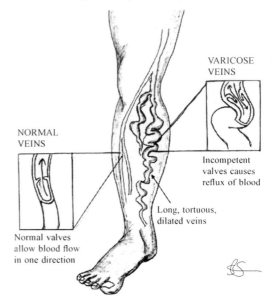

Figure 10.7: Normal veins and varicose veins.

Top tips

• A handheld Doppler ultrasound is a useful tool when assessing peripheral circulation.

Peripheral vascular examination (lower limb)

1. Wash hands/clean hands with alcohol hand wash

2. Introduction yourself appropriately (full name and role)

3. Explain the examination and gain verbal consent

4. Expose the patient as required ensuring privacy and dignity is maintained

5. Ensure the patient is comfortable, and encourage them to ask questions at any point during the consultation. Reiterate to the patient if they feel uncomfortable at any point or have any concerns you will be happy to stop the examination

6. When examining females it is always best to have a chaperone

7. ***Perform adequate examination:***

    a. Adequately expose the patient (entire lower limbs)

    b. General inspection of the patient:

        i. Ensure the patient is comfortable at rest

        ii. Look for mottling, duskiness, necrosis, and missing toes

        iii. Ulceration: note the site, size, shape, edge, presence of slough, and whether the ulcer is venous (painless, varicose veins, eczema) or arterial (painful and punched out lesions).

        iv. Hands: note any discolouration, tar staining and temperature.

        v. Document any scars from previous operations

    c. Palpation

        i. Temperature (using the back of your hands, comparing both sides)

        ii. Tenderness

        iii. Capillary refill time

        iv. Peripheral pulses (femoral, popliteal, posterior tibial, dorsalis pedis)

    d. Auscultation

        i. listen for bruits over the femoral and aorta

    e. Specific Tests

        i. Buerger's Angle can be identified by raising the leg and noting the angle at which the leg becomes white. (Ask about hip pain prior to performing the test!)

           • $\geq 90°$ = Normal angle

           • $20° - 30°$ = Ischaemic leg

           • $< 20°$ = Severe ischaemia

        ii. Buerger's test is where the patient lies supine, and one leg is lifted up for 2-3 minutes. The patient then sits up and hangs the leg over the side of the bed. The leg is observed and the time taken for the foot to become pink is noted.

            • Foot stays pink = Normal

            • Turns pink slowly + reactive hyperaemia = Ischaemic leg

            • Takes 30 seconds = Severe ischaemia

        iii. Ankle-Brachial Pressure index

            • The systolic blood pressure in the arms should be the same or slightly above the systolic blood pressure in the legs.

            • The ABPI is the value given for the ratio of the systolic BP of the legs to the systolic BP of the arms.

            • This is calculated using a Doppler probe.

    f. Complete the examination by performing a neurological and locomotor examination. Do not forget to ask the patient to walk.

8. Reposition patient to ensure dignity and comfort, thank the patient

9. Attend to patient's dignity and privacy throughout the examination

10. Communicate well with the patient throughout

11. Present findings in a logical and appropriate manner

Further reading and references

➢ Douglas D, Nicol F, Robertson C (2009). *Macleod's Clinical Examination* (12 Ed.). Churchill Livingstone.

➢ Epstein O, Perkin GD, Cookson J (2008). *Clinical examination* (4 Ed.). Mosby

➢ Hall T (2008). *PACES for the MRCP: With 250 Clinical Cases* (2 Ed.). Churchill Livingstone

➢ National Institute for health and Clinical Excellence (2006). *Parkinson's Disease. National clinical guideline for diagnosis and management in primary and secondary care (CG35).*

INTRODUCTION

The Foundation Year 2 (FY2) is the final part of the Foundation Programme. By this stage a doctor has successfully completed 12 months, and is fully registered with the General Medical Council (GMC). The Foundation Year 1 (FY1) will have improved your general medical and surgical knowledge, as well as allowed you to develop and learn new skills. These attributes will aid and support your overall professional development.

The FY2 year has been specifically designed to expose you to a number of different specialties. These specialties tend to be specialist areas of medicine and surgery where one would require specialist knowledge or experience to progress. Each specialty has limited places for FY2 doctors, however if you are interested in a particular specialty your educational supervisor can help you to arrange a taster week, allowing you to explore your interest.

The following include summaries of a few of the potential specialties that you may be interested in.

SPECIALTIES

General practice

This placement will be different to all the settings you will have worked in during your FY1 year. It is the environment of primary care medicine. Here you will gain experience in caring for patients where there is more continuity of care, and initiate further referrals. This will enable you to follow the care of a patient from the acute illness to their investigations, diagnosis, and recovery. By actively being involved in this pathway you will gain better understanding of the patient and therefore provide good quality care.

When starting your placement you will initially have an induction to general practice, which will include working with General Practitioners (GPs) and other primary health care workers. During this attachment you will have the opportunity to see patients in the surgery and at their homes (under supervision). Other aspects of this placement will include working on a project, completing assessments and attending formal FY2 teaching sessions.

Academic placements

If you are an individual who is interested in research, teaching or education, an academic clinical attachment may be for you. The academic field involves participating in innovative research, training both undergraduates and postgraduates, whilst maintaining a clinical role. During this rotation you will therefore have the opportunity to combine a research project in a specialty of your choice with clinical work. This will inevitably allow you to develop and improve your research skills whilst, at the same time gain your foundation competencies. It may also allow you to fully immerse yourself into the world of academia and its trials and tribulations as well as its excitement.

There are a number of different academic rotations available. A career as an academic offers a wide range of opportunities which will undoubtedly prove to be challenging and at the same time a satisfying career pathway.

Paediatrics

Paediatrics is a specialty involved in the care of children up to the age of 16 years, within which there are a number of sub-specialties. At the start of the rotation you will be given a specific role with responsibilities. You will have the opportunity to take an active role on the children's ward, neonatal unit (and attending neonatal resuscitation), outpatient clinics, children's day unit and paediatric accident and emergency. When seeing new patients for the first time you will be encouraged to assess the patient and make a management plan. This should then be discussed with a senior member of the team before initiating any treatment.

During the rotation you will receive training on neonatal and paediatric life support. Further training will help to develop your skills in confidently performing newborn examinations, as well as practical procedures such as venepuncture, cannulation and lumbar punctures.

This rotation will provide many opportunities to perform an audit, be involved in teaching, and participate in clinical presentations. These activities will be integral to help you to achieve your foundation competencies and provide an invaluable insight into a career in paediatrics.

Obstetrics and Gynaecology

Obstetrics and Gynaecology is a specialty encompassing the care involved in 'women's health'. During this rotation you will gain an accurate insight into this specialty by developing your Obstetrics and Gynaecology knowledge and related basic skills. Both of these will develop when exposed to areas such as gynaecology theatre, labour ward, early pregnancy unit, and outpatient clinics (antenatal clinic, gynaecology clinic and urodynamics).

To continue to develop as a junior doctor, you will be given the opportunity to perform an audit or presentation, and attend educational courses (e.g. Basic Surgical Skills and Advanced Life Support in Obstetrics).

This rotation will successfully provide you with an overview of the life of an Obstetrician and Gynaecologist. This rotation encompasses both medicine and surgery, which is often what attracts junior doctors to this field.

Psychiatry

Psychiatry is a field of medicine that incorporates the psychological and social aspects of patient care. It is a specialty in which patients with mental health illnesses are treated; such as learning disabilities, anxiety, depression and schizophrenia. This specialty confronts the issues of the impact of mental health disease on the lives of patients and their friends and families. Health professionals working within this field work closely in a multidisciplinary team both in hospital and in the community.

During your psychiatric rotation you will definitely be given the opportunity to improve your communication skills, as this is one of the only fields of medicine in which a diagnosis is made solely on history, mental state and physical examination. Your responsibilities as an FY2 doctor will involve the daily management of all the patients on the ward, reviewing patients in the community, attending outpatient clinics, attending multidisciplinary meetings, and sometimes assessing patients in the accident and emergency department.

Currently, basic specialist training will take a minimum of three years and involve rotations in general practice, accident and emergency and general medicine. You will then enter higher specialist training (after completing the Royal College of Psychiatrist exams). This will involve teaching in general psychiatry for adults, which lasts three years.

Ophthalmology

Ophthalmology is a specialty involved in the management of disorders of the eye. It is another specialty that encompasses many aspects of medicine and surgery. This rotation will endeavour to broaden your knowledge on the anatomy and physiology of the visual system. It will also illustrate the diagnosis and management of common ophthalmological conditions and acute ophthalmological emergencies.

During this rotation you will build upon your examination skills by practicing ophthalmoscopy, testing for visual acuity, intra-ocular pressure measurement, slit lamp use, and many others. By attending clinics you will improve your knowledge on eye disease associated with other medical conditions, such as diabetes and hypertension. When attending theatre sessions you will gain an understanding of basic surgical skills and the effectiveness of laser treatment.

Throughout this and all other rotations you will be assessed using your foundation learning portfolio. Try to use the portfolio to document interesting cases and learning points from the rotation. This will aid your decision when applying to a training post in this specialty.

Other specialties that you may be exposed to as an FY2 include:

- Accident and Emergency
- Ears, Nose, and Throat (ENT)
- Pathology
- Microbiology
- Radiology
- ITU
- Public Health Medicine
- Clinical genetics

Often as a Foundation Year doctor you may feel overwhelmed with the many options available. There will be those who already know exactly what specialty they want to enter and there will be others who remain unsure. This is why it is essential to have thought about your options early.

Study leave

When starting the FY2 year you will be entitled to study leave. In most trusts this is approximately 30 days, out of which ten days will be used as part of your formal foundation year teaching. This time can often be difficult to arrange, as cover must be arranged for your clinical duties. It is therefore imperative that you try to plan in advance when you would like to take this leave. Study leave can be used for attending educational courses (e.g. Advanced Life Support (ALS), Advanced Trauma Life Support (ATLS)), simulation courses, and performing projects.

Foundation learning portfolio

During the FY2 year you will have to complete a number of assessments, which are of a similar format to those assessments completed in the FY1 year. These assessments should be added to your foundation portfolio. The foundation portfolio should be kept up to date throughout the year. It should contain all of your educational meetings, personal development plan, educational agreements, teaching sessions and reflective practice.

At the end of the year your postgraduate Dean will decide whether you have gained all of your foundation competencies, and therefore have successfully completed the Foundation Programme. You will receive a Foundation Achievement of Competency Document (FACD), as evidence for completion of the Foundation Programme.

Specialist Training

When starting the foundation programme you will inevitably be overwhelmed with the transition from being a medical student to a junior doctor. You will be introduced to a variety of medical and surgical specialties.

It is important to consider early which specialty you may want to pursue and enter the training programme. There is a lot of help available to assist you; talk to senior members of your team, your educational and clinical supervisors. In addition, you may wish to discuss this with a careers advisor.

Once you have decided on a future career choice it will not be long before you will have to apply for the specific training. Usually this occurs after working for at least four months as an FY2 doctor. This requires you to be prepared early so as to be in line with national recruitment specifications for your specialty.

Further reading and references

➤ www.foundationprogramme.nhs.uk
➤ www.mmc.nhs.uk

INTRODUCTION

Towards the end of the first Foundation Year 2 (FY2) rotation, the application round for specialist training will begin. Application forms and questions vary between each specialty and sometimes, the grade of ST applied for as well. It is essential to check the dates at which specific specialty application rounds are open, bearing in mind that this may differ between individual deaneries.

Currently, a national recruitment scheme exists for specialties such as medicine, paediatrics and obstetrics and gynaecology. Hence, only one application form needs to be completed and this can be utilised for each deanery you are applying to. However, with certain specialties such as surgery, individual applications need to be made to each deanery applied to, and these may vary greatly in content between the deaneries.

Often the deaneries give a limited time period within which the application forms must be completed, and therefore preparation in advance is key in order to ensure success.

Each specialty has a person specification which outlines the features required for short listing in a particular specialty. These specifications tend to be similar within each specialty, with some particular differences such as an emphasis on communication skills in specialties such as paediatrics. There is often also a guide to how the applications are scored, and if available this can be found on the deanery website. This is very helpful when structuring your answers in order to focus on the specific areas which will ensure you score highly. In this chapter we hope to provide an insight into the core generic specifications for ST applications so that a candidate may be better equipped to maximise his/her potential score.

GENERAL ADVICE

In general, it is essential to include examples of personal experience and reflection within your answers as this is the only way in which recruiters can differentiate your answers from those given generically by applicants. It is also important to have a structure within your answers in order to make it easier for the recruiters to recognise your achievement and score you appropriately.

The first part of the application form will most likely ask for your personal details and any previous work experience. It will also require information such as your qualifications (both undergraduate and postgraduate), courses you have been on and details of at least two referees whom you wish to nominate; think carefully about whom you choose as your reference needs to support your application.

Why our specialty?

Every application form is bound to ask why you are applying for the specific specialty and how you can demonstrate your commitment to the specialty. It is important not to list generic reasons here; your answer will be much more effective if you outline three to four specific reasons for your chosen specialty and expand upon these. For example, you may enjoy the challenge posed by the different levels of communication required in paediatrics or the mixture of surgical and medical skills required in obstetrics and gynaecology. In terms of demonstrating your commitment, examples include specific audit work or research conducted within the specialty, undertaking postgraduate examinations, and attending courses in order to enhance your skills relevant to your chosen specialty, such as the basic surgical skills course for surgery, and advanced trauma life support for emergency/ trauma surgery.

Skills

Often within the application there will be at least one question asking for an example from your own experience which illustrates a quality or skill which you possess. It is important to carefully consider all of your options and choose an example which appropriately displays your skills and includes an element of personal experience and reflective practice. This will ensure you score maximal points. In terms of structuring these types of answers, it is best to start your answer with a concise description of the situation or example which you are using. You can then continue by describing what you did and how you did it, after which a conclusion can be made where you can outline what you learnt from the situation or experience and highlight the skills which you developed as a result.

You will most certainly have a question enquiring into the specific skills which you possess making you suitable for your chosen specialty. It is important to use personal examples here which highlight how your experiences enabled you to develop specific skills. In your answers, you can include examples of feedback from your colleagues which have enabled you to build upon and develop your skills.

When asked for examples of the skills and qualities you possess which make you suitable for the specialty, it is important to discuss the particular skills which are relevant to your field, such as organisation and decision making.

There is often a question asking for an example of your communication skills. Situations which can be used include speaking to patients or relatives about medical information such as consenting or bereavement, an experience of an acute situation where communication skills were paramount to the clinical outcome and relevant communication skills courses that you have attended which have improved your clinical practice.

For example, you may have kept a log book of performed procedures (surgery, anaesthetics). You can also give evidence of directly observed procedures for clinical procedures performed. You can discuss experience of working in appropriate departments and skills or competencies achieved during this time.

Non-academic achievements

It is important to illustrate a good work-life balance with examples of achievements and commitment to activities outside the world of medicine. For example, sporting achievements and charity work as well as hobbies. Ensure you discuss the achievement itself, what makes you particularly proud of it and what skills you gained from it which will be relevant in your working life. The highest points will be scored where the achievement was within the context of a high level of competition as well as where you have shown your level of commitment. Always include some personal reflection of the achievement.

Audit

It is important to both demonstrate your understanding of the audit process and give an example of an audit in which you had a significant role. A good example will be where the audit resulted in a change and hence improvement in clinical practice.

Start your answer by giving a brief description of the audit, the reasoning behind initiating it, for example if there was a deficit in clinical practice, and what your specific aims were. Describe the level at which you contributed to data collection, analysis and presentation. Highlight your role within the audit, emphasising exactly what you did. Discuss the results and how they were applied into clinical practice. Also, show awareness of the importance of completing the audit cycle in particular if you performed a re-audit which shows an improvement in practice as a result of your audit. Often, maximal points can potentially be scored where the audit has been presented regionally or published.

Research

Many applicants will have done an intercalated BSc and hence will have undertaken a research project. Ensure you describe your specific role in the research and the skills which you developed, as well as their relevance to your clinical practice. Any presentation or publications resulting from the research should be highlighted.

Publications and presentations

You will often need to list any publications in a peer-reviewed journal and any presentations which you have done. You will score highly if the presentation is at a national or international level. Your role must be highlighted in particular if you were the first author of a publication.

List relevant publications that are already in print or that you are currently working on, in the standard format 'Author, Title, Journal, Issue, Book number, pages, date'. List presentations/posters in order starting with those performed at international, national, regional and local department levels.

Teaching experience

Teaching is important. Try to structure your answer by dividing it into teaching experience of both a formal and an informal nature as well as any experience outside of medicine. Examples include teaching to undergraduates and being an Objective Structured Clinical Examiner (OSCE) examiner, being a course examiner (Advanced Life Support (ALS)/Advanced Trauma Life Support (ATLS)), and educating medical, social or charitable organisations (e.g. elective).

Discuss the different teaching methods you have used as well as the content of your teaching sessions. You will score highly if you have had formal training in teaching methods and hence it would be useful to attend a teaching course. Teaching at a regional level will also score higher than that at a local level.

Management/leadership

Pick a good example which illustrates your skills best, which may be medical or non-medical. You can use more than one example ensuring you describe the activity and how it enabled you to develop leadership/management skills as well as how these are relevant clinically. Roles include the running of medical committees and societies, involvement in rota co-ordination and sports team captain or local magazine editor.

Teamwork

This is relevant to every specialty and you must be able to discuss examples where you have shown you are able to understand your role within a team and worked in coordination with others in order to achieve a common aim. Emphasise the importance of good communications skills, appreciation of the work performed by others and responsibility to perform your own role. In particular, demonstrate your involvement in multidisciplinary teams within clinical practice where optimal patient care is most important. Highlight your achievements as a result of effective teamwork.

CONCLUSION

In order to score highly it is essential to make your answers structured and focussed, illustrating personal examples and reflection where relevant. Ensure you are familiar with the scoring system and person specification for your speciality as well as the skills and qualities which are most relevant to it.

Good luck!

Further reading and references

➢ www.foundationprogramme.nhs.uk
➢ www.mmc.nhs.uk

Index

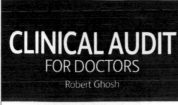
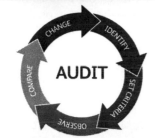

More Titles in the Progressing Your Medical Career Series

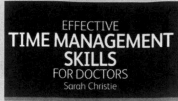

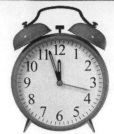

January 2009

176 pages

Paperback

ISBN 978-1-906839-08-6

£19.99

Do you find it difficult to achieve a work-life balance? Would you like to know how you can become more effective with the time you have?

With the introduction of the European Working Time Directive, which will severely limit the hours in the working week, it is more important than ever that doctors improve their personal effectiveness and time management skills. This interactive book will enable you to focus on what activities are needlessly taking up your time and what steps you can take to manage your time better.

By taking the time to read through, complete the exercises and follow the advice contained within this book you will begin to:

- Understand where your time is being needlessly wasted

- Discover how to be more assertive and learn how to say 'No'

- Set yourself priorities and stick to them

- Learn how to complete tasks more efficiently

- Plan better so you can spend more time doing the things you enjoy

In recent years, with the introduction of the NHS Plan and Lord Darzi's commitment to improve the quality of healthcare provision, there is a need for doctors to become more effective within their working environment. This book will offer you the chance to regain some clarity on how you actually spend your time and give you the impetus to ensure you achieve the tasks and goals which are important to you.

develop medica

www.developmedica.com

More Titles in the Progressing Your Medical Career Series

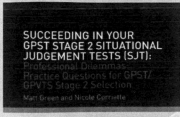

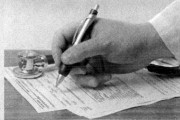

SUCCEEDING IN YOUR GPST STAGE 2 SITUATIONAL JUDGEMENT TESTS (SJT): Professional Dilemmas Practice Questions for GPST/ GPVTS Stage 2 Selection

Matt Green and Nicole Corriette

Situational Judgment Tests (SJTs) or Professional Dilemmas form a significant part of the GPST recruitment process and yet many doctors will not have experienced questions of this type under examination conditions. It is therefore essential that candidates sitting the GPST Stage 2 exam have a clear understanding of how to approach questions of this type as poor performance in this section will almost certainly result in not progressing to the Stage 3 selection day.

This interactive book, which contains detailed guidance, and over 70 practice questions (including detailed explanations of all the answers), aims to help doctors prepare for and successfully complete their GPST Stage 2 exam. In this book, Nicole Corriette and Matt Green:

- Describe the context of Situational Judgement Tests within the GPST Stage 2 selection process

- Explore the various ethical principles that you must consider when answering these types of questions

- Set out how to approach the various question types you will be faced with

- Provide over 70 questions to put into practice everything that you learn

- Detailed explanations of the correct answers are also provided to aid your preparations

This engaging, easy to use and comprehensive book is essential reading for anyone serious about excelling in their GPST Stage 2 examination and successfully progressing to Stage 3 of the GPST selection process.

December 2008

200 pages

Paperback

ISBN 978-0-9556746-9-3

£19.99

develop medica

www.developmedica.com

More Titles in the Progressing Your Medical Career Series

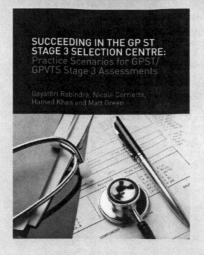

SUCCEEDING IN THE GP ST STAGE 3 SELECTION CENTRE: Practice Scenarios for GPST/ GPVTS Stage 3 Assessments

Gayathri Rabindra, Nicole Corriette, Hamed Khan and Matt Green

January 2009
392 pages
Paperback
ISBN 978-1-9068390-3-1
£24.99

This step-by-step guide to the GP ST Stage 3 Selection process is full of valuable advice and practice questions, with an emphasis on the type of scenarios that candidates can expect to face on the assessment day.

In this book, which has been written by experts with first hand experience in this assessment, the following are addressed:

- Detailed description of the consultation, discussion and prioritisation tasks and how to approach them

- Cross reference to the person specification and markscheme - describing what the selectors are looking for, and the different ways to approach the tasks

- Ten practice scenarios for each of the three tasks to reinforce your learning together with detailed discussion of possible answers for each scenario

- Personal perspectives - with tips from individuals who have successfully completed the selection process

- Discussion of the key concepts and terms that you will be faced with including amongst others significant event analysis and GP contracts.

Written by GPs who have first-hand experience of the process, this guide is a must have resource for any doctor serious about succeeding in their application to the GPST training scheme.

develop
medica

More Titles in the Progressing Your Medical Career Series

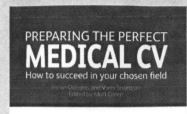

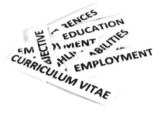

Are you unsure of how to structure your Medical CV? Would you like to know how to ensure you stand out from the crowd?

With competition for medical posts at an all time high it is vital that your Medical CV stands out over those of your fellow applicants. This comprehensive, unique and easy-to-read guide has been written with this in mind to help medical students and doctors of all grades prepare a Medical CV of the highest quality. Whether you are applying to medical school, currently completing your medical degree or a doctor progressing through your career (foundation doctor, specialty trainee in general practice, surgery or medicine, GP career grade or Consultant) this guide includes specific guidance for applicants at every level.

This time-saving and detailed guide:

- Explains what selection panels are looking for when reviewing applications at all levels.

- Discusses how to structure your Medical CV to ensure you stand out for the right reasons.

- Explores what information to include (and not include) in your CV.

- Covers what to consider when maintaining a portfolio at every step of your career, including for revalidation and relicensing purposes.

- Provides examples of high quality CVs to illustrate the above.

- Templates to help you create your own high impact CV.

This unique guide will show you how to prepare your CV for every step of your medical career from Medical School right through to Consultant level and should be a constant companion to ensure you secure your first choice post every time.

January 2009
176 pages
Paperback
ISBN 978-0-9556746-3-1
£19.99

develop
medica

www.developmedica.com

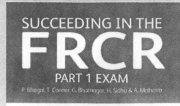
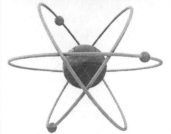

Lightning Source UK Ltd.
Milton Keynes UK
13 April 2010

152704UK00002BA/2/P